THE SECRETS OF GENERATION

EDITED BY RAYMOND STEPHANSON
AND DARREN N. WAGNER

The Secrets of Generation

Reproduction in the Long Eighteenth Century

UNIVERSITY OF TORONTO PRESS
Toronto Buffalo London

Toronto Buffalo London
www.utppublishing.com

ISBN 978-1-4426-4696-4 (cloth)

Printed on acid-free paper

Library and Archives Canada Cataloguing in Publication

The secrets of generation : reproduction in the long eighteenth century/edited by Raymond Stephanson and Darren N. Wagner.

Includes bibliographical references and index.
ISBN 978-1-4426-4696-4 (cloth)

1. Human reproduction – Europe – History – 18th century. I. Stephanson, Raymond, editor II. Wagner, Darren N., 1984–, author, editor

QP251.S42 2015 612.609409'033 C2015-905130-4

Publication of this book was made possible with the help of a grant from the Scouloudi Foundation in association with the Institute of Historical Research.

Publication of this book was also made possible by a subvention from the University of Saskatchewan.

University of Toronto Press acknowledges the financial assistance to its publishing program of the Canada Council for the Arts and the Ontario Arts Council, an agency of the Government of Ontario.

Canada Council for the Arts Conseil des Arts du Canada

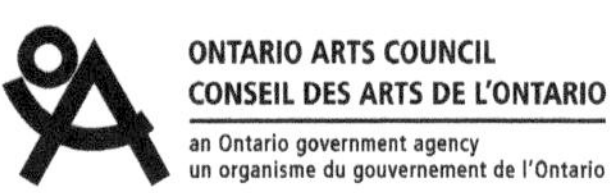

Funded by the Government of Canada Financé par le gouvernement du Canada

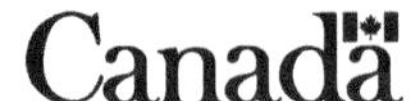

Contents

Illustrations

Acknowledgments

It is no secret that preparing a collection, especially one as lengthy and diverse as this, is a truly collaborative effort. Our twenty-four contributors have been irreproachable in their professional outlook and cooperative spirit. Because of them, and their excellent scholarship, editing this book has been wholly worthwhile and enlightening. Thanks also go to our three anonymous reviewers, whose helpful and articulate suggestions have improved the volume. In a world where nothing comes free, we duly thank those who have made this project possible through generous publication grants: the Scouloudi Foundation in association with the Institute of Historical Research, and the University of Saskatchewan in conjunction with the College of Arts and Science and the Department of English. Our editors at the University of Toronto Press, Richard Ratzlaff and Miriam Skey, are well-deserving of our final note of gratitude, as their support and guidance have been indispensable helps in carrying this book from conception to full term.

Preface

One of the most profoundly creative of all natural processes, reproduction fascinates us. It always has, from ancient creation myths poeticizing the birth of the cosmos and all life forms, to the breathtaking colour photographs by Lennart Nilsson in the 1960s dramatically rendering dead fetuses as though they were alive in outer space; from the 1978 birth of Louise Brown – the first IVF baby – whose conception took place in a petri dish, to the cloning of Dolly the sheep in Scotland in 1996. The mysteries of life and its begetting are always around us in real time, in the glorious shooting forth of the crocus from the cold spring ground, the teeming bustle of ant hills, the frenzied spawning runs of salmon, our family pets, and of course in our own species of now over seven billion people. Little wonder that the birth of organisms claims our attention, each of us playing key roles in the drama of reproduction, either as participants or witnesses.

The acceleration of knowledge in early twenty-first-century reproductive biology has been extraordinary, and we are easily captivated by technologies that dazzle with promises of human control over nature's ancient birthing regimes. In the spring of 2013 a particular pregnancy – one of millions around the world – marked an important new chapter in human reproduction: a twenty-two-year-old Turkish woman, having received the world's first successfully transplanted uterus in 2011, was impregnated after fertilized embryos were placed in her transplanted womb. The popularization of imaging technologies: 3D and 4D ultrasound images of the fetus, with parents-to-be now able to share such images with expectant grandparents by e-mail. The commercialization of reproductive vanities: a Japanese company will print a life-size 3D resin model of your fetus for $1250 US. In vitro fertilization has given us "Octomom," the Californian who birthed octuplets in 2009, creating a tabloid feeding frenzy and much criticism. The artificial human womb appears to be just around the corner, perhaps a possibility by mid-century. In the early 1990s an artificial placenta successfully kept mid- to late-stage goat fetuses alive until term. Artificial amniotic fluid has been developed at Temple University. In 2002 tissue samples were grown from endometrial cells removed from a human donor; fertilized eggs attached after six days. In 2013 the engineering of artificial ovaries looked possible, giving hope to women who had lost ovarian function. New freeze-drying techniques allowing cow oocytes to be stored indefinitely as a powder open the possibility that women may one day be able to achieve pregnancy by simply adding water and sperm to their powdered eggs, which would then be implanted. In 2006 scientists in Japan demonstrated the transformation of adult skin cells into pluripotent stem cells, a technique that in essence promises to extend our lives by inserting reprogrammed living material into our bodies; that same discovery has led more recently to the cloning of embryos from skin cells. One can only marvel at where such technologies might take us a generation from now. Perhaps a benign version of Mary Shelley's *Frankenstein* will be at hand, with humans able to create human life outside wombs or even bodies.

We are fascinated and unnerved, too, by the onerous ethical and political challenges that come with the surge in technological capacity. In 2012 the British government sought advice about how to develop policies for three-parent embryos in which offspring would have genetic material from father, mother, and a female donor so as to bypass inherited mitochondrial diseases. Another remarkable development, to be sure, but the complex procedure also raised moral questions about designer babies. There is the biology of fertility as commercial enterprise and those who profit from it. What about surrogacy, or wombs for rent? One can go online and buy fashion model ova or the sperm from talented athletes or handsome men to improve the odds of beautiful, smarter children. There is the shady underground of reproductive tourism, with desperate people seeking countries in which they can quietly pay for technologies designed to produce children for them. And there are many other vexed ethical implications thrown into relief by technology. Preimplantation genetic diagnosis with its difficult range of moral choices. Abortion. The medical use of human embryonic stem cells. And the touchy question about education: some public schools will teach children a little bit about the birds and the bees; other schools won't touch it at all. Eliciting tremendous curiosity and requiring billions of dollars annually, reproduction as a technology, as a social, medical, commercial, or political issue also pushes buttons and raises alarm.

But all of this has a history, and many of the roots of our present preoccupations in the Western world can be traced back to the seventeenth and eighteenth centuries in western Europe when reproduction – "generation" as it was then usually called – was being ushered into the new empirical enthusiasms of the Scientific Revolution, becoming a subject within which we can now detect precursors of some modern structures and concepts. A few parallels and connections are instructive here, not to argue some direct historical cause-and-effect but rather to suggest the continuity of human interests over time. Take the reproductive connections between the brain and groin. For we moderns, it is the hypothalamic-pituitary-gonadal axis; for the early moderns, it was (for males) an inverse hydraulic relationship between animal spirits in the brain and sperm use. Of course the details are obviously very different, as is the terminology, but remarkably the conceptual scaffolding is similar, with the earlier model offering an intriguing antecedent for how we explain the intricate interplay of hormonal secretions. Or compare Enlightenment notions that the maternal imagination could have direct (and usually negative) impact on the fetus to its parallel in modern myths such as the "Mozart effect" or the heavily moralized policing of pregnant-mom behaviour meant to prevent deleterious effects on the fetus caused by what a woman consumes or experiences. A different kind of foreshadowing lurks in the pop-culture publication titled *Procreation Refin'd: A New Method for the Begetting Children with Handsome Faces* (1710) – an advice manual whose current manifestation can be discovered in recent sites such as BeautifulPeople.com with its sperm and egg bank section promising handsome babies. Our modern MRI and ultrasound image-captures of hidden structures and processes find their counterpart in the skilled engravers and artists of three centuries ago who used their creative imaging technologies to offer stunning illustrations of women's bellies revealing the living fetus or the floating fetal subject within a womb abstracted from the female body – both then and now evidence of the powerful human drive to reveal the invisible mechanisms of reproduction. Parallels such as these reflect something about the abiding human interests in certain structural principles or interrelationships that appear to have existed over many centuries, but they also call attention to the curiosity we all have about how to measure the past in terms of the present, and also how to read the present *from* the past. It is this kind of curiosity that the chapters in this collection are meant to stimulate.

We believe that a major strength of this collection is its interdisciplinary expositions of reproduction, from theories of conception and concepts of species to pathological ovaries and museum displays of male genitalia; from Italian, German, and British to French and American experience; from the literary metaphor to the art historical to the satirical; from the fetus and childhood disability to maternal experience. The twenty-two essays collected here represent not only the scholarly state-of-the-field for the past quarter century but also how such a diverse and culturally implicated subject might be understood in new ways not only as a history of reproductive biology, but also as feminist history, as a history of theories of heredity, as pathology, as a pro-nuptial and pro-natal ideology, as a history of subjectivity, as a history of fetuses and babies, of technology, of literary history, and as a birds-and-bees commercial publishing industry.

Reproduction will continue to fascinate us as it always has, and successive generations will have to engage with the intricate realities of what that always-present force entails, not only in its present manifestations or future horizons, but also in relation to the past, from whence so many of its enduring interests and worries will have come. We invite readers of all kinds to explore "the secrets of generation" in the long eighteenth century.

THE SECRETS OF GENERATION

Introduction

RAYMOND STEPHANSON AND DARREN N. WAGNER

"Generation" in the eighteenth century has received all manner of interesting research over the past quarter century, with important publications by historians of science and medicine; cultural and social historians of various kinds; literary, feminist, and art historians; sex and gender historians; historians of human embodiment. *The Secrets of Generation* adds to this important scholarship, offering a wide-ranging collection of essays that reflects the various thematics, methodologies, geographies, and subdisciplinary interests that now inform what is a very complex and broad subject. Some chapters offer expert surveys of the state of the field for certain areas, while others tackle new possibilities intended to advance our understanding of cutting-edge research frontiers. Both retrospective and forward-looking, the present collection of twenty-two chapters is in part an assessment of how historians have approached "reproduction in the eighteenth century" thus far, and in part a redefinition of some major issues that promise to revise our understanding of the subject in important ways.

We imagine readers of this book to be of several kinds, coming from quite different base camps – medical history, art history, biomedicine, literary history, sex and gender, culture and the body, medical humanities, reproductive science, social anthropology – but willing to engage in the energizing forays into other disciplinary territories and time periods where encounters with different analytical tools used by others allow one to bring back new insights and concepts into one's home subject. The intended primary reader here is the specialist or graduate student in eighteenth-century studies, but this collection is also designed to appeal to the non-specialist reader with a general interest in the history of reproduction or the intersection of reproductive bodies and social context. What will be familiar subject areas to some readers will be foreign to others; familiar interpretive terrain for the literary or art historian may very well be new ground for the medical historian, just as obvious questions to the social anthropologist might strike new sparks for someone in the medical humanities. The editors hope that the diversity of subjects and approaches will make this book a helpful and enduring resource for experts in eighteenth-century studies as well as for graduate-level history of science courses, cultural studies approaches to the eighteenth-century, and interdisciplinary seminars with a strong medical humanities-history conjunction.

With our non-specialist readers in mind, we begin with the three keywords in the title of this book: "secrets," "generation," and "reproduction." There is no precise modern-day equivalent to the eighteenth-century term "generation," which is a somewhat larger concept than what we would now call "reproduction." But there is an important historical connection between the two. In late seventeenth- and eighteenth-century usage, "generation" included ideas of human procreativity but also notions of plant propagation and animal reproduction, as well as embryology and heredity. The word sometimes also carried with it an implication of divine agency, the edict to increase and multiply. But "generation" and its various connotations would gradually be replaced by "reproduction" – and other specialized terms – as searches for biological mechanisms and material causes in the second half of the eighteenth century ousted older explanatory models. Although the use of "reproduction" to describe the subject matter in this book is in some respects anachronistic, it is also meant to reflect the historical shift from the older and somewhat more inclusive senses of "generation" to the newer disciplinary subsets heralded by that new profession – biology – and its creation of the "life" sciences at the end of the eighteenth and into the nineteenth centuries (Jacob 1973, 72–3). Throughout this book, the two terms will be present and, while not exactly equivalent, they serve as reminders that the long eighteenth century is witness to this paradigm shift (Muri 2010).

Samuel Johnson – that gifted figure of *A Dictionary of the English Language* (1755) fame – offered a concise but provocative digest of the meaning of the third term, "secrets": "1. Something studiously hidden. 2. A thing unknown; something not yet discovered. 3. Privacy; secrecy" (1755/1979, s.v. "Secrets"). In these few words, Johnson captured much of what we need to know about attitudes towards human reproduction for the long eighteenth century. Studiously hidden secrets took various forms, from the private reproductive behaviours of ordinary women and men to birds-and-bees knowledge not proper in polite conversation. And there were other contexts. For midwife Jane Sharp in the 1670s, "the secrets of the Female sex" were their genitalia, necessitating polite prose but blunt and no-nonsense discussion (1671/1999, 38). For French accoucheur Pierre Dionis in the early eighteenth century, a proper understanding of "how a Child is form'd" required "the modern Anatomists [who] ... have enter'd into the hidden Secrets of Nature" (1719, 1). For the physician-poet John Armstrong, the hormonal rush of puberty in teenaged girls was "urg'd with secret Flames" and awkward self-consciousness (1739, 2). For quack James Graham in the 1780s, one of the most horrific but common causes of infertility and weakened progeny was masturbation, what he called "secret pollutions" (1780, 22). In Mary Shelley's famous early nineteenth-century novel Victor Frankenstein recounts his surprise "that I alone should be reserved to discover so astonishing a secret ... as the cause of generation and life; nay, more, I became myself capable of bestowing animation upon lifeless matter" (1818/2012, 79). The secrets of generation could indeed be private acts, or private parts, or inappropriate conversation matter, or special knowledge owned by the modern doctor and sequestered from the eyes of the hoi-polloi or the vulgar. But generation was also in another sense an open secret, announced everywhere by new plant growth, calving seasons, and new babies – part of the divine order of things and nature's marvellous way of sustaining life over time. "See, through this Air, this Ocean, and this Earth, / All Matter quick, and bursting into birth": the brilliant couplet artistry of Alexander Pope in *An Essay on Man* (Tillotson, Fussell, and Waingrow 1969, 639) enjoined his readers to see what was obvious about all living matter up and down the great chain of being: birth, life, coming into existence.

Secret but everywhere. Mysteriously hidden and yet ubiquitous. Impolite, profane, and obscene, but natural and good. The cultural logic that permitted the eighteenth century to have it both ways was simple enough: the human duty to reproduce was part of the divine dispensation, and that meant that such mysteries *required* investigation and invited the dissemination of such knowledge. Multiplying the species was a desired potential for all humans not only as a biblical injunction but also as a nation-building concept of power and wealth represented by population growth. These contexts made it easy to argue that a respectful explanation of private and impolite matters was acceptable and desirable, but typically with the following caveat: knowledge about the "secrets of generation" should be available only for adults who were married, about to be married, and who wished to make babies (Porter and Hall 1995, 11).

There was another cultural phenomenon – a material development – that encouraged a public peekaboo access to these otherwise private secrets. As is well known, the combination of a quickly expanding print culture at the end of the seventeenth century in addition to an escalating consumer interest in printed matter about sex and reproduction produced a body of materials whose quantity and availability were unlike anything before. Secrets, in other words, were also being made public. There would remain the first and third Johnsonian connotations of that which is known but hidden, and that which is none of your business, but thanks to the new print culture – sexual advice literature, midwifery manuals, popular sexologies, erotica, publications warning of venereal disease or masturbation, medical treatises in the vernacular, even the novel – Johnson's second sense comes into play in a manner convenient for the quarry we pursue here: that which is unknown and sought after (Johnson's implication) became publicly available for an unprecedented number of readers (Porter and Hall 1995, 33). This entrance of reproductive "secrets" into a public marketplace of printed materials, and the various cultural effects of their subsequent circulation, are fundamentally important developments to the history examined in this collection of essays.

This public entry was sometimes accompanied by a careful authorial rhetoric designed to clarify the narrative contract that would exist between author/text and reader. In this new milieu in which woodcuts, engravings, and explicit prose promised to open up impolite realities to public view, there were new protocols to be established for how these secrets should be received. Take for example one of the first of many sexual advice treatises that began to be published from the late seventeenth century – *Aristotle's Master-Piece* – an anonymous compilation of theories and recommendations about procreation that would be revised and reprinted well into the nineteenth century (Porter and Hall 1995, 33–64; and see M.D. Nichols's chapter in this volume). The subtitle for these editions included the idea of "secrets," as in *Aristotle's Compleat Master-Piece ... Displaying the Secrets of Nature in the Generation of Man* (1733), and importantly, prefatory materials typically set the conditions for the "display" to follow: "What is there more common than the begetting of Children? And yet what is there more wonderful and mysterious than the plastick Power of Nature, by which they are form'd? ... [S]ince it is our Duty to be acquainted with our selves, and to search out the Wonders of God in Nature, I need not make any Apology for anatomizing the secret Parts of Generation" (9, 12). As the subtitle suggests, the visual "display" of secrets became an important feature in many of these publications (see chapters by Pranghofer, McTavish, D.N. Wagner, and Lieske in this volume), offering graphic illustrations of the organs of generation (both male and female, external and internal), images of the fancied embryo in situ, the position and growth of the fetus, delivery techniques, the new-fad obstetrical instruments, or realistic images of the gravid uterus starkly opened to view. Taken together, the newly public imaging combined features of the alien or macabre item in a cabinet of curiosities, the specialized technical image for medical instruction, and the prurience of the pornographic gaze.

Little wonder, then, that some authors (at least in the early going of this publication history) were careful to declare their high-minded intentions. But making visible what was otherwise invisible or forbidden also confronted the reader-viewer with the action and tendency of his or her own imagination, and these tendencies were textually formalized by authors in projections of different types of readers. Writing in Latin in the late seventeenth century, the gifted reproductive biologist Regnier de Graaf would sternly caution his readers about how they might respond to his treatise on the male organs of generation: "If, however, anyone has a nature so disrespectful and lascivious as to try to seize upon what I have made public concerning the genital parts for lewd imaginings and scurrilous jokes, let him pay the penalty for his own wickedness" (1668/1972, 7). The pious and well-meaning de Graaf was typical in his differentiation of reader profiles, although such distinctions were not always sincere. Quack John Marten's STD compendium – *Gonosologium Novum: or, a New System Of all the Secret Infirmities and Diseases, Natural, Accidental, and Venereal in Men and Women* (1709) – would use the same rhetorical formula (including "*Secret*" in the subtitle) even though his intentions were money-grubbing and his treatise a curious mélange of medical description, cures for sale, mountebank flourishes, and smutty inset tales: "But if any should complain the Discourse is too plain, or that it may sully the Minds of them that read it, my advice is, that such would lay it aside, for if those that read it, cannot manage or subdue their Passions, they are not fit to be acquainted with such Matters" (A4). In the first wave of "secrets of generation" publications from the late seventeenth and early eighteenth centuries, the apparent dilemma of impolite subject matter and reception was flagged many times in prefaces and introductions, but these defences, apologias, and warnings were also the product of a larger set of social values and anxieties about reproduction: after all, how was one to write about a subject filled with the potential for excess when one's key moral point was moderation within pro-natal and pro-nuptial contexts? Secrets had been made publicly available but prefaces often suggested there needed to be a collective understanding of who would read such materials and how they would be used. Many of these publications typically housed an underlying set of cultural constraints and moralized treatments of their materials meant to control and discourage the free play of libidos, fantasy, and the uncensored energies of the reproductive body. But the human imagination – then as now – is unruly and difficult to control, and it is likely that the proliferation of printed materials about generation aided the pornographic imagination as much as it articulated a range of cultural norms about the proper function of sex and reproduction. And although intended for married folk or those about to enter into such reproductive formalities, there is little doubt that eager teenagers – then as now – found out ways to have access to "secrets" about their own bodies.

One thing is certain: the number of categories related to the secrets of generation multiplied in extraordinary fashion as reader consumerism increased into the eighteenth century (Jordanova 1986; Porter and Hall, 1995; Cody 2005; Davidson 2009). From how to beget boy or girl babies, to diet and preparations for pregnant moms-to-be, to cures and charms for barrenness – the topics covered in the printed materials were considerable, reflecting the interests and curiosities of a readership keen to find answers to secrets and questions such as the following: the differences between male and female bodies (Laqueur 1990); how to produce beautiful children (Quillet 1710); signs of the onset of puberty; whether it is better to copulate on an empty or a full stomach (Venette 1740, 37); dangers of the maternal imagination (Todd 1995); tips for increasing healthy male seed (Graham 1780); the function of pleasure; enhancing fertility (McLaren 1984); questions of where the embryo originated; fetal nutrition; questions of when the fetus acquired a soul; how to handle newborns; birth abnormalities (see Turner's chapter); the production of maternal milk from blood; how to choose a wet nurse (see Boon's chapter); the problem with hymens and signs of virginity; the dangers of masturbation (Laqueur 2003); at what age to marry and reproduce; ideas about heredity and the transmission of traits (Jacob 1973; Müller-Wille and Rheinberger 2012); false conceptions and stillborns; difficult labour and birthing (see Lieske's chapter); learned discussions by midwives and man-midwives as their turf-war developed (Lieske 2007; King 2007; see chapter by Peakman and Watkins); the fashionable new man-midwives (Cody 2005, 152–97); pathologies of the pelvis or the ovary (see chapters by Lieske and Frampton); the obstetrical atlas (Jordanova 1985); reproduction tropes in erotica (Peakman 2003; Harvey 2004). As well, popularized sex-lit gave non-specialist readers knowledge of prevailing reproductive theories such as preformationism, which dominated explanatory models until the mid-century (McLaren 1984, 13–29; Porter and Hall 1995; Pinto-Correia 1997; see Dal Prete's chapter).

Other printed materials were quite technical and commanded a smaller readership, although their impact would also be felt over time (Cole 1930; J. Needham 1959; Roger 1963/1997; Gasking 1967; Roe 1981; McLaren 1984; Pinto-Correia 1997; Cobb 2006; Smith 2006). After the work of William Harvey on generation (*De Generatione Animalium*, 1651, translated in 1653 as *Anatomical Exercitations Concerning the Generation of Living Creatures*), Regnier de Graaf's treatises on the organs of generation of males and females (*Tractatus de Virorum Organis Generationi Inservientibus*, 1668; *De Mulierum Organis Generationi Inservientibus Tractatus Novus*, 1672), Antonie van Leeuwenhoek's microscopic imaging of sperm in *Philosophical Transactions* (1678), studies of chicken embryo development by Marcello Malpighi (*Dissertatio Epistolica de Formatione Pulli in Ovo*, 1673), studies of insect reproduction by Jan Swammerdam (*Historia Insectorum Generalis*, 1669) – to mention only a few of the important figures – there was also a sharply increased specialist interest in ideas about reproduction. One need only thumb through the indices of *Philosophical Transactions* and other learned journals of this period to get a sense that, in Elizabeth Gasking's words, "far from being a casual interest, it was in fact a central issue" (15). Indeed, the materialist underpinnings of the new science as it concerned generation – from studies of genitalia, to nerve and blood supplies, to the roles played by females and males in conception, to embryogenesis, to fetal nutrition – offered the tantalizing possibility of truths about the origins of life itself, or at least, about that generative moment and biological sequence that might unlock some of the secrets of life-giving. In the new paradigm of the human body as machine, with accurate mechanical blueprints perhaps only one experiment away, the elusive mysteries of generation seemed to many to be within reach.

Little wonder that reproduction in its broadest senses should have claimed so significant a space in the public imaginary, often blurring distinctions between specialist interests and the curiosity of non-experts. Witness the Mary Toft hoax of 1726, her claim of having given birth to rabbits engaging both learned and popular interests, with lampoons and satires competing with the serious (and credulous) comments by some of the medical elite (Todd 1995, 1–63). The interest in generation was wide ranging, both popular and scientific, informing a tremendous amount of material being published and consumed.

Reproduction in the long eighteenth century had important sociosexual, familial, legal, and political aspects as well. Modern feminist scholars have already devoted much attention to the gendered aspects of this complex history in which questions of identity and agency were always present (Schiebinger 1986; Perry 1991; Fissell 1995; Nussbaum 1995; Fissell 2004; Crawford 2004; Park 2006; Keller 2007; Klepp 2009). From the passivity of female bodies increasingly subject to the medical gaze of the male obstetrician, to the reproductive female body as site of cultural anxieties, or the succession crisis surrounding Charles II's efforts to reproduce a legitimate male heir, or the ways in which notions of the family were structured, generation also served variously as a symbol for values and concerns defined differentially by social contexts, professional practice, and politics. Legal and economic distinctions, too, hovered near the birthing room: illegitimacy and inheritance; foundlings and Poor Laws (see D.W. Nichol's chapter); infanticide (see C. Wagner's chapter). From a personal vantage point, pregnancy might have provoked the joys, hopes, or worries of individual moms-to-be (see chapters by Meek, Boon, Golightly, Toulalan, Lieske, and C. Wagner), or conjured up individual fantasies about impending motherhood or fatherhood, but from a retrospective view over two hundred years later reproduction in the eighteenth century is a vast subject, an extraordinarily diverse receptacle of human value systems, social practices, and ideological outlines.

We do a disservice to this history, however, if we limit the "secrets of generation" only to humans. Accompanying the new fascination with reproduction was a notion that accurate accounts of generation might participate in larger ordering paradigms within the divine creation, and that reproductive processes of all kinds might have a common structure or a set of uniform biological systems. As Shirley A. Roe has remarked, in the Enlightenment search to find the laws of nature there was "a need to unify the life sciences" (2003, 416), and this required attention to the full range of living beings on the *échelle des êtres.* Not just humans, but also animals and plants. Perhaps there were parallels and correspondences linking the reproductive physiologies and mechanisms of the Two Kingdoms. The "analogy of nature" – as it was sometimes called – encouraged all manner of detailed comparisons of plants and animals, often framed with reference to human biology. From the late seventeenth century on – as the new empiricism impacted botanical investigations – natural philosophers looked for resemblances and equivalences in systems of nutrition, growth, circulation of fluids, respiration, and reproduction. The result was a wide range of assumptions that plants and animals shared similar or identical features, either structurally or functionally (J.T. Needham 1749; Parsons 1752). Plant propagation and animal generation became strongly linked once the idea of *sexus plantarum*, or the "sexes of plants," came into the conceptual range of attention among botanists from the seventeenth century on. After Nehemiah Grew's *The Anatomy of Plants* (London, 1682), it was widely agreed that plant propagation involved male and female parts corresponding to the genitalia of animals or humans; that pollen from the anther and stickiness on the stigma would be equivalent to sperm and vaginal (or uterine) readiness; that this sexual exchange or transmission was required in order for fructification to occur; and that seeds and germs formed within the plant's ovary would become the vegetative correspondents to embryos, fetuses, or offspring (Bradley 1717, 13, 14, 18; Jussieu 1719).

There were secrets, too, in the generation of plants. As gardener Richard Bradley put it in 1717, "I think myself obliged to declare that the first Hint of this Secret was communicated to me several Years ago by a worthy member of the *Royal Society*, *Robert Balle*, Esq; who has had this Notion for above Thirty Years, that *Plants* had a Mode of *Generating* somewhat analogous to that of *Animals*" (12). Of course the most famous botanist was Carl von Linné (1707–78), arguably the first to personify the sexes of plants directly as a complete system. Plant propagation had intrigued him since his early twenties, and as a university student at Uppsala in 1729 he had written the dissertation *Præludia Sponsaliarum Plantarum* (Prelude to the Betrothal of Plants) in Swedish, developing what some would later object to as an obscene analogy between plant sexuality and that of humans. According to the poetically inclined young Linnaeus,

> [T]hese few pages deal with the great analogy that exists between plants and animals in terms of their similar means of propagating their species ... In springtime when the delightful Sun comes closer to our Zenith, it awakens life in all living things that have lain low ... Love assails the very plants, since among them both *mares* [males] and *foeminæ* [females], and Hermaphrodites too, hold their nuptials. And this is what I have now set out to describe and demonstrate from the genitalia of the plants themselves: which are male, which female and which hermaphroditic ... The actual petals of the Flower ... contribute nothing to generation. Instead, they serve only as Bridal beds that the great Creator has so gloriously provided, adorned with generous Bed curtains and perfumed with many delightful fragrances, where the bridegroom and his bride may celebrate their Nuptials with so much greater solemnity. Now that the bed has been thus prepared, it is time for the Bridegroom to embrace his beloved Bride, and offer her his gifts. By this I mean that one sees how the testicles open and pour forth *pulverem genitalem* [the generative powder], which falls on the *tubam* [the tube] and fertilises ovarium [the ovary]. (Linnaeus 1729/2007, 65, 67–8, 81)

Despite the almost pornographic personification here, the supposed parallels of generation in the Two Kingdoms would prevail into the late eighteenth century, and Linnaeus's work would be translated several times for polite readerships that included women, and would receive verse popularization in Erasmus Darwin's "The Loves of the Plants," which became the second part of his *The Botanic Garden* (1791). In a curious way, the impolite secrets of generation/propagation in plants entered fashionable society, allowing a collective fantasy, as it were, in which sexual arrangements, congress, and male and female genitalia were made politely available through a new fad of botany as popular pastime (Shteir 1996, ch. 1).

And nature, as it turned out, also had odd mysteries of its own, challenging or confounding common-sense notions about generation. In 1740, Swiss naturalist Charles Bonnet discovered parthenogenesis in aphids. He was able to rear ten generations without any males (Gasking 1967, 64). The implications were significant: traditional explanations requiring male and female conjunction, the merging of fluids, or egg and sperm, were challenged by these findings, although the lack of male suggested that perhaps ovist preformationism was the correct theory. At about the same time, in the early 1740s, Bonnet's relative Abraham Trembley discovered something remarkable about fresh water polyps. Not only did these hydra appear to have both plant-like *and* animal qualities, but when cut apart, either horizontally or vertically, the parts would regenerate into completely new individuals, somehow able to reproduce missing head, tail, or other parts. What was there in this tiny organism that could recreate a new polyp? It appeared that somehow matter itself might contain an autonomous reproductive energy that did not require a sexual act or an egg. The self-regeneration of these zoophytes challenged the neat pattern of preformationism (Dawson 1984, 55). There were other oddities, as well, such as questions about whether spontaneous generation could occur. In 1749 John Turberville Needham, the English Roman Catholic and colleague of Buffon, claimed that there was a kind of universal semen from which all generation originated, and at microscopic levels one could see this in the spontaneous generation of animalcula in boiled meat infusoria (Roe 1981, 18–19). While many disagreed – his experiment inadvertently let in micro-organisms; matter itself could not flip the reproductive life-switch on – he was nevertheless one of several experimentalists in the 1740s who was convinced that generation was somehow the property of matter itself. The philosophical and theological implications of such discoveries and theories were complex (Dawson 1987; Vartanian 1950): had God made all organisms in advance at the beginning? could matter contain within itself the power to develop life, or did it need a divine "push" for it to reproduce? could generation be explained as preformed individuals waiting to be sparked into growth by sexual congress or was there a sequential development of different parts from an unformed mass (known as epigenesis)? why were males sometimes irrelevant to generation (see Rousseau's chapter)?

Interest in self-generating life and regeneration was also related to the possibility of artificial reproduction. There were those who wondered whether nature's generative work could be imitated, controlled, or even improved. Richard Bradley wrote rather proudly of common greenhouse practices by which fellow-gardener "Mr. Thomas Fowler" was able "to cut Cucumbers on *New Year's Day*"; indeed, if he wished, he could eat cucumbers any month of the year (1726, 199–200). Assisted reproduction through heat was a means of artificially bringing life into being, and such techniques were deployed with success in another context by French polymath René Antoine Ferchault de Réaumur, whose *Art de faire éclorre et d'élever en tout saison des oiseaux Domestiques de toutes espèces* (1749; translated in 1750 as *The Art of Hatching and Bringing Up Domestick Fowls of All Kinds, at any Time of the Year*) offered a detailed account of experiments with Egyptian techniques for using artificial heat to incubate chicks. This work had quite an impact, and references to Réaumur's practices are routinely indexed in scientific dictionaries under "hatching" and "stoves." The fundamental premise is one we now take for granted, but which in the mid-eighteenth century was brand new to most: using artificial means to sustain chick development until hatching and beyond without the hen. Réaumur refers to the interior of his incubation device as "the artificial mother" (1749/1750, 249). We need an act of historical imagination here to appreciate the powerful implications of Réaumur's demonstrations that human interventions could mimic the necessary conditions for life to come into being, and one of the memorable features of his painstaking accounts is his excitement in the recognition that his experiments have generated life outside nature's normal course: "I could hardly let the first four and twenty hours pass without attempting to view the effect which a well proportioned and well managed heat had produced in the eggs; I broke two, in which I had the pleasure to see the beating of the little heart ... this was a sight which a naturalist cou'd not be tired of, were it to last much longer than it does" (61). In his prize-winning dissertation on the sexes of plants (sponsored by the Imperial Academy at Petersburgh), Linnaeus, too, would wax eloquent about the transport of pollen from a male date-palm in Leipzig to fertilize a female palm in Berlin (Linnaeus 1786, 50–1). The point to be taken from these examples is that the eighteenth century also developed technologies not only to better understand generation in plants, animals, and humans, but also to harness and control these natural biological processes for economic and social reasons. Being able to produce vegetables by artificial heat at any time of the year, or to fertilize plants at long distance by human intervention, or to dramatically increase available food resources through mass incubation were not inconsiderable advances.

There were other developments in what we would now call assisted reproductive technology, such as the famous first successful attempt at human artificial insemination in 1776 by the Scottish surgeon John Hunter, who advised a linen-draper with hypospadias on how to use a syringe to impregnate his wife (McLaren 1984, 13; see Rousseau's chapter). Hunter was successful, as were Lazzaro Spallanzani's experiments with artificial insemination in dogs. One of the Italian biologist's curiosities about what he called "artificial fecundation" was whether one could "substitute the electrical fluid in the stead of the semen." Karl Achard had earlier used electricity to hasten the development and hatching of chickens, causing Charles Bonnet and Spallanzani to wonder whether electricity might be able to cause fertilization in frogs (Spallanzani 1784, 2:185). Of course Spallanzani's attempts did not work, but the very concept is an indication of the intricate and sophisticated experimental levels at which human and animal reproduction were being researched. In the 1780s quack James Graham fancied a direct connection between fertility and electricity, offering his insulated, electrified bed for couples who were willing to pay for fertility (1780, 70–1). In his view, electrically enhanced copulation not only produced prolonged and glorious male orgasms (he seemed disinterested in female pleasure) but also guaranteed conception. Indeed, for Graham the very friction of copulation was inherently electrical: "I am clearly and decidedly of opinion, that even the venereal act itself, at all times, and under every circumstance, is in fact no other than an electrical operation!" (1783, 19). Human technologies to repair infertility, or to replace natural processes where nature had failed, or to discover the underlying energy forces (such as electricity) that might be present in reproduction (and therefore to be isolated, replicated, and deployed artificially) – these technical ventures were also part of the larger industrialization of the sciences, particularly in the second half of the century, where technologies of various kinds were being tested and developed for economic, social, or practical benefits.

Take the notion of improving the breed: could selective breeding and hybrids allow humans to engineer new kinds, new species, or improvements to a population (Davidson 2009, 86–99)? As preformationist views were overtaken by more complex epigenetic approaches in which both maternal and paternal fluids or matter somehow acted together to produce specific combinations of traits in offspring, newer notions of heredity also entered the scene: perhaps species were not fixed but rather malleable or subject to inherited variation. Plant and animal breeders had long known that they could manipulate outcomes by controlling reproductive combinations in particular ways. Famous livestock breeder Robert Bakewell of Dishley in Leicestershire (see Lehleiter's chapter) experimented from the 1760s with selective breeding of sheep so as to produce a brand new hybrid that would mature and fatten more quickly than any other – the secret of which Bakewell would never divulge (Wood and Orel 2001, 66). But could such manipulations be applied to human populations? In the mid-1740s Pierre-Louis Moreau de Maupertuis pondered the production of new species: "We find new breeds of dogs, pigeons, canaries appearing on the market, though they did not exist in nature. At first they were individual freaks, but art and repeated generations turned them into new species .... Why is this art restricted to animals?" (1745/1966, 72). Theories about improving or altering human populations through various means – race/class mixing, purification of blood by limiting reproductive partners, selecting for desirable characteristics, health regimes, fertility enhancements – also entered the larger context of generation, leading to a variety of eugenics theories (see chapters by Waller and Lettow). The political economy of generation and governmental interest in controlled reproduction was also on the horizon, with its predictable agendas about racial hierarchies, gender, and colonialist interests soon to follow. At the end of the century Thomas Malthus's *An Essay on the Principle of Population* (1798) would offer a dramatic mathematical model that projected the social miseries of unrestrained fertility among the poor.

But what about generation over the longer haul of earth's history (see chapters by Bowler and Müller-Wille)? Did living things each have some primordial form repeated over again through the centuries, or did they change and mutate over time? Did the processes of generation ensure the continuity of species or did accident and contingency play a role in changing the structure and function of organisms? Fossil records suggested that perhaps some species went out of existence never to return. Did that suggest that new species might also come into being? Before Darwin and his intellectual predecessors towards the end of the eighteenth century, there were several competing concepts: species were fixed essences; mutations and hybrids problematized such claims; the language used to differentiate species was artificial and only individuals existed (Mayr 1982, 251–97). When one stood back and took the longer view, the secrets of generation seemed also coeval with the history of the planet, and therefore intimately tied up with the mysteries of the origins of life itself. Benoît de Maillet's *Telliamed* (1748; English translation 1750) had entertained the idea that over time one species might well be changed into another. His notion was that the earth was about two billion years old, and at some point marine life had transformed into terrestrial life, and that even humans had come out of the sea. Once temporality was factored in, the grand query about the reproduction of species over the earth's history confronted the scientific and philosophical imagination with newer questions complicating older views: what were the effects of time, environment, and chance, and what was God's work in all this?

We must not forget the poets, novelists, and satirists who incorporated so many of these new interests and subjects, offering an important commentary as both review-of and cultural-response-to the secrets of generation and their public proliferation. Literary and artistic works carried their own impact, often shaping the collective perceptions of a reading population. The scores of novels that included reproductive themes – maternity and foundlings, to mention only two – reflected but also helped to fashion ways of thinking about the status quo or fantasizing some disruption or challenge to it (see chapters by Meek and Golightly). Daniel Defoe's monstrous mothers – Moll Flanders and Roxana – or Henry Fielding's gentlemen-in-disguise foundlings – Joseph Andrews and Tom Jones – offered different narrative responses by which readers could calibrate their own feelings about the personal and social protocols of generation. But the sexual and reproductive economies of some fictions were hardly unproblematic, confronting readers with fictional characters whose actions cut against the grain of expectations or decorum (Erickson 1986; Bowers 1996). These literary statements – the fictionalized what-ifs of sex and reproduction – captured the vexed personal and social aspects of generation in ways that the detached treatises of natural philosophers never could. Poetry such as Elizabeth Boyd's mournful heroic couplets in 1733 "On the Death of an Infant of five Days old, being a beautiful but abortive Birth" (Lonsdale 1989, 135), or Anna Barbauld's touching poem in 1795 "To a Little Invisible Being who is Expected Soon to Become Visible" (ibid., 307–8) represented a new kind of attention to individual experience or what we might understand as the psychologizing of generation. The literary record gives us an important glimpse of how people in the eighteenth century might have imagined their own reproductive bodies, and how they fantasized the social implications of generation.

Perhaps the most famous eighteenth-century novel about reproduction – from the moment of conception to difficult birthing to damages caused by the man-midwife's forceps – was Laurence Sterne's *Life and Opinions of Tristram Shandy* (1759–67). Deeply affected by the scientific debates about how human life was formed, his satirical handling of the preformationist origins of baby Tristram included a comically detailed account of the moment of conception in the very first chapter, situated – as the reader soon learns – in the marriage bed of Walter and Elizabeth Shandy:

> I wish either my father or my mother ... had minded what they were about when they begot me; had they duly consider'd how much depended upon what they were then doing ... "*Pray, my dear*, quoth my mother, *have you not forgot to wind up the clock? – Good G – !* Cried my father, making an exclamation, but taking care to moderate his voice at the same time. *Did ever woman, since the creation of the world, interrupt a man with such a silly question?*"... Then let me tell you, Sir, it was a very unseasonable question at least – because it scattered and dispersed the animal spirits, whose business it was to have escorted and gone hand-in-hand with the HOMUNCULUS, and conducted him safe to the place destined for his reception. (Sterne 2004, 1–2)

Opening his novel with father Walter's interrupted ejaculation was a cheeky, risky, and outrageous gambit, but the huge popularity of Sterne's serially published narrative pointed to the extraordinary interest in and knowledge of generation among readers, who clearly relished the author's artful deployment of such matters. Satirically adapting older mechanical explanations of conception, and adding sly nods towards the doubtful efficacy of the male organ of generation, tussles between midwife and man-midwife, debates about forceps, and the effects of birth canal contractions on the baby's skull, Sterne took a handful of reproductive themes and theories and playfully plugged them into the new culture of nervous sensibility and sentimentalism (Stephanson 2012).

There were other notable literary versions of the secrets of generation, from the passing mention in Swift's *Gulliver's Travels* (1726) that one of the king of Brobdingnag's "great Scholars ... seemed to think that I might be an Embrio, or abortive Birth" (Swift 1726/2008, 93) to the more remarkable attempt in Shelley's *Frankenstein* to frame the possibilities of human intervention by which electricity and other contemporary developments in chemistry might be able to reproduce life outside nature's normal course: "Whence, I often asked myself, did the principle of life proceed? ... It was with these feelings that I began the creation of a human being ... A new species would bless me as its creator and source" (Shelley 1818/2012, 78,

80). But generation was also at the core of important symbolic configurations, both positive and negative, and some literary artefacts prompted deep reflection about the relationship of the human to the divine, of the origins of human creativity, or even of the horrors of urban civilization. Milton's *Paradise Lost* took as one of its many subjects the complex relationship between two reproductive modes: God's parthenogenetic creation of preformed living beings in Eden as opposed to the inevitable fallen world within which the reproductive labour of Eve would proceed epigenetically in time (see chapter by Harol and MacQueen). Decades later, in his beautiful "Ode on the Poetical Character" (1747), William Collins presented his legend of the origins of literary creativity itself as a reproductive result issuing from the congress of male and female divinities: "The Band [girdle of poetry], as Fairy Legends say, / Was wove on that creating Day, / When He [God], who call'd with Thought to Birth / Yon tented Sky, this laughing Earth ... And she [Fancy], from out the veiling Cloud, / Breath'd her magic Notes aloud: / And Thou, Thou rich-hair'd Youth of Morn, [Phoebus Apollo, god of poetry] And all thy subject Life was born!" (Tillotson, Fussell, and Waingrow 1969, 919). Nearly a generation later William Blake used the reproductive trope to frame the sad cultural and social effects of the new industrialism in his bleak poem "London": "But most thro' midnight streets I hear / How the youthful Harlot's curse / Blasts the new born Infant's tear, / And blights with plagues the Marriage hearse" (ibid., 1504). Metaphors of conception, labour, birth (or abortion) also became part of a common figurative vocabulary when male authors referred self-consciously to the nature of their creative processes or to the book-object itself, which they likened to an embryo, offspring, brain child, or foundling (Stephanson 2004, 93–158).

Predictably, the satirists loved the secrets of generation because the collision of the fleshy truths of biology with the polite veneer of culture afforded all manner of risible subjects, from garden-variety hypocrisies or euphemisms to social satire and personal lampoons of the bedroom antics of the rich and famous (see D.W. Nichol's chapter). Parodies of the political economy of reproduction and population were most famously undertaken by Swift's deadly impersonation in *A Modest Proposal* (1729) and then again in Daniel Maclauchlan's *An Essay Upon Improving and Adding to the Strength of Great Britain and Ireland, by Fornication, Justifying the Same from Scripture and Reason* (1735). The satirical logic of the latter was that if God had ordained reproductive sex as a natural good for personal pleasure and the maintenance of the species, then surely unmarried folks (men in particular) ought to pursue a morally unconstrained erotic career in the interests of the national good. Social and gender issues were always close to the scene of these satirical remixes, holding forth the dangerous possibility of unrestrained sexual desiring while thumbing the nose at propriety and decorum. But reproductive theories and technologies were also subject to the satirist's sting, as in John Hill's *Lucina Sine Concubitu* (1750) (see chapters by Rousseau and Peakman and Watkins), an outrageous spoof of parthenogenesis in which a mechanical device filtered out sperm floating in the air, which was then used as a kind of dietary supplement to produce a pregnancy without men. This far-fetched proposal was a stalking horse for a variety of satirical targets, but it was also part of an interesting fictional trend in the 1740s and early 1750s that experimented with the potential outcome of new reproductive technologies. The most complex of these literary applications is Vincent Miller's *The Man-Plant: Or, Scheme for Increasing and Improving the British Breed* (1751). There are satirical objects here, but Miller (a pseudonym) adapts then-current science and technology to write a remarkable mock-treatise on the artificial womb. Using greenhouse techniques, Réaumur's incubation methods, electricity, and selective breeding as his narrative materials, Miller invents a fictional science about reproduction a full generation before Mary Shelley's gothic approach to the artificial creation of human life. In some cases, as here, the literary could often imagine and articulate what the science could not yet see.

Reproduction – "generation" – in its various eighteenth-century manifestations – biological, literary, technological, cultural, economic, medical – is a huge subject: from science fictions about the artificial generation of humans to botany and the sex lives of plants; from theories about species from the beginning of time to novels of sensibility and poetry about birthing and maternity; from animal breeders to human birth abnormalities; from museum displays of dried and inflated male genitalia to how-to-make-babies manuals for ordinary folk; from the philosophical and religious implications of reproduction to diseased ovaries and mercenary wet nurses; from parthenogenesis in aphids to breeding and bloodlines in humans; from literary satires and erotica to scientific treatises; from Antonie van Leeuwenhoek to John Milton; and more. The twenty-two chapters collected here reflect this remarkable variety of subjects, and they also call attention to the many interconnections and overlapping issues that bring together otherwise seemingly disparate dimensions and modes.

No collection of essays on so vast a subject can ever hope to be complete or exhaustive, however, and the editors are well aware that there are gaps. Invitations to contribute were extended to many specialists in the field, and the scholars who agreed to offer their expert knowledge have marked the scope and range of materials and subjects treated here. It would have been desirable to have had chapters dealing more fully with the male reproductive system, for instance, or with pleasure, reproductive deviants (masturbators, mollies, lesbians, impotent males), fetal-maternal-placenta feedback loops, population debates, contraception, or the commercialization of fertility, but there are also considerations of the publisher's space limitations in what is an already lengthy volume. Despite inevitable gaps, this collection comprises a wide-ranging treatment, and the twenty-four authors – from Canada, the United Kingdom, Italy, Germany, and the United States – have engaged deeply and diversely in an immense historical subject, offering new perspectives and approaches that define many of the most significant avenues of research for reproduction in the long eighteenth century.

Sections

This collection is divided into four subject-centred sections intended to emphasize common threads and themes. The following editorial overviews explain the common ground and shared interests of each section.

I Generation, Species, Breeding

Connecting this section's general themes of fetal development, species categorization, and breeding practices is a fundamental question that was of particular moment in the eighteenth century: how does generation work? The reader today will find it useful to keep in mind the following classical ideas about generation that – with diminishing influence – informed learned discussions and debates throughout the period. Seed was the essential material parents contributed to the creation of their progeny. Aristotelians held that males contributed seed and women matter, Galenists that both sexes contributed seed. In terms of development after conception, Aristotelian epigenesis was the general understanding until the late seventeenth century. The historian Joseph Needham offered a useful, although crude, shorthand account of the study of antenatal development before the early modern period: after Aristotle and until the Renaissance, "embryology has very little history" (Needham 1934, 41). A definitive human quality is endowed during this early development, which point was known as "quickening," or the moment of ensoulment. With genetics a distant future, an offspring's traits "were not linked to a hereditary substance" (Müller-Wille and Rheinberger 2012, 2), but were believed to reflect qualities endowed to parental seed, affected by a parent's thought, constitution, and behaviour, while leaving significant space for divine interventions and any number of environmental factors, which included "everything from nutrition to weather" (Davidson 2009, 3). Yet, more broadly controlling the form of developing progeny was the overarching organization of living beings: the great chain of being.

It was a significant change when, in the late seventeenth and eighteenth centuries, theories about generation came under scrutiny, particularly by experimental anatomists or, as Jacques Roger specified, a new kind of medical men who "devoted themselves entirely to research" (Roger 1963/1997, 138). Watershed moments like William Harvey's proclamation of "Ex Ovo Omnia" or Antoni van Leeuwenhoek's microscopic observation of seminal sperm were also disputed grounds for eighteenth-century medical men, natural philosophers, and cultural critics. With experiments, observations, and debates about generation came different theories that defined eighteenth-century thought. Preformation held that living things develop from miniature versions, whereas epigenesis held that living things develop through the sequential unfolding of parts. Pre-existence was the idea that souls exist before conception and are endowed during fetal development. That idea related to *emboîtement*, which considered living things to develop from pre-existing germs since the beginning of the world. With eggs and sperm known, which contained the fundamental substance necessary for life? Spermists contended male sperm contain the germ material; ovists contended female ova contain the germ material. New optic instruments made viewable a microscopic world teeming with life. Many asserted that these animalcules, or microscopic animals, contained the germ material, as in spermism. These theories, in various forms and combinations, proved to be unusually fertile soil for speculation, argument, prejudice, and learning about the nature of generation throughout the period.

The first three essays deal explicitly with how theories of generation were formulated, discussed, and disseminated among learned, primarily male, circles, but within varying national, political, and religious contexts. Moving from the gardens of Padua and Pisa to those of Oxford and Uppsala, Staffan Müller-Wille's chapter explores how translating ideas from garden experiments to printed page signalled a shift from the intellectual and practical modes of natural history to those of modern biology. In particular, Linnaeus's theories of reproduction derived in part from the epistemic practices of collecting, cataloguing, and circulating specimens and names. The conclusion Müller-Wille draws is that this form of knowledge creation inspired a theory of organic reproduction. The subsequent chapter by Ivano Dal Prete offers a nuanced study of theories and arguments about generation advanced by eighteenth-century Italian philosophers. While focusing specifically on discussions of preformationism and epigenesis, Dal Prete carefully details how scholastic traditions, theological doctrines, empirical limitations, clerical agendas, and Venetian politics significantly influenced debates about pre-existence. The Catholic Church, as Dal Prete contends, resisted preformationism as promoting mechanical philosophy, whereas the late eighteenth-century Republic of Venice supported that theory as a separation of natural philosophy from theology. Those kinds of theoretical debates about generation are also the topic of Peter J. Bowler's chapter. Bowler challenges traditional scholarly accounts that tidily separate pre-existence and materialism as supporting notions of stability and mutability, respectively, in life forms. His close examination of the ideas of comte de Buffon and Charles Bonnet, among other mid-eighteenth-century thinkers, reveals the short-fallings and oversights of that binary interpretation. One major consideration in the theoretical discussions highlighted by these first three authors, and which the following chapters scrutinize in detail, was inheritance.

Human breeding and heredity were topics with profound implications for eighteenth-century European social and political structures. Late eighteenth-century contexts of military conflict, increasing urbanization, blooming industrialization, and nascent demography cast breeding and population into sharp relief. John C. Waller's chapter demonstrates how aristocratic pedigrees were maintained through ideas of "noble blood" in Europe, its colonies, and America. Each country's hereditary classes underwent different changes; however, as Waller points out, they similarly used the language and ideas of generation in making biological claims and, ultimately, began mixing with bourgeois values and blood. Narrowing in on French and German discussions, Susanne Lettow analyses late eighteenth-century ideas about breeding for improvement in animals and humans. Her chapter compellingly demonstrates that European philosophers considered and promoted "race-mixing" with exotic peoples as a way of improving population. These philosophical discussions, Lettow suggests, reflected colonial experiences, but also political attitudes about intervening in reproduction and social perspectives on gender and ethnic others. Yet, as this section's closing chapter illustrates, not all types of breeding were seen in a positive light. Through a close reading of the *Wilhelm Meister* texts written by the German savant Johann Wolfgang von Goethe, Christine Lehleiter argues that incest was tabooed on the grounds of reproductive principles derived from experiments in animal husbandry. In Goethe's depictions, social censure and medical curiosity centre on the body of the incest child, Mignon. As Lehleiter concludes, eighteenth-century experiments in generation powerfully altered the way in which sex and reproduction were understood, and ushered in the biological perspectives that dominate our modern perceptions of these topics.

Resonant throughout the section's chapters is the idea that learned understandings of generation both meaningfully absorbed and influentially permeated broader eighteenth-century concerns and discussions. Taken together, these essays especially illuminate what historian Shirley A. Roe has described as the "extrascientific components" (Roe 1981, 148) – the wider political, social, religious, and philosophical considerations – that moulded understandings and discussions about generation in the eighteenth century.

II Fetus, Child, Mother

Cultural historians and literary scholars of eighteenth-century generation pay much attention to reproductive bodies and gender, with far greater focus falling on female, rather than male, bodies. Major discussions in this historiography include the influence of anatomical study on gender, most notably in Thomas Laqueur's one-sex/two-sex model; the meanings of different kinds of medical language, such as tropes, the vernacular, and technical jargon; the different technologies, techniques, perspectives, and "visual idioms" (Jordanova 1999, 214) that communicated scientific and cultural ideas about the body and reproduction; the dramatically changing medical vocations and practices that created "a new kind of corporeality" for birthing women (Duden 1991, 17); the sexual and reproductive science that "followed broader political struggles" (Schiebinger 1993, 183); the political "imperative to control women's sexuality and fecundity" that arose with empire (Nussbaum 1995, 1). This scope most frequently focuses on pregnant and birthing bodies, but also often encompasses non-parturient female, fetal, or infant bodies. The authors of this section examine eighteenth-century perceptions of these subjects, particularly highlighting such issues as fetal personhood, maternal status, health, and gender as variously represented by medicine, law, and literature. The first three essays concentrate on fetuses and infants, the latter three on perspectives about and from mothers.

Fetuses embody a sense of hidden growth and unknown outcomes, spurring curiosity and anxiety. Visualization, as Sebastian Pranghofer's chapter discusses, has been instrumental in knowing about fetuses and creating a sense of fetal personhood. Through examining eighteenth-century images of the unborn, Pranghofer richly details how such visual portrayals of fetuses in medical works influenced the social, scientific, religious, and legal standing of those otherwise little-seen entities. Corinna Wagner's chapter also considers fetuses and infants in law and medicine, but while exploring late eighteenth-and early nineteenth-century cases of maternal violence reported in court trials, newspapers, and medical texts. There was, Wagner argues, an increasing responsibility assumed by medics to give anatomical testimony about such crimes, and provide biological and psychological reasons for such seemingly unnatural acts by mothers. These medical explanations of maternal violence accommodated a broad cultural perspective that women were inherently good mothers. Also raising the topic of parental culpability, David M. Turner's chapter looks at congenital deformity, infant disability, and ideas of monstrosity. By examining explanations of physical defects and birth anomalies, Turner shows how parental responsibility for those occurrences changed from being an act of divine intervention, to maternal impressions, to more empirical perspectives about hereditary patterns. He contends that the unwanted social and economic burden associated with disability, combined with perceptions about abnormalities as hereditary, powerfully informed eighteenth-century attitudes and choices about reproduction.

A theme that both Wagner and Turner emphasize, and which figures prominently in the latter three essays of this section, is the connection between women's minds and their reproductive body parts or functions. Heather Meek's essay explores this connection through the figure of the hysteric, which, as she argues, changed dramatically mid-century. Meek describes a shift in understandings of hysteria from a condition common among females to one that was reserved for a marginal few sufferers. Late eighteenth-century hysterics were cast as "unnatural"; yet, as Meek reveals, that pathology provided both escape from mounting social strictures connected to motherhood and a space for the creative expression of women writers. One particularly controlled and debated maternal practice in the eighteenth century was breastfeeding. Through examining the writings of the Swiss physician, Samuel-Auguste Tissot, Sonja Boon's chapter unfolds the varied medical, social, and moral pros and cons associated with different ways of nursing or not nursing. As Boon shows, wet-nursing had important implications for the physical health, moral standing, and social status of the mother, nurse, and child. Boon argues that lactation became linked to understandings of self and identity, which reflected class, gender, race, and sexuality. Capping this section, Jennifer Golightly's chapter analyses the reproductive themes in the novels of late eighteenth-century female writers, Mary Wollstonecraft, Mary Hays, and Eliza Fenwick.

Golightly clearly demonstrates that these women's fictional narratives and radical politics were bound up with their reflections on, experiences of, and attitudes towards reproduction and maternity. As a whole, this section offers a wide array of scholarly perspectives – based on visual, medical, legal, and literary materials – that detail how eighteenth-century fetuses, children, and mothers were complexly involved in the changing ideas and practices related to generation.

III Pathologies, Body Parts, Display

The phrase "secrets of generation" partially refers to the shame and modesty connected to sexual body parts in Western culture. To what degree did medicine and science transform the "quite lax" attitudes towards sexuality that Michel Foucault described in his gloss of the history of sexuality (Foucault 1976/1998, 3)? Was the early modern period, as his opening account suggests, "a time of direct gestures, shameless discourse, and open transgressions, when anatomies were shown and intermingled at will" (ibid.)? Over the long eighteenth century particular contexts developed in which private parts could be publicly viewed. The chapters of the third section consider how reproductive and sexual bodies or body parts came under public inspection, especially within specific medical and anatomical frameworks, which included wider cultural, artistic, and literary participations. The first three essays explore the scrutinizing medical gaze aimed at pathological and abnormal bodies/parts, whereas the subsequent two essays take a more concerted look at the anatomical, aesthetic, and literary display of bodies/parts. Certain perceptions and themes about sex and generation recur throughout this section: normal and abnormal; the mind and the body; noteworthy and inconsequential; displayable and unviewable. These value-laden categories informed medical diagnoses, patient concerns, anatomical curatorial choices, and viewer/reader responses. This section contains diverse explorations of the different approaches – the considerations, values, practices, and anxieties – involved in determining how female and male reproductive body parts were shown and examined, and by whom.

Body consciousness, as we know it today, involves social expectations – largely concerning our age and sex – and our modern, innately gendered sense of self, which scholars like Dror Wahrman have argued emerged in the late eighteenth century (Wahrman 2004, 44). Yet, as Sarah Toulalan's chapter argues here, perceptions of appropriate body sizes, especially for sexual and procreative purposes, loomed large in early modern medical discourse. Toulalan intricately details how perceptions of fat and lean bodies of females and males related to fertility, sexual desire, the logistics of lovemaking, and general health, and all in keeping with significant changes in physiological thinking. Turning from obese and slim bodies to stunted and contorted bones, Pam Lieske's chapter examines how deformed female pelvises were cast into medical and public attention as an impediment to "the mechanism of birth" (Wilson 1995, 1). Misshapen pelvises were a real and present danger in the eighteenth-century world of widespread rickets, rare Caesarean sections, and experimental obstetric instruments. Lieske gathers the written and visual discourse about pelvic bones and delineates the various tactics and strategies medics deployed – such as demonstrations, measurements, models, and experiments – to cope with such deformities during birthing. Sally Frampton's chapter considers another female reproductive body part, the ovary, and how it figured in pathology. Diseased ovaries, as Frampton discusses, inspired especially ambivalent reactions and interpretations from practitioners and patients. These responses ranged from showcasing dropsical ovaries as monstrous spectacle to explanations of molar pregnancies as little more than generation gone wrong. Understandings of how reproduction worked, as these three essays suggest, were often gathered from times when reproduction did not work.

The last two chapters in this section deal specifically with how anatomical techniques and displays intersected with generation. Lianne McTavish explores how preparations of cadaveric materials were the site of continued generation, as smaller organisms proliferated on the dead, organic remains. Eighteenth-century French medics and anatomists, particularly Honoré Fragonard, theorized about and defended against the human body as a breeding ground for everything from parasitic insects to microscopic animalcules. McTavish's analysis shows how preserving bodies was a creative art intent on perpetuating lifelikeness while resisting the encroachment of parasitical reproductivity. In these aesthetic preservations, procreativity became male creativity. The section's last chapter, by Darren N. Wagner, focuses on the anatomical preparation and display of male genitalia. Wagner reveals how penises and testicles were significantly involved in developing specialized techniques, vocational identities, select markets, and general discussions characteristic of eighteenth-century British anatomy. His principle argument is that male genital preparations demonstrated a specific physiology of animal spirits and nerves, which centred on understandings of how body and mind interacted in sex and reproduction. Like other discussions in this book, these two chapters announce eighteenth-century anatomy as a special discipline for thinking about human and non-human generation; they also distinguish the role of aesthetic and literary domains in eighteenth-century generation. The section taken as a whole highlights certain kinds of mediations with bodies and body parts hitherto little noticed in the historiography of eighteenth-century reproduction, although meaningful then and deserving of attention now.

IV Attitudes, Tropes, Satire

This final section explores further one of the most influential, sophisticated, and varied aspects of this book's topic: generation and print. The manifold and rapid changes that transpired in generation would not have happened had not eighteenth-century print culture been so robust. Texts about generation circulated in all manner of marketplaces and public/private spheres: from transnational communities of learned medical men, to libraries in metropolitan aristocratic houses, to bedside tables in colonial rural homesteads. Diverse genres entered into discussions about what conception entailed, how intercourse should be performed, or who should deliver babies. Generation as an important topic circulated among specialists and non-specialists, practitioners and patients, women and men, medics and literati. The boundaries of such groups, however, were regularly blurred, subverted, or merely feigned in print. Literati doubled as doctors, men wrote as women, non-specialists preceded specialists, and practitioners invented patient biographies. Generation was also often bound in print with sex. Tim Hitchcock reminded his reader that the "range of eighteenth-century literatures in which sex formed a prominent part is extensive" (Hitchcock 1997, 17). One should further remember that who read what varied tremendously. As Mary Fissell observed, "Very few English men and even fewer women ever read a Latin anatomical text, but almost everyone encountered models of the body in the ballads, jokes, religious works, and popular medical books" about sex and reproduction (Fissell 2004, 1–2). A cornerstone of eighteenth-century society, print culture says much about generation in both practice and theory.

The section's first two chapters each focus on a specific text, both of which were hugely influential yet of entirely disparate genres and purposes. The first book is *Aristotle's Masterpiece* (1694/1986), which Marcia D. Nichols shows to be a text that represents the anomalous and the quotidian through its long, complex print history yet common, everyday accounts of generation. This text is, as Roy Porter described it, "evidence of what literate Europe encountered by way of 'all you need to know about sex but never dared to ask'" (Porter 1994, 136). By analysing this book's history in eighteenth-century America, Nichols argues that the different versions printed, sold, and circulated reflected changing gender politics. Moving from a prosaic domestic book to an iconic epic poem, Corrinne Harol and Jessica MacQueen probe *Paradise Lost* to decipher John Milton's depiction of generation theories and gender politics. Eve's proclivity to labour, Harol and MacQueen argue, reflects her epigenesist bearing, which lies in stark opposition to God's and Eden's preformationist design. In the postlapsarian world, as the authors incisively detail, Eve knowingly exercises her choice to reproduce, thereby exerting female agency over human procreation.

The final three chapters, all authored by scholars interested in how discussions about generation and literary ideas were mutually informed, particularly consider the satiric. In an expansive study that includes domestic manuals, midwifery treatises, and John Hill's satires, Julie Peakman and Sarah Watkins investigate how different genres promoted different attitudes towards reproduction. Their survey reveals that among the competing printed claims within the medical marketplace, satire frequently – and influentially – occupied a moderate position. What Peakman and Watkins describe is a special type of erotic satire that took issue with learned discussions about conception, pregnancy, and birth. The penultimate chapter, by Donald W. Nichol, explores a vastly different kind of poetic tradition, one which included the mid-eighteenth-century versions of the *Foundling Hospital for Wit*. Borrowing their titles and themes from the London charitable institution for unwanted newborns, the Foundling Hospital (founded 1741), these verse satires, as Nichol unveils, engaged a wider politics about reproductive tropes, London's literary culture, and the eye-opening sex-lives of noteworthy persons in the social circle of the original version's author, Hanbury Williams. A fitting conclusion, George Rousseau's chapter returns to John Hill to elaborate how his satire on generation, *Lucina Sine Concubitu*, was also a serious commentary on science, technology, politics, and ideology. Although *Lucina* was marginalized as strange and lewd, it offered sophisticated syntheses of contemporary ideas about generation, and homed in on certain scientific realities that were just on the horizon. Rousseau further shows that *Lucina*'s ideas of panspermism (sperm free-floating in the air) and asexual reproduction resonated with later discussions about generation and even revolutionary and post-revolutionary politics.

In sum, this section maps the intricate ways that ideas were communicated through different genres and among various reading and writing circles. Print significantly participated not only in disclosing the secrets of generation but in how generation – once disclosed – was understood, approached, and handled, especially as a topic in eighteenth-century "popular culture." Literature, particularly satire, offers a helpful refraction of the history of reproduction, allowing sharp readers now a better glimpse at how generation was understood then.

REFERENCES

Aristotle's Compleat Master-Piece. 1733. 19th ed. London.

Aristotle's Masterpiece. (1694) 1986. Edited by Randolph Trumbach. New York: Garland.

Armstrong, J. 1739. *The Oeconomy of Love*. 3rd ed. London: T. Cooper.

Bowers, T. 1996. *The Politics of Motherhood: British Writing and Culture 1680 – 1760*. Cambridge: Cambridge University Press.

Bradley, R. 1717. *New Improvements of Planting and Gardening*. London.: W. Mears.

Bradley, R. 1726. *A General Treatise of Husbandry and Gardening; Containing a new System of Vegetation*. Vol. 2. London: T. Woodward.

Cobb, M. 2006. *Generation: The Seventeenth-Century Scientists Who Unraveled the Secrets of Sex, Life, and Growth*. New York: Bloomsbury.

Cody, L.F. 2005. *Birthing the Nation: Sex, Science, and the Conception of Eighteenth-Century Britons*. Oxford: Oxford University Press.

Cole, F.J. 1930. *Early Theories of Sexual Generation*. Oxford: Oxford University Press.

Crawford, P. 2004. *Blood, Bodies and Families in Early Modern England*. Harlow: Pearson Longman.

Davidson, J. 2009. *Breeding: A Partial History of the Eighteenth Century*. New York: Columbia University Press.

Dawson, V.P. 1984. "Trembley, Bonnet, and Réaumur and the Issue of Biological Continuity." *Studies in Eighteenth-Century Culture* 13:43–63.

Dawson, V.P. 1987. *Nature's Enigma: The Problem of the Polyp in the Letters of Bonnet, Trembley, and Réaumur*. Philadelphia: American Philosophical Society, Memoir 174.

De Graaf, R. (1668) 1972. *Regnier De Graaf on the Human Reproductive Organs*. Translated by H.D. Jocelyn and B.P. Setchell. Oxford: Blackwell Scientific Publications.

Dionis, P. 1719. *A General Treatise of Midwifery*. London: A. Bell.

Duden, B. 1991. *The Woman Beneath the Skin: A Doctor's Patients in Eighteenth-Century Germany*. Translated by T. Dunlap. Cambridge, MA: Harvard University Press.

Erickson, R. 1986. *Mother Midnight: Birth, Sex, and Fate in Eighteenth-Century Fiction (Defoe, Richardson, and Sterne)*. New York: AMS.

Fissell, M. 1995. "Gender and Generation: Representing Reproduction in Early Modern England." *Gender & History* 7 (3):433–56. http://dx.doi.org/10.1111/j.1468-0424.1995.tb00035.x.

Fissell, M. 2004. *Vernacular Bodies: The Politics of Reproduction in Early Modern England*. Oxford: Oxford University Press.

Foucault, M. (1976) 1998. *The Will to Knowledge: The History of Sexuality*. Vol. 1. Translated by R. Hurley. London: Penguin.

Gasking, E. 1967. *Investigations into Generation 1651–1828*. Baltimore: Johns Hopkins University Press.

Graham, J. 1780. *A Lecture on the Generation, Increase and Improvement of the Human Species*. London: M. Smith.

Graham, J. 1783. *A Lecture on the Generation, Increase, and Improvement of the Human Species*. London: printed and sold at the Temple of Health.

Harvey, K. 2004. *Reading Sex in the Eighteenth Century*. Cambridge: Cambridge University Press.

Hitchcock, T. 1997. *English Sexualities, 1700–1800*. Basingstoke: Macmillan Press.

Jacob, F. 1973. *The Logic of Life: A History of Heredity*. Translated by Betty E. Spillmann. Princeton: Princeton University Press.

Johnson, S. (1755) 1979. *A Dictionary of the English Language*. New York: Arno.

Jordanova, L.J. 1985. "Gender, Generation and Science: William Hunter's Obstetrical Atlas." In *William Hunter and the Eighteenth-Century Medical World*, edited by W.F. Bynum and R. Porter, 385–412. Cambridge: Cambridge University Press.

Jordanova, L.J. 1986. "Naturalizing the Family: Literature and the Bio-Medical Sciences in the Late Eighteenth Century." In *Languages of Nature: Critical Essays on Science and Literature*, edited by L.J. Jordanova, 86–116. New Brunswick, NJ: Rutgers.

Jordanova, L.J. 1999. *Nature Displayed: Gender, Science and Medicine 1760–1820*. New York: Longman.

Jussieu. A. de. 1719. Du rapport des plantes avec les animaux tiré de la différence de leurs sexes. MS. 284, 1721, Bibliothèque du Muséum d'histoire naturelle.

Keller, E. 2007. *Generating Bodies and Gendered Selves: The Rhetoric of Reproduction in Early Modern England*. Seattle: University of Washington Press.

King, H. 2007. *Midwifery, Obstetrics and the Rise of Gynaecology: The Uses of a Sixteenth-Century Compendium*. Aldershot: Ashgate.

Klepp, S. 2009. *Revolutionary Conceptions: Women, Fertility and Family Limitation in America, 1760–1820*. Chapel Hill: University of North Carolina Press. http://dx.doi.org/10.5149/9780807838716_Klepp.

Laqueur, T. 1990. *Making Sex: Body and Gender from the Greeks to Freud*. Cambridge, MA: Harvard University Press.

Laqueur, T. 2003. *Solitary Sex: A Cultural History of Masturbation*. New York: Zone Books.

Lieske, P. 2007. *Eighteenth-Century British Midwifery*. London: Pickering & Chatto.

Linnaeus, C. (1729) 2007. *Carl von Linné/Linnaeus, "Praeludia Sponsaliarum Plantarum."* Translated by Xtina Wootz and Krister Östlund. Uppsala: Universitetsbibliotek.

Linnaeus, C. 1786. *A Dissertation on the Sexes of Plants.* Translated from the Latin of Linnaeus by James Edward Smith. Dublin: L. White.

Lonsdale, R. 1989. *Eighteenth-Century Women Poets: An Oxford Anthology*. Oxford: Oxford University Press.

Maclauchlan, D. 1735. *An Essay Upon Improving and Adding to the Strength of Great Britain and Ireland, by Fornication: Justifying the Same from Scripture and Reason*. Dublin .

Marten, J. 1709. *Gonosologium Novum: Or, a New System Of all the Secret Infirmities and Diseases, Natural, Accidental, and Venereal in Men and Women*. London: S. Crouch.

Maupertuis, P.-L.M. de. (1745) 1966. *Vénus physique (1745)"The Earthly Venus" by Pierre-Louis Moreau de Maupertuis*. Translated from "Vénus physique" by S.B. Boas, with notes and introduction by G. Boas. New York: Johnson Reprint Collection.

Mayr, E. 1982. *The Growth of Biological Thought: Diversity, Evolution, and inheritance*. Cambridge, MA, and London: Belknap Press of Harvard University.

McLaren, A. 1984. *Reproductive Rituals: The Perception of Fertility in England from the Sixteenth to the Nineteenth Century*. London and New York: Methuen.

Miller, V. 1751. *The Man-Plant: or, Scheme for Increasing and Improving the British Breed*. London: M. Cooper.

Müller-Wille, S., and H.-J. Rheinberger. 2012. *A Cultural History of Heredity*. Chicago: University of Chicago Press. http://dx.doi.org/10.7208/chicago/9780226545721.001.0001.

Muri, A. 2010. "Imagining Reproduction: The Politics of Reproduction, Technology and the Woman Machine." *Journal of Medical Humanities* 31 (1):53–67. http://dx.doi.org/10.1007/s10912-009-9102-8.

Needham, J. 1934. *A History of Embryology*. Cambridge: Cambridge University Press.

Needham, J. 1959. *A History of Embryology*. New York: Abelard-Schuman.
Needham, J.T. 1749. *Observations Upon the Generation,Composition, and Decomposition of Animal and Vegetable Substances*. London.
Nussbaum, F. 1995. *Torrid Zones: Maternity, Sexuality and Empire in Eighteenth-Century English Narrative*. Baltimore and London: Johns Hopkins University Press.
Park, K. 2006. *Secrets of Women: Gender, Generation, and the Origins of Human Dissection*. New York: Zone Books.
Parsons, J. 1752. *Philosophical Observations on the Analogy between the Propagation of Vegetables and That of Animals*. London: C. Davis.
Peakman, J. 2003. *Mighty Lewd Books: The Development of Pornography in Eighteenth-Century England*. London: Palgrave. http://dx.doi.org/10.1057/9780230512573.
Perry, R. 1991. "Colonizing the Breast: Sexuality and Maternity in Eighteenth-Century England." *Journal of the History of Sexuality* 2 (2):204–35.
Pinto-Correia, C. 1997. *The Ovary of Eve: Egg and Sperm and Preformation*. Chicago: University of Chicago Press. http://dx.doi.org/10.7208/chicago/9780226669502.001.0001.
Porter, R. 1994. "The Literature of Sexual Advice before 1800." In *Sexual Knowledge, Sexual Science: The History of Attitudes to Sexuality*, edited by R. Porter and M. Teich, 134–58. Cambridge: Cambridge University Press.
Porter, R., and L. Hall. 1995. *The Facts of Life: The Creation of Sexual Knowledge in Britain, 1650–1950*. New Haven and London: Yale University Press.
Quillet, C. 1710. *Callipaedia: Or, the Art of Getting Pretty Children*. London: B. Lintott.
Réaumur, R.A.F. (1749) 1750. *The Art of Hatching and Bringing Up Domestick Fowls of All Kinds, at any Time of the Year.* Trans. 1750. London: C. Davis.
Roe, S.A. 1981. *Matter, Life, and Generation: 18th-Century Embryology and the Haller-Wolff Debate*. Cambridge: Cambridge University Press.
Roe, S.A. 2003. The Life Sciences. In *The Cambridge History of Science.* Vol. 4, *Eighteenth-Century Science*, edited by Roy Porter, 397–416. Cambridge: Cambridge University Press. http://dx.doi.org/10.1017/CHOL9780521572439.018.
Roger, J. (1963) 1997. *The Life Sciences in Eighteenth-Century French Thought*. Translated by Robert Ellrich. Stanford: Stanford University Press.
Schiebinger, L. 1986. "Skeletons in the Closet: The First Illustrations of the Female Skeleton in Eighteenth-Century Anatomy." *Representations* (Berkeley, Calif.) 14:42–82. http://dx.doi.org/10.1525/rep.1986.14.1.99p01227.
Schiebinger, L. 1993. *Nature's Body: Gender in the Making of Modern Science*. Boston: Beacon Press.

Sharp, J. (1671) 1999. *The Midwives Book*. Edited by E. Hobby. New York: Oxford University Pess.
Shelley, M. (1818) 2012. *Frankenstein*. Edited by D.L. Mcdonald and K. Scherf. Peterborough: Broadview.
Shteir, A.B. 1996. *Cultivating Women, Cultivating Science: Flora's Daughters and Botany in England, 1760–1860*. Baltimore: Johns Hopkins University Press.
Smith, J.E.H., ed. 2006. *The Problem of Animal Generation in Early Modern Philosophy*. Cambridge: Cambridge University Press. http://dx.doi.org/10.1017/CBO9780511498572.
Spallanzani, L. 1784. *Dissertations Relative to the Natural History of Animals and Vegetables.* Translated from the Italian of the Abbe Spallanzani. Vol. 2. London: J. Murray.
Stephanson, R. 2004. *The Yard of Wit: Male Creativity and Sexuality, 1650–1750*. Philadelphia: University of Pennsylvania Press.
Stephanson, R. 2012. "*Tristram Shandy* and the Art of Conception." In *Vital Matters: Eighteenth-Century Views of Conception, Life, and Death*, edited by H. Deutsch and M. Terrall, 93–108. Toronto: University of Toronto Press.
Sterne, L. 2004. *The Life and Opinions of Tristram Shandy, Gentleman*. Edited by Robert Folkenflik. New York: Modern Library.
Swift, J. (1726) 2008. *Gulliver's Travels*. Edited by C. Rawson. Oxford: Oxford University Press.
Tillotson, G., P. Fussell, and M. Waingrow, eds. 1969. *Eighteenth-Century English Literature*. New York: Harcourt, Brace & World.
Todd, D. 1995. *Imagining Monsters: Miscreations of the Self in Eighteenth-Century England*. Chicago: University of Chicago Press.
Vartanian, A. 1950. "Trembley's Polyp, La Mettrie, and Eighteenth-Century French Materialism." *Journal of the History of Ideas* 11 (3):259–86. http://dx.doi.org/10.2307/2707732.
Venette, N. 1740. *The Pleasures of Conjugal-Love Explain'd … Done from the French, by a Physician*. London: P. Meighan.
Wahrman, D. 2004. *The Making of the Modern Self: Identity and Culture in Eighteenth-Century England.* New Haven: Yale University Press.
Wilson, A. 1995. *The Making of Man-Midwifery: Childbirth in England 1660–1770*. London: University College London Press.
Wood, R.J., and V. Orel. 2001. *Genetic Prehistory in Selective Breeding: A Prelude to Mendel.* Oxford: Oxford University Press.

PART ONE

Generation, Species, Breeding

1 Reproducing Species

STAFFAN MÜLLER-WILLE

Hardly any originary moment in the history of the life sciences can be dated as precisely as the origin of the term "biology." In 1802, two leading theoreticians, Jean-Baptiste de Lamarck (1744–1829) and Gottfried Reinhold Treviranus (1776–1837), coined this term to designate a new science (Baron 1966).[1] And yet it remains nebulous what this new term designated exactly. Clearly not a new discipline – it was only around 1900 that biology acquired the usual insignia of a scientific discipline like dedicated chairs, associations, journals, textbooks, and teaching programs (Coleman 1971, ch. 1; Pauly 1984; Caron 1988). There is also no clear-cut paradigmatic achievement – an experiment, a theoretical proposal – that one can point out as ushering in the age of biology. All that one is left with is the vague but unavoidable impression that "around 1800" all the concepts that have to do with life and living beings change their meaning. Reproduction itself is a key example, alongside organization, generation, heredity, species, history (Rey 1989; Jacob 1970/1993; Jordanova 1995; Roger 1963/1998; Müller-Wille and Rheinberger 2012, ch. 2). Reinhard Koselleck has called this time a "saddle period," in which socio-political discourse underwent a total "transformation of the premodern usage of language to our usage" (Koselleck 2002, 5). The same can be said about the life sciences in the same period, as Michel Foucault did long ago with the usual aplomb. It is worth quoting him at length:

> At the institutional level, the inevitable correlatives of this patterning [of nature, by taxonomy; the original has *découpage*] were botanical gardens and natural history collections. And their importance, for Classical culture, does not lie in what they make it [*sic*] possible to see, but in what they hide and in what, by this process of obliteration, they allow to emerge: they screen off

> anatomy and function, they conceal the organism, in order to raise up before the eyes of those who await the truth the visible relief of forms, with their elements, their mode of distribution, and their measurements. They are books furnished with structures, the space in which characteristics combine, and in which classifications are physically displayed. One day, towards the end of the eighteenth century, Cuvier was to topple the glass jars of the Museum, smash them open, and dissect all the forms of animal visibility that the Classical age had preserved in them. This iconoclastic gesture ... does not reveal a new curiosity directed towards a secret that no one had the interest or courage to uncover, or the possibility of uncovering, before. It is rather, and much more seriously, a mutation in the natural dimension of Western culture [*mutation dans l'espace naturel de la culture occidentale*]: the end of history in the sense in which it was understood by Tournefort, Linnaeus, Buffon, and Adanson ... and it was also the beginning of what by substituting anatomy for classification, organism for structure, internal subordination for visible character, the series for tabulation, was to make possible the precipitation into the old flat world of animals and plants, engraved in black and white, of a whole profound mass of time to which men were to give the renewed name of *history*. (Foucault 1966/1974, 137–8)

In this chapter I would like to suggest that it is time to revisit Michel Foucault's thesis, but with a twist. To remain in his imagery, I want to raise the question how the "glass jars" of classical natural history gradually came to be filled with exactly the kind of life that would later on become the subject of "biology" according to Foucault. I address this question in three steps: first, casting the net widely, by reviewing the history of botanical gardens from the Renaissance to the "classical" age of natural history (first section); second, by highlighting how the circulation of specimens and names among naturalists developed into an essential tool of knowledge accumulation during the seventeenth century (second and third sections); and finally, now narrowly focusing on the work of Carl Linnaeus (1707–78), by showing how these tools impacted on the earliest attempts to formulate a theory of organic reproduction (fourth section).

From Theatre to Tableau

Some time around 1545, the first botanical gardens were founded at the universities of Padua and Pisa (priority remains under dispute to this day). Let us take a closer look at what these institutions contained. Figure 1.1 shows a ground plan of the garden in Padua from its first printed guide, published in 1591. What strikes the beholder is its strictly geometrical, and yet involute layout: a circular perimeter contains four square areas, which in turn are occupied by flower beds laid out according to more complex geometrical patterns. Garden historians have paid a lot of attention to this striking design, which appears in aerial photographs of Padua to this day like a tattoo on the city's skin. Interpretations range from a design following natural philosophical pinciples, according to which each plant is assigned a place in the garden according to planetary constellations and associated combinations of the four primary qualities hot, cold, dry, and wet (Schiller 1987); to a design in the hermetic tradition, according to which the geometric patterns invest the garden with a multitude of hidden meanings, decodable for the initiated (Tongiorgio Tomasi 1983); to the relatively straightforward interpretation, that the four squares simply represent the four corners of the world, and hence the geographic distribution of plants (Prest 1981, 46–8). All of these interpretations share the assumption that the garden design should be understood as resulting from attempts at representing topological relationships, be they cosmological, magical, or geographic. The rationale of such attempts, according to historian of Renaissance art and science Lucia Tongiorgi Tomasi, was that botanists and gardeners tried to emulate the conditions of natural environments from which the plants were taken (Tongiorgio Tomasi 1983, 23).

Historical sources provide scant evidence for these modern interpretations, however. If they engage in a discussion of the garden design at all, they hint at a representation of the four corners of the sky and the ideal layout of an ancient Roman city (Ubrizsy Savioa 1995, 173). I believe there is a reason for this diffidence. In the end, the garden primarily served the practical purpose of teaching medical students the knowledge of pharmaceutic drugs. The courses, or "demonstrations" (*demonstrationes*) as they were called, followed a strict routine: the demonstrator pointed out plants to the students, whereas the "professor" pronounced their names and added information on distinctive features, medical uses, and literary records (Reeds 1976; Ogilvie 2006, ch. 3). Essentially, a demonstration thus associated a name with a plant growing at a certain place in the garden through the simple act of pointing at it, while the name at the same time provided access to oral and literary traditions supposedly dealing with the plant in question (on the fundamental epistemological significance of pointing, see Barnes, Bloor, and Henry 1996, 47–59).

This didactic function of early botanical gardens suggests that the garden design served as a mnemonic device. Names were inscribed into a concrete arrangement of the plants they referred to, and this arrangement

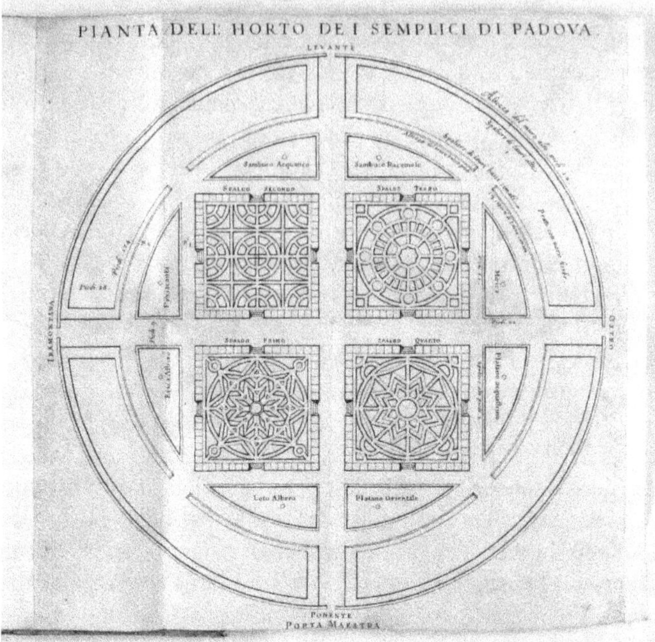

Figure 1.1 The garden as a world theatre. Ground view of the botanical garden in Padua. Copper engraving from Girolamo Porro, *Horto dei semplici di Padova* (Venice 1591). Source: Wikimedia Commons.

was saturated with representations of cosmological, physical, and geometrical relationships. Each name corresponded to a place defined by its topological relationships with other such places; and each place had a name that evoked its proper traditions. It is in this sense that the guide of 1591 talks of the garden as a "small theatre, almost a little world" (Rippa Bonati and Dal Piaz 1995, 42). And it is in this sense, also, that Foucault (1974, 131) spoke of natural history in the Renaissance as "the circular procession of the 'show'" (*montre* in the original, which rather means "pointer" or "indicator"). One curious feature that the garden of Padua possessed in the Renaissance brings this character to the fore particularly well. We know from historical documents and meticulous reconstructions which plants grew in which beds in the first few years of the garden. And it turns out that plants of the same species were often grown at different places in the garden, bearing different names (Ubrizsy Savioa 1995, 179 and 197). The protagonists of Padua's garden "theatre" could play different roles, depending on context, without becoming "duplicates" (cf. Olmi 1992, 152–61; Swan 2001, 118).

The gardens at Padua and Pisa served as models for the foundation of similar gardens at European universities, first in Northern Italy, later, at the beginning of the seventeenth century, elsewhere in Europe as well – Leiden, Oxford, Paris, to name just the most important. Teaching "materia medica" remained the chief function and the courses continued to follow the established pattern of "demonstrations." And yet one can observe from quite early on drastic changes in garden design: the garden at Leiden, founded in 1587, basically consisted of long, numbered flower beds arranged in parallel to form squares, and the plants seem to be distributed at random in these beds. The garden at Oxford presented itself in a similarly plain manner. All one can still glean from these plans is the motif of the "four corners of the world." But even this motif should eventually go. In the botanical garden of Uppsala, brought to international fame in the mid-eighteenth century by Linnaeus, all floral design is absent (see figure 1.2). Plants were distributed on the one hand according to their needs into hot houses, basins with running and still water, and two large areas with perennial plants on one side, and annual plants on the other. The two areas, in turn, divide into twenty-four parallel beds, corresponding to the classes of Linnaeus's sexual system. The order of plants within each area, that is, is purely taxonomic, solely depending on the number and arrangement of male and female flower parts, with no reference to pharmaceutic virtues, geography, or habitus. This design was introduced by Linnaeus into the university garden in 1731 already, when he served as "demonstrator" there.[2]

Even this order resulted in a concrete arrangement of plants, and Linnaeus always emphasized the pedagogic prerogatives of such an arrangement (e.g., Linnaeus 1738, "Lectori" [unpag.]). But this arrangement had no connection anymore with the cosmic order of nature or geographic space. If at all, the arrangement according to the sexual system pointed on a metaphorical level to the follies of human sexuality. Linnaeus liked to explain his system by referring to "husbands" and "wives" and their various amorous liaisons, which included polygamy, adultery, prostitution, homosexuality, and incest – certainly to the delight of his students, but causing indignation in many of his colleagues (Schiebinger 1991). If one abstracts from this metaphorical level – and thus takes the fun away – what one is left with is an abstract grid of taxonomic identities in which each plant species – in contrast to the garden at Padua in its early years – takes on a strictly defined, unambiguous position that corresponds to a unique

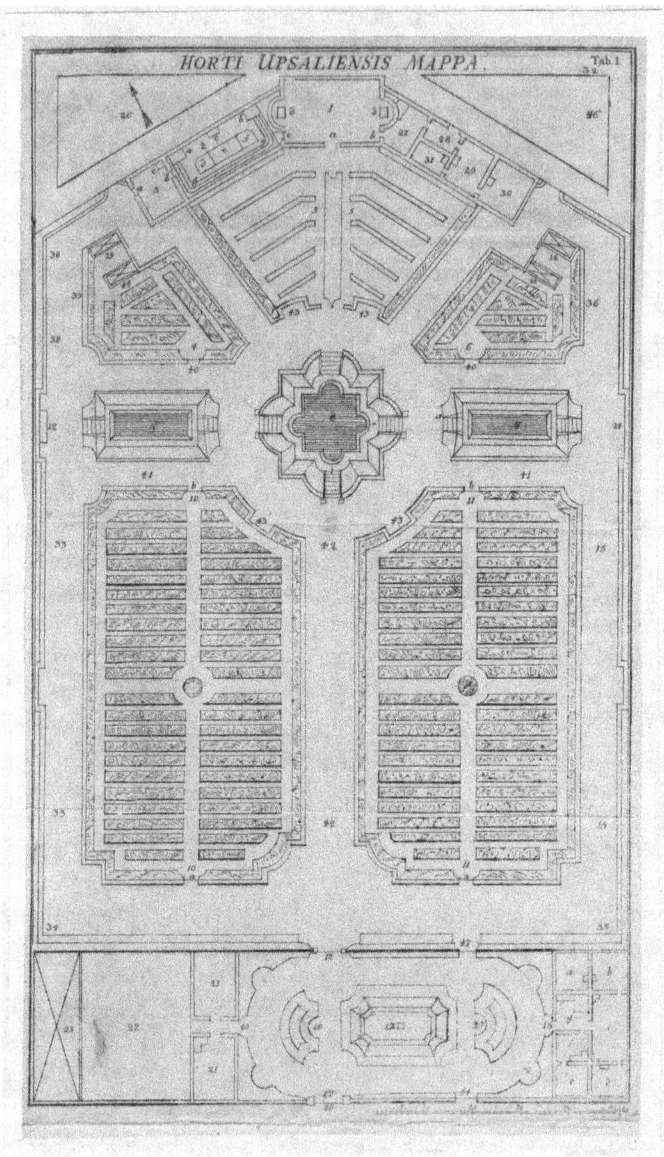

Figure 1.2 The garden as tableau. Ground view of the botanical garden in Uppsala. Copper engraving from Carolus Linnaeus, *Hortus Upsaliensis* (Uppsala 1745). Courtesy Uppsala University Library.

name. This is what Foucault called the "tableau," a "non-temporal rectangle in which, stripped of all commentary, of all enveloping language, creatures present themselves one beside another, their surfaces visible, grouped according to their common features, and thus already virtually analysed, and bearers of nothing but their name" (Foucault 1974, 131).

Names and Lists

The linear arrangement of flower beds in Linnaeus's botanical garden has a surprising parallel in a feature of the garden guide published for Padua in 1591. This guide contained not only the ground plan discussed above, but it also displayed the four areas separately once more. A clearer picture of the individual beds thus emerges, and each of the beds is inscribed with a unique number. These numbers correspond to a numbered series of blank rectangles to the right of the plan, which provided space for entering the names of plant species growing in respective beds. The names in turn could be found in an alphabetical index at the end of the guide. To connect this index with the beds of the garden one had to visit the garden, however, and attend a demonstration (Rhodes 1984, 329; Ubriszy Savioa 1995, 183–4; for a similar guide published in 1601 for the botanical garden in Leiden, see Swan 2001, 124–5).

It is the linear series of blank spaces that provides the surprising parallel with Linnaeus's garden. While the numbers do refer to the elements of floral garden design, the series itself assumes the simplest form of a "tableau," the form of a list (on the significance of lists for early modern natural history, see Delbourgo and Müller-Wille 2012). Individual copies of the guide have survived in libraries that contain plant names entered in script and thus show that the guide was indeed used as just indicated. The guide hence provided students and other visitors of the garden with a template that helped them to make annotations during demonstrations in such a way that they could identify names and specimens on their own when revisiting the garden at a later date. The guide, or more precisely, the numbers it contained, replaced the wooden pointer of the demonstrator.

If this had been the sole function of the guide, its usefulness would have been quite restricted, however. Plant specimens were continually rearranged in the garden of Padua (Ubrizsy Savioa 1995, 176–81). A guide that had been filled out during one year would therefore not necessarily give an accurate picture of the arrangement of specimens in the next year anymore. Yet similar lists abound in other contexts as well. Garden directors undertook far-reaching excursions to collect specimens and seeds, and would exchange these, in addition to drawings and dried specimens, with other botanists to complete their "world theatres." Routinely, this exchange was accompanied by letters containing lists detailing the names of exchanged materials (on botanical exchange see Stearn 1961; Wijnands 1988; Bourguet 1996; Spary 2000, 61–78; Dauser et al. 2008; on the use of lists in this context, Heniger 1971; Pugliano 2012). Whole garden plans, with plant names meticulously entered into the beds, were sent to inform correspondents about the specimens growing in one's garden (Masson 1972), and there also existed printed instructions for building up these "paper gardens" (*horti papyricaei*; Ferrarius 1638, 211). Such lists and maps, finally, could also be published to make them known among a wider audience. These "catalogues" of individual gardens and certain regions covered by botanical excursions constituted a distinct and characteristic genre in the seventeenth century, and set into train a process of iteration, as the listed names were routinely complemented with references to earlier catalogues (Cooper 2007, ch. 2). Manuscript lists and plans, in turn, could make use of these printed enumerations. A garden plan sent by Ulysse Aldrovandi to one of his correspondents, for example, referred to Pietro Andrea Matthioli's *Commentarii in Libros Sex Pedacii Dioscoridis Anazarbei* (1554) (Ubriszy Savioa 1995, 181).

Such lists, plans, and catalogues cannot have possessed a value of their own. Taken individually and by their plain words, they referred to an extremely local and ephemeral setting – a set of plant specimens, growing here and there, in this year, or another (many catalogues went into several editions). What gave them value was not their actual content, but that they could be used to reiterate the references they contained elsewhere (through citation) and thus to intercalate these references into new contexts (other letters, especially response letters; new lists and catalogues addressing others). One is beginning to get a sense that the "tableau" of classical natural history was not at all as static as common lore has it.

Circulation of Words and Things

The establishment of correspondence networks and new genres of natural history went hand in hand with the formation of new social identities of collectors and naturalists. Natural history became a means of communicating across social and religious divides and opened routes for vertical mobility (Cook 2007). "Collectors depended on resources of learned culture to complete their personal mosaics," as Paula Findlen expressed this for the Italian Renaissance (Findlen 1994, 304). Bibliography in particular served as a genre to depict these new social identities and relationships, and to trace the increasing division of labour. Linnaeus, for example, portrayed botany in his *Bibliotheca Botanica* (1736) as a "free republic," the subjects of which differed by their function only for the overall purpose of botany, and in which recognition was distributed strictly according to merit. The primary distinction that Linnaeus drew was that between "collectors" and "systematists" (*methodici*). Collectors contributed to the "number of species," either by sending specimens or seeds, or by producing descriptions or drawings of "new" species. "Systematists" on the other hand presided over the institutions where this material accumulated, botanical gardens in particular, and hence were in a position to adjudicate on claims to discovery and digest the new material through classification and proper naming. They were thus epistemically privileged, but at the same time highly dependent on exchange with collectors outside their institutions. Hence the language of equality and disinterested friendship that speaks from natural history correspondences. Without fair compensation and recognition, a systematist would risk seeing his sources for "new" species run dry (Müller-Wille 2003).

This formation of a system of exchange in botany had important consequences for the delineation of its epistemic object. Discourse began to articulate itself on two levels that were connected again and again in countless transactions, but increasingly began to appear as logically and objectively independent of each other: on one level representatives and representations of species circulated, be it in the form of living exemplars reproduced by seed, in the form of dried herbarium specimens, or in the form of detailed descriptions and drawings produced from such specimens; on another level names, or numbers, referring to these representations circulated, be it in lists, tables, catalogues, classification systems, or more discursive descriptions and accounts.[3] It is this articulation of discourse into a level of circulating representations and a level of circulating designations that Foucault seems to have had in mind when he spoke about a "duplicated representation," and a reduction of signs to their signifying function only, in the transition from the Renaissance to the classical age (Foucault 1974, 63–7).

Let me illustrate this further by contrasting the practice of teaching by demonstration with the practice of botanical exchange. In demonstrations, both teacher and student belong to the same local tradition, or rather, their relationship constitutes that very same local tradition. It is the teacher who points at, or calls out, an object to produce an impression on the mind of the student (this is the original, pedagogic meaning of lat. *informatio*). In botanical exchange, the relationship is more symmetrical and constitutes a continual back and forth of disclosure, acknowledgment, correction, and further inquiry between people who belong to different local traditions. References, names, or simply numbers would therefore serve recipients of information primarily to get back to the author (or someone else) with confirmations, criticisms, or amendments. For this, the relationship between name and object established at the author's end at a certain place and time needs to be reconstituted, or reproduced, at the recipient's end, and hence in another context, at another place and time.

Context matters, of course, and a whole range of things may happen as a consequence of exchanging names, representations, and associated bits of factual knowledge among distant transactors. Two of them are especially salient:

1. On the level of representations, it not only becomes apparent that certain attributes vary with context, but also mandatory for the sake of communication to note which of the attributes vary with context, and in what manner, and which remain constant. This distinction is at the core of Linnaeus's famous species definition: "There are as many species as there were different forms produced by the Infinite Being in the beginning. Which forms afterwards produce more, but always similar forms according to inherent laws of generation; so that there are no more species now than came into being in the beginning. Hence, there are as many species as there are different forms or structures of plants occurring today, setting aside those which place or accident exhibits to be less different (varieties)" (Linnaeus 1737b, "Ratio operis," aph. 5 [unpag.]; translation quoted from Müller-Wille and Reeds 2007, 565). Botanical gardens and collections became places where differences were "reduced" locally, to use a term frequently employed by Linnaeus. Here, as presumably in paradise, species would stand out against each other in their original and characteristic features. At the same time, however, botanical gardens will produce certain differences. *Betula nana*, the dwarf birch, is a small shrub in its native tundra environment, but grows into a bush or even tree when imported into botanical gardens in more temperate regions. What begins to unfold in the system of gardens is a history of reproducing species and varieties (Müller-Wille, 2001).
2. On the level of plant names one can observe a parallel shift towards reducing their meaning to pure reference. The more names served to communicate information, the less one could rely on their relationship

with other words and propositions in a given idiom. This trend becomes most apparent in the development of so-called synonymies in the seventeenth century. In place of an explicit definition of a species, botanists began to provide long lists of names previously employed in botanical literature. Each of the names in a synonymy list thus constituted a reference to a particular representation of the species in question. One name stands in for the other, while the synonymy list at the same time constitutes a series of instances of the species that again highlights diversity rather than unity. At the same time, juxtaposed in this manner, names turn out to be entirely conventional in nature, lacking intrinsic meaning beyond their capacity to denote or point out. "Names have the same value on the market of botany as the coin has in the commonwealth, which is accepted at a certain price without necessitating a metallurgic examination," as Linnaeus put it in a famous metaphor (Linnaeus 1737a, 204; if not otherwise stated, all translations are my own).

Species in the pre-Darwinian era, as one can see from these two points, did not at all present themselves to naturalists as static entities, as the historiography of the life sciences commonly assumes.[4] Quite on the contrary, they presented themselves as reservoirs productive of a bewildering diversity. The early modern term *copia*, meaning learned profusion with both negative and positive connotations, nicely captures this (Ekedahl 2005; on early modern "information overload" see Ogilvie 2003; Blair 2010).

Economy of Nature and the Organism

John Prest has traced back the history of botanical gardens to the medieval idea of a *hortus conclusus*, a place of private reclusion and religious contemplation (Prest 1981, 22). And indeed, such gardens were usually enclosed by walls and access was more or less strictly regulated (with separate entrances for the public, the gardeners, and the professor). One can look at these walls as an effective means to produce the real abstractions discussed in the previous section: inside the garden, the clean world of systematically arranged and clearly distinguished plant species, each carrying its name; outside of it, the chaotic world of natural and cultivated varieties with their vernacular names and associated lore. "Earth does not bring forth everything everywhere, and the various families of plants are scattered all over the world," as Linnaeus claimed in 1737. In order to reverse this situation, and have access to the productions of nature at a single place, the botanist therefore depended "on global trade (*commercia per totum orbem*), libraries with all books published on plants, gardens, hothouses and gardeners" (Linnaeus 1737c, "Dedicatio" [unpag.]).

Linnaeus's description of what could be demanded of a botanical garden as a place of study, especially his mention of global trade, stands in a certain tension with the idea of a closed garden, however. And indeed, with regard to their legal status the gardens of Padua and Pisa were distinguished from private gardens right from the start as "public gardens" (*horti publici*; Ubrizsy Savioa 1995, 173). The gardens included a "spezzieria," that is an apothecary's workshop, in which plants were distilled and the products tested with respect to their pharmaceutic efficacy (Rhodes 1984, 327). In addition, the gardens served as a reference collection for Venetian spice traders (Ubrizsy Savioa 1995, 181). From early on, botanical gardens grew into centres of a "plant mercantilism" (Bourguet 1996, 95) – the Dutch East India Company founded a garden at the Cape of Good Hope in 1652 (Prest 1981, 43) – and they would turn into an essential instrument of colonial expansion in the nineteenth century (Miller and Reill 1996; McCracken 1997; Drayton 2000; Schiebinger and Swan 2005; Schaffer et al. 2009). This instrument could also be used for the shaping of national territories and their subjects. Botanical gardens offered a space to appropriate foreign nature through acclimatization, to explore the national fauna and flora for species that could serve as substitutes for expensive imports, and to set standards for national production and trade (Osborne 1994; Mukerji 1997; Barrera-Osario 2006). It comes as no surprise, therefore, to find that the paper-tools discussed in the previous section show similarities with practices of annotation common in the commercial world (te Heesen 2004).

Botany as a scholarly enterprise was therefore always part of the sphere of manufacture and mercantile activities. The walls of botanical gardens did not so much constitute a sharp dividing line between an inside world of pure science and an outside world saturated by economic and political interests. Rather, they functioned in the manner of a membrane, mediating a standardized reproduction of plant specimens under highly controlled conditions on the inside with the outside distribution of plants on a range of natural and artificial (horti- and agricultural) habitats. One can witness this in Linnaeus's tireless (and at times tiring) emphasis on the "utility" of natural history for the nation, his many "patriotic" projects – research trips through various provinces of Sweden, popular treatises on edible and poisonous domestic plants or on exotic consumer goods like coffee or tobacco, and countless projects striving for the acclimatization of plants like tea or the mulberry to the harsh winters in Sweden (Koerner 1999). The botanic garden at Uppsala was both a catch basin of local experiences and a fountain for new experimental objects.

Interestingly, one finds this membrane function reflected in two dichotomies that structure Linnaeus's natural philosophy. The first of these dichotomies pertains to what he called the "economy of nature," which he defined as "the all-wise of the Creator in relation to natural things, by which they are fitted to produce general ends and reciprocal uses." The economy of nature was not simply upheld, according to Linnaeus, by mutual relations of consumption and production. Rather, as he explained in 1749, it encompassed relations in two dimensions: first, the dimension of a "continued series" (*continuata series* in the Latin original), in which individuals generate their like; and second, the spatial dimension of a "mutual connection" (*nexus inter se* in the Latin original), in which individuals "lend a helping hand to each other, so that the death and destruction of one would serve the restitution of the other" (Linnaeus 1749b, 1–2; translation based on Linnaeus 1775, 39–40).

"Continued generation" (*generatio continuata*) was a technical term Linnaeus had introduced to set himself apart from all those theories of generation that focused on the original moment of creating an individual, be it divine, or more mundane, and thus allowed for the possibility of equivocal generation. "Continued generation" extended beyond the production of an individual, and was strictly regulated by "laws of generation" (*leges generationis*) (Linnaeus 1737b, "Ratio operis," aph. 5; see Müller-Wille and Rheinberger 2012, ch. 2, for a detailed discussion). With this concept of generation he came very close to what Buffon, at about the same time, addressed as reproduction. And as in Buffon, a temporal, if not historical, dimension thus opened in Linnaeus's philosophy of nature. This dimension becomes most palpable in the monographic descriptions of particular species that Linnaeus produced occasionally. In a separate section that was often entitled *Historia*, he would deliver an account of when specimens of the species in question were first introduced into a botanical garden, how they travelled to other gardens from there, who produced descriptions and drawings from these specimens, and which changes they would undergo in the course of their translations. The most famous of these monographs is perhaps *Peloria*, in which Linnaeus put forward the idea that species originated in time from hybridization among a few original forms (Müller-Wille 2008).

The second dimension, the mutual *nexus* (a term with the juridical connotation of contractual obligations), in contrast to the diachronic dimension of *series*, relates to the synchronic, trophic relationships that organisms depend on for their reproduction. In this dimension, members of a species are distributed across a range of habitats, forming different varieties depending on local food supply and climatic conditions. That this distribution does not end up in degeneration and eventual decay is due, according to Linnaeus, to the exact "proportion" with which reproduction according to the "laws of generation" ensures that each lost individual is replaced by a new one. As the twelfth edition of the *Systema Naturae* had it, "Thus hunger distributes those, which Venus reunites" (Linnaeus 1766–8, 1:18). And in *Politiae Naturae* he formulated the same thought using a striking economic metaphor. At first sight, Linnaeus argued, nature might appear to consist of a war of all against all; on closer inspection, however, one sees that

> it is difficult, if not impossible, to discern beginning and end in divine works. In a circle, namely, runs everything. Not less than on weekly markets (*in nundinis*). At first one only sees how a great mass of people spreads out in this or that direction, while nevertheless each of them has his home (*domicilium*), from where he approached and to which he will proceed. (Linnaeus 1760, 17–18)

The second dichotomy in Linnaeus's natural philosophy that reflects the membrane function of the walls of botanical gardens pertains to the individual body, rather than nature at large. All organisms, according to Linnaeus, are composed from two substances, the medullar and the cortical substance. The former is characterized by a capacity for infinite growth. It is represented by the pith in plants, and the nervous system in animals, and is passed on to offspring along the maternal line. The latter surrounds the former and provides nutrition and protection from noxious, environmental influences. It is passed on along the paternal line. Both substances depend on each other for their proper function. It is the antagonistic relationship between medullar expansion and cortical constraint that gives organisms their specific form.[5] This is how the twelfth edition of *Systema Naturae* expresses this relationship, now calling the cortical substance "corporeal":

> The plant machine consists of two contrary substances:
>
> the outer, corporeal substance, that enwraps, nourishes, descends, adheres to the earth, tries eagerly to enclose the medulla, slightly hard, but grows into a tender point; the inner, medullar substance, enwrapped, vivifying, melting downwards, striving upwards, unlimited with respect to multiplication and divisibility, agitated with creation, from the beginning steadily moving up along the path of least resistance, [where it finds] its exit; once the corporeal

> substance engulfing it grows weaker, [the medulla] breaks its clasp, and undergoes a metamorphosis, and weds itself after this escape to the corporeal substance again, so that the circle continues in new lifes being dispersed. (Linnaeus 1766–8, 1:7)

The language employed in this passage echoes the iatromechanical model of organisms as hydraulic machines, composed of vessels filled with circulating humours. Linnaeus always inserted himself into that tradition; for example, in 1737 he described how he had brought a banana tree to flower and fruit in a Dutch merchant-banker's private botanical garden by excessive watering and heating (Müller-Wille 2007, 62–4). But Linnaeus projects an antagonism of reproductive and environmental forces onto this model that clearly derives from his own daily toil of "reducing" local varieties to their proper species, be it in his garden at Uppsala, on paper, or in print. This antagonism brought him as close as he could get to later notions of a continuous struggle for life, and it also motivated him to develop a highly gendered theory of hybridization as a source for new species (Stevens and Cullen 1990; Müller-Wille and Orel 2007, 177–82).[6] For him, living "hydraulic machines" – in Swedish lectures he would sometimes also use the term "organism" (*organismus*) – were therefore categorically distinct from non-living objects. Plants and animals were not just a conglomerate of matter (*congesta*) but organized (*organisata*) for the purpose of restoring themselves from exhaustion and dispersal (Linnaeus 1766–8, 1:15–16; cf. Müller-Wille 1999, 124).

Conclusion: From Natural History to Biology

It is a well-known fact that it was the French naturalist Georges-Louis Leclerc Comte de Buffon who first introduced the term "reproduction" into the life sciences in 1748 when he inquired after the "secret cause," by which nature "enables beings to propagate their kinds" (Buffon 1780, 2:29). Buffon, director of the Jardin du Roi in Paris and author of a natural history in thirty-six volumes, borrowed the expression from contemporary theology, where it referred to the resurrection of the dead on doomsday. In this context, reproduction literally meant the re-creation of bodies that had fallen apart into their constituent parts, at another time and another place (McLaughlin 2001, 174–9). Buffon's metaphorical move highlights two things: first, that what he referred to as reproduction had previously been the domain of the divine; and second, that reproduction, or the restitution of organisms *at a distance*, is actually a highly improbable idea.

Linnaeus did not employ this metaphor, and preferred to stick to the term "continuous generation" (*generatio continuata*). The alternation of dispersal and restitution of organic form, always with a potential for added difference, was as much emphasized by Linnaeus as it was by Buffon though. This was a perspective, as I have tried to argue in this chapter, that could only be gained because naturalists themselves engaged in a quasi-economy of long-distance collection and exchange, both on the level of specimens, and on the level of written information, be it in script or print. Categories like species or genera ceased to be rungs on the scale of nature, and began to appear as repositories of a burgeoning, if not exploding, potential for new forms of life. Throughout his career, Linnaeus struggled to find means to contain this potential, and his manuscripts and printed output clearly bear witness of this struggle. Interestingly, he hit upon serial publication of ever-amended and corrected catalogues of life as the solution (Müller-Wille and Charmantier 2012).

What does this mean for the emergence of biology around 1800, with which this chapter opened? Long before naturalists of the nineteenth century found an apposite language to speak about organic reproduction in general, it seems, cultural techniques had been developed that brought the corresponding phenomena to the fore. To borrow an expression from economic history, biology, like captalism, was preceded by a long phase of "primitive accumulation" in natural history. This relationship between biology and natural history is difficult to see because there exists a long tradition in biology of viewing natural history as its opposite. Refraining from intervention and being preoccupied with description and classification only, natural history produces static and particularist views of life, and is therefore inherently unable to throw light on the dynamic laws that govern life in general. As I hope to have shown in this chapter, by focusing on the history of botanical gardens, nothing could be further from the truth. By enclosing and mobilizing life on a global scale, it was natural history itself that moved reproduction into the centre of the life sciences.

NOTES

1 Occasional earlier usages of the term "biology" did usually not relate to a science of life, but to writings of a biographic nature, e.g., necrologues (Kanz 2002). For one earlier usage of "biologia" in the sense of a science of general laws of the living, see McLaughlin (2002).

2 A detailed description of the garden can be found in Linnaeus (1749a); for a historical account of the garden under Linnaeus's directorship, see Broberg, Ellenius, and Jonsell (1983).
3 Cf. Swan (2001, 109) who contrasts "naturalistic figuration (mimetic pictures)" with "schematic representation (grids)."
4 See Mayr (1982) for a classic account of the history of biology that builds on this notion, and Winsor (2006), for a recent, forceful critique. See Bowler, this volume, for a similar critique with respect to early modern theories of generation.
5 On the emerging model of gender roles on which Linnaeus built his theory, see Meek, this volume.
6 On eighteenth-century discussions about hybrids, see the chapter by Lettow in this volume.

REFERENCES

Barnes, B., D. Bloor, and J. Henry. 1996. *Scientific Knowledge: A Sociological Analysis.* Chicago: University of Chicago Press.

Baron, W. 1966. "Gedanken über den ursprünglichen Sinn der Ausdrücke Botanik, Zoologie und Biologie." In *Medizingeschichte im Spektrum*, edited by G. Rath and H. Schipperges, 1–10. Wiesbaden: Steiner (= Sudhoffs Archiv, Beihefte, vol. 7).

Barrera-Osorio, A. 2006. *Experiencing Nature: The Spanish American Empire and the Early Scientific Revolution.* Austin: University of Texas Press.

Blair, A.M. 2010. *Too Much to Know: Managing Scholarly Information before the Modern Age.* New Haven: Yale University Press.

Bourguet, M.-N. 1996. "Voyage, collecte, collections: Le catalogue de la nature (fin 17e – début 19e siècles)." In *Terres à decouvrir, terres à parcourir: exploration et connaissance du monde, XIIe–XIXe siècles*, edited by D. Lecoq and A. Chambard, 185–207. Paris: Publications de l'Université Paris 7- Denis Diderot.

Broberg, G., A. Ellenius, and B. Jonsell. 1983. *Linnaeus and His Garden.* Uppsala: no pub.

Buffon, G.L.L. Comte de. 1780. *Natural History, General and Particular, by the Count de Buffon.* Translated by W. Smellie. 8 vols. Edinburgh: William Creech.

Caron, J.A. 1988. "'Biology' in the Life Sciences: A Historiographical Contribution." *History of Science* 26:223–68.

Coleman, W. 1971. *Biology in the Nineteenth Century: Problems of Form, Function, and Transformation.* New York: Wiley.

Cook, H.J. 2007. *Matters of Exchange: Commerce, Medicine, and Science in the Dutch Golden Age*. New Haven: Yale University Press. http://dx.doi.org/10.12987/yale/9780300117967.001.0001.

Cooper, A. 2007. *Inventing the Indigenous: Local Knowledge and Natural History in Early Modern Europe*. Cambridge: Cambridge University Press.

Dauser, R., S. Hächler, M. Kempe, F. Mauelshagen, and M. Stuber, eds. 2008. *Wissen im Netz: Botanik und Pflanzentransfer in europäischen Korrespondenznetzen des 18. Jahrhunderts*. Berlin: Akademie Verlag (= Colloquia Augustana, vol. 24). http://dx.doi.org/10.1524/9783050055893.

Delbourgo, J., and S. Müller-Wille. 2012. Introduction to Focus Section: Listmania. *Isis* 103 (4): 710–5. http://dx.doi.org/10.1086/669045.

Drayton, R. 2000. *Nature's Government: Science, Imperial Britain, and the Improvement of the World*. New Haven: Yale University Press.

Ekedahl, N. 2005. "Collecting Flowers: Linnaean Method and the Humanist Art of Reading." *Symbolae Botanicae Upsalienses* 33:47–59.

Ferrarius, Johann Baptista. 1638. *Flora s. de Florum cultura*. Amsterdam: Jansson.

Findlen, P. 1994. *Possessing Nature: Museums, Collecting, and Scientific Culture in Early Modern Italy*. Berkeley: University of California Press.

Foucault, M. (1966) 1974. *The Order of Things: An Archeology of the Human Sciences*. London: Routledge.

te Heesen, A. 2004. "Accounting for the Natural World: Double-Entry Bookkeeping in the Field." In *Colonial Botany: Science, Commerce, and Politics in the Early Modern World*, edited by L. Schiebinger and C. Swan, 237–51. Philadelphia: University of Pennsylvania Press.

Heniger, J. 1971. "Some Botanical Activities of Hermann Boerhaave, Professor of Botany and Director of the Botanic Garden at Leiden." *Janus* 58:1–78.

Jacob, François. (1970) 1993. *The Logic of Life: A History of Heredity*. Princeton, NJ: Princeton University Press.

Jordanova, L. 1995. "Interrogating the Concept of Reproduction in the Eighteenth Century." In *Conceiving the New World Order*, edited by F.D. Ginsburg and R. Rapp, 369–86. Berkeley: University of California Press.

Kanz, K.T. 2002. "Von der BIOLOGIA zur Biologie. Zur Begriffsentwicklung und Disziplingenese vom 17. bis zum 20. Jahrhundert." In *Die Entstehung biologischer Disziplinen II: Beiträge zur 10. Jahrestagung der DGGTB in Berlin 2001*, edited by U. Hoßfeld and T. Junker, 9–30. Berlin: VWB (= Verhandlungen zur Geschichte und Theorie der Biologie, vol. 9).

Koerner, L. 1999. *Linnaeus: Nature and Nation*. Cambridge, MA: Harvard University Press.

Koselleck, R. 2002. *The Practice of Conceptual History: Timing History, Spacing Concepts*. Translated by T.S. Presner. Stanford, CA: Stanford University Press.

Linnaeus, C. 1736. *Bibliotheca Botanica Recensens Libros Plus Mille de Plantis.* Amsterdam: Schouten.
Linnaeus, C. 1737a. *Critica Botanica in quo Nomina Plantarum Generica, Specifica, & Variantia Examini Subjicuntur.* Leiden: Wishoff.
Linnaeus, C. 1737b. *Genera Plantarum Eorumque Characteres Naturales Secundum Numerum, Figuram, Situm, Proportionem Omnium Fructificationis Partium.* Leiden: Wishoff.
Linnaeus, C. 1737c. *Hortus Cliffortianus Plantas Exhibens Quas in Hortis Tam Vivis Quam Siccis, Hartecampi in Hollandia, Coluit Vir Nobillissimus & Generosissimus Georgius Clifford.* Amsterdam: no pub.
Linnaeus, C. 1738. *Classes Plantarum seu Systemata Plantarum Omnia a Fructificatione Desumta.* Leiden: Wishoff.
Linnaeus, C. 1749a. "Hortus upsaliensis." In *Ammoenitates Academicae, seu Dissertationes Variae Physicae, Medicae, Botanicae antehac Seorsim Editae.* 10 vols. 1:172–210. Stockholm and Leipzig: Kiesewetter.
Linnaeus, C. 1749b. *Oeconomia Naturae.* Dissertation. Respondent D. Biberg. Uppsala: No pub.
Linnaeus, C. 1760. *Politiae Naturae.* Dissertation. Respondent H.C. D. Wilcke. Uppsala: No pub.
Linnaeus, C. 1766–8. *Systema Naturae per Regna Tria Naturae.* 12th ed. 3 vols. Stockholm: Salvius.
Linnaeus, C. 1775. "The Economy of Nature." In *Miscellaneous Tracts in Physick and Husbandry*, edited and translated by B. Stillingfleet, 39–40. London: R and J. Dodsley, S. Baker, and M. Cooper.
Masson, G. 1972. "Italian Flower Collectors' Gardens in Seventeenth-Century Italy." In *The Italian Garden*, edited by D.R. Coffin, 63–89. Washington, DC: Dumbarton Oaks.
Mayr, E. 1982. *The Growth of Biological Thought: Diversity, Evolution and Inheritance.* Cambridge, MA: Belknap Press.
McCracken, D.P. 1997. *Gardens of Empire: Botanical Institutions of the Victorian British Empire.* London: Leicester University Press.
McLaughlin, P. 2001. *What Functions Explain: Functional Explanation and Self-Reproducing Systems.* Cambridge: Cambridge University Press. http://dx.doi.org/10.1017/CBO9780511498510.012.
McLaughlin, P. 2002. "Naming Biology." *Journal of the History of Biology* 35 (1): 1–4. http://dx.doi.org/10.1023/A:1014535811678.
Miller, D.P., and P.H. Reill, eds. 1996. *Visions of Empire: Voyages, Botany, and Representations of Nature.* Cambridge: Cambridge University Press.
Mukerji, C. 1997. *Territorial Ambitions and the Gardens of Versailles.* Cambridge: Cambridge University Press.

Müller-Wille, S. 1999. *Botanik und weltweiter Handel: Zur Begründung eines natürlichen Systems der Pflanzen durch Carl von Linné (1707–1778).* Berlin: Verlag für Wissenschaft und Bildung.

Müller-Wille, S. 2001. "Gardens of Paradise." *Endeavour* 25 (2): 49–54. http://dx.doi.org/10.1016/S0160-9327(00)01358-2.

Müller-Wille, S. 2003. "Nature as a Marketplace: The Political Economy of Linnaean Botany."In *Oeconomies in the Age of Newton,* edited by M. Schabas and N. De Marchi, 154–72. Durham, NC: Duke University Press (= History of Political Economy, Supplement, Vol. 35).

Müller-Wille, S. 2007. Introduction. In C. Linnaeus, *Musa Cliffortiana/Clifford's Banana Tree*, translated by S. Freer, 15–67. Vienna: International Association for Plant Taxonomy (= Regnum Vegetabile, Vol. 148).

Müller-Wille, S. 2008. "History Redoubled: The Synthesis of Facts in Linnaean Natural History." In *Philosophies of Technology: Francis Bacon and His Contemporaries*, edited by G. Engel, N. Karafyllis, R. Nanni, and C. Zittel, 2 vols, 2:515–38. Leiden: Brill (= Intersections: *Yearbook for Early Modern Studies*, vol. 11). http://dx.doi.org/10.1163/ej.9789004170506.i-582.134.

Müller-Wille, S. and I. Charmantier. 2012. "Natural History and Information Overload: The Case of Linnaeus." *Studies in History and Philosophy of the Biological and Biomedical Sciences* 43:4–15.

Müller-Wille, S., and V. Orel. 2007. "From Linnaean Species to Mendelian Factors: Elements of Hybridism, 1751–1870." *Annals of Science* 64 (2): 171–215. http://dx.doi.org/10.1080/00033790601111567.

Müller-Wille, S., and K. Reeds. 2007. "A Translation of Carl Linnaeus's Introduction to *Genera Plantarum* (1737)." *Studies in History and Philosophy of the Biological and Biomedical Sciences* 38 (3): 563–72. http://dx.doi.org/10.1016/j.shpsc.2007.06.003.

Müller-Wille, S., and H.-J. Rheinberger. 2012. *A Cultural History of Heredity*. Chicago: University of Chicago Press. http://dx.doi.org/10.7208/chicago/9780226545721.001.0001.

Ogilvie, B.W. 2003. "The Many Books of Nature: Renaissance Naturalists and Information Overload." *Journal of the History of Ideas* 64 (1): 29–40. http://dx.doi.org/10.1353/jhi.2003.0015.

Ogilvie, B.W. 2006. *The Science of Describing: Natural History in Renaissance Europe*. Chicago: University of Chicago Press. http://dx.doi.org/10.7208/chicago/9780226620862.001.0001.

Olmi, G. 1992. *L'inventario del mondo: Catalogazione della natura e luoghi del sapere nella prima età moderna.* Bologna: Società editrice il Mulino.

Osborne, M.A. 1994. *Nature, the Exotic, and the Science of French Colonialism: Science, Technology and Society*. Bloomington: Indiana University Press.

Pauly, P. 1984. “The Appearance of Academic Biology in Late Nineteenth-Century America.” *Journal of the History of Biology* 17 (3): 369–97. http://dx.doi.org/10.1007/BF00126369.

Prest, J. 1981. *The Garden of Eden: The Botanic Garden and the Re-Creation of Paradise*. New Haven: Yale University Press.

Pugliano, V. 2012. “Specimen Lists: Artisanal Writing or Natural Historical Paperwork?” *Isis* 103 (4): 716–26. http://dx.doi.org/10.1086/669049.

Reeds, K. 1976. “Renaissance Humanism and Botany.” *Annals of Science* 33:527–33.

Rey, R. 1989. “Génération et hérédité au 18e siecle.” In *L’ordre des caractères: Aspects de l’hérédité dans l’histoire des sciences de l’homme*, edited by J.-L. Fischer, 7–41. Paris: Vrin.

Rhodes, D.E. 1984. “The Botanical Garden of Padua: The First Hundred Years.” *Journal of Garden History* 4 (4): 327–31. http://dx.doi.org/10.1080/01445170.1984.10444105.

Rippa Bonati, M., and V. Dal Piaz. 1995. “The Design and Form of the Padua *Horto medicinale*.” In *The Botanical Garden of Padua 1545–1995*, edited by A. Minelli, 33–54. Venice: Marsilio.

Roger, J. 1998. *The Life Sciences in Eighteenth-Century French Thought*. Edited by K.R. Benson. Translated by R. Ellrich. Stanford, CA: University of California Press.

Schaffer, S., L. Roberts, K. Raj, and J. Delbourgo, eds. 2009. *The Brokered World: Go-Betweens and Global Intelligence, 1770–1820.* Sagamore Beach, MA:. Science History Publications.

Schiebinger, L. 1991. “The Private Life of Plants: Sexual Politics in Carl Linnaeus and Erasmus Darwin.” In *Science and Sensibility: Gender and Scientific Enquiry, 1780–1945*, edited by M. Benjamin, 121–43. Oxford: Blackwell.

Schiebinger, L., and C. Swan, eds. 2005. *Colonial Botany: Science, Commerce, and Politics in the Early Modern World*. Philadelphia: University of Pennsylvania Press.

Schiller, P. 1987. *L’Orto botanico di Padova: Geografia astrologica e scienza della botanica moderna*. Venice: Centro Tedesco di Studi Veneziani.

Spary, E. 2000. *Utopia’s Garden: French Natural History from Old Regime to Revolution*. Chicago: University of Chicago Press. http://dx.doi.org/10.7208/chicago/9780226768700.001.0001.

Stearn, W.T. 1961. “Botanical Gardens and Botanical Literature in the Eighteenth Century.” In *Catalogue of Botanical Books in the Collection of Rachel McMasters Miller Hunt*. Vol. 1, edited by J. Quinby and A. Stevenson, xli–cxl. Pittsburgh: Hunt Library.

Stevens, P.F., and S.P. Cullen. 1990. “Linnaeus, the Cortex-Medulla Theory, and the Key to His Understanding of Plant Form and Natural Relationships.” *Journal of the Arnold Arboretum* 71:179–220.

Swan, C. 2001. "From Blowfish to Flower Still Life Paintings." In *Merchants and Marvels: Commerce, Science, and Art in Early Modern Europe*, edited by P. Smith and P. Findlen, 109–36. London: Routledge.

Tongiorgi Tomasi, L. 1983. "Projects for Botanical and Other Gardens: A 16th Century Manual." *Journal of Garden History* 3 (1): 1–34. http://dx.doi.org/10.1080/01445170.1983.10412420.

Ubrizsy Savioa, A. 1995. "The Botanical Garden of Padua in Guildano's Days." In *The Botanical Garden of Padua 1545–1995*, edited by A. Minelli, 173–84. Venice: Marsilio.

Wijnands, D.O. 1988. "Hortus auriaci: The Gardens of Orange and Their Place in Late Seventeenth-Century Botany and Horticulture." *Journal of Garden History* 8:61–86, 271–304.

Winsor, M.P. 2006. "The Creation of the Essentialism Story: An Exercise in Metahistory." *History and Philosophy of the Life Sciences* 28:149–74.

2 Cultures and Politics of Preformationism in Eighteenth-Century Italy

IVANO DAL PRETE

Scholarship on eighteenth-century embryology has maintained that the debate on generation was fraught with political and social implications. In particular, preformationism has been regarded as the philosophical underpinning of conservative policies. Peter Reill has remarked that preformation "was very easily adapted during the early eighteenth century to serve as a support for the status quo – for political absolutism, religious orthodoxy, and established social hierarchies" (Reill 2005, 5). As Peter Bowler argues in this volume, however, the intellectual sophistication and diversity of eighteenth-century reproductive theories makes it difficult to draw definite lines between preformationism and epigenesis. In this chapter, I will further complicate the framework of Enlightenment embryology by showing that preformation and epigenesis did not even have fixed political and social roles. On the contrary, they could be used to support either conservative or progressive policies, according to local cultural traditions, contingencies, and political agendas.

The Italian case that I examine here is a compelling example of this complexity. I will first outline the uneasy development of Italian preformationism and of its alleged manifesto, Antonio Vallisneri's *History of Generation* (1721). Second, I will argue that in eighteenth-century Italy preformationism was usually associated with progressive policies, while epigenesis was identified with conservative views. Preformationism was employed to modify the attitude of the Church on issues such as the status of early embryos, and to foster jurisdictionalism and political reformism. On the contrary, conservative Catholics often regarded epigenesis as closer to the traditions of the Church, and they considered mechanist philosophies as a danger to the moral values that supported the society of the Old Regime.

The Controversy on Generation in Late Seventeenth-Century Italy

> The controversy [on preformationism] should be decided in Italy, because it had its beginning here.
>
> Vallisneri 1721, 233

In a 1712 letter to the naturalist Antonio Vallisneri, the Venetian philosopher Antonio Conti thus epitomized the expectations of a growing part of the Italian learned community. Although William Harvey first conceived of the egg, his idea would have been of little consequence if Italian naturalists such as Francesco Redi and Marcello Malpighi had not investigated with the "utmost accuracy and perspicacity the existence, fecundation, and structure of ovaries and eggs" (233, my translations). In spite of their head start, the philosopher complained that his fellow countrymen had later been overtaken by the "ultramontanes," who corroborated the discoveries of those great Italians with sound observations and related them "to the general laws of nature." Meanwhile, in Italy, "certain philosophers out of reverence, laziness or excessive faith, being unable to part from the texts of the ancients, got lost into their metaphysics instead of pursuing the secrets of nature into the bowels of the animals" (233).

In short, Italian natural history had not been spared by the economic, political, and intellectual crisis the country seemed to have fallen into by the early eighteenth century. The country was being marginalized by the growing penetration of "ultramontane" (in particular, French) culture and language, a trend that Conti – together with other leading Italian intellectuals – was determined to reverse. His account readily identified the main obstacle to the modernization of Italian scientific culture: the persisting strength of the epigenesist tradition. Fortunately for Italy's reputation, Vallisneri's work had convinced almost everyone to abandon at least the Aristotelian theory of spontaneous generation from putrescent matter (*ex putri*). "No one questions now the egg and the first envelope, barring those who do not want or cannot provide themselves with a microscope, and trust more the words and authority of the ancients than the faithful and sincere witnessing of their own eyes" (233).

Natural philosophers were thus left with two final tasks: to investigate the first part of generation that still escapes our senses; and to demonstrate once and for all that the embryo does not take shape through the "combination of different parts of matter," but that it pre-exists since the creation of the world as a minuscule, perfectly outlined animal that becomes visible as it begins growing (233).

Conti's anticipation of the forthcoming triumph of pre-existence in Italy proved optimistic, just like the alleged preformationist faith of some of his heroes did. While Nicolas Malebranche and others often quoted Malpighi's observations of chick embryos as evidence for preformation, Malpighi never argued for the *emboîtement* of successive generations, as many preformationists maintained (Roe 1981, 3–4; Bernardi 1986, 46–60; Bertoloni Meli 2011, 208–27). In his correspondence, he actually rejected this radical form of pre-existence (Bertoloni Meli 2011, 226). His restraint was, in fact, a typical trait of post-Galilean Italian science: experimenters favoured the description of phenomena over potentially hazardous theoretical elaborations, and were often wary of extending the validity of empirical data through analogy and "general laws of nature."

Redi's *Experiments on the Generation of Insects* (Redi 1668), one of the most widely read and reprinted scientific works of its time, presented solid experimental evidence for the thesis that living beings can only be generated by parents of the same species. Yet, it also reported uncanny and seemingly contradictory conclusions, in particular about the galls of certain plants which later gave origin to insects. Accustomed to examining natural specimens in his laboratory rather than in the field, Redi missed the swarms of insects depositing eggs in those same places where galls would later develop. He thus attributed their formation to the plant itself (47). Far from an entirely mechanistic conception of life and generation, Redi credited plants not only with a vegetative soul but also with a sensitive one, which could produce animal life. While the Italian naturalist was a firm advocate of the procreation *ex ovo*, his main concern was to demonstrate that life can never arise from inorganic matter. The generation of insects from plants did not violate this principle (16–17).

By 1679 Malpighi had already clarified the origin *ex ovo* of the insects of the galls, but Redi never publicly disavowed his previous conclusions. Redi's "great sin" (Redi 1668, 127) was deftly exploited by the supporters of spontaneous generation, particularly influential at the Roman College (the central Jesuit University) and at the "Sapienza," the University of Rome. Among them, botanist Giovan Battista Trionfetti and the Jesuit naturalist Filippo Buonanni (see Fazzari 2005) could hardly be described as hopeless Aristotelians who only studied nature in the books of the Master. Buonanni, in particular, was an up-to-date experimental philosopher and an accomplished instrument maker. As a matter of fact, the microscopes that he made himself, or could purchase from prestigious Roman opticians such as Tortoni, Cellio, or Campani, far surpassed those used by Malpighi (Fazzari 1999, 116–17; Fazzari 2007).

Buonanni argued that Redi's discussion of the galls of plants uncovered the contradictions into which the detractors of spontaneous generation fell: eventually, they had to acknowledge the existence of generative forces in nature, capable of producing "insects" without the intervention of parents of the same species. The Jesuit naturalist's criticism expanded into a broad attack on the very foundations of modern science. Buonanni questioned in particular the viability of Redi's experimental method (based on the repetition of the experiment) as a viable tool to decide scientific controversies. He ruled out the possibility of determining invariable laws of nature from a given set of observations. A skilled and innovative microscopist himself (Fazzari 2007), Buonanni insisted nonetheless on the irreproducible nature of the experiment and on the difficulty of interpreting unequivocally its results (Fazzari 1999, 107; Fantini 1994, xii).

As evidenced by Buonanni's skilled criticism of Redi, Conti's description of epigenesists as backward and scientifically irrelevant was not entirely true. Many of them regarded themselves as Aristotelians, but seventeenth-century Aristotelianism was, in fact, a constantly evolving field that incorporated and fostered many aspects of modern experimental philosophy, particularly within the Society of Jesus (Schmitt 1983; Martin 2011, 106–24). Italian culture was particularly receptive to the writings of the Genevan "journalist" Jean Le Clerc, who between 1703 and 1706 re-elaborated and spread Henry More's and Ralph Cudworth's epigenetic theses. In his widely read "Bibliothèque choisie," Le Clerc surmised that a vital principle (or "plastic force") of divine origin supervises the mechanical laws of nature. By maintaining the notion of a living nature, while at the same time depriving it of potentially irreligious implications (Monti 2009, XXII), Le Clerc's epigenetic ideas were welcomed by many of his Italian readers.

The Qualms of an Empiricist: Vallisneri's *History of Generation*

When he obtained a chair of medicine at Padua University in 1700, Vallisneri was the rising star of Italian natural history and the undisputed heir to his late master Malpighi. Vallisneri acquired a reputation as a naturalist in the late 1690s thanks to his studies of the anatomy of "insects," aimed to support reproduction *ex ovo* ("insects" meant a vast range of small animals, including worms, crabs, and snails). In 1712–13 he was still correcting Redi's observations, to show that his mistakes did not undermine the epistemological validity of induction from experiment (Vallisneri 2005, 5–16). As Conti pointed out, Vallisneri's work was instrumental in persuading the last supporters of spontaneous generation.

Until the early 1710s, Vallisneri remained close to Malpighi's positions and methodology. While a supporter of mechanistic explanations in natural philosophy, the Paduan naturalist was also a staunch empiricist. In particular, he refused to accept the idea that preformed germs might be enveloped one into the other since the creation – a theory that no observation could conceivably confirm (Vallisneri 2009, v). His later "conversion" to orthodox preformationism was due to a combination of factors, besides strictly scientific considerations. New empirical results played a significant role, but so did pressures from other influential intellectuals, personal ambition, commitment to the prestige of Italian culture, and the identification of preformationism with the cause of the moderns.

Vallisneri's observations of spermatic worms no doubt contributed to the evolution of his embryological ideas. Leeuwenhoek's momentous finding (1677) had been readily put in the service of the preformationist views of the discoverer. As Jim Bennet notes, Hooke's or Leeuwenhoek's microscopical observations reveal "major assumptions about what we need to see but cannot. Hooke was explicit that this was the micro-mechanical world postulated by the mechanical philosophy" (Bennett 2007, 71–2). Malpighi's and Vallisneri's approach was quite different, as they regarded microscopy more as a tool to sharpen and extend the senses; they retained the pragmatic attitude "of the practicing anatomist," rather than that of the "Democritean philosopher" (Bennett 2007, 71–2). Besides, the very existence of the worms was still disputed in early eighteenth-century Italy: together with other naturalists, Vallisneri for a long time could not find any evidence of animalculi in the spermatic fluid, to the point that in 1710 he still regarded them as optical aberrations. Their visibility was indeed far from trivial, as it depended not only on adequate instruments but even on appropriate observing techniques (Luzzini 2007, 74; Generali 2007, 252–62; Monti 2009, XLVIII–LVIII); both became available to Vallisneri only around 1713, thanks to the support of a local network of naturalists and instrument makers, and to the access to English microscopes acquired in Venice (Generali 2007; Luzzini 2007).

In the same years, Vallisneri strengthened his relations with a variegated group of leading intellectuals in the Venetian area and outside. In 1708 he made his acquaintance with Conti, who had just moved to Padua from Venice where he took part in the meetings of a group of "Cartesian philosophers" (Romagnani 2009, 115). While deeply interested in the problems of generation, Conti had little familiarity with medicine and anatomy. But his philosophical and mathematical competences, combined with his vast European acquaintances, perfectly complemented Vallisneri's medical and naturalistic expertise. In 1710 Vallisneri was one of the founders and the scientific adviser of the *Giornale de' Letterati d'Italia* (*Journal of Italian Literate Men*), conceived as an instrument for the renewal of Italian culture and the revival of its waning influence in Europe. Though its stance was definitely anti-Aristotelian and anti-Jesuitical, the new journal held a moderate editorial line which was acceptable both to the censors and to its public, made up of clergymen, rationalistic intellectuals, and orthodox Catholics who sided with the moderns (Generali 1984, 244–8). After 1710 Vallisneri began to turn towards preformationism. After the defeat of spontaneous generation, Vallisneri's considerable skills as a polemicist were now mainly directed against Le Clerc's "plastic forces" and other attempts to revive "occult" forces in natural philosophy (Dal Prete 2009, 101). Under Conti's influence, the Paduan naturalist recognized that any antagonist system would require an appropriate philosophical frame; in contemporary Europe this was usually provided by preformationism, which was undermining the last vestiges of "Aristotelianism, hermeticism and natural magic" (Reill 2005, 34). Furthermore, preformationism was increasingly presented as the only viable modern mechanical philosophy, thus calling for a stark choice between the pre-existence of the germs and sticking with the ancients. Vallisneri's own recent observations of spermatic worms and of countless, small animals in the blood of infected cattle (Vallisneri 2005, 57) seemed to confirm that it was hardly possible to set a lower limit to the size of perfectly formed, functional organisms. As Conti explained to him, this was perfectly compatible with the infinite divisibility of matter which underlay the whole theory of the pre-existence.[1]

From 1712 on, Vallisneri became actively involved in the polemic against epigenesis and the numerous "unorthodox" variants of preformationism that were being pursued in Italy. One of them was the theory of the "seminal light" elaborated by the Ferrarese physician Francesco Nigrisoli, which Conti considered a dangerous concession to spontaneism. According to Nigrisoli, the "seminal light" is created by God in the male sperm to help organize the germ in the maternal ovaries; while fecundation acted upon an already formed germ, its formation did not pre-exist the female body. At first, Vallisneri did not judge Nigrisoli's work negatively, but the harsh reply that Conti published a few years later was clearly written with Vallisneri's assistance in the parts dealing with embryological observations. The Venetian philosopher insisted that, as the most authoritative Italian physician and naturalist, only Vallisneri could eradicate this "scandal of Italy" with a comprehensive discussion of the problem of generation (Monti 2009, XX–XXI).

Conti was joined by one of the leading European intellectuals, Wilhelm Gottfried Leibniz – also a supporter of pre-existence – who urged Vallisneri to solve the long-debated problem of whether preformed bodies resided in the female eggs ("ovism"), or in the male spermatic worms ("spermism"). Leibniz and Vallisneri never corresponded directly, their exchanges always taking place through a network of intermediaries. In any case, the German philosopher's appreciation of his work removed Vallisneri's remaining hesitations (Monti 2009, LXXVII–LXXX; Generali 1987). Last but not least, the reticence towards a system that was triumphing all over Europe seemed to emphasize Italy's backwardness. In order to recover its place in modern European culture, Italian natural history had to be preformationist. To secure his own scientific leadership in the country, Vallisneri needed to write its preformationist manifesto.

Conceived as the long-awaited, major Italian contribution to European preformationism, the *History of Generation* was written in the national literary language rather than in Latin. Vallisneri's choice was in line with his support of Italian culture, and his efforts towards the creation of a modern terminology for natural history in Italian (Scotti Morgana 1981; Rinaldi 2008; Vallisneri 2013). Following Leibniz's suggestion, the two sections of the book were devoted respectively to the history of spermism and to that of ovism, with Vallisneri decidedly taking side with the latter. The Italian naturalist ridiculed the alleged observations of "little men" enshrined in the head of the spermatic worms, such as those of Dalempatius, and the "nonsensical slaughter" that every ejaculation would imply. On the contrary, Vallisneri described the ovist hypothesis as "the simplest, the clearest … and finally, the worthiest of the boundless omnipotence, and wisdom of God: hence, the truest" (Monti 2009, LIX).

In spite of such declarations, however, ovists had been unsuccessful in finding the preformed embryo in the female body. In his treatise Vallisneri conveyed to the reader the impression that his choice was based on mere likelihood, rather than on solid evidence, and he did little to hide this uncomfortable fact. As he wrote to the Swiss naturalist Louis Bourguet, he was determined to state: "What is certain as certain, and what is uncertain as uncertain. It is a great fact … that I was never able to see an egg."[2] Vallisneri did not refrain from searching for theoretical frameworks for the phenomena he observed, but the laws of nature had to be rooted into solid observations. Yet, the defence of preformationism – on which so much seemed to depend – required that he accept the existence of what he could neither see nor touch. The naturalist thus acknowledged that the preformed germs could, and should be seen through the "eyes of reason," but his concession was always a half-hearted one, taken – according to his own admission – after decade-long hesitations (Vallisneri 2009, 215).

Even though Vallisneri sanctioned the preformation of germs, he balked at the idea of bestowing his authority upon the most radical tenets of the preformationist orthodoxy, where experimental philosophy yielded to metaphysics and theology: the pre-existence of germs, their encasement into one another, and their primeval creation, not to mention the pre-existence of their souls endorsed by Leibniz. While he asserted that pre-existence was the "logical conclusion, of what has been said so far," little in the experimental history of generation he presented actually led to that conclusion (Monti 2009, LIX). Instead of discussing the subject of pre-existence, he preferred to publish anonymously in his treatise the long letter that Conti had written to him in 1712. In that letter the Venetian philosopher dismissed "plastic forces" and "seminal lights," trying to demonstrate instead that "animals are already perfectly formed before they become visible; and that they become visible, inasmuch as they develop" (Vallisneri 2009, 225). Finally, he showed that all living beings "were perfectly formed in the Beginning, so that every animal was enshrined in the ovaries of the first of its species, and in the progress of time they just developed and grew" (Vallisneri 2009, 238).

Conti's theory rested on the notion of the instantaneous creation of all things, which Vallisneri strongly favoured over the six days of the biblical account "since He had no need to rest, and Moses wrote that because of the limited understanding of men."[3] Once again, this was no matter for an experimental philosopher, who willingly left the floor to the theologian: in this case, the Augustinian monk Giacinto Tonti, an Aristotelian, and a supporter of spontaneous generation. A colleague of Vallisneri at Padua University, Tonti wrote in 1714 a book endorsing Augustine's theory of the instantaneous creation. In his *History of Generation*, Vallisneri published numerous excerpts from Tonti's work, without adding any original remarks. As he wrote in his correspondence, "The only difference between us is that Tonti believes God created every future living being virtually and *in potentia*; while I think the Almighty made them *in actu*, and they are all encased."[4] Furthermore, Tonti refuted Leibniz's idea that not only the bodies of every living creature, but even their souls pre-existed and were created in the Beginning – a statement whose religious orthodoxy appeared doubtful, and from which Vallisneri preferred to distance himself (Monti 2009, 49–51, 76).

The *History of Generation* was meant to prove the modernity of Italian culture by reinforcing the preformationist orthodoxy. In fact, Vallisneri's work could not help showing the resilience of the Galilean empiricist tradition, and the unwillingness of its leading Italian representative to meddle in the philosophical and theological issues that were part of the preformationist doctrine. Readers of the *History of Generation* could have easily justified the many Italian "shy preformationists," who endorsed mechanical explanations in natural philosophy and maybe even preformation, but regarded the pre-existence of the germs and their encasement as a simple conjecture (Bernardi 1986, 233–9). Conti's judgment of Vallisneri's treatise was paradoxical and telling at the same time. The philosopher did not approve the insertion of his 1712 letter on generation, which was published without consulting him. Indeed, the intellectual who more than anyone else pressured a reluctant Vallisneri to embrace radical preformationism had since become much more cautious. After censuring for years "spontaneists" as well as "shy" and unorthodox preformationists, Corti preferred now to "balance the theories according to their degrees of probabilities,"[5] because he could not find any compelling reason to side with a particular one.

The *Sacred Embryology*: or, the Parish Priest in the Delivery Room

In spite of its awkward results, the *History of Generation* considerably reinforced the appeal of preformationism and its circulation in Italian society. Indeed, the historical significance of Vallisneri's work could hardly be understated. Early 1700s preformationism has always been touted as the philosophical support for the entrenched religious beliefs and hierarchies; yet, Vallisneri was a lukewarm Catholic, critical in his correspondence of the influence of "monks" and "priests" on Italian science and society, and inclined to libertine views. He was not an atheist, as the pre-existence of germs required an act of intelligent creation. It is doubtful though, whether his Creator coincided with that of the Catholic tradition. While discussing with Conti his ideas on the "great chain of beings" and the necessary continuity between each species and the next, he dared hint that the same principle could apply to their souls:

> If this is how things go, farewell Cartesian machines, farewell to the clocks which fool our eyes! Every organic body that can feel, is born, grows, develops, and begets, will have its soul, like us ... If we consider this chain and

> progression of souls ... it seems a legitimate inference that souls all share the same nature. Here is a confession that my beneficial Jesuit confessor has never heard.[6]

Conti, Vallisneri, and their acolytes envisioned preformationism as an element of modernization and progress, not as a support of the status quo. By adopting and disseminating preformationism, they actually challenged the long-standing stance of Catholic theologians on problems such as the time of the ensoulment (i.e., the infusion of the immortal soul) in the fetus, with its immense moral and social implications. The church is today adamant that the fetus is endowed with an immortal soul from the very moment of conception; that doctrine, however, was only defined between the late nineteenth century and the early twentieth century (Betta 2006, 313–25). Before preformationism became influential in Italian culture, Catholic theologians generally held a very different view, which was rooted in the Aristotelian epigenetic theory of generation endorsed by Thomas Aquinas.

It was commonly held that a fetus could only receive its immortal soul when it acquired a distinct human shape. According to Aristotle, the embryo is at first an undifferentiated mass of flesh, which does not reach that stage until forty to eighty days from conception. Therefore, an embryo could not be considered a human being during the first weeks of pregnancy. Although voluntary abortion was a serious sin, abortions in the early stages of pregnancy could not be seen as homicides. Consequently, they were neither treated nor punished as such.

While it was the prevalent doctrine, "late ensoulment" was not undisputed. From a theological point of view, the debate on the time of ensoulment was especially linked to the problem of the baptism of aborted fetuses. In line with the emphasis placed on baptism by post-Tridentine Catholic theology and Jansenist rigorism, their salvation could only be guaranteed by administering the sacrament on their bodies, while they were still alive. By denying them human status in the first weeks of pregnancy, the Aristotelian theory of late ensoulment put at risk – according to some theologians – the eternal life of the embryos. During the seventeenth century, authors such as Girolamo Fiorentini or Paolo Zacchia strongly endorsed the instantaneous or early ensoulment of the embryo and, therefore, the necessity to baptize aborted or imperilled fetuses of any age. Their views met with the firm rebuttal of the Congregation of the Index. Accordingly, Fiorentini was only allowed to publish milder, more cautious versions of his original work. He was required to make it clear that his theses must not be regarded as the doctrine of the church; that instantaneous ensoulment was a problematic issue; and he was not allowed to argue that a mortal sin is committed by those who do not baptize early miscarriages (Cangiamila 1748, 40; Betta 2006, 37).

In the early 1700s, late ensoulment was not only the traditional position of the church, but plain common sense. To procure an abortion within the first weeks of a pregnancy was widely regarded as a light sin at most. After all, no human life was suppressed in the process and no soul was deprived of potential salvation. The moment of the ensoulment was often delayed until birth, a belief so widespread that in 1679 Pope Innocent XI had to issue a decree reminding people that such "laxity," along with abortions practised by unmarried women, was unacceptable (Filippini 1993, 160). Midwives, barbers, surgeons, and university-trained physicians alike considered "lawful at least the abortion of inanimate fetuses" (Cangiamila 1748, 10–11). The Aristotelian-Thomistic orthodoxy was defended by orders as powerful and influential as the Society of Jesus, whose members were often judged to be rather tolerant when it came to abortive and contraceptive practices (Monti 1996, 429–34).

Around the turn of the century, the growing success of preformationism emboldened the supporters of early ensoulment. Since the preformed embryo had a complete and perfectly defined human shape, which simply started to grow after fecundation, it was deemed suitable to receive a human soul from the moment of conception. In 1702 the Milanese physician Bartolomeo Corte published the resounding *Letter on the likely time of the infusion of the rational soul in the fetus* (Corte 1702), claiming that modern microscopical observations demonstrated the "perfect" organization of the fetus immediately after fecundation (if not before). This claim made it very likely that the rational soul could incarnate well before the traditional forty days from conception. In spite of Corte's well-known piety, his *Letter* was not only condemned outright but even added to the list of the forbidden books (De Ferrari 1983, 693). Among other issues, the ecclesiastic censor argued that in order to support his claims the author misinterpreted, misrepresented or – even worse – surreptitiously falsified the writings of several Fathers of the Church and of Thomas Aquinas. On the contrary, their opinions had been very far from those of Corte whose *Letter* threatened to spread a dangerously wrong interpretation of their teachings (Monti 1996, 429–34). In spite of noticeable exceptions and a lively debate, in the early eighteenth century the only individual considered as a full human being during the first weeks of pregnancy was the mother (Monti 1996, 416).

The years of Benedict XIV's pontificate (1740–58) marked a turning point in the controversy. Benedict XIV is well known for his reformism, his scientific interests, and for the 1757 edition of the Index of forbidden books, which no longer mentioned Copernicanism. He also maintained that science could be a useful tool for theology (Rosa 1966). In the new climate, the Sicilian priest Emanuele Cangiamila felt encouraged to make preformationism the scientific basis of his *Sacred Embryology*: "a crucial text for the Catholic doctrine on the regulation of birth" (Betta 2006, 23), as well as for the theological movement that, a century and a half later, eventually led the Holy Office to legislate on the *vexata questio*. First published in 1745 and explicitly approved by the pope in 1756 (Forleo 2001, preface), Cangiamila's work was translated by the 1770s into Latin, Italian, Spanish, French, and Portuguese in both abridged and unabridged versions.

In its many vernacular, abridged versions the *Sacred Embryology* appeared as a practical guide for parish priests having to deal with problematic pregnancies and abortions, difficult deliveries, or parishioners trying to stop an unwanted pregnancy in its early stages, whether suspect or real. Like Bartolomeo Corte before him, but in a more favourable context and backed by more authoritative sources, Cangiamila explained to his readers that modern science had almost proved the early ensoulment of the fetus: "Modern philosophers found the ovary in women, and observed with countless experiments ... that the organs of plants and animals preexist in seeds and embryos ... it seems therefore extremely likely that the soul is infused in the human embryo since the time that immediately follows conception" (Cangiamila 1748, 45–6).

Malpighi and Vallisneri were among the moderns – identified by Cangiamila with the preformationists – who showed that the embryo "is always perceptible in the fecundated egg, and that it exists already before fecundation, even though before that event it can only be seen, and obscurely, with the microscope" (Cangiamila 1748, 45–6). Like Vallisneri, Cangiamila sided with the ovist version of preformationism and rejected the notion that all souls were created at the same time as that of Adam's (Cangiamila 1756, 19). Once proved that embryos were endowed with a human soul since conception, their eternal salvation must come before every other consideration – including the earthly life and health of the mother. Fetuses must absolutely be baptized in cases of difficult deliveries, or at any other stage of the pregnancy if their lives seemed to be in serious danger.

The Sicilian theologian recommended carrying out the rite with the use of the intrauterine syringe, even though the validity of this method was sometimes questioned by theologians. When the syringe could not be used – as was often the case – a C-section on the body of the mother appeared as a viable alternative, even if the mother was still alive. C-sections on a living mother had traditionally been discouraged by the church, as they were considered the equivalent of a death sentence "and the same as killing the mother to save the fetus, which is obviously illicit" (Cangiamila 1748, 136). Nonetheless Cangiamila argued that, thanks to modern advances in medicine and surgery, the survival of the mother should no longer be considered unlikely.[7] It was therefore acceptable to endanger the temporal life of the mother, in order to save the eternal soul of the fetus.

The enforcement of Cangiamila's program required the eradication of long-established beliefs and practices, as well as a strengthened control of the church over the female body; indeed, it may be seen as part of the "obstetric revolution" that brought traditionally female practices under direct male control. The parish priest had to "preach, and inculcate that abortion is illicit, whether the fetus is animated or not, and even though the intention is to save a woman from infamy, and death" (Cangiamila 1748, 10–11). While midwives were already expected to be approved and instructed by parish priests (Filippini 1993, 158–60), Cangiamila warned that they should not be trusted when it came to the administration of baptisms because of their "ignorance," "superstition," or "wickedness." He thus encouraged parish priests to be present in person during deliveries or complications that took place in their area of responsibility, and to be ready to perform C-sections themselves if the need arose and a surgeon or a barber was not immediately available (Cangiamila 1748, 144). The mother's approval is always required, but the priest should do everything he can in order to obtain it and in extreme cases, remind the mother that not to give her consent would be a mortal sin.

Cangiamila's program was supported by the reforming wing of the church, which believed in the collaboration between Catholic theology and modern science – even when the latter was represented by mechanist philosophies. On the contrary, it was opposed by more conservative groups whose approach to pregnancy control and abortive practices tended to be less restrictive. Even though preformationism implied an act of intelligent creation, epigenesis was in fact more readily identified with the tradition of the church. A machine-like universe left little or no room for direct divine intervention, and did not appear particularly appealing to many conservative Italian Catholics. In eighteenth-century Italy, preformationism tended to identify with the independence of natural philosophy from theology, the limitation of ecclesiastical jurisdictions, and social and political reformism.

Generation and Politics in the Twilight of the Republic of Venice

The political dimension of the struggle between preformationism and epigenesis was particularly evident in late eighteenth-century Republic of

Venice. Around 1760, the government undertook a series of reforms that, among other things, limited the boundaries of the ecclesiastic jurisdiction. The reformist movement was welcomed in the progressive circles of Verona, the second largest town in the Venetian state (with a population of about 45,000) and a fertile ground for Jansenist rigorism and anti-curialism. Among the reformers, the professors and graduates of the school for military engineers established in town asked for increased social mobility, and for a more prominent role in the administration of the Venetian state for the rising technocracy they represented (Farinella1993). The professor of theology at the local seminary, Father Scudellini, was close to the city's progressive circles. When in 1761 he dealt with the problem of the baptism of aborted fetuses, he followed Cangiamila's example by turning the theological problem into a scientific one.

Scudellini's starting point was Vallisneri's *History of Generation*, which still retained considerable influence in northern Italy forty years after its publication. Drawing from the Paduan naturalist, the Veronese theologian claimed that the progress of science offered information that had not been available in previous centuries, so as to put the truth of preformationism beyond any doubt. The early ensoulment of fetuses was therefore extremely likely, and their baptism absolutely necessary (Scudellini 1761). Scudellini's theses were not new, and did not elicit strong reactions at first. In the late 1760s, however, the political and cultural climate became less favourable to reformist views, as the curialist party of the Venetian aristocracy increased its influence in the government. Conservative Catholics, who perceived preformationism as a sign of the ongoing secularization of the society, took advantage of the changed political situation to attack Scudellini's work.

The controversy brought to light the fracture existing between the conservative and the progressive wings within the local church itself, as Scudellini's main critic was his predecessor in the chair of theology at the Veronese seminary. By 1769, generation had become the talk of the town. Verona was flooded with an unusual production of books, leaflets, pamphlets, and satirical poems. Public letters were affixed to street walls. Prominent naturalists became involved in the polemic and the gazettes published their reactions, which were heatedly discussed in the city coffeehouses. Aristocratic salons and local academies resonated with warnings against the "abuses of reason" represented by mechanist theories (Dal Prete 2008, 359–74).

To its critics, preformationism appeared not only irrational and unproved, but also a product of French materialism that had long been undermining the traditional religious values and the very foundations of society. As the

Jesuits retained a firm control over the local educational system, many educated citizens were still raised within the Aristotelian and Thomistic tradition (Gecchele 2000). They considered natural knowledge as a set of ever-changing theories whose value was probabilistic at best. Science was therefore an unreliable base for the establishment of moral and religious issues, which deal with eternal truths. Drawing from Le Clerc and John Needham, they interpreted Newtonian gravity as a phenomenon that attested to the existence in nature of immaterial, active forces. It was generally agreed that the Aristotelian spontaneous generation of insects and lower animals had been finally refuted. But a "vital" or "plastic" force similar to gravity could well account for the growth of fetuses from undifferentiated matter, without any need to stick to a soulless universe and to socially dangerous theories.

On the preformationist side, the involvement of well-known naturalists such us Lazzaro Spallanzani and the geologist Alberto Fortis shows that more was at stake than a local dispute. Fortis, in particular, perceived the Veronese controversy as a crucial test for the faltering reforming will of the government. His appointment to the chair of natural history at Padua University was vetoed by the curialist party of the Venetian senate, because of his "lack of respect for the Bible" (Ciancio 1996, 504–5). Fortis now perceived criticisms of the preformationist doctrine as assaults on the authority of modern science. The intrusion of religious considerations in scientific matters, and the interference of clergyman and theologians with natural history, was unacceptable to him. His claim that natural history should be left to the specialists provoked harsh replies. Fortis represented a technocracy that began to claim an exclusive control over the scientific discourse, to the exclusion of amateurs who practised and discussed natural philosophy in private houses and academies. Fortis's attitude was deemed arrogant and dangerous by the local aristocracy, which intended to take part in (and retain some control over) the elaboration and spread of scientific ideas and practices.

Fortis strenuously defended Vallisneri's work (Fortis 1768), but it was all too easy for the Veronese epigenesists to point at the patent inconsistencies in the *History of Generation*. While the Paduan naturalist constantly asserted that he was "satisfied to know what little" he could "touch, and see," he actually endorsed the existence of preformed machines that no microscope had ever shown (Dal Prete 2008, 370). The epigenesists claimed that preformationist doctrines were being imposed for ideological reasons, when a growing corpus of observations and discoveries seemed to confirm, rather than dispel, many basic tenets of traditional epigenetic theories.

Even Vallisneri Jr, professor of natural history at Padua University, resoundingly disavowed his father's preformationist ideas, and his later recantation was partial and reluctant (Contardi 1994, 3; Bernardi 1986, 399–410). Lazzaro Spallanzani termed the works of the Veronese epigenesists "trash, regurgitations of occultism, irrationalism and pseudo-science," but in spite of his derogatory tones "preformationism found in Italy increasing difficulties; and Spallanzani himself had to face an increasing number of epigenesists ... each one endorsing vital principles modeled after Newtonian principles, such as the 'organizing force,' the 'generating virtue,' or the 'vital force'" (Bernardi 1989, 74).

As the century drew to a close, the conservative elites of the Republic explicitly linked the political turmoil that led to the French Revolution to the spread of mechanist philosophies. The refusal to recognize the existence of invisible, imponderable forces in nature resulted in materialism, scepticism, and in the destruction of the religious and moral basis of Old Regime society (Ciancio 1992, 281). The French physician Pierre Thouvenel, who after 1789 found refuge in the Venetian territory together with many aristocratic emigrants, placed Alessandro Volta and Spallanzani among the "incredulous men, commonly called materialists," who regarded every "occult cause" as "unnatural, or against nature" ([Gazola] 1802, 215). The Veronese patrician Gian Battista Gazola, one of his hosts and a well-known naturalist and collector (Dal Prete 2007, 2013), concluded indeed that mechanist naturalists were one and the same with "free masons, Jacobins, and modern philosophers" ([Gazola] 1802, 13).

Conclusions

Preformationism was adopted by leading Italian naturalists, such as Vallisneri, from the early decades of the century; its dependence on deductive models proved nonetheless difficult to reconcile with the empiricist traditions of Italian natural history. In fact, epigenesis maintained a strong foothold in the country throughout the century. In spite of the fact that preformationism called for an act of intelligent creation, conservative Italian Catholics considered epigenesis much closer to the traditions of the church and rejected the notion of a soulless, mechanical universe. Preformationism underpinned the rise of the doctrine of "instantaneous ensoulment," which was used in turn to foster a tighter ecclesiastical control over the female body. That was considered a departure from the theological (and social) status quo and conservative Catholics opposed it. Likewise, in late eighteenth-century Republic of Venice preformationism was the system of choice for the supporters of political and social reforms, the independence of natural philosophy from theology, and the limitation of the ecclesiastical prerogatives. The established elites, on the other hand, often regarded preformationism as the epitome of the modern mechanical philosophies that removed God from the world and, with Him, the religious and moral values that held together society.

NOTES

I am especially grateful to Dario Generali and Maria Teresa Monti, whose work on Antonio Vallisneri and eighteenth-century Italian embryology has been invaluable to my own research.

1 A. Conti to A. Vallisneri, 16 May 1710. Livorno, Autografoteca Bastogi, Cass. 30 ins. 2185.
2 A. Conti to L. Bourguet, 6 April 1714. Neuchâtel, Bibliothèque Publique et Universitaire, Ms. 1282, 160–1.
3 A. Vallisneri to L.A. Muratori, 17 April 1714. Modena, Biblioteca Estense; Archivio Muratori, filza 81, fasc. 55, letter 39.
4 A. Vallisneri to L. Bourguet, 2 January 1714. Neuchâtel, Bibliothèque Publique et Universitaire, Ms. 1282, 145–6.
5 A. Conti to A. Vallisneri, 13 May 1727. Livorno, Biblioteca Labronica. Autografoteca Bastogi, Cass. 30, ins. 2185.
6 A. Vallisneri to A. Conti, 18 April 1727. Livorno, Biblioteca Labronica. Autografoteca Bastogi, Cass. 30, ins. 2185.
7 Available statistics are in fact appalling: mortality rates lay anywhere between 50 per cent and 80 per cent, and did not start to improve until the late 1800s (Betta 2006, 135).

REFERENCES

Bennett, J. 2007. "Malpighi and the Microscope." In *Marcello Malpighi: Anatomist and Physician*, edited by D. Bertoloni Meli, 63–72. Florence: Olschki.
Bernardi, W. 1986. *Le metafisiche dell'embrione: Scienze della vita e filosofia da Malphighi a Spallanzani (1672–1793)*. Florence: Olschki.
Bernardi, W. 1989. "Influssi newtoniani nella biologia del settecento." *Giornale di Fisica* (30): 71–6.
Bertoloni Meli, D. 2011. *Mechanism, Experiment, Disease: Marcello Malpighi and Seventeenth-Century Anatomy*. Baltimore: Johns Hopkins University Press.

Betta, E. 2006 *Animare la vita: Disciplina della nascita tra medicina e morale nell'Ottocento*. Bologna: Il Mulino.

Cangiamila, E. 1748. *Compendio dell'Embriologia Sacra: Ovvero dell'Uffizio de' Sacerdoti Medici, e Superiori circa l'Eterna Salute de' Bambini racchiusi nell'Utero*. Palermo: Francesco Valenza.

Cangiamila, E. 1756. *Compendio dell'embriologia sacra*. Livorno: Paolo Fanteschi e Compagni.

Ciancio, L. 1992. "La resistibile ascesa della rabdomanzia: Pierre Thouvenel e la Guerra di Dieci Anni." *Intersezioni* (Bologna, Italy) 2 (12): 267–90.

Ciancio, L. 1996. "Geologia e ortodossia: L'eredità galileiana nella geologia veneta del secondo Settecento." In *La politica della scienza: Toscana e stati italiani nel tardo Settecento*, edited by G. Barsanti, V. Becagli, and R. Pasta, 491–507. Florence: Olschki.

Cogrossi, C.F 2005. *Nuova idea del male contagioso de' buoi*. Edited by M. De Zan, 51–83. Florence: Olschki.

Contardi, S. 1994. *La rivincita dei "filosofi di carta": Saggio sulla filosofia naturale di Antonio Vallisneir junior*. Florence: Olschki.

Corte, B. 1702. *Lettera nella quale si dinota da qual tempo probabilmente s'infonde nel feto l'anima ragionevole*. Milan.

Dal Prete, I. 2007. "Giovan Battista Gazola." In *Storia della Società Letteraria di Verona tra Ottocento e Novecento*, edited by G. Romagnani and M. Zangarini, 61–77. Verona: Cierre.

Dal Prete, I. 2008. *Scienza e Società nel Settecento Veneto: Il caso veronese 1680–1797*. Milan: Franco Angeli.

Dal Prete, I. 2009. "I carteggi Conti-Vallisneri." In *Antonio Conti: Uno scienziato nella République des Lettres*, edited by G. Baldassarri, S. Contarini, and F. Fedi, 97–111. Padua: Il Poligrafo.

Dal Prete, I. 2013. "The Gazola Family's Scientific Cabinet: Politics, Society and Scientific Collecting in the Twilight of the Republic of Venice." In *Making Science Public in 18th-Century Europe: The Role of Cabinets of Experimental Philosophy*, edited by J. Bennett and S. Talas, 155–72. Leiden: Brill.

De Ferrari, A. 1983. "Corte (Curtius), Bartolomeo." In *Dizionario Biografico degli Italiani*. Vol. 29. Rome: Treccani.

Fantini, B. 1994. "Francesco Redi e il metodo sperimentale in biologia." In F. Redi, *Esperienze intorno alla generazione degl'insetti*, edited by B. Fantini, VII–XXIX. Rome: Teknos.

Farinella, C. 1993. *L'Accademia Repubblicana: La Società dei Quaranta e Anton Mario Lorgna*. Milan: Franco Angeli.

Fazzari, M. 1999. "Redi, Buonanni e la controversia sulla generazione spontanea: Una rilettura." In *Francesco Redi: Un protagonista della scienza moderna*, edited by W. Bernardi and L. Guerrini, 91–127. Florence: Olschki.

Fazzari, M. 2005. "Filippo Buonanni: un caso di invisibilità creata dai contemporanei, ovvero come si diventa invisibili." In *Figure dell'invisibilità: Le scienze della vita nell'Italia d'Antico Regime*, edited by M.T. Monti and M. Ratcliff, 21–82. Florence: Olschki.
Fazzari, M. 2007. "Incredibili visioni: Roma e i microscopi alla fine del '600." In *From Makers to Users. Microscopes, Markets, and Scientific Practices in the Seventeenth and Eighteenth Centuries*, edited by D. Generali and M. Ratcliff, 3–42. Florence: Olschki.
Filippini, N.M. 1993. "The Church, the State and Childbirth: The Midwife in Italy during the Eighteenth Century." In *The Art of Midwifery: Early Modern Midwives in Europe*, edited by H. Marland, 153–76. London: Routledge.
Forleo, R., ed. 2001. *Embriologia sacra, overo, Dell'uffizio de' sacerdoti, medici, e superiori, circa l'eterna salute de' bambini racchiusi nell'utero*. Rome: CIC edizioni internazionali.
[Fortis, A.] 1768. *Difesa del Celebre Sig. Antonio Vallisnieri dagl'Insulti dell'Autore delle Lettere d'un Curato di Campagna, uscite in Verona l'anno 1767*. Padua: Conzatti.
[Gazola, G.B.] 1802. *La guerra di dieci anni: Raccolta polemico-fisica sull'elettrometria Galvano-organica*. Verona.
Gecchele, M. 2000. *Fedeli sudditi e buoni cristiani: La "rivoluzione" scolastica di fine Settecento tra la Lombardia austriaca e la Serenissima*. Verona: Mazziana.
Generali, D. 1984. "Il 'Giornale de' letterati d'Italia' e la cultura veneta del primo settecento." *Rivista di Storia della Filosofia* (Milan, Italy) 2:243–81.
Generali, D. 1987. "Antonio Vallisneri 'corrispondente' leibniziano." In *Rapporti di scienziati europei con lo Studio bolognese fra '600 e '700*, edited by M. Cavazza, 125–40. Bologna: Istituto per la storia dell'Università.
Generali, D. 2007. "L'uso del microscopio in Vallisneri." In *From Makers to Users: Microscopes, Markets, and Scientific Practices in the Seventeenth and Eighteenth Centuries*, edited by D. Generali and M. Ratcliff, 231–70. Florence: Olschki.
Luzzini, F. 2007. "Antonio Vallisneri e la questione dei vermicelli spermatici." In *From Makers to Users: Microscopes, Markets, and Scientific Practices in the Seventeenth and Eighteenth Centuries*, edited by D. Generali and M. Ratcliff, 73–89. Florence: Olschki.
Martin, C. 2011. *Renaissance Meteorology: Pomponazzi to Descartes*. Baltimore: Johns Hopkins University Press.
Monti, M.T. 1996. "Politica della scienza nella Milano spagnola: Considerazioni in margine a una questione medico-teologica." In *Per una storia critica della scienza*, edited by M. Beretta, F. Mondella, and M.T. Monti, 405–37. Bologna: Cisalpino.
Monti, M.T. 2009. "La scrittura e i gesti dell'Istoria." In *Antonio Vallisneri: Istoria delle Generazione*, edited by M.T. Monti, XV–CIV. Florence: Olschki.

Redi, F. 1668. *Esperienze intorno alla generazione degl'insetti.* Florence: All'insegna della Stella.

Redi, F. 1996. *Esperienze intorno alla generazione degl'insetti.* Edited by W. Bernardi. Florence: Giunti.

Reill, P. 2005. *Vitalizing Nature in the Enlightenment.* Berkeley: University of California Press.

Rinaldi, M. 2008. "Nel 'vasto impero delle parole.' Il 'Saggio alfabetico' di Vallisneri e il linguaggio della conoscenza." In *Antonio Vallisneri: La figura, il contesto, le immagini storiografiche*, edited by D. Generali, 317–38. Florence: Olschki.

Roe, S. 1981. *Matter, Life and Generation: Eighteenth-Century Embryology and the Haller-Wolff Debate.* Cambridge: Cambridge University Press.

Romagnani, G.P. 2009. "Antonio Conti e Scipione Maffei." In *Antonio Conti: Uno scienziato nella République des Lettres*, edited by G. Baldassarri, S. Contarini, and F. Fedi, 113–40. Padua: Il Poligrafo.

Rosa, M. 1966. *Benedetto XIV: Dizionario Biografico degli Italiani.* Vol. 8. Rome: Treccani.

Schmitt, C. 1983. *Aristotle and the Renaissance.* Cambridge, MA: Harvard University Press. http://dx.doi.org/10.4159/harvard.9780674432819.

Scotti Morgana, S. 1981. *Esordi della lessicografia scientifica italiana: Il "Saggio alfabetico 'Istoria medica e naturale" di Antonio Vallisneri.* Florence: La Nuova Italia.

Scudellini, A. 1761. *De Abortivis Baptizandis Dissertatio, habita in Collegio Episcopali Veronensi anno 1761.* Verona.

Vallisneri, A. 1721. *Istoria della Generazione dell'Uomo, e degli Animali, se sia da' Vermicelli spermatici, o dalle Uova.* Venice: Giovanni Gabriele Hertz.

Vallisneri, A. 2005. *Miglioramenti, e correzioni ecc.* Edited by I. Dal Prete. Florence: Olschki.

Vallisneri, A. 2009. *Istoria della Generazione dell'Uomo, e degli Animali, se sia da' Vermicelli spermatici, o dalle Uova.* Edited by M.T. Monti. Florence: Olschki.

Vallisneri, A. 2013. *Che ogni italiano debba scrivere in lingua purgata italiana, o toscana, per debito, per giustizia e per decoro della nostra Italia.* Edited by D. Generali. Florence: Olschki.

3 Theories of Generation and the History of Life

PETER J. BOWLER

A long time ago – in 1971 to be precise – I completed a PhD thesis at the University of Toronto on the relationship between theories of generation and ideas about the stability of species in the eighteenth century. Two articles were published from this project (Bowler 1973a and 1973b), but my interests then switched to evolution theories in the nineteenth and eventually early twentieth centuries. After a gap of over forty years I have now been invited to return to my original topic, and in this chapter I will try to provide a survey of the ideas I first cut my historical teeth on, supplemented by some additional research. In my article contrasting the ideas of the comte de Buffon and Charles Bonnet, I showed that the simple dichotomies often employed to depict the wider implications of the rival theories of generation were unworkable when evaluated at a detailed level. For all his reputation as a pioneer transformist, Buffon ultimately seems to have concluded that the basic forms of animal life were predetermined by the laws of nature. Conversely, Bonnet was able to adapt the theory of pre-existing germs – admittedly in a highly idiosyncratic manner – to the possibility that life on earth had advanced through a series of progressive steps towards the modern situation. These two examples undermined the conventional assumption that pre-existence was invariably used to bolster belief in the stability of natural forms, while the new materialist theories of generation favoured a belief in the mutability of nature. In this chapter I hope to reinforce that message by appealing to a wider range of examples.

Traditional histories of evolutionism focused on the eighteenth century as a prelude to the emergence of Darwinism, often seeking apparent anticipations of later developments – a technique encapsulated in the title of the collection *Forerunners of Darwin* (Glass, Temkin, and Strauss 1959). Much attention quite rightly focused on the discovery of fossils and the emergence of a sense that the earth was much older than implied by the biblical story of creation and had passed through a series of revolutions in which its inhabitants had changed. New ideas about the classification of species were also important for creating a sense that there was some form of genuine "relationship" between groups of allied forms. It was recognized that some figures conventionally seen as precursors of transformism, notably Buffon and P.L.M. de Maupertuis, were also interested in generation (to the extent that Maupertuis was also depicted as a precursor of Mendel). My own thesis drew on the magisterial work of Jacques Roger (1963, trans. 1998), which showed the complexity of the debates over generation and linked those debates to wider issues including the emerging doubts about the stability of nature and the decline of natural theology.

It seemed to me, then as now, that there must be a link between views about how the succession of new organisms is ensured within species and ideas about the origin of the first members of the species and the possibility that successive generations might not conserve the same form as the originals. But to the extent that such a relationship had been acknowledged in the era of *Forerunners of Darwin*, historians had presumed a relatively simple link between models of generation and openness to the possibility of transformism. The theory of pre-existing germs, especially in the form known as *emboîtement* or encapsulement, was linked to belief in design by God and the assumption that his actions at the creation predetermined and fixed the form of each species. Those savants who insisted that material nature was incapable of generating complex living forms were forced to imagine that God originally created the germs – miniatures which served as the basis for each new generation – encapsulated one within the other like a series of Russian dolls. They were enclosed within either the male sperm or, more probably, the female ovum, so that the whole human race was enclosed originally in the ovaries of Eve. In the late seventeenth century when this theory first emerged, it seemed natural to assume that the series of germs was designed to a single pattern for each species to ensure the stability of creation as a whole. On this basis C.O. Whitman had described Bonnet, perhaps the leading exponent of pre-existence in the eighteenth century, as committed to the absolute fixity of nature (Whitman 1895; see also Glass 1959b).

As Staffan Müller-Wille shows in this volume, the work of taxonomists and collectors had begun to suggest that species should be seen not as static entities, but as reservoirs of variety. But how free was the potential for variation, and to what extent was it restrained by the laws governing reproduction? Traditionally, historians have seen the focus on variety as reaching its climax in the radical opponents of the argument from design who argued that material nature could generate living forms de novo and saw no reason why the original or the presently existing forms should be perpetuated intact from one generation to the next. Materialist writers such as Denis Diderot and the baron d'Holbach used the new theories of generation to argue for the spontaneous generation of new species and their subsequent instability, and Buffon was widely seen as an associate of this program. Here was a neat dichotomy: pre-existence implied design and stability, materialist theories of generation promoted spontaneous generation and transformism.

Roger's work showed the difficulty of maintaining such a dichotomy into the middle decades of the eighteenth century. My thesis was written to explore the complexity he revealed from the viewpoint of someone interested in early ideas about the possibility that living forms may have changed in the course of the earth's history. Even in the existing literature there was some recognition of the potential for old ideas to be interpreted in new ways. Arthur O. Lovejoy's study of the chain of being (1936) outlined the somewhat bizarre modifications of the theory of pre-existing germs that allowed Bonnet to "temporalize" the chain into a vision of progress in the history of life. But most of the earlier literature was locked into the assumption that the materialist theories of generation were the chief agents responsible for creating an openness to the possibility of change. To challenge this my article contrasting the positions of Bonnet and Buffon was written to show that for all the superficial elements of "degeneration" introduced by Buffon, his world view retained an underlying element of stability because he believed that the possible combinations of organic particles were limited to certain predetermined forms corresponding to the species we know. Change was thus largely predetermined, as was Bonnet's vision of progress. I now propose to extend this point by giving other examples where acceptance of pre-existing germs did not preclude a willingness to allow at least a superficial element of change, while new theories of generation retained the principle that if change occurred it must be predetermined.

Several preliminary observations are necessary before proceeding. Most obviously, the ideas discussed below should not be treated in any simple-minded sense as anticipations of nineteenth-century evolutionism (Bowler 2009, ch. 3). There were indeed occasional suggestions of transformations within species, possibly but not necessarily recognizing that relationship might indicate descent from a common ancestor. Nor should we forget the extent to which nineteenth-century transmutationists were reluctant to accept the Darwinian notion of open-ended, non-predetermined evolution. But in the eighteenth century, materialist speculations often focused more on the idea that new living forms might appear by spontaneous generation, with the possibility of subsequent instability being used more as a weapon to attack the argument from design than as a working hypothesis for the study of natural history. Where something resembling transformism was postulated, it was more likely to be seen as the unfolding of a predetermined pattern than as a trial-and-error process anticipating the logic of natural selection. What we are dealing with here is at best the prehistory of transformism, the emergence of a climate of opinion which made it possible to contemplate some form of development in the history of life on earth. Closer analogues to what emerged in the era of Darwinism do not appear until the end of the century with the work of Erasmus Darwin and J.B. Lamarck.

In the area of generation, we must also be wary of using terms such as "preformation" and "epigenesist" when describing the rival theories (Bowler 1971). One could imagine the embryo to be preformed at the point of conception without believing that the structure existed earlier, let alone that a whole series of miniatures was encapsulated within the female ovum. For this reason it is preferable to use the term "pre-existing germs" to denote those theories in which the miniature organism exists long prior to conception. Nor was the theory of *emboîtement* the only explanation of where the germs resided before conception, since the rival panspermist view postulated germs floating freely around in space waiting for a chance to enter a living body and begin the process of growth. The preformed or pre-existing embryo was not necessarily thought of as a potentially visible miniature – it could be an outline or pattern folded up so that it did not become obvious until expanded. On such a model the parts might unfold sequentially, making it hard to establish an observational test to distinguish between preformation and epigenesis. Furthermore, if "epigenesist" is defined in the terms established by William Harvey, i.e., as the sequential formation of the parts of the embryo, some of the new materialist theories of generation were not epigenetic because they postulated the formation of a complete pattern for the embryo immediately after conception. In that case, no observations of the embryo after conception could decide between the new hypotheses and preformation/pre-existence.

At a more fundamental level, any attempt to portray these debates in terms of alternative world views defined by materialism and vitalism, or design and instability, founders on the complexity of the issues as they developed. The theory of pre-existing germs was formulated in the late seventeenth century to resolve the problem created by the Cartesian model of a world composed solely of inert matter and motion. If matter were really inert, it seemed implausible that motion alone could assemble particles into complex structures such as living bodies. Natural processes could expand an existing structure, but not create one, hence the need for pre-existing germs to explain (or explain away) the process of generation. Theories of genuine epigenesis required that matter be governed by more active or purposeful forces than mere motion, a view that certainly re-emerged in the late eighteenth century under the name of vitalism.

A number of scholars have now demonstrated that depicting these debates solely in terms of the conflict between the mechanical philosophy and vitalism obscures the complex development of Enlightenment ideas about the nature of matter (Reill 2005; Roe 1981; see also Dal Prete in this volume). Materialists were increasingly willing to admit that matter did have powers normally attributed to life itself, thus implying that it did have the capacity to organize itself into complex bodies. True epigenesis was still a problem since the sequential development of parts would require extended purposeful activity, but an initial act of complexification was credible, hence the new theories of generation. This "vitalization" of material nature is often attributed to the influence of Leibniz's philosophy and influenced a number of the thinkers discussed in this chapter (Duchesneau 2006, 2010; Rieppel 1988). There were radical materialists in the broader sense who used the new ideas to undermine the argument for an initial act of divine creation, but others were willing to see the active powers of nature as representing a dispensation of the Creator intended to achieve his goals indirectly in the course of time. J.B. Robinet's belief that all matter is composed of germs represents one manifestation of the latter view, but John Turberville Needham's contribution to the new theory of generation was also inspired by a religious motivation.

I begin my survey with the theory of pre-existing germs in order to show that the idea could be adapted to allow for an element of development in the history of life on earth. Bonnet and Robinet's efforts to temporalize the chain of being form one strand of this story, but it is often forgotten that one of the more radical thinkers who pioneered the idea of an extended earth history – Benoît de Maillet – still retained this approach to generation. I then move on to the new theories, acknowledging their influence on radical thinkers such as Diderot and d'Holbach, but showing how it was still possible to argue that the creative activity of material nature operated within fixed limits which look remarkably like the old idea of permanently fixed species. Buffon falls into this category, while his one-time collaborator Needham shows how the new theories could be adapted to give a materialized interpretation of the Genesis story of creation.

Pre-existence and Mutability

When the theory of pre-existing germs was first mooted it was simply assumed that God created germs corresponding to all of the known species, thus ensuring their fixity. On the principle of *emboîtement*, the successive generations of the human race were enclosed one inside the other within the ovaries of Eve, and the same was true for all other species. Bonnet adopted this view, and statements in his *Considérations sur les corps organisés* of 1762 have been taken as classic illustrations of the static vision of nature:

> Nature is surely admirable in her conservation of individuals, but she is especially so in the conservation of species ... The centuries transmit this magnificent spectacle from one to another; and they transmit exactly that which they receive. Nothing changes, nothing alters; perfect identity. Victorious over the elements, time and death, the species are conserved, and the period of their duration is unknown to us. (Bonnet 1779, 5, 231–2, my translation)

But the theory could be adapted to allow for an element of change, even if this was necessarily predetermined by the germs formed at the creation. Bonnet himself later allowed for the progressive appearance of new forms in the course of time, as did Robinet. Meanwhile more radical thinkers such as de Maillet and La Mettrie openly postulated major developments in the history of life, in part by appealing to the alternative panspermist version of pre-existence in which the germs float freely about in nature.

Several techniques could be used to allow for the appearance of new forms in the course of time. On the panspermist model, it was possible to assume that under certain circumstances nature might provide conditions in which germs could start to grow without a parental host, thus a new species would appear in what would look superficially like an act of spontaneous generation. These first forms would then absorb other germs of the same type to initiate the normal process of reproduction. Even on the principle of *emboîtement*, one could suppose that the sequence of germs was not identical throughout, so that God could allow for revolutions in the history of life by predesigning new sets of germs corresponding to new forms of life.

An equally promising line of attack was to limit the extent to which the germs dictated the final form of the adult organism. Initially, some exponents of the pre-existence theory seem to have thought that every individual peculiarity was preformed in the germ. But this would make the Creator responsible for every deformity and monstrosity, so later supporters of the theory tended to assume that the germ defined only the basic specific form of the individual, all personal characteristics being the outcome of parental or environmental influences on the growing embryo. As Bonnet delared: "The germ carries the original imprint of the species, and not that of the individual. It is a man, a horse, a bull etc., but it is not a certain man, a *certain* horse or a *certain* bull" (Bonnet 1762, 2:256; 1779, 6:392–3; my translation) This move transfers most of the issues later incorporated into the concept of heredity to the developmental process, making it hard to find observational tests to distinguish between the old theory of generation and the new. More important for the present topic, it allows for the possibility that external influences might have at least some effect on the form of the species.

Bonnet's preferred way of introducing an element of change into the history of life on earth involved fundamental transformations predetermined in the actual sequence of germs as originally created. In theory, one might simply suppose that God had created a developmental sequence in the germs encapsulated into the first created life forms. But Bonnet came to the scheme outlined in his *Palingénésie philosophique* of 1769 via his psychological theories and his religious convictions (Bowler 1971). He was attracted to the idea of reincarnation and postulated that this might be possible if every human, and indeed every organism, contained within itself a germ that would allow its soul to be reawakened in a new body some time after the death of the first. The renewal would follow some great revolution on the earth's surface, but it would also be in a more perfect form, allowing the higher present-day animals to be reincarnated in human form (Bonnet 1769, 1:176–7; 1779, 15:177). He then generalized the process to include a whole series of previous revolutions by which living things have successively progressed towards their present states (1769, 1:257; 1779, 15:275–6). This was the process described by Lovejoy (1936) as the temporalization of the chain of being. But it should be noted that Bonnet also linked his theory to the growing realization that there may have been catastrophic revolutions in the earth's physical environment, requiring new adaptations in each period (1769, 1:257; 1779, 15:275–6).

Because Bonnet's theory required numerous interlocking sequences of germs, it can hardly be counted as a straightforward modification of the *emboîtement* principle. Jean-Baptiste Robinet's later ideas were equally idiosyncratic – he was a philosopher rather than a naturalist and his views seldom addressed the technical issues that obsessed other students of generation. His four-volume *De la nature* (1761–6) often developed themes that attracted ridicule, for instance his claim that minerals and even the planets reproduce themselves (1:210–17 and 224–5). Nevertheless, his was a dynamic vision of nature and in the end this included an element of historical progress. He accepted the theory of germs and assumed that these entities were miniature organisms (1:255 and 4:136). Like others at the time he thought that both males and females produced semen containing animalcules (spermatozoa) but he thought these tiny creatures were actually composed of germs (1:141, 156). In his fourth volume he argued that all matter was composed of germs, so that one germ developed by absorbing masses of other germs (4:83, 103). He portrayed all matter as active and sensitive, responding on this point to Diderot (4:11, 115; see Roger 1963, 651).

Initially, Robinet had insisted that all this dynamism was constrained within limits defined by stable species (1761–6, 1:49, 64). But in his fourth volume he attacked both Buffon and Bonnet on this point, insisting now on the complete continuity of the chain of being (4:5–11). He proposed the idea of a single "prototype" of which all living things were variants (4:2–17), although this was evidently more a property of animalism than a structural prototype in the evolutionary sense (4:55 and 76). His vision of natural process again fits Lovejoy's model of the temporalized chain of being because he suggests that at first only the germs of the simplest organisms were able to develop, after which these in turn served as hosts to allow germs of the next highest type to form, and so on up the chain to humankind (4:6). There was little effort to relate this vision to new ideas about the earth's history, but Robinet evidently assumed that it would take vast amounts of time.

> As for the order of the development, I am sure that nature has always proceeded from the least composite to the more composite. The most complex organization that we know, and that which produces most phenomena, is that of man. There would thus have been times when no human germ had developed. But how many millions of years or centuries were necessary to bring the human seed to maturity? We are no longer in a position to say. There are no intervals, small or large, between the successive and neighbouring developments. Nature passes from one to the other without discontinuity. (4:128, my translation)

Here what is, in effect, the panspermist version of the theory of pre-existing germs becomes the basis for a model of historical progress predetermined by the forms prefigured in the germs that were created as the foundation for the universe itself.

In another work (1768) Robinet attracted ridicule for suggesting that lower forms of life could be found anticipating the human form, mermen or aquatic humans being an example. But this idea was by no means uncommon at the beginning of the century and was incorporated into what was probably the most influential text expounding an extended vision of earth history, Benoît de Maillet's *Telliamed* (1748, but written much earlier, see the translation 1968 and Cohen 2011). Where Robinet sought to modify traditional ideas of design and creation, de Maillet clearly intended to undermine the credibility of Genesis through his vision of an earth formed and developed through natural causes over vast periods of time. Presented as the teaching of an eastern sage (whose name just happened to be his own, spelled backwards) *Telliamed* linked the cosmological views of Descartes to the new geological thinking and then challenged the conventional view of human origins in a manner that inspired Buffon and many later writers. Yet de Maillet was not really a materialist, because he still accepted that all life develops from pre-existing germs – he merely evaded the implication that the germs must have been designed by declaring that the universe was eternal. As we shall see, his system was taken up by the radical materialist La Mettrie, suggesting that the concept of pre-existing germs had become so pervasive that it took time before materialist thinkers could really come to grips with the need to formulate an alternative model of generation.

De Maillet's scheme of earth history saw the planet gradually drying up after initially being completely covered with water. Life appeared from minute and hence invisible germs or seeds that pervade the whole universe (1748, 2:218–19; 1968, 225). In normal generation these are prepared for fertility in the male, but in the earth's early history "the waters surrounding the globe became at certain times and under certain circumstances, proper for fecundity" (1748, 2:22, translation 1968, 227). This would look like spontaneous generation, and de Maillet suggests that the process still occurs as in the animalcules found in vegetable infusions. But the new organisms were actually derived from germs, not generated from unformed matter. Since the earliest of these events occurred before the first dry land appeared, the first forms of life were all aquatic. They included equivalents of all the terrestrial animals with which we are now familiar, including humans. De Maillet insisted that these aquatic equivalents are still to be found in the oceans, hence his belief in the reality of mermen (1748, 2:151–71; 1968, 192–200). He insisted that the transition from the aquatic to the terrestrial form would not be difficult once dry land appeared – the fins of flying fish, for instance, could easily be transformed into legs (1748, 2:137–9; 1968, 186–7). Nevertheless, "the appearance of the original shape remains in the whole, and it will always be easy to recognize" (1748, 2:140; 1968, 187). The transformation seems to involve something like the inheritance of acquired characteristics, but de Maillet also saw a role for trial and error: "If a hundred million individuals perished in contracting the habit, it is only necessary that two should succeed in order to start the species" (1748, 2:142; 1968, 188).

These last points have frequently been seen as anticipations of transformism, but de Maillet's reliance on the panspermist version of the germ theory ensured that the changes were unable to produce genuinely new species. The species were defined by the germs, and although a huge modification in each was required to produce the terrestrial form, the underlying specific type remained. A section not printed in the first edition suggested that new species could appear from time to time, but only because there were some types of germs that had not undergone the initial equivalent of spontaneous generation in earlier periods (1968, 228–31). In the end, for all the massive amount of change de Maillet postulated in the history of the earth and its inhabitants, his inability to think of a materialist alternative to the germ theory ensured that his speculations contained an underlying element of predictability in the sequence of events.

Telliamed had some influence on the later naturalists who sought to extend the age of the earth, but it also seems to have impressed one of the most significant materialist thinkers of the period, Julien Offray de La Mettrie. In his *L'homme machine* of 1748, La Mettrie drew inspiration from Abraham Trembley's discovery of the regenerative powers of the polyp or freshwater hydra to argue that all matter had the capacity to produce the functions of life – including the mental and moral powers of humanity (La Mettrie 1991; see Dawson 1991; Vartanian 1950). Curiously, Trembley himself was not very interested in theories of generation, but seems to have been inclined towards the idea of pre-existing germs (Baker 1952, 180–6). La Mettrie insisted that the polyp made nonsense out of the existing theories, by which he presumably meant the *emboîtement* version of pre-existence (La Mettrie 1960, 181; 1774, 1:333). Normal generation occurred by an epigenetic process from the "worm" of the male semen after it found its way into the female ovum (La Mettrie 1960, 349; 1774, 1:192). But this reference to epigenesis was somewhat misleading, since La

Mettrie went on to say that the actual arrangement of the parts had always existed in the germ within the male spermatozoa (1960, 194; 1774, 1:352). The germ was thus not an actual miniature of the organism but some sort of framework whose parts would become unfolded sequentially to give the appearance of epigenetic development.

It was in his *Système de l'Epicure* of 1750 that La Mettrie addressed the question of the origin of life on earth, explicitly acknowledging the influence of *Telliamed* (La Mettrie 1774, 1:241). He now accepted the panspermist version of pre-existence, assuming that the freely floating germs normally have to find their way into the male of an appropriate form in order to begin the process of development: "There are, therefore, eggs or seeds in the air, as much for animals as for vegetables; they have been there and they will always be there. Each individual attracts to himself those of his type, or those which are proper to him; unless one prefers that the seeds seek bodies where they can mature, germinate, develop." He immediately goes on to suppose, however, that the first steps in the process occur in the air itself: "Their first womb was thus the air, whose heat started their preparation" (1774, 1:231–2, my translation). This in turn allowed him to speculate that in the earth's early history the first germs were able to develop without parents: "The earth must have served as a uterus to man; it must have opened its womb to the human germs, already prepared, so that given certain laws, this superb animal could hatch out" (1774, 1:232).

Like de Maillet, La Mettrie thought that the human (and presumably other) species had not first appeared in their present form. There was a gradual development over a long period of time, but La Mettrie seems to have had no interest in the idea that there would need to be a transition from aquatic to terrestrial forms. In a much bolder challenge to the argument from design he insisted that the first generations had been imperfect, often lacking organs, and that only the most perfect survived and reproduced. Monstrosities showed that this process still took place to a limited extent. In the past this gradual process of trial and error (one hesitates to say natural selection, given the very different context) was crucial to allow the human race to progress towards its present form: "perfection could no more be the work of a day for nature than for art" (1774, 1:234). Here we see La Mettrie making the best effort he could to escape the traditional link between the theory of pre-existing germs and the assumption that the germs were created by God. De Maillet had evaded the issue of design by making the germs eternal, but La Mettrie went one step further by limiting their effect and throwing the emphasis onto a natural process of perfection operating through the epigenetic forces responsible for development. This was perhaps as far as a materialist could go to challenge the traditional belief in divine creation without throwing out the germ theory altogether. Later writers in this tradition turned to the new theories of generation to complete their move towards a world view that excluded the argument from design altogether.

Materialism and Stability

The new theories of generation devised in the late 1740s by Maupertuis, Buffon, and Needham were intended to provide an explanation of how natural processes could form complex living bodies. Their proponents insisted that the concept of pre-existing germs was no explanation at all – it denied the reality of generation by supposing that all structures were created by God at the beginning of the universe. The new theories were an attempt to resolve the problem that had led to the emergence of the concept of germs in the seventeenth century. They sought to show how natural processes driven by the laws governing matter could generate complex structures – even if this required the postulation of natural forces that looked remarkably like the powers normally attributed to living things. Normal generation involved the coming together of material particles from the male and female reproductive systems, which were somehow able to recognize the place they needed to take up in the new organism. It was widely assumed that this assembly took place immediately after conception, producing a complete miniature organism that subsequently grew by expansion, as did the hypothetical pre-existing germs.

One crucial difference between the new theories and the old was that now it became possible to imagine the spontaneous generation of new organisms from an unstructured mass of particles. Buffon and Needham claimed to have observed the spontaneous generation of animalcules in vegetable and animal infusions, sparking a debate with Bonnet and Lazzaro Spallanzani that dragged on for decades. On a wider scale, the revival of the idea of spontaneous generation gave a new impetus for radical thinkers who wanted to undermine the Genesis story of creation and the argument from design. Materialist thinkers such as Diderot and d'Holbach could claim that natural processes were responsible for the origin of life on earth. By insisting that there was nothing to impose any absolute or pre-existing order on the products, they could also undermine the argument from design. The claim that the existence of monstrosities illustrated the lack of any stable forms defining the species could be used to argue that the origin of life itself was a process of trial and error. The species we now see cannot be truly stable – but more important, the same lack of a stable order could be seen in the processes that originally generated the first forms of life on earth. Open-ended spontaneous generation seemed a more potent weapon against the argument from design than transformism.

Yet whatever the wide-ranging speculations of the materialist philosophers, the savants and naturalists who were the real architects of new theories of generation found it hard to throw off the belief that the assembly of living species we now observe was somehow predetermined. There might be spontaneous generation, but it was not an equivocal or unplanned production of new structures. Buffon famously allowed for a significant degree of modification within species in the course of time, but in the end he seems to have thought that the basic forms of the species are somehow predetermined by the laws of nature – only certain combinations are stable and these will emerge wherever life is allowed to flourish. Needham too, still firmly committed to a Christian view of the world, took on board the new ideas about earth history only to the extent of providing a modified understanding of the sequence of creation described in Genesis. The potential of the new theories to serve as foundations for a truly materialist philosophy was freely exploited by those thinkers who were not directly involved in the technical debates, but seems to have been less attractive to savants who had to deal with issues of concern to working naturalists. Needham's case also illustrates that the new theories were not necessarily products of a desire to throw off the Christian world view altogether. Materialism was by no means incompatible with the belief that the universe had a stable or predictable underlying structure.

The more radical implications of the new system were explored most enthusiastically by Denis Diderot and the baron d'Holbach. Diderot's use of the idea of spontaneous generation to undermine the credibility of the argument from design is well known (see, for instance, Roger 1963, 585–682). In his *Lettre sur les aveugles* of 1749 he presented matter as the source of all organization, including that of living things. But imagining the deathbed ruminations of the blind Nicholas Saunderson allowed him to visualize the natural creation of living things as a process of trial and error along the lines pioneered by Lucretius. Saunderson portrays himself as a monstrosity, lacking vital organs, thus illustrating the inability of nature to conserve the type. In the distant past the eternal motion of matter created living forms blindly, many being unable to survive or reproduce, although a few by chance were able to establish themselves as the founders of the species we know (Diderot 1964, 121–3). *De l'interpretation de la nature* of

1753 notes the ideas of Maupertuis and Buffon and suggests that the particles of matter have a kind of sensitivity which prompts them to assume a particular place in a living body (229–31). There are hints that all forms of life may have diverged from a common prototype in a progressive sequence (186–8, 241). But in *Le rêve de d'Alembert* Diderot returned to the idea of a blind creative process, citing Needham's observations as evidence that this can still be observed in action (289–90, 299). Even large animals may be created this way, given time and the right circumstances (302). Once formed, the new types are by no means stable. As animals seek to satisfy their needs they can change their structure in a way that may permanently affect their offspring (1964, 308–10). The appearance of monstrosities is again cited as an obvious challenge to the idea of a stable, orderly creation (324–5).

The baron d'Holbach's *Système de la nature*, published in 1770 under an assumed name, became one of the most notorious symbols of the new materialism. D'Holbach's world view was more mechanistic than Diderot's and his model for how material particles combine into complex structures was based on analogies with chemical combination. The affinities of the various particles allowed them to form even living bodies, with Needham's observations again being presented as evidence (d'Holbach 1821, 1:27). In normal generation the parts of the embryo would be assembled by epigenesis, although no details were given of how this would work (1:87). D'Holbach did not explicitly suggest that the original spontaneous generation by which animals and humans were formed would be a process of trial and error, but he clearly did not believe that the existing species were stable or permanent. Species are adapted to their circumstances, which are always subject to change, and the appearance of monsters that are not coordinated with their surroundings is a clear indication that the process is not perfectly coordinated (1:99–101). Nor was transmutation the only source of change in the world of life – in the past some species were produced before humankind, and even now nature might be assembling in her great laboratory "the elements suitable for hatching out new generations which have nothing in common with the species presently existing" (1:104). Here again, an apparently open-ended process of spontaneous generation plays a greater role than transformism in the assault on the idea of a stable, orderly world.

Diderot and d'Holbach were obviously exploiting the new theories of generation to promote their image of nature as a scene of constant unplanned change. But the architects of the new theories did not necessarily intend them to be used in this way; indeed Needham went out of his way to insist that he did not think that the spontaneous generation of organisms occurred at random. Buffon too after much vacillation concluded that only certain forms corresponding to the species we know could be formed. Maupertuis is the only one of the three principal figures who gave some credence to the image of a hugely prolific nature generating forms that might not correspond to those we know. His best-known work, the popularly written *Venus physique* of 1745 (translation Maupertuis 1968), attacked the theory of pre-existing germs and proposed that the embryo was formed from particles contained in the mixture of male and female semens after intercourse. His reflections on the implications of the phenomena of inheritance are well documented because they seem to anticipate modern views (Glass 1958a; Sandler 1983). His study of how polydactyly ran in families was used to argue that an accident in the generation of one individual could be transmitted to later generations, something that seemed incompatible with the germ theory. The second part of the book speculated about the origin of the human races, arguing that the Black races were also the products of accidents of generation in their first ancestors, after which they migrated to the tropics where the climate was better suited to them.

If new races could be produced by new combinations of the particles in semen, did this imply that new species could appear in the same way? Could there be circumstances in which new forms could appear by spontaneous generation? These were the implications that interested the radical philosophers, and Maupertuis himself addressed them briefly in his other works. His *Essai de cosmologie*, published in 1751 but probably written in the early 1740s, was an attack on the traditional argument from design. It explicitly raised the possibility of new forms appearing through spontaneous generation and implied that many of these would be unable to survive (1768, 1:11). An alternative suggestion was that there had originally been a more or less continuous range of living forms, many of which were subsequently wiped out in a catastrophe, leaving only the species we know (1768, 1:71–2). Maupertuis's *Système de la nature*, originally a Latin thesis published under the name of Baumann in 1751, again supported the idea that living forms could be produced by the attraction of material particles, just as in chemical combinations. He suggested that after a global disaster "New animals, new plants, and perhaps even completely new things could be produced" (1768, 2:170). Nor would the species be stable over time, since they could be transformed by accumulated errors in the process of generation (1768, 2:164–5).

Here Maupertuis seems to join with Diderot and d'Holbach in undermining the notion of a stable organic creation. His views may not have been quite as radical, however, since although he rejected the traditional view that species were designed by a Creator, he was willing to accept that the properties which allowed material particles to "know" how to fit together to form living structures were inherent to their very nature (1768, 2:183). Maupertuis had always recognized that to make the new theories of generation work, it would be necessary to suppose that the particles in the semen had some element of sensitivity that would guide them to assemble in a purposeful way. Perhaps this line of thought would allow the retention of a more basic notion of design confined to the underlying properties of matter itself.

Buffon's views on generation and the stability of species have been widely discussed (for my own views see Bowler 1973a). After some vacillation he came to believe that the various species within each genus have been produced by "degeneration" from a single parent form. He now supposed the Linnaean species to be merely well-marked varieties of a single more basic form, produced by modifications within the generative process in the course of time. His earlier notion of an "internal mould" which guided the organic particles in the semen to arrange themselves in an orderly pattern now seems to represent the basic form of the species, modifiable to a significant but still limited extent. Buffon had worked with Needham on the spontaneous generation of microorganisms, and in his *Epoques de la nature* of 1778 (a supplementary volume to his *Histoire naturelle*) he postulated two acts of spontaneous generation in the earth's history in which more complex forms were produced from unorganized organic matter. The first corresponded to a period when the earth was much hotter, the second – using the organic matter freed when the first species eventually died out – produced the species we know today. These degenerated in size as the earth cooled further, but Buffon is quite explicit that they retain the basic structure of the original forms (1774–89, 5:168, 185–6).

Buffon's clearest statements about the spontaneous generation of new species came in earlier supplementary volumes, especially the fourth (1774–89, 4:357–64). At first sight, he seems to be following the materialist view that particles assemble at random and only a few viable forms survive and reproduce. But he then makes it clear that the successful forms are always the same wherever and whenever the process occurs, and these correspond to the species we know. If all life were annihilated, new forms would be generated and "these new beings would in some manner resemble the old, because brute and living matter are always the same and would give the same general plan of organization and the same varieties in the particular forms" (4:365). It is in this context that we can understand the suggestion made in the second supplementary volume that as the planets in the solar system cool down, they will all become populated by animals similar to those now found on earth (2: 509). It seems evident that for all his repudiation of the traditional argument from design, Buffon thought that matter had been created with properties which predisposed it to form only certain combinations which thus define the basic forms of life.

Buffon's collaborator on the experiments that seemed to confirm the spontaneous generation of microorganisms was John Turberville Needham, a Catholic priest who retained his faith and sought to reconcile it with his studies. He too opted for a twin-semen theory of generation based on the idea of a vegetative force in nature (Roe, 1983). He adopted a metaphysic in which nature was a balance between constructive and destructive tendencies, which led to a certain amount of flexibility in his thinking, displayed in his letters to Bonnet (Mazzolini and Roe, 1986). On one point Needham was absolutely consistent: spontaneous generation was not a random process working through trial and error. It operated according to laws and produced only predetermined forms corresponding to fixed species (see his notes in Spallanzani 1769, 1:206 and 228). His "Recherches physiques et metaphysiques sur la nature et le religion" (forming the second volume of Spallanzani 1769) extended his ideas to give a complete history of nature paralleling those of Buffon and Bonnet.

Like Bonnet, Needham was anxious to preserve the spirit if not the letter of the Genesis story of creation, allowing more time than the traditional interpretation while resisting calls for a vast increase in the timescale. Where Bonnet saw the sequential appearance of new forms in the course of time as a consequence of pre-existing germs, Needham invoked spontaneous generation – while anxiously distancing himself from the account in Diderot's *Lettre sur les aveugles* (Spallanzani 1979, 2:32–8). The process was predetermined by the laws of nature and led to increasing levels of perfection, perhaps best understood by analogy with the development of an egg (2:56). He adopted Linnaeus's view that life appeared on a single mountainous island, which gradually extended into the present land surface as the oceans retreated. The increasing heat from the sun rendered nature "prolific," allowing the generation of plants in the third period, fish and birds in the fourth, lower animals in the fifth, and quadrupeds in the sixth (2:187–92). Here we have the "days" of the Genesis account interpreted as a sequence of distinct periods of creation, all predetermined by the laws imposed by God to govern the spontaneous generation of life from active matter. For all the disputes between Needham and Bonnet over the basic process of generation, their efforts to reconcile their theories with the new ideas about the history of life on earth were thus remarkably similar in outline.

Conclusion

This brief outline of the various efforts made by eighteenth-century savants to link theories of generation with the emerging sense that the earth and its inhabitants have an extended history has shown that we must be very careful not to fall into the trap of assuming one-to-one links between positions in the two areas. Bonnet and Needham fell out completely on the topic of generation, but shared a Christian world view that allowed them to come up with remarkably similar ways of reinterpreting the Genesis story of creation. De Maillet and La Mettrie retained the basic principle of the concept of pre-existing germs, but modified its implications to allow them to challenge Genesis and the traditional argument from design. Far from being a barrier to acceptance of a natural history of creation, the germ theory could be interpreted by both atheists and traditionalists to allow for the successive appearance of new forms in the course of time. Radicals and conservatives differed only on the extent to which the germs could be modified and on how the sequence of new forms was determined. Conversely, the new theories of generation – while forming the perfect basis for materialists to argue for a complete rejection of the argument from design – could equally well be modified to allow for the law-bound predetermination of the forms that would be generated. What we see is a widespread recognition by proponents of rival philosophical positions and rival views of generation that there was a need to adapt their views to provide a natural explanation of how life unfolded in the course of the earth's history. The sheer variety of positions they came up with confirms the strength of the new perception of history, but warns against any attempt to draw direct lines between these early efforts and later theories of evolution.

REFERENCES

Baker, J.A. 1952. *Abraham Trembley of Geneva: Scientist and Philosopher*. London: Arnold.

Bonnet, C. 1762. *Considérations sur les corps organisés*. 2 vols. Amsterdam: Marc-Michel Rey.

Bonnet, C. 1769. *Palingénésie philosophique, ou idées sur l'état passé et sur l'état future des êtres vivans.* 2 vols. Geneva: Claude Philibert et Barthemi Chiroi.
Bonnet, C. 1779. *Oeuvres d'histoire naturelle et de philosophie.* 19 vols. Neuchatel: Samuel Fauche. http://dx.doi.org/10.5962/bhl.title.51265.
Bowler, P.J. 1971. "Preformation and Pre-existence in the Seventeenth Century: A Brief Analysis." *Journal of the History of Biology* 4 (2): 221–44. http://dx.doi.org/10.1007/BF00138311.
Bowler, P.J. 1973a. "Bonnet and Buffon: Theories of Generation and the Problem of Species." *Journal of the History of Biology* 6 (2): 259–81. http://dx.doi.org/10.1007/BF00127610.
Bowler, P.J. 1973b. "Evolutionism in the Enlightenment." *History of Science* 12:159–83.
Bowler, P.J. 2009. *Evolution: The History of an Idea.* 25th anniversary edition. Berkeley: University of California Press.
Buffon, G. 1749–67. *Histoire naturelle, générale et particulière.* 15 vols. Paris: Imprimerie Royale.
Buffon, G. 1774–89. *Histoire naturelle, générale et particulière, supplément.* 7 vols. Paris: Imprimerie Royale.
Cohen, C. 2011. *Science, libitinage et clandestinité à l'aube des lumières: Le transformisme de Telliamed.* Paris: Presses Universitaires de France.
Dawson, V.P. 1991. "Regeneration, Parthenogenesis and the Immutable Order of Nature." *Archives of Natural History* 18 (3): 309–21. http://dx.doi.org/10.3366/anh.1991.18.3.309.
De Maillet, B. 1748. *Telliamed, ou entretiens d'un philosophe indien avec un missionare français sur la diminution de la mer, la formation de la terre, l'origine de l'homme etc.* Amsterdam: L'Honoré et Fils.
De Maillet, B. 1968. *Telliamed, or Conversations between an Indian Philosopher and a French Missionary on the Diminution of the Sea.* Translated by A.V. Carozzi. Urbana: University of Illinois Press.
d'Holbach, P.-H.T. 1821. *Système de la nature: ou des lois du monde physique et du monde moral.* 2 vols. Paris, reprinted Hildesheim: Georg Olms, 1966.
Diderot, D. 1964. *Oeuvres philosophiques.* Edited by P. Vernière. Paris: Classiques Garnier.
Duchesneau, F. 2006. "Charles Bonnet's Neo-Leibnizian Theory of Organic Bodies." In *The Problem of Animal Generation in Early Modern Philosophy,* edited by J.E.H. Smith, 85–314. Cambridge: Cambridge University Press. http://dx.doi.org/10.1017/CBO9780511498572.014.
Duchesneau, F. 2010. *Leibniz: Le vivant et l'organism.* Paris: Vrin.

Glass, B. 1959a. "Maupertuis, Pioneer of Genetics." In *Forerunners of Darwin, 1745–1859*, edited by B. Glass, O. Temkin, and W.L. Straus, Jr, 51–83. Baltimore: Johns Hopkins University Press.

Glass, B. 1959b. "Heredity and Variation in Eighteenth-Century Concepts of the Species." In *Forerunners of Darwin, 1745–1859*, edited by B. Glass, O. Temkin. and W.L. Straus, Jr, 144–72. Baltimore: Johns Hopkins University Press.

La Mettrie, J.O. 1960. *L'homme machine.* Edited by Aram Vartanian. Princeton: Princeton University Press.

La Mettrie, J.O. 1774. *Oeuvres philosophiques.* 2 vols. Berlin.

La Mettrie, J.O. 1991. *Man a Machine and Man a Plant.* Translated by R.A. Watson and M. Rybalka. Indianapolis: Hackett.

Lovejoy, A.O. (1936) 1960. *The Great Chain of Being: A Study in the History of an Idea.* Reprinted New York: Harper.

Maupertuis, P.L.M. 1768. *Oeuvres philosophiques.* 4 vols. Lyon: J.-M. Bruyset. Reprinted Hildesheim: Georg Olms, 1968.

Maupertuis, P.L.M. 1968. *The Earthly Venus.* Translated by S.B. Boas. New York: Johnson Reprint.

Mazzolini, R.G., and S.A. Roe, eds. 1986. *Science against the Unbelievers: The Correspondence of Bonnet and Needham, 1760–1780.* Oxford: Voltaire Foundation.

Reill, P.H. 2005. *Vitalizing Nature in the Enlightenment.* Berkeley: University of California Press.

Rieppel, O. 1988. "The Reception of Leibniz's Philosophy in the Writings of Charles Bonnet." *Journal of the History of Biology* 21 (1): 119–45. http://dx.doi.org/10.1007/BF00125796.

Robinet, J.-B. 1761–6. *De la nature.* 4 vols. Amsterdam: E. van Harrevelt.

Roe, S.A. 1981. *Matter, Life and Generation: Eighteenth-Century Embryology and the Haller-Wolff Debate.* Cambridge: Cambridge University Press.

Roe, S.A. 1983. "John Turberville Needham and the Generation of Living Organisms." *Isis* 74:159–84.

Roger, J. 1963. *Les Sciences de la vie dans la pensée française du XVIIIe siècle.* Paris: Armand Colin.

Roger, J. 1998. *The Life Sciences in Eighteenth-Century French Thought.* Translated by R. Ellrich. Stanford: Stanford University Press.

Sandler, I. 1983. "Pierre Louis Moreau de Maupertuis – A Precursor of Mendel?" *Journal of the History of Biology* 16 (1): 101–36. http://dx.doi.org/10.1007/BF00186677.

Spallanzani, L. 1769. *Nouvelles récherches sur les découvertes microscopiques et la génération des corps organisés … avec des notes par M. Needham.* 2 vols. London and Paris: Lacombe.

Vartanian, A. 1950. "Trembley's Polyp, La Mettrie, and Eighteenth-Century French Materialism." *Journal of the History of Ideas* 11 (3): 259–86. http://dx.doi.org/10.2307/2707732.

Whitman, C.O. 1895. "Bonnet's Theory of Evolution." In *Biological Lectures Delivered at the Marine Biological Laboratory* of *Woods Hole 1894*, 225–40. Boston: Marine Biological Laboratory.

4 Born to Virtue: Ideas of Generation and the Eighteenth-Century Elites

JOHN C. WALLER

"I never can recommend any but a gentleman to serve with gentlemen. There is little prospect of a low dog's doing any shining act" (Wright 1864, 416). General James Wolfe's statement from a letter of 1758 reeks of aristocratic disdain for men of ignoble birth. He was expressing the same contempt for lesser blood delightfully sent up by Jane Austen's *Pride and Prejudice* in which Lady Catherine de Bourgh asserts that she and her daughter have a "natural taste" for music. It matters not to Lady Catherine that neither she nor her child actually knows how to play the pianoforte. Her ladyship simply assumes that, given their exalted blood, they would outperform anyone born to a lower social grade should they ever be inclined to learn (Austen 1813). This essentialist doctrine is traceable in a continuous thread from the eighth-century BC *Odyssey* of Homer to the elaborate genealogies of which eighteenth-century aristocrats were so enamoured. These fictions of noble blood were articulated a lot more crudely than discussions of generation by physicians, natural philosophers, and animal breeders. But few ideas related to sex and heredity in the Enlightenment were anywhere near as enduring or culturally salient as the belief that honour is dependent on being fashioned from the right kind of seed. This chapter looks at how eighteenth-century elites drew on notions of generation to rationalize their status and at how the utilitarian demands of fiscal-military states affected how they deployed ancient ideologies of special blood. Appreciating how and when nobles invoked their pedigrees is obviously relevant to understanding how they saw themselves and were seen by others. It is also crucial for grasping the depth and variety of eighteenth-century ideas about sexual generation. Perhaps most significantly, the elitist concern for blood purity reveals that Europeans and colonial Americans could think of heredity as a relatively fixed force long before the emergence of eugenic movements in the late nineteenth century.

Blood Matters

In *The Logic of Life* the French historian François Jacob argued that until the later Enlightenment ideas about generation were quite different from those that ultimately fed into the science of genetics and the practice of eugenics. He explained that "the generation of every plant and every animals was, to some degree, a unique, isolated event, independent of any other creation, rather like the production of a work of art by man" (Jacob 1989, 7). What Jacob appears to have meant is that sexual generation was believed to be a highly adventitious process without predictable outcomes. Even if a specific quality were believed to be transmissible via the parental seed, physicians and parents could agree that it might be enhanced, tempered, or subverted by factors operating after conception but before birth such as climatic conditions, maternal nutrition, the mother's imagination, the consistency and quantity of the seed, the quality of breast milk, heavenly perturbations, and astral emanations (see Davidson 2009). Jacob's argument neatly complements one of the master narratives in the history of science according to which the harsh biological doctrines that underpinned later eugenic laws were the product of intellectual developments of recent provenance (Kevles 1985). Other historians of the life sciences have reached similar conclusions about the dominance of soft hereditarianism in the eighteenth century (Müller-Wille and Rheinberger 2007). Yet although Jacob was quite right to emphasize how capricious the act of procreation often appeared to be, he neglected to mention prevalent views about breeding that already assumed a high level of continuity from parents to children. In particular, the manner in which large numbers of people in the Enlightenment thought about the biology of caste presupposed a belief that ancestral qualities can be transmitted virtually unchanged for many generations.

Men and women of the eighteenth century routinely acted and spoke as if certain people were born with essences that placed them permanently lower in a hierarchy of human worth. This chapter is concerned with the nobility but it is important to point out that in the slave societies of the Caribbean and the Americas many whites expressed an equivalent sense of superiority over those of African descent. This feeling of supremacy was so taken for granted that it was expressed less often through words than in an unthinking (and self-serving) moral indifference to slavery. Europe's born aristocrats habitually behaved as if the same kind of unbridgeable gap separated their own kind from the peasantry and bourgeoisie. Racism and social elitism both depend on the same psychological capacity to divide the world into categories of "them" and "us" according to self-interest, acculturation, and tradition. But when the dominant social or ethnic groups of the Enlightenment elected to verbalize this almost visceral sense of superiority they often used the language of procreation. In doing so they stressed not the fickle effects of diet, mind, weather, and cosmos that were identified by Jacob, but the simple idea that generation is a process by which like nearly always reproduces like. And so, whites in the Americas dehumanized their slaves by insisting that they had inherited inferior essences from their racial progenitors, while aristocrats fetishized their pedigrees as testaments to the apparent immutability of their inherited virtues (Jordan 1968; Davis 2006; Devyver 1973; Aubert 2004; Dewald 1996). This kind of essentialism flourished as elite Europeans and white colonists in the Americas rationalized and strove to uphold their ascendancy.

Aristocrats did not have to rely on biological concepts of any sophistication in asserting their intrinsic superiority. Few hazarded an attempt to explain how gentility might be physiologically transmitted and those who did hardly broke new conceptual ground. According to Gilles André de la Roque in his *Traité de la Noblesse*, "There is in the seed I know not what force and I know not what principle which transmits and continues the inclinations of fathers in their descendants" (Aubert 2013, 178; La Roque 1734). Few writers supplied a more detailed description. Most just assumed that a purified form of arterial blood carried the essence of nobility into seeds and embryos. Fluid and vivifying, it seemed an obvious vehicle for the conveyance of noble qualities. Some may also have been aware of the Aristotelian tradition of identifying blood as both the matter supplied by the mother and the medium by which fathers stamped their qualities on the unborn. But for most born gentlemen it was no less than a truism, requiring neither reflection nor further elaboration, that aristocratic parents passed to their children the aptitudes for virtue that they too had supposedly inherited. Nor were aristocrats obviously troubled by basic contradictions in how they talked about the inheritance of nobility, for while they extolled the power of ancestral blood they were paradoxically willing to accept new men into their order and to expel born gentlemen if they engaged in tawdry activities like trade. All that seems to have mattered to the majority of nobles was that they were able, if called upon to do so, to identify a credible biological substrate to the transmission of gentility (Devyver 1973). Of course, no eighteenth-century aristocracy defined itself exclusively in terms of blood. Maintaining noble status usually required not only actual power but a capacity to live with the ostentation of a noble. Moreover, wise parents appreciated the need to provide their offspring with the right kinds of example and education. Nevertheless, nobilities relied on the prestige of belonging to an exclusive caste, and birth had always been a key criterion by which they sought both to prevent the dilution of their caste and reduce outside competition for royal patronage and local renown.

Throughout the eighteenth century aristocrats invested in lavishly illustrated pedigrees, the classic expression of their belief that pedigree matters. Gentlemen had been making bold and fanciful assertions about the primeval origins of their putative virtues since at least the early 1500s (Stone 1967; Heal and Holmes 1994; Dewald 1996). Genteel families invested in family trees proudly sporting medieval or biblical progenitors at the apex, interlocking lines connecting the blood of heroes from a misty past with their modern descendants. The French author Henri de Boulainvilliers, one of the eighteenth century's most eloquent noble ideologues, wrote wistfully from his Norman château of the birth of the French aristocracy among Frankish warriors of the fifth century AD (Devyver 1973; Jouanna 1977; Ellis 1988). True nobles, said Boulainvilliers, are descendants of those early conquerors and they have retained a different essence to the commonality. In reality, noble lineages were neither so ancient nor so biologically pure, but the more remote in time a progenitor the more respect his modern heirs could expect to elicit. As a result, on the eve of the Revolution French genealogists had never been so busy trying to track down long-forgotten forbears for eager clients. In fact, in the decade before 1789 more aristocratic family histories were published in France than at any time since the mid-1600s (Smith 1996, 59). Nor was this surge of family pride the strangled whimper of a dying order (Higonnet 1981). Hence, to many nobles, says William Doyle, the ending of French nobility in 1790 "seemed nothing less than an attempt to change biology" (Doyle 2009, 6).

British gentlemen developed an equally keen sense of identity as a caste of blood in addition to wealth and power. One can read it in the innumerable recorded examples of brutal put-downs and contemptuous brush-offs aimed at men of lower birth. The British peerage was never a closed elite and always made room for some of those who had made professional or commercial fortunes. But it usually took a few generations before those with bourgeois ancestors could marry into this highest rank of British gentility (McCahill 1998; Wasson 1998; Spring and Spring 1985: Stone and Fawtier Stone 1984). John Carteret, second Earl of Granville, once remarked that when the daughter of the Duke of Richmond married the grandson of a yeoman farmer, he felt as if "our fleet or our army were beat, or Mons betrayed into the hands of the French" (Habakkuk 1953, 19). We find the same essentialist idioms in the arch remarks of British noblemen to the genteel pretensions of the colonial elites of the West Indies and North America. Like other English gentlemen, the governor of Virginia, Francis Nicholson, mocked the shallow pedigrees of the American gentry in his midst. They "derive their originals," he sneered, "either as from themselves or at farthest their fathers, but very few Grandfathers." When the wealthy Virginia planter William Byrd II visited England to find a suitable heiress to marry, he was astounded by the contempt elicited by his naive aspiration (Evans 2009, 24). Indeed, the arrogant rejection of the social pretensions of rich colonials by the English elites may have provided fuel for the American Revolution (Rozbicki 1998).

The mythology of blood did gain some traction in British North America where in the northern, middle, and southern colonies there emerged a Creole elite of merchants, landowners, and government officials who dressed and acted in ways that set them apart and who stereotyped their social inferiors as belonging to a "common herd." These elites derided the "obscure and inferior persons" who sometimes got elected to the House of Burgesses, adopted the studied manners and Latin tags of the educated gentleman, and sometimes dispatched letters to the Herald's Office in London seeking evidence of eminent forbears. The Carter family of Virginia, for instance, had their arms carved on every conceivable item of silverware in their possession (Rozbicki 1998, 45; Wood 1992; Evans 2009; Fischer 1989). The New Yorker Ephraim Paine later spoke of the "Southern Nabob's who behave as thoug [*sic*] they viewed themselves a superior Order of animals when Compared with those of the other end of the Confederacy" (Rozbicki 2011, 63). The northern states had their own equivalents to these pedigree-proud southern planters. In parts of the Hudson River Valley north of New York City there were powerful families like the Philipses, Livingstons, and the Van Rensselaers, some of whom boasted of their descent from Dutch settlers of the 1600s (Clark 2006). Not even the Revolution could wholly crush the desire of successful colonial families to dignify their status with fables of noble descent. George Washington used his family's ancestral seal on letters, corresponded with a London herald, and aspired to turn Mount Vernon into an English-style manor house.

In Europe, those born outside the nobility were often the most enamoured of noble birth and covetous of getting in on the act. The desire of the newly ennobled and the upwardly mobile bourgeoisie to marry into the ranks of old aristocracy reveals a widespread acquiescence with the claim that virtue was at least partly acquired from parental seed. Right up until the Revolution, rich financiers and officials in France were willing to trade some of their wealth for the prestige that marrying into the sword or court nobility could confer on their offspring (Chaussinand-Nogaret 1985). This kind of clamouring for old blood inevitably reinforced the mystique of pedigree. Equally telling is the fact that commoners who rose to illustrious state position in Prussia had to be made into hereditary nobles in order for them to be able to exercise authority. Newly minted noble titles were needed to give officials of "vulgar" origin the kudos without which the commons tended to ignore them (Rosenberg 1966, 138–9).

To those aspirant gentlemen for whom a noble marriage or official letters of ennoblement were out of the question there remained the option of acquiring a counterfeit pedigree. The English author and journalist Daniel Defoe described in his 1726 essay *The Complete English Tradesman* "the tradesmen of England, as they grow wealthy, coming every day to the Heralds' Office, to search for the Coats of Arms of their ancestors" (377). Even some of those who openly regarded genealogy as ludicrous and self-serving vanity were not above inventing connections to exalted bloodlines. Defoe had lampooned the aristocratic taste for pedigrees, but he could not resist changing his name from "Daniel Foe" to "Daniel Defoe" and making the bogus claim of a lineal descent from the great De Beau Faux family (Defoe 1703). Eighteenth-century literature betrays the same popular appreciation for noble stock. Georgian novelists recapitulated the ancient plotline known as the "Foundling Tale" according to which an incongruously virtuous man raised as peasant or servant is later discovered to carry the blood of kings or gentlemen (Fielding 1749; Davidson 2009, 15; Perry 2004, 399). These were implicit affirmations of the idea that courage and moral probity rely upon a person having the best kind of blood. The Anglo-Irish satirist Jonathan Swift was more forthright. Even the noble horses, or Houyhnhnms, of *Gulliver's Travels* were differentiated into castes on the basis of innate inequalities. "A pearl holds its Value although it be found in a Dunghill," Swift wrote elsewhere, but "that is not the most probable place to search for it" (Swift 1711, 1).

If non-nobles in Europe showed a widespread willingness to accept the aristocracy's belief in innate inequality they had a number of pragmatic reasons for doing so. A stable and hierarchical system seemed to be a necessary guarantor of social order without which the property of both high and low might be imperilled (Bush 1988). In addition, the doors to the nobility could be kept open just enough to allow in the wealthier bourgeoisie and thereby mute criticism of aristocratic exclusivity (Wasson 1998). Meanwhile, lower down the social scale there were many forms of patronage and clientship by which able men were hitched to the aristocratic system. In addition, there were psychological benefits for non-nobles of having a nobility of birth occupying prestigious positions in the church, state, and army. First, those at nearly every rank could comfort themselves with the thought that they too had social inferiors upon whose ancestry they could look with condescension. In this "hierarchy of disdain" a husbandman would refuse to let his daughter marry a tanner with much the same zeal as an earl would forbid his daughter from marrying into the minor gentry. Second, a man entitled to rule by dint of his birth did not engender a sense of relative failure among those over whom he presided as did the parvenu who left his old peers in the dust. The French jurist Gaspard de Réal de Curban made this point in his *La science de la gouvernement* (1551–64), arguing that it was preferable to assign power on an arbitrary basis like birth because there "is no shame in yielding when I may say 'I owe this to my birth"' (Palmer 1959–64, 62).

Those who regarded aristocracy as outmoded or who disliked the conceitedness of individual nobles knew how much the credibility of nobility relied on vague notions of generation. This is why explicit denials of the heritability of mental and moral traits became central to critiques of the eighteenth-century nobility. When Claude Helvétius insisted on complete human equality in his 1758 book, *On Mind*, copies were seized and burned by the Paris hangman. But Helvétius was drawing on ideas developed and expressed in the most fashionable Parisian salons by leading intellectuals of the French Enlightenment (Carson 2002). In the decades before the Revolution a collection of Parisian thinkers formed a radical talk-shop called the Society of Thirty that took careful aim at what they saw as an insufferable arrogance bred by the ideology of noble descent. The Abbé Sieyès, in a pamphlet of 1789, complained that it is an "absolute fact that the privileged class look upon themselves as another species of beings" (Doyle 2009, 182). Subsequently the leaders of the Revolution were every bit as convinced that normative beliefs about generation lay at the heart of the nobility's kudos. Waves of attacks on the genealogical mentality accompanied the Terror. Deeply troubled by the preserved memories of long-dead nobles, the Jacobins hunted down and incinerated books about nobility and destroyed any manuscript bearing coats of arms (Doyle 2009).

Egalitarian themes were also developed by generations of English journalists, poets, and playwrights. "Nobility of Blood," wrote the English poet Edward Bysshe in 1710, "Is but a glitt'ring and fallacious Good" (Bysshe 1762, 85). Alexander Pope's *Essay on Man* contains a similar rebuke to the blood-obsessed lord:

> Worth makes the man, and want of it, the fellow;
> The rest is all but leather or prunella ...
> What can ennoble sots, or slaves, or cowards?
> Alas! Not all the blood of all the HOWARDS. (Pope 1736, lines 203–4, 215–16)

Taking advantage of the weakening of censorship laws, London's Grub Street journalists inveighed against the blind respect paid to dissipated nobles of long descent. Mocking the genteel delusions of superior blood became a virtual stock in trade for the early eighteenth-century satirist. Emboldened by the revolutionary fervour in France, William Godwin later argued for the complete abolition of all social distinctions based on birth. The heritability of power, he wrote, presents the gravest "insult upon reason and justice." "Examine the new-born son of a peer, and of a mechanic," he went on, "Has nature designated in different lineaments their future fortune?" (Godwin 1798, 86). The differences between a peer and a peasant were for Godwin utterly artificial, for a "generous blood, a gallant and fearless spirit is by no means propagated from father to son" (86). In his 1791 *Rights of Man*, Thomas Paine declared that the descendants of hereditary rulers are usually "below the average of human understanding": for among the progeny of great men we find "one is a tyrant, another an idiot, a third insane, and some all three together" (1792, 92).

Although at one level these critiques of noble essentialism reveal a growing egalitarianism, at another they indicate that a belief in the special contents of aristocratic loins had a pervasive hold. Opponents of the nobility were convinced that dismantling the "gothic debris" of genealogy was a precondition for bringing aristocrats to their senses if not necessarily to their knees.

Generation and Status Consciousness

Enlightenment critiques of inherited nobility resonate so strongly in the present that it can be hard to imagine why so many people once colluded in the belief that high birth entails an innate superiority. To a large extent the idea flourished simply because it seemed to provide an explanation for something that remained true across much of Europe during the eighteenth century: wealth, power, and privilege were largely concentrated in the hands of families claiming ancient descent. To be sure, without regular incursions of commoners into the nobility the order would have become rapidly extinct due to the sterility of heirs or early deaths caused by disease and warfare. Many nobles were also no richer than yeoman farmers or even well-to-do peasants (Bush 1988). But, as the members of social and political castes, European aristocrats still exercised enormous authority. And, accustomed from childhood to pre-eminence, it was inevitable that many of them should have come to see themselves as intrinsically special. What is merely conventional has a strong tendency to be seen as ordained by God or nature. This is especially true, of course, where there are substantial rewards in income and status for accepting a false prospectus.

Nobles enjoyed a range of advantages that nurtured their collective sense of innate superiority. By inheritance they held disproportionate shares of the land and wealth in most kingdoms. In France, for instance, nobles comprised about 1 per cent of the population and yet owned between a quarter and third of the land (Swann 1995, 151). Noble landownership also conferred a variety of legal and customary rights, entitling the well-born to exercise authority over their tenants as well as to participate in the government of the realm (Cannon 1984). And even though the rise of fiscal-military states had allowed monarchies to curb nobles and to insert their own agents between crown and populace, it often paid for them to rely on the traditional elites to administer civil and criminal jurisdiction, to oversee the implementation of tax collection, and to raise troops when the king required them (Scott 1995). Moreover, centralized states offered nobles opportunities to gain in respect and riches from state service (Beik 1985). The British aristocracy emerged as an official governing class during the eighteenth century (Habakkuk 1953). In France, too, large sections of the traditional aristocracy learned to profit from a stronger monarchy. Presentation at court required that a nobleman prove his nobility back until before 1400 and these "immemorial nobles" dominated life at the Palace of Versailles (McManners 1953). Aristocrats throughout Europe also monopolized the higher echelons of the church and the military (Bush 1988). Wielding such substantial powers inevitably helped to sustain the conviction that they were innately fitted to govern.

The importance of social inequalities in sustaining the innatist mindset is demonstrated by the lesser appetite for ancestor worship where disparities in wealth were relatively modest. Although we have seen that some wealthy Creoles in North America boasted of their stock, the idea that nobility is a hereditarily transmissible trait gained much less purchase in the thirteen colonies. Rich Americans lacked the opulence required to instil the fawning deference for inborn rank that prevailed across the Atlantic Ocean. The egalitarian ethos found rural New England to be an especially conducive environment due to the absence of social extremes. Richard Montgomery, who led an expedition in 1775 to try to capture Quebec from the British, complained that the "New England troops are the worst stuff imaginable. There is such an equality among them, that the officers have no authority" (Clark 2011, 55). Much the same applied to rural Pennsylvania, dubbed "the best poor man's country in the world" (Lemon 1972, xiii). While a landed gentry did exist in New York, New Jersey, and in the slave states of the southern colonies, most of the land was divided into modest lots farmed by individual family units. And, where most wealthy dynasties were of recent provenance, many poorer settlers were convinced that they could realistically aspire to riches: white Americans of the later 1700s were already on the way to anointing the self-made man as the ultimate home-grown hero. Furthermore, the planter elites of the south, living in dread of slave rebellion, also saw the need to keep low-ranking whites on side by ideologically smoothing over the cleavages of white society (Morgan 1972). In these circumstances even members of the colonial elites were willing to echo Thomas Paine in attacking the "Vanity of Birth and Title" as another kind of English tyranny to be defeated. John Adams, for instance, wrote that true gentility was to be found just as often among "husbandmen, merchants, mechanics, or labourers" as "magistrates and officers of government" (Wood 1992, 195).

Biology as Ideology

Ideas about the special qualities of noble blood did more than just rationalize the place of the aristocracy. They also actively helped to legitimate the existence of powerful castes defined by birth. As one might expect, nobles trumpeted the alleged value of their stock most vehemently where their ancient privileges were felt to be in jeopardy (Devyver 1973; Bitton 1969). And many an eighteenth-century noble fetishized his ancestry because his order did confront an unprecedented level of threat.

The chief danger to Europe's nobilities arose from monarchs recruiting growing numbers of commoners into the higher echelons of the state. Kings did this in part because nobles of long pedigree often lacked the knowledge, temperament, and appetite for hard work that bureaucratic states required. Men hailing from the lower nobility, commerce, or finance, in contrast, were frequently adept at law, bookkeeping, and arithmetic. Often they were ennobled in return for effective service. The once headstrong Danish nobles found that they had to become faithful civil servants or retreat back to their estates: rank became largely a function of office (Jesperson 1995). Likewise, Spain's grandees had to make room for a bureaucracy of trained jurists selected for ability over birth (Carr 1953; Thompson 1995). Much the same is true for Prussia where Frederick William I had a policy of passing over indigenous aristocrats for posts in his administration. The stigma of low birth was "surprisingly surmountable" (Rosenberg 1966, 147–8). Among the older nobility of pre-Revolutionary France the selling of state offices caused particular grievance. Men who had made or inherited fortunes were able to buy government posts that brought automatic and heritable ennoblement. Somewhere between eight and ten thousand new French nobles were created between the early 1700s and 1789 (Doyle 2009). Tensions developed between an immemorial "sword" nobility and the often landless "nobles of the robe" who had considerable influence within the machinery of the state but whose noble status was only one or a few generations old (Stone 1975). The result was a profoundly divided nobility with little sense of common purpose.

Eighteenth-century kingdoms also valorized the non-noble talents required to make the commercial fortunes that were enriching the more successful states. French writers upbraided aristocrats for their snobbish contempt for trade. They argued that the nation could only counter the fast-rising wealth and power of England by encouraging nobles to take an active role in buying, selling, and manufacturing. Sympathetic to such arguments, the crown mandated in 1767 that two men be ennobled every year for success in industry and commerce (Doyle 2009, 55). When Napoleon rehabilitated the idea of nobility in the early nineteenth century a majority of his creations had never been noble before 1789. A similar respect for the money to be generated by trade and industry developed in eighteenth-century Spain. Desperate to reverse what they saw as a humiliating economic decline, Spanish intellectuals and officers of the state mounted a campaign to change the aristocratic conception of honour to embrace bourgeois achievements. They mocked the poor hidalgo who had little left of which to boast than his Visigothic blood and chided the lack of education of great lords who expected a place close to the king. A decree of 1783 granted ennoblement to Spanish families that remained committed to commerce or manufacturing for three generations rather than trading in their capital for land and the trappings of gentility (Thompson 1990, 228). By the early 1700s a majority of those applying for noble status did not even bother to claim to have inherited noble blood. Traditional values were colliding with the ideology of bourgeois "utility" (Callahan 1972).

Confronted by changing values and so many new men, large numbers of European noblemen defensively deployed the language of generation and heredity. With almost the predictability of a physical law, born gentlemen who had sunk into provincial obscurity or felt that they had been passed over for promotion in favour of those of lower birth loudly proclaimed that commoners were unfit by nature for high office (Devyver 1973; Jouanna 1977). Nobles seized on birth as a key criterion for exercising power because the one thing the upwardly mobile could not change was his parentage. Hence, fearing for the survival of his order in what he saw as an age of venality and bourgeois ambition, the duc de Saint-Simon condemned "plebeian lawyers," repeating the timeworn mantra that "Kings create ennobled persons but not nobles" (Mousnier 1974, 261). In the summer of 1790, during the debate in the National Assembly that led to the abolition of the French nobility, Alsatian Count Landenberg-Wagenbourg stripped his defence of aristocracy down to the same core principle. The special blood of the nobility, he avowed, renders its members timelessly superior to the third estate. Gentility can never be legislated into oblivion because nothing can efface the virtues immanent in aristocratic bloodlines (Doyle 2009, 5).

The inherited qualities identified by the nobility were also explicitly selected to distinguish them from the bourgeoisie. Gentlemen were said to be born with generous spirits that lessened their capacity for selfish, ambitious, or venal behaviour. They boasted that their blood fortified them against the narrow-minded pursuit of position and profit and impelled them to loyalty and self-sacrifice (Smith 1996). In 1762 an embattled Swedish count rehearsed the argument that nobles were naturally disposed to political and martial virtue, stressing the qualities that made rule by aristocrats just and wise: "the Noble mind, the zealous ardour, and the eminent inclinations for liberty, for manliness, virtue and wit" (Wolff 2008, 83). Insisting that these moral virtues were also inherited had the added advantage for the nobleman of allowing him to assert that they were so integral to his physical and spiritual nature that they could never be subverted. Gentlemen, the logic went, are naturally virtuous whereas the loyalty of the newly ennobled is contingent on them getting the cash they selfishly crave (Smith 2005).

Rhapsodizing about blood and seed also became a form of palliative nostalgia for nobles who retired to their estates smarting at what they saw as the elevation of the vulgar at the expense of the truly noble. Perhaps half of pre-Revolutionary French noblemen, says William Doyle, clung doggedly to an ancestral pride as they saw men whose grandfathers had been plebeians gain political clout and desirable state posts (Doyle 2009, 25). One Spanish writer remarked, with a certain amount of exaggeration, of the poor hidalgos, "How nourishing was the crust of black bread eaten beneath the genealogical tree" (Carr 1953, 55).

But there were many eighteenth-century nobles who perceived that trusty dogmas about breeding were no longer sufficient or appropriate. Plenty were driven to downplay or eschew biological doctrines. Some Spanish noblemen began to engage in mercantile affairs (Thompson 1995, 229; Carr 1953). In France, born gentlemen acquired a more bourgeois outlook after socializing with successful capitalists in clubs, theatres, and salons (Chaussinand-Nogaret 1985). Wealth was dissolving old distinctions. Marriages between nobles of the sword and robe were nowhere near so scandalous in the later 1700s as they had been in the 1600s (Swann 1995, 147). Similarly, in Berlin, differences of rank were played down in salon culture. By the late 1700s the nobles who attended Berlin's salons shared at least some commitment to meritocratic principles (Dewald 1996, 51). Meanwhile, in England a "landed invasion" of towns by rural gentlemen wishing to enjoy the superior entertainments of urban life meant that they too now mixed routinely with the professional and mercantile elites (Clark 2000, 6; Borsay 1989). Apprenticeships to physicians and apothecaries also offered routes to wealth that many a younger son of gentry birth simply could not afford to resist. In the process the definition of gentility increasingly stressed qualities other than birth and pedigree (Rogers 1979, 444).

The demands of state service also helped to close the gap in mentalities between pedigreed nobles and the newly ennobled and bourgeois arriviste. In Prussia those men of exalted ancestry who rose to high position often felt more kinship with powerful parvenus than with those members of their own caste who remained on their estates (Rosenberg 1966, 147). More and more European nobles were also attending academies or universities. In fact, nobilities concerned about losing their pre-eminence as a caste had been sending their sons to gain a formal education since the early 1500s (Dewald 1996, 152; Hexter 1961). They knew that embracing the ethos of utility and civic virtue could win lucrative government posts. Academies in Austria and Bohemia offered the specialized skills young noblemen needed to be appointed as courtiers or diplomats. Spanish grandees also began to send their children overseas to gain a formal education. In Britain the sons of the nobility attended public schools in which they were expected to acquire the love for classical examples and the manliness of character which would mould them into fine statesmen (Cannon 1984, 43). Similarly, long before the crises of the 1780s, a vocal section of the French nobility had embraced the language of virtue and merit. Rather than always falling back on a mania for the right kind of blood, they celebrated the ideals of civic humanism expounded by Cicero and Plutarch (Smith 2005, 33).

Even so, the ideology of noble birth remained a lot more than an analgesic for the marginalized, bitter, and reactionary. Few aristocrats felt there was a necessary contradiction between the lexicons of blood and merit. They did not define "merit" in the same way as the bourgeoisie, but they did feel that they had utility as a caste that could be refined by education and effort. So European nobles frequently charted a middle course which combined an appreciation for cultivating moral qualities and practical knowledge with a belief that their blood gave them a special aptitude to acquire what they needed in order to become useful servants of the state. Their innate virtues were channelled and reinforced by schooling within an aristocratic household or noble college. In Britain, for example, gentlemen aspiring to careers in government found that they could combine the language of heredity with a commitment to an education conducive to acquiring political competence. From a selective reading of Greek and Roman literature those destined for high government office derived an affirmation of the patrician's right to rule, but they nonetheless felt that reading Horace, Polybius, and Aristotle gave them the knowledge to govern with wisdom and good sense (Cannon 1984, 35).

In military service Europe's nobilities of birth found the perfect milieu in which to assert that they were the best leaders by virtue of both breeding and instruction. The days of the mounted warrior operating virtually independently on the battlefield were long gone, but monarchs still had good reason to turn to the nobility for good officer material. They needed men who could get soldiers to act with the robotic obedience necessary for charging through hails of cannon fire towards columns or squares bristling with rifles and bayonets (Melton 1995). The honour codes of the nobility, fuelled by beliefs about blood and family destiny, proved just the thing for getting genteel officers to go unflinchingly into battle while the soldiery's respect for pedigree made them more likely to follow. Under Frederick I, the Prussian Junker nobility adopted a code of honour in which even so much as to duck at the sound of an incoming cannon ball was to be guilty of cowardice (Melton 1995, 98). At the same time, these well-bred sons were attending colleges in order to learn about modern strategy (Wilson 2009, 99). In 1781 the French high command mandated that only those with three generations of nobility could enter the army's officer corps. The architects of this policy were motivated in part by the environmentalist belief that aristocratic households were especially good at inculcating a warrior mentality (Bien 1979), but this assessment was grafted onto the existing belief in the innate fittedness of noblemen to lead lesser men into battle with courage and honour (Smith 1996). So long as Europe's nobles were willing to make sacrifices of life and leisure, the modern fiscal-military state was prepared to enhance their appearance of constituting an inherently special caste.

Blood Lives On

Most nobilities survived the turmoil of the eighteenth century with power and prestige intact. There were exceptions: Danish and Swedish aristocrats saw much of their authority in government eclipsed and the French aristocracy would never recoup its earlier political influence. Other nobilities were more resilient. In central and eastern Europe they mostly entered the 1800s strong and confident. In Britain, too, gentlemen still exercised enormous power. As Hamish Scott points out, the nobilities of most European states were to maintain "social leadership and their dominance over public life into the twentieth century" (Scott 1995, 274). And, having held on to their wealth and adapted to the demands of modernizing states, they also preserved much of their old esteem. This is not to say that aristocracies could be quite as boastful of their blood as their predecessors. There appears to have been a growing feeling that a gentleman should be educated and cultured and that obsessing about one's blood connoted a lack of sophistication. The English journalist William Cobbett was on to something when he explained in 1811 that the previous decades had seen "an insurrection of talents and courage and industry against birth and rank" (Cobbett 1811, 587). The old distinction between gentlemen and non-gentlemen was being challenged by an alternative antithesis between the polished man of low or high birth and the coarse, uneducated man who might very well be represented by a squire fixated on hunting and genealogy (Dewald 1996, 51).

Even so, powerful nobilities still rationalized and justified their pre-eminence in terms of ancestry. They also discovered that the middle and working classes of the dawning industrial age were prepared to defer to high birth and even to fawn over ancient pedigrees. The cult of individual character coexisted with a traditional respect for blood. Many a British industrialist sent his sons to public school to shed their coarseness and acquire the accent and manners of the rural upper class. New and old families in mid-century Britain were willing to pay heavy taxes in order to display armorial bearings on their writing paper, family silver, and cutlery. In many other parts of Europe the rich bourgeoisie continued to seek noble wives. The sons of the Prussian bourgeois elites even took up dueling (Spring 1977). And in France thousands of non-nobles adopted the particle 'de' to lend their names a genteel mystique: the novelists Guy Maupassant and Honoré Balzac both ennobled themselves in this way (Higgs 1987).

In consequence, the men of science who promoted the idea of selective human breeding in the later nineteenth century were in a position to draw on traditional and salient concerns about aristocratic blood and misalliance. The difference is that eugenicists were usually the scions of an upper middle class that prided itself on its intellectual and utilitarian achievements and identified its own rank as the true repository of useful, heritable aptitudes (Norton 1981; Szreter 1996). In his 1865 article "Hereditary Talent," Francis Galton mocked the pride in Norman ancestry of English lords as a mathematical absurdity, but he happily availed himself of the ancient aristocratic belief in the inherent inequality of humankind (100). Eugenics made sense to Galton and to sympathetic contemporaries in part because they belonged to cultures fully accustomed to imagining that ancestry largely maketh the man.

REFERENCES

Aubert, G. 2004. "'The Blood of France': Race and Purity of Blood in the French Atlantic World." *William and Mary Quarterly* 61 (3): 439–78. http://dx.doi.org/10.2307/3491805.

Aubert, G. 2013. "Kinship, Blood, and the Emergence of the Racial Nation in the French Atlantic World, 1600–1789." In *Blood & Kinship: Matter for Metaphor from Ancient Rome to the Present*, edited by Christopher H. Johnson, Bernhard Jussen, David Warren Sabean, and Simon Teuscher, 175–95. New York: Berghahn Books.

Austen, J. 1813. *Pride and Prejudice*. London: T. Egerton.

Beik, W. 1985. *Absolutism and Society in Seventeenth-Century France: State Power and Provincial Aristocracy in Languedoc*. Cambridge: Cambridge University Press. http://dx.doi.org/10.1017/CBO9780511583797.

Bien, D. 1979. "The Army in the French Enlightenment: Reform, Reaction and Revolution." *Past & Present* 85 (1): 68–98. http://dx.doi.org/10.1093/past/85.1.68.

Bitton, D. 1969. *The French Nobility in Crisis, 1560–1640*. Stanford: Stanford University Press.
Borsay, P. 1989. *The English Urban Renaissance: Culture and Society in the Provincial Town, 1660–1770*. New York: Oxford University Press.
Bush, M. 1988. *Rich Noble, Poor Noble*. Manchester: Manchester University Press.
Bysshe, E. 1762. *The Art of English Poetry*. London: Printed for Hitch and Hawes.
Callahan, W.J. 1972. *Honor, Commerce, and Industry in Eighteenth-Century Spain*. Boston: Baker Library.
Cannon, J.A. 1984. *Aristocratic Century: the Peerage of Eighteenth-Century England*. New York: Cambridge University Press. http://dx.doi.org/10.1017/CBO9780511607998.
Carr, R. 1953. "Spain." In *The European Nobility in the Eighteenth Century*, edited by A. Goodwin, 44–60. London: A.C. Black.
Carson, J. 2002. "Differentiating a Republican Citizenry: Talents, Human Science, and Enlightenment Theories of Governance." *Osiris* 17 (1): 74–103. http://dx.doi.org/10.1086/649360.
Chaussinand-Nogaret, G. 1985. *The French Nobility in the Eighteenth Century: From Feudalism to Enlightenment*. Translated by William Doyle. Cambridge: Cambridge University Press. http://dx.doi.org/10.1017/CBO9780511622236.
Clark, C. 2006. *Social Change in America: From the Revolution through the Civil War*. Chicago: Ivan R. Dee.
Clark, P., ed. 2000. Introduction. In *The Cambridge Urban History of Britain*, Vol. 2, *1540–1840*, edited by Peter Clark, 1–24. Cambridge: Cambridge University Press. http://dx.doi.org/10.1017/CHOL9780521431415.002.
Cobbett, W. 1811. *Cobbett's Weekly Political Register*. Saturday, 9 November, 587.
Davidson, J. 2009. *Breeding: A Partial History of the Eighteenth Century*. New York: Columbia University Press.
Davis, D.B. 2006. *Inhuman Bondage: The Rise and Fall of Slavery in the New World*. New York: Oxford University Press.
Defoe, D. 1703. *A Collection of the Writings of the Author of the True-Born English-Man*. London.
Defoe, D. 1726. *The Complete English Tradesman*. London: Charles Rivington.
Devyver, A. 1973. *Le sang épuré: les préjugés de race chez les gentilshommes français de l'Ancien Régime, 1560–1720*. Brussels: Editions de l'Université de Bruxelles.
Dewald, J. 1996. *The European Nobility, 1400–1800*. Cambridge: Cambridge University Press.
Doyle, W. 2009. *Aristocracy and Its Enemies in the Age of Revolution*. New York: Oxford University Press. http://dx.doi.org/10.1093/acprof:oso/9780199559855.001.0001.

Ellis, H.A. 1988. *Boulainvilliers and the French Monarchy: Aristocratic Politics in Early Eighteenth-Century France*. Ithaca: Cornell University Press.
Evans, E.G. 2009. *A "topping people": The Rise and Decline of Virginia's Old Political Elite, 1680–1790*. Charlottesville: University of Virginia Press.
Fielding, H. 1749. *The History of Tom Jones, a Foundling*. London: A. Millar.
Fischer, D.H. 1989. *Albion's Seed: Four British Folkways in America*. New York: Oxford University Press.
Galton, G. 1865. "Hereditary Talent and Character." *Macmillan's Magazine* 12:157–66.
Godwin, W. 1798. *An Enquiry Concerning Political Justice, and Its Influence on General Virtue and Happiness*. Vol. 2. Dublin: for Luke White.
Habakkuk, H.J. 1953. "England." In *The European Nobility in the Eighteenth Century*, edited by A. Goodwin, 1–22. London: A.C. Black.
Heal, F., and C. Holmes. 1994. *The Gentry in England and Wales, 1500–1700*. Basingstoke, Hampshire: Macmillan.
Hexter, J.H. 1961. *Reappraisals in History*. London: Longman.
Higgs, D. 1987. *Nobles in Nineteenth-Century France*. Baltimore: Johns Hopkins University Press.
Higonnet, P. 1981. *Class, Ideology, and the Rights of Nobles during the French Revolution*. New York: Oxford University Press.
Jacob, F. 1989. *The Logic of Life: A History of Heredity.* Translated by Betty E. Spillmann. Harmondsworth: Penguin.
Jesperson, K. 1995. "The Rise and Fall of the Danish Nobility 1600–1800." In *The European Nobilities in the Seventeenth and Eighteenth Centuries*, edited by H.M. Scott, 41–70. London: Longman.
Jordan, W.D. 1968. *White over Black: American Attitudes toward the Negro, 1550–1812*. Chapel Hill: University of North Carolina Press.
Jouanna, A. 1977. *Ordre social: mythes et hiérarchies dans la France du XVIe siècle*. Paris: Hachette.
Kevles, D.J. 1985. *In the Name of Eugenics: Genetics and the Uses of Human Heredity*. New York: Knopf.
Lemon, J.T. 1972. *The Best Poor Man's Country: A Geographical Study of Early Southeastern Pennsylvania*. Baltimore: Johns Hopkins UniversityPress.
La Roque, G.A. de. 1734. *Traité de la noblesse, et de toutes ses differentes especes*. Rouen: P. Le Boucher et Jore pere & fils.
McCahill, M.W. 1998. "Open Elites: Recruitment to the French Noblesse and the English Aristocracy in the Eighteenth Century." *Albion: A Quarterly Journal Concerned with British Studies* 30 (4): 599–629. http://dx.doi.org/10.2307/4053851.
McManners, J. 1953. "France." In *The European Nobility in the Eighteenth Century*, edited by A. Goodwin, 23–42. London: A.C. Black.

Melton, E. 1995. "The Prussian Junkers, 1600–1786." In *The European Nobilities in the Seventeenth and Eighteenth Centuries*, edited by H.M. Scott, 79–101. London: Longman.

Morgan, E.S. 1972. "Slavery and Freedom: The American Paradox." *Journal of American History* 59 (1): 5–29. http://dx.doi.org/10.2307/1888384.

Mousnier, R. 1974. *Les institutions de la France sous la monarchie absolue: 1598–1789*. Paris: Presses universitaires de France.

Müller-Wille, S., and H.-J. Rheinberger. 2007. *Heredity Produced: At the Crossroads of Biology, Politics, and Culture, 1500–1870*. Cambridge, MA: Massachusetts Institute of Technology Press.

Norton, B. 1981. "Psychologists and Class." In *Biology, Medicine and Society 1840–1940*, edited by Charles Webster, 280–314. New York: Cambridge University Press.

Paine, T. 1792. *Rights of Man: Being an Answer to Mr. Burke's Attack on the French Revolution*. London: James Watson.

Palmer, R.R. 1959–64. *The Age of the Democratic Revolution: A Political History of Europe and America, 1760–1800*. Princeton: Princeton University Press.

Perry, R. 2004. *Novel Relations: The Transformation of Kinship in English Literature and Culture, 1748–1818*. New York: Cambridge University Press. http://dx.doi.org/10.1017/CBO9780511484438.

Pope, A. 1736. *An Essay on Man*. London: J. Witford.

Rogers, N. 1979. "Money, Land and Lineage: The Big Bourgeoisie of Hanoverian London." *Social History* 4 (3): 437–54.

Rosenberg, H. 1966. *Bureaucracy, Aristocracy, and Autocracy: The Prussian Experience, 1660–1815*. Boston: Beacon Press.

Rozbicki, M. 1998. *The Complete Colonial Gentleman: Cultural Legitimacy in Plantation America*. Charlottesville: University Press of Virginia.

Rozbicki, M. 2011. *Culture and Liberty in the Age of the American Revolution*. Charlottesville: University Press of Virginia.

Scott, H.M., ed. 1995. *The European Nobilities in the Seventeenth and Eighteenth Centuries*. London: Longman.

Smith, J.M. 1996. *The Culture of Merit: Nobility, Royal Service, and the Making of Absolute Monarchy in France, 1600–1789*. Ann Arbor: University of Michigan Press.

Smith, J.M. 2005. *Nobility Reimagined: The Patriotic Nation in Eighteenth-Century France*. Ithaca: Cornell University Press.

Spring, D. 1977. *European Landed Elites in the Nineteenth Century*. Baltimore: Johns Hopkins University Press.

Spring, E., and D. Spring. 1985. "The English Landed Elite, 1540–1879: A Review." *Albion: A Quarterly Journal Concerned with British Studies* 17 (2): 149–66. http://dx.doi.org/10.2307/4049213.

Stone, B. 1975. "Robe against Sword: The Parlement of Paris and the French Aristocracy." *French Historical Studies* 9 (2): 278–303. http://dx.doi.org/10.2307/286129.

Stone, L. 1967. *The Crisis of the Aristocracy, 1558–1641*. New York: Oxford University Press.

Stone, L., and J.C. Fawtier Stone. 1984. *An Open Elite? England, 1540–1880*. New York: Oxford University Press.

Swann, J. 1995. "The French nobility, 1715–1789." In *The European Nobilities in the Seventeenth and Eighteenth Centuries*, edited by H.M. Scott, 142–73. London: Longman.

Swift, J. 1711. "The Virtue of Parents is a Large Dowry to Their Children." *Examiner* 1 (May number 41): 1–2.

Szreter, S. 1996. *Fertility, Class, and Gender in Britain, 1860–1940*. New York: Cambridge University Press.

Thompson, I.A.A. 1995. "The Nobility in Spain, 1600–1800." In *The European Nobilities in the Seventeenth and Eighteenth Centuries*, edited by H.M. Scott, 191–255. London: Longman.

Wasson, E.A. 1998. "The Penetration of New Wealth into the English Governing Class from the Middle Ages to the First World War." *Economic History Review* 51 (1): 25–48. http://dx.doi.org/10.1111/1468-0289.00082.

Wilson, P.H. 2009. "Prussia as a Fiscal-Military State." In *The Fiscal-Military State in Eighteenth-Century Europe: Essays in Honour of P.G.M. Dickson*, edited by Christopher Storrs, 95–124. Farnham: Ashgate.

Wolff, C. 2008. *Noble Conceptions of Politics in Eighteenth-Century Sweden (c. 1740–1790)*. Helsinki: The Finnish Literature Society.

Wood, G.S. 1992. *The Radicalism of the American Revolution*. New York:. Knopf.

Wright, R. 1864. *The Life of Major-General James Wolfe*. London: Chapman and Hall.

5 Improving Reproduction: Articulations of Breeding and "Race-Mixing" in French and German Discourse (1750–1800)

SUSANNE LETTOW

The idea that processes of propagation can be regulated and improved has a long history since it builds on experiences of animal breeding, which is one of the most fundamental economic practices of human societies. A famous example of an ancient politicalization of this idea is certainly Plato's suggestion for human breeding in *The Republic* where he articulates politics as herding. However, ideas of breeding and cross-breeding that were formulated in the second half of the eighteenth century were highly specific as they acquired their meanings within the scientific, cultural, and political contexts of the period. In particular the shift from "generation" to "reproduction" (Roger 1997, 19), through which propagation was less understood as a process that required divine intervention and increasingly "became recognizable as a domain governed by laws of its own" (Müller-Wille and Rheinberger 2007, 6), constituted a new epistemic horizon. It was of utmost importance that the concept of reproduction – which surfaced mid-century in the context of the disputes over epigenesis and preformation – constituted a new sense of temporality, and in particular the idea of an open future in which really "new" individuals emerge. This sense of futurity gave rise to new attempts to know, calculate, and regulate future events, including the emergence of human beings.

Part of the new epigenetic understanding of reproduction was the idea that the outcomes of reproduction result from the very specific combinations of maternal and paternal substances. This view constituted an enormous scientific interest about how the "mixing" and transmission of parental traits worked. Particularly interesting objects of speculation and research were cases in which anomalies like diseases or disabilities were transmitted from one generation to the next, or cases in which the parents were of different skin colour. These cases proved that the new individual had not existed prior to the coupling of the parents, and that it was shaped only in the process of reproduction. "Race-mixing" – as it was called by authors of the period who mused about the variations of skin colour and other physical traits that resulted from the joint reproduction of individuals from different global regions and physical shape – was thus one of the main issues dealt with in scientific debates on reproduction in the second half of the eighteenth century. It became a paradigmatic case for reasoning about and calculating the outcomes of reproduction by naturalists such as Pierre-Louis Moreau de Maupertuis or George-Louis Leclerc, comte de Buffon, who were among the most prominent critics of preformationism. Their epigenetic understanding that highlighted the practical contingency of reproductive processes was closely entwined with political strategies for managing and improving reproduction, as the example of Charles-Augustin Vandermonde makes clear.

Certainly, the interest that scientists and the wider audience took in issues of race-mixing and the transmission of visible traits through reproduction was not only motivated by epistemic concerns.[1] Another reason why race-mixing played such an important role in the scientific, philosophical, and political debates has to do with the colonial situation. Since the sixteenth century, the European expansion had led to an enormous colonial mobility, and thus to historically new reproductive relations. These globalized forms of reproduction met with various attempts to regulate and manage them, to draw lines between accepted and unaccepted, legal and illegal relations, and to stabilize colour-based hierarchies. According to the *castas*-system that was developed in the Spanish and Portuguese colonies in the late sixteenth century, individuals were legally and socially classified according to a combinatorial analysis of the skin colours of their ancestry. The calculation of reproductive acts and their outcomes in terms of physical shape thus played a major role in stabilizing power relations in these colonies.

In the European context, the genealogical knowledge produced by the *castas*-system received great interest for several reasons. First, it seemed to provide knowledge about hereditary processes, an issue that was raised by epigenesists such as Maupertuis. Second, the abstract form of reasoning about the different forms of "mixing" facilitated the creation of a European gaze on global populations or a "new planetary consciousness" that subsumed global populations to Eurocentric ordering patterns.[2] In addition, theoretical reflections on race-mixing came to play a central role in the debates on strategies for the improvement of reproduction and the perfectibility of humans, which were geared towards the populations of

European states.[3] The "quantifying spirit" that spread during the last decades of the Ancien Régime contributed much to the formation of demography and population politics in so far as numbers of births, deaths, and diseases now were counted and calculated on a national scale (Frängsmyr, Heilbron, and Rider 1990).[4] According to Emma Spary, the perspective of improvement "became immensely popular in the latter half of the eighteenth century, as Europe's monarchs and ministers came to see natural history and the introduction of new species of plants and animals as a certain way to increase national revenues and private wealth" (Spary 1996, 179). Human breeding and race-mixing in this context were mostly addressed, as I show in this chapter, as strategies for improving the population and increasing power.

Although debates on "reproduction," "heredity," and "race" in the eighteenth century differ from later biopolitical discourses and politics in many respects, there are also striking similarities that are hard to ignore. Some scholars emphasize continuity with eugenic programs and policies of the nineteenth and twentieth centuries. Sara Figal (Eigen), for example, states that "at the end of the eighteenth century, the policing of morals and manners was specifically extended – for the most part only in theory – to the policing of reproduction for the improvement of the bodies and minds of future members of the species" (Eigen 2008, 85). According to her, these theories that referred to "the 'facts' of heredity to improve the human race (or parts thereof) have a history that we now identify as eugenic" (Eigen 2008, 85). Jenny Davidson, who focuses on the British context, also diagnoses the emergence of a "growing interest in what we would call selective breeding" (Davidson 2009, 3) and a set of "proto-eugenic arguments" in the period (5). Anne Carol, in her history of eugenics in France, explicitly defends the idea of a "specific medical pre-Galtonian eugenics" (Carol 1995, 10).[5] In her view, the discursive coherence between eugenics after Galton and earlier forms is established through the three concepts of degeneration, heredity, and race (11). Although the continuities these authors draw on are indeed highly relevant, my aim in this chapter is not to engage in a debate about discontinuity and continuity but rather to explore the specific political-epistemic constellations of the period when "reproduction" became a domain of human intervention and improvement to a formerly unknown extent.[6]

In what follows, I first focus on Pierre-Louis Moreau de Maupertuis, George-Louis Leclerc de Buffon, Charles-August Vandermonde, and Denis Diderot, whose ideas circulated widely in the European debates on reproduction and race-mixing. In the second part of the chapter, I turn to the German context where, by the end of the century, authors such as Immanuel Kant, Johann Gottfried Herder, Johann Friedrich Blumenbach, Christoph Meiners, and Johann Peter Frank adopted and re-articulated many of the ideas formulated by the French authors. These debates, in particular Kant's definition of race and the objections and adaptations it provoked, were highly important for the constitution of greatly influenced modern race discourse and biopolitics. With regards to the specific issue of race-mixing, the enthusiasm for strategies of breeding and improvement is, in the German context of the late eighteenth century, clearly subdued in comparison to the mid-century French debates. Authors such as Kant, Herder, and Meiners expressed reservations. However, positive attitudes toward human breeding and race-mixing as strategies for the improvement of society did not vanish entirely, as is the case with Johann Peter Frank, whose plans for the management of reproductive relations recalled the political proposals of Vandermonde.

Race-Mixing and the Speculative Experimentalization of Reproduction: Scientific, Philosophical, and Political Debates in France around 1750

One of the first authors who used the terms "to reproduce" and "reproduction," and who linked the new understanding of reproduction to reflections on hereditary transmission and racial diversity, was Pierre-Louis Moreau de Maupertuis.[7] Against preformationism, he emphasized that both sexes play an equally important role in reproduction, and that children inherit traits from fathers as well as from the mothers. He made this argument by pointing to the transmission of abnormal traits, such as polydactyly, over several generations and to racial "mixtures" (*mélange d'espèces*).[8] The case of albinism in Africans – which Maupertuis discussed at length – might not, at first glance, seem to be a good example for the transmission of parental traits. However, Maupertuis argued that if we assume that "white is the colour of the first humans" while "black has become an inheritable colour only by accident" because of climatic circumstances, one can understand that sometimes the "primitive colour ... reappears" (1745/1780, 142–3). Such a hazardous reappearance of hereditary characteristics, which can disappear for generations, could also be observed in families, and thus did not contradict the rule that both parents contribute equally to the transmission of traits. In contrast, the observation of hereditary processes showed that inheritance works over long periods of time and occasionally produced "variations" so that races or species could not be understood as fixed entities but, in principle, were malleable. As Staffan Müller-Wille puts it, "the concept of heredity, when it entered biology ... did not refer to the fixity of species ... It was geared rather towards a much more specific phenomenon – namely, that of 'heritable variation'" (Müller-Wille 2014, 218).

This epistemic interest in variation was closely linked with a breeding perspective: namely, the perspective of practical intervention into processes of human reproduction. This is clearly the case in Maupertuis's *Vénus physique*. In the chapter "The Production of New Species," he first referred to dog breeding, which was geared at the "correction" of forms and the intentional "variation" of colours, which led to the "invention" of dog-races like the *Arlequin* or the *Mopse* (Maupertuis 1745/1780, 122–3). Then Maupertuis proposed transferring these practices to the domain of human breeding: "Why," he asked, "is this art confined to animals? Why do the smug Sultans in their seraglios, who keep women of all known species, not make new species?" (123). The fact that he presented the Oriental harem as the perfect breeding place is, however, in no way accidental but reveals a gendered and eroticized subtext of the debates on race-mixing in the eighteenth century. John Chardin's travelogues from the Caucasus, which were published more than half a century earlier and circulated widely, are a most important example in this respect.

Chardin had claimed that "while the original Persian stock is extremely ungainly," the Persian aristocracy had "improved their collective beauty through a century of consistent and deliberate interbreeding with Georgian and Circassian women," who were said to be of extreme beauty (Figal 2014, 172). Maupertuis, too, drew a link between a male erotic desire for reproducing with a beautiful and exotic female slave and a population-oriented argument for improvement.[9] However, he re-articulated this fantasy within a new context. Figal, who reveals the significance of Chardin's eroticized travelogues for the paradoxical constitution of the concept of the Caucasian race, emphasizes that Chardin did not make any scientific claims. He "simply presumed as common knowledge that physical characteristics unique to a particular people are transmitted – and transmuted – through patterns of reproduction" (172). Maupertuis's reflections on breeding, in contrast, were coherently interwoven with his critique of preformationism, thus with a specific theoretical position vis-à-vis the contemporary scientific debates on reproduction. In addition, it is important to notice that in Maupertuis's writings speculation and experiment are closely connected. "The practice of breeding animals and collecting evidence from human families," Mary Terrall states, "played a positive part in articulating the role of the two sexes in reproduction, as well as in theories about the forces driving the process" (Terrall 2007, 253). Accordingly, Maupertuis's use of a breeding vocabulary, including his comparisons among plant, animal, and human breeding, was not just metaphorical but refers to experiences and experiments. In particular, Maupertuis's examples are from the domains of gardening or pet breeding, practices that were fashionable in polite culture. In his discussion of black albinism, for instance, Maupertuis referred to gardeners who said "that all these species of plants and bushes consisting of mixed elements (*panachés*), which we admire in our gardens, result from varieties that have become hereditary and that disappear if one neglects to take care of them" (Maupertuis 1745/1780, 132). Hereditary varieties in plants or in humans thus depend on active attention and "care." Like many of his contemporaries, and in particular the learned women of the salon, Maupertuis himself carried out experiments on dogs (Terrall 1996, 225). In a letter from 1752 he reported on the inheritance of an abnormal colour characteristic over several generations in his breeding experiments with a female Icelandic dog, and he mused about the results of forced cross-breeding among animals. Such experiments, he speculated, "would result in plenty of curiosities" (Maupertuis 1752, 420–1, quoted in Terrall 2007, 266), or in "new animals, perhaps even species that nature has not yet produced" (267). Here, and likewise in the example of the sultans who could breed new species, Maupertuis's perspective is clearly constituted by a fascination with diversity, multiformity, and most of all newness.

However, with respect to envisioning human breeding, Maupertuis was far from unique. Even proponents of preformationism such as Charles Bonnet and Lazzaro Spallanzani mused over experiments in plant and animal breeding and their applicability to human reproduction.[10] Bonnet, writing to Spallanzani, referred to the latter's plans for cross-breeding cats, dogs, and rabbits, and concluded that from these experiments "the most important and unexpected discoveries" would follow (Spallanzani 1784, 242, quoted in Davidson 2009, 88). He further wondered whether these discoveries would "one day be applied in the human species to purposes we little think of, and of which the consequences will not be trivial" (Spallanzani 1784, 242, quoted in Davidson 2009, 88). Improving the species and society at large through intervening in the processes of human reproduction was thus an issue that loomed large in the scientific debates in the second half of the eighteenth century. Another example is Julien Offray de La Mettrie who, with reference to Maupertuis, asked: "Do we not, so to speak, prune a man like a tree?" (La Mettrie 1748/1996, 82). At the same time, expectations of improvement, progress, and increasing perfection of human life did not go uncontested. The sense of an open, non-determined future that was to be shaped by human action also implied the possibility of negative developments, decline, and decay. Ideas of improving reproduction therefore went hand in hand with fears about degeneration. This, in particular, is the case in Buffon, whose ideas were to circulate widely in the subsequent debates on breeding and race-mixing.

According to Buffon's theory of reproduction, which shares many insights with Maupertuis, male and female fluids belong to unspecified "organic matter" and consist of "organic molecules" that are "mixed" in reproduction. The specific shape of the assemblage of the mixed molecules from which the new organism results is due to what Buffon calls the "inner mould" (*moule intérieure*). This "inner mould" guarantees order and organic structure. However, despite its stabilizing power, species are not reproduced perfectly unchanged. Varieties, according to Buffon, emerge due to changes in climate, nutrition, and morals. Nature, and in particular human nature, is flexible, which means that it has the potential for improvement or degeneration. In his article "The Horse," published in volume 4 of the *Histoire naturelle* in 1753, Buffon expressed his conviction that breeding practices could prevent degeneration, and breeding in this context meant race-mixing.

> In order to have beautiful horses, good dogs, etc., it is necessary to give foreign males to the native females, and reciprocally to the native males, foreign females; failing that, animals will degenerate ... In mixing the races, and above all in renewing them constantly with foreign races, the form seems to perfect itself and Nature seems to revive herself. (Buffon 1753, 215–17, quoted in Terrall 2007, 268)

Some years later, in the article *The Degeneration of Animals* (1766), Buffon's view was more pessimistic. In contrast to his earlier suggestions, he argued that domestication is a main reason for degeneration. Animals that are subjected to the "tyranny" of man, Buffon stated, have been particularly "degraded" and "disfigured" (Buffon 1766, 317): "We will find on all enslaved animals the stigmata of their captivity and the imprint of their shackles" (317). Buffon was aware the fact that what might look like improvement might not actually be. With regards to Nature herself, to improve or to spoil oneself (*se perfectionner ou se vicier*) means the same thing: "denaturalization" (318). For humans, he thought, the utility of animal products – like Angora wool – is a strong motivation to modify and to improve certain characteristics of animals; for the animals, however, this process means degeneration. So, in contrast to Maupertuis, Buffon's position on breeding was at least ambivalent.

This, however, does not mean that he was not interested in breeding experiments. On the contrary, in his view, such experiments can lead to new knowledge about the "degeneration of species through mixing" and thus about the "unity or diversity of each kind (genre)" (338). Although Buffon addressed "mixing" as a process of degeneration instead of improvement he did not reject it but, in the same article, referred to it as an epistemic practice when he discussed "race-mixing" (*mélange des races*). Buffon calculated and compared the effects of long-term reproductive processes under the condition of geographic dislocation. He concluded that it takes only "one hundred and fifty or two hundred years for cleaning the skin of a Negro by way of mixing it with the blood of a White" (313). At the same time, scientific curiosity also inspired a complementary experiment, namely, that of hindering race-mixing through enforced isolation. Like Maupertuis, Buffon assumed that "white" is the primordial colour of humans, and that "black" skin colour is a variation that can be retracted.[11] Africans, he suggested, could be brought to a Nordic country such as Denmark and then be deprived of any possibility to reproduce with the local population. "One has to lock up the Negroes with their females, and meticulously preserve their race without allowing them to crossbreed" (314). This he concluded, is the "only means which we can employ in order to know how much time would be needed to reintegrate in this respect the nature of man, and ... how much was needed to change her from white to black" (314). Read against the backdrop of his reflections on degeneration and race-mixing it becomes clear that Buffon's definition of the species – the idea that within a species all male and female members can reproduce with each other and bring forth fertile offspring – contributes to an interventionist understanding of reproduction. It opens up the horizon for enquiries and interventions into the specific reproductive arrangements among the various members of the human species.

These scientific speculations and musings on race-mixing and breeding resonated with the political discourse. In particular, Charles-Augustin Vandermonde, who referred to Maupertuis's and Buffon's theories of reproduction in his *Essai sur la manière de perfectionner l'espèce humaine* (*Essay on the Method of Improving the Human Species*, 1756), discussed race-mixing as a means for improving the population. Like Maupertuis, La Mettrie, or Buffon, he formulated his project of improvement by comparing it to animal breeding. "Since one has been able to perfect the races of horses, dogs, cats, fowl, pigeons," he wrote, "why not try some attempts with the human race?" (Vandermonde 1756, 94). In contrast to earlier recommendations on how to produce "good" offspring, Vandermonde addressed a new object of concern, the human species, and he directed his advice to a new subject. It is, as Anne Carol argues, no longer the married couple who wants to have good and beautiful children but the legislator who is in charge of his population (Carol 1995). Vandermonde drew on the opposition between degeneration and perfection, and articulated it as the task of political sovereigns to promote the latter. In his view, perfection means to "populate ... [the] state with subjects capable of defending them and of causing the arts to flourish there" (Eigen 2008, 92). Wealth and military strength are the main effects he envisaged. Among his positive examples of intermarriage on a large scale that produced such positive effects, are great cities such as Paris, coastal populations, and the Ottoman Empire, one of the most powerful states of the period. Vandermonde attributed its political success to the mixture of the population, in particular the "mixture" with a "prodigious quantity of Georgian, Mingrelian, and Circassian slaves" (Vandermonde 1756, 111). This, again, resonates with Chardin's reports from Oriental peoples who improved their beauty through the appropriation of the superior blood of Circassians by way of reproduction with female slaves. Certainly, race-mixing here is part of an imperial narrative in which competing states and their rulers try to augment power through the incorporation of foreign "blood." The enslaved women of the Caucasus in this imperial narrative function as breeding stock, a source of "endless supply" that remains untouched by the surrounding processes of mixing, as Figal has shown (Figal 2014, 181). The fascination with race-mixing as a means of improving populations and augmenting the power of European states thus relied on the assumption of a pure unmixed female stock that serves as a resource. "Mixing" thereby was not meant as a mutual exchange but as strategic appropriation of foreign women.

As I show in the following section, this idea of race-mixing as an imperial strategy of improving the population circulated widely and was also adopted in the German context. However, it did not go uncontested, although reasons for the reluctance toward race-mixing varied. Diderot's anti-colonial, ironic critique of calculated improvement through reproduction is certainly unique. He dismantled the colonial European perspective by inversing positions in his *Supplément au voyage de Bougainville*. In his fictional dialogue, written as a critique of Bougainville's *Voyage around the World* (1771), the non-Europeans, the Tahitians, confront the European intruder with their own project of improving their blood through race-mixing. The clerk of Bougainville's expedition is assigned to Ourou, a Tahitian family head, after the Tahitians have appropriated the whole crew. He is heavily pushed by Ourou to have a baby with one of his daughters. His refusal is not accepted and his astonishment is met with the following answer:

> While being more robust and healthier than you, we have realized at first glance that you are superior to us in terms of intelligence; and immediately we have destined some of our most beautiful women and girls to collect the seed of a better race like yours. It is an experiment that we have tried and which can succeed. We have taken from you and your people the only part that we are able to extract; and believe me, we savages also know how to calculate. (Diderot 1792/2007, 62)

Obviously, Diderot's Tahitians try to manage and improve their "race" by way of inter-racial reproduction as European writers envisaged it for their own countries. The erotic fantasy of the *Supplément,* which is predominantly geared towards challenging religious constraints of sex and desire, ridicules these attempts. By addressing race-mixing as more or less enforced and calculated appropriation of the "seed" – the precious male reproductive substance – from the European intruder, colonial and gender hierarchies are simultaneously inversed. In Diderot, instead of the blood of the exotic female slave, the sperm of the male European elite becomes a reproductive resource that has to be appropriated.

Despite Diderot's irony, the enthusiasm for human breeding as a means for improving society at large prevailed in the late eighteenth century. Condorcet, in his posthumously published *Sketch of a Historical Picture of the Progress of the Human Mind* (1793), claimed that the moral and physical improvement of humans are just two aspects of the same process, and the "natural organization" of humans – like that of plants and animals – can be successfully subjected to breeding strategies in order to avoid degeneration. "The perfectibility or the organic degeneration of races of plants, of animals can be regarded as one of the general laws of nature" (1793/1988, 293), he wrote. This law, he added "also applies to the human species" (293). His friend and admirer Cabanis repeated this contemplation by transforming it in an interpellation on active breeding practices:

> After we have occupied ourselves so minutely with the means of making better and stronger races of animals and useful and agreeable plants; after we have done a hundred times over the races of horses and dogs; after we have

> transplanted, grafted, worked over fruits and flowers in every manner, why is it not shameful to have totally neglected the human race! As though it were more distant! – As if it were more essential to have large strong cattle than healthy vigorous men; good smelling peaches and speckled tulips, than wise and good citizens. (Cabanis quoted from Hilts 1984, 266)

This enthusiasm for human breeding that to a great extent went hand in hand with a positive view of race-mixing certainly helped to shape modern biopolitics although it was not part of a coherent political strategy.

Race-Mixing, Diversity, and "Pure Descent": German Debates in the Late Eighteenth Century

Many of the ideas that were formulated in the French context circulated widely within the German debates on race, human variation, and improvement during the last decades of the century. Kant's essays on race made a peculiar contribution to these debates because his definition of race gave rise to sharp critiques as well as to subsequent adaptations. Kant built on Buffon's definition of the species and then introduced several sublevels: "races" (*Rassen*), "varieties" (*Varietäten*), "variations" (*Spielarten*), and "special sorts" (*Schläge*). These are distinguished by the ways in which parental traits are transmitted to the next generation. Races, Kant claimed, are defined by "hereditary differences" that "persistently preserve themselves ... over prolonged generations" that are always transmitting half-breeds (*halbschlächtig*) (Kant 1775/2007, 85). The issue of race-mixing is thus at the heart of Kant's definition in so far as races are "in large measure defined by the production of hybrids" (Bernasconi 2002, 156).

Throughout his discussion of the concept of race, Kant frequently referred to practices of "mixing" and calculated the outcomes of different reproductive arrangements, similar to the combinational analyses of the *castas*-system: "Through mixing with the White," he wrote, "the East Indian yields the *yellow Mestizo*, just as the American with the white yields the *red Mestizo,* and the White with the Negro the *Mulatto*, the American with the Negro the *Kabugl,* or the black *Caribbean*" (Kant 1775/2007, 89). He was, however, quite reluctant when it came to the desirability of race-mixing. This is very much in line with his rejection of Maupertuis's suggestion of "raising in some province a naturally noble sort of human beings in which understanding, excellence and integrity would be hereditary" (Kant 1775/2007, 86). Kant argued that this would not be wise, first, because perfection works through the "intermingling" (*Vermengung*) of good and evil, and that the latter is an important incentive (*Triebkraft*) for human action. Second, according to Kant, human breeding would hinder nature which by working "undisturbed" (without transplantings or foreign mixings) over many generations produces a "lasting sort" that marks "ethnic groups" (*Völkerschaften*) forever. These could, according to Kant, be called races if "what is characteristic" is not "too insignificant and ... not too hard to describe to ground a special division on it" (Kant 1775/2007, 87). Nature, in short, aims at the production of stable forms and characteristics that must not be destroyed by human intervention. The concept of nature in Kant thus functions as a barrier against any breeding project.

In addition, for Kant, races are relatively fixed entities because they developed from a primordial "stem race" that contained the "germs" of the now existing races.[12] These germs unfolded in different geographical regions, and in this way the human species was made suitable for different environments. Once established, this development of the races cannot be reversed or changed otherwise. Reproduction among members of the different races is thus, in Kant's view, possible but the very idea of "half-races" or "mixed-races" (Kant 1775/2007, 88) presupposes that there are clearly distinguished groups that transmit their characteristics by way of heredity. Alexis Philonenko and Robert Bernasconi have therefore argued that Kant "was opposed to the mixing of races" (Bernasconi 2002, 154). Indeed, in a text not published in the *Akademie-Ausgabe*,[13] Kant warned, as Bernasconi puts it, "that race mixing degrades 'the good race' without lifting up 'the bad race' proportionally" (155) and claimed that "the Governor of Mexico has wisely rescinded the order of the court of Spain favoring this mixing of race" (quoted from Bernasconi 2002, 155). However, although Kant was clearly opposed to the idea of race-mixing as a means of human breeding and improvement, his position is ambivalent.

Of course, his idea that nature aims at the production of lasting differences and the preservation of manifoldness (*Mannigfaltigkeit*) seems to suggest that Kant rejected race-mixing in so far as it could lead to dissolving racial diversity by merging all differences. He advanced this argument with regards "to the melting together" of varieties (1788/2007, 202) and also in the *Anthropology from a Pragmatic Point of View* with regards to the mixing of what he called "natural characters."[14] However, at the same time, Kant conceded that nature with regard to the races "seems at least to permit melting together, though it does not favor it" (202). The reason is that such melting-together of racial traits makes the creature "fit for several climates" (202), although these adaptations are far from being as perfect as the initial development of the races from the primordial "stem." Kant was thus not strictly opposed to race-mixing. And yet, Kant's theory of race, which acknowledges the reality of globalized reproductive relations, at the same time emphasizes the idea that races are lines of "pure descent" (*reine Abstammung*).[15] Defending his concept of race against one of his most prominent opponents, Georg Forster, Kant claimed that races are not just distributed on the earth according to climatic differences but that they are dispersed "cycladically in unified heaps (*Haufen*) ... within the confines of a country" (Kant 1788/2007, 211). They form specific reproductive communities in so far as "each of these races," according to Kant "is, as it were, isolated" (212). This idea of isolation and "pure descent," although it surfaces only at the margins of Kant's theory of race, resonates with Herder's equally ambivalent position.

Herder, like Forster, was one of the most outspoken critics of Kant's concept of race that, according to him, construes difference and segregation where we only find "changeable and unnoticeable" transitions (Herder 1784–91/2002, part 2, book 7, 231). Instead of clearly distinguishable races, we only find "shades" within one big picture (231). Similar to Kant's, Herder's position oscillates between a political-ethical preference for the preservation of "primordial characters" (233) or the "character of the earthly region" (234), and, on the other hand, the acknowledgment of the reality of interracial reproductinve relations. Such relations, in Herder's view, happen because "all or at least most nations of the earth sooner or later migrated" (254). The Mongols, for example, degenerate (*verarten*)[16] or improve (*veredeln*) in every region of the earth, but only in their own country "they are what they have been for thousands of years and will remain the same" (232). Certainly there is a prevailing nostalgia in Herder's description of the Mongols or the native inhabitants of California for their primordial adaptation to the climate in which they lived. The process of departure from the primordial type by migration and mixture with peoples from other regions of the earth for Herder was not without risks, in particular, if it happened too rapidly.[17] Still, it is unavoidable that species and types change to a certain degree according to their environment so that "the rose degenerates and the dog acquires something of a wolf" (254). This process is well "in accordance with history" (254). Like Buffon before him, Herder in addition wondered about the possibilities of changing skin colour, and compared climatic influences with processes of reproduction. The mixing of "foreign nations," he claimed, produces such changes much more quickly than dislocations from geographical regions: "Within a few generations all Mongol, Chinese, American traits disappear" (250).

In contrast to Kant, human nature, for Herder, was absolutely malleable, and he accounted for this without much regret. Human nature has been altered throughout history, and Herder's suggestion was to set up a "physical-geographical history of the descent (*Abstammung*) and degeneration (*Verartung*) of our race (*Geschlecht*) that accounts for the most important results of these changes" (255).

A third author, who advanced an ambivalent position towards the issues of race-mixing, purity, and breeding, was Christoph Meiners. As a university professor in Göttingen, he was at odds with his colleague Johann Friedrich Blumenbach, who in 1795 also introduced the concept of the Caucasian race. Meiners is of particular interest here because in his *Sketch of the History of Mankind* (*Grundriss der Geschichte der Menschheit*, 1785) he problematized the "purity" of the people from the Caucasus from which all other "Caucasians" are supposed to be descendants (*Abkömmlinge*). He regretted that this "ethnic stem" (*Völkerstamm*) was "no longer entirely pure and unmixed" (Meiners 1785/1793), but nevertheless claimed that the "Caucasians and in particular their women are the most beautiful peoples of the whole earth" (§12, 13).[18] Although he did not elaborate on this issue, a preference for the "purity" of races surfaces in this passage.

This resonates with Meiners's anti-egalitarian essay *Über die Natur der afrikanischen Neger* (*On the Nature of African Negros*, 1790),[19] in which he formulated a pro-slavery position. He rejected all emancipatory claims that had been formulated in the wake of the French Revolution and parallelized Africans and Jews, for both in his view had made unjustified claims to equality. Although Meiners adopted Kant's concept of race he did not share Kant's reluctance towards breeding. On the contrary, Meiners who drew on the opposition of "degeneration" (*Ausartung*) and "improvement" (*Veredelung*) repeated the breeding enthusiasm of the French authors by comparing, again, human breeding to plant and animal breeding. If one "inoculates a noble branch into an ignoble stock and allows an animal of a better kind to mix with one of a worse," he wrote, "the fruits of the former and the brood of the latter are inevitably improved" (Meiners 1790, 11). His argument is that the causes and effects that are at work in animals and plants also apply to humans where these phenomena are "even more flamboyant" (11). Although Meiners did not elaborate much on the issues of racial purity and human breeding, it follows from the context that he did not associate human improvement with race-mixing. In his theory of race, he established clear distinctions and hierarchies between the superior race of the "Caucasians" and the inferior "Mongols" as well as among the various subgroups that certainly, in his perspective, could not and should not melt into each another. The perspective of human breeding and population politics that surfaces in his writings is no longer based on the idea of an imperial appropriation of others but seems to be a strategy of internal improvement in the interests of populating a nation. This strategy of preserving the purity of a supposedly superior race can be understood as another form of an imperial regulation of reproduction, distinct from the appropriation of foreigners through race-mixing.

However, at the turn of the nineteenth century, it was by no means a hegemonic idea. Meiners's views were part of a broader cultural and political-ethical controversy about human differences and hierarchies and were criticized and ridiculed by contemporaries such as Georg Foster, Christoph Martin Wieland, and Georg Christoph Lichtenberg.[20] They coexisted with opposing views. Johann Peter Frank, for example, a major proponent of the program of the "medical police" (*medizinische Policey*), which was geared towards improving the health and well-being of the population, re-articulated ideas that had been expressed by Vandermonde about three decades earlier. In his *System einer vollständigen medicinischen Policey* (1779–1819), Frank developed a plan for strategic human breeding. In particular he "outlines a policy for the regulation of marriage and the production of offspring specifically in order to eliminate targeted diseases, mitigate individual suffering, lessen the public burden of the orphaned and infirm, and proactively generate a healthier and generally more productive population" (Eigen 2008, 99). Thereby he emphatically re-articulated Vandermonde's claim that populations that do not reproduce with foreigners degenerate. If they "continue to sow the same fruit upon the same acre" (Frank 1779–1819, 452), he suggested, perfection declines. Mixing, by contrast, can help to improve the "race," and according to Frank, such improvement is sustained by the exotic drift of male desire. European men, according to Frank, "wished to marry Mongol girls because ... they are 'hot-blooded.' Conversely, wealthy Mongol men wished to marry Russian (Caucasian, Georgian) girls from poor families because of their superior beauty" (Eigen 2008, 224). Again, race-mixing appears to be a strategy that was driven by two converging ends, namely the fulfilment of male desire for exotic but "inferior" women and the augmentation of the power of the nation state. The positive reference to reproductive relations of Europeans with non-Europeans, which contrasts ideas of "pure descent," thus remained a discursive and political option at the turn of the century.

Conclusion

In the second half of the eighteenth century, race-mixing and human breeding were of central interest in the epistemic debates that dealt with questions of reproduction and heredity and in the political debates on the improvement of populations. In both respects, these debates built on the experiences of globalized reproductive relations that came with the colonial mobilization of humans since the sixteenth century. Reproductive relations between humans of different skin colour and physical shape were thus an object of scientific curiosity that gave rise to speculations about scientific and political modes of intervention into reproduction. To a great extent, race-mixing in this context was articulated as a power strategy of the improvement of European populations. As the repeated articulation of the figure of the beautiful Circassian female slave reveals, race-mixing as a breeding strategy also had a gendered subtext. This highly imaginative figure constituted the idea of a "foreign" female, part of a subordinated population, who is ready for appropriation and destined to contribute to the strengthening of the power of those who appropriate her. With the invention of the Caucasian race, this exotic figure was familiarized and transformed into the core figure of European identity, as Figal has argued. This discursive annexation of the Other resonated with growing concerns about the vanishing of racial differences through reproductive processes. However, these concerns did not lead to clear rejections or prohibitions of race-mixing. The preservation of "purity" as a hegemonic strategy of "improving" or then "securing" the population was yet to be invented.

NOTES

1 On the process of "[v]isualizing 'race' in the 18th century" and the various cultural, political, and scientific meanings of "race" see Gissis 2011.
2 See Pratt 1992. For an analysis of the meaning of the *castas*-system see Mazzolini 2007.
3 Ann Laura Stoler has argued that "you could not get from eighteenth- to nineteenth-century technologies of sex in Europe without tracking them across colonial ground" (2002, 143). This argument holds with regards to population politics, as well instanced by race-mixing.
4 It is noticeable that the term "perfectibility," which was later widely used by the ideologues, and in particular Condorcet, was first coined by Turgot. "In 1772, just before Turgot came to power as controller-general of finance,

his predecessor ordered that the intendants forward every year, retrospective to 1770, the numbers of births, deaths, and marriages that took place in their jurisdictions. Turgot then demanded that they make a head count in the leading towns and a few neighbouring country parishes. Division of this head count by the average number of births in the same regions over the preceding decade ... would give a coefficient ... by which all the data about birth for all France could be converted into a figure that might be defined as the French population" (Heilbron 1990, 12).

5 All translations in this text, if not stated otherwise, are mine.

6 John C. Waller, in his contribution to this volume, explores another set of thoughts to which eugenic programs in the nineteenth century also referred, namely aristocratic ideas of "noble blood" that were especially important for the concept of race in France.

7 For the emergence and the circulation of the concept of reproduction in the eighteenth and early nineteenth centuries, see Lettow 2014.

8 Like most of his contemporaries, Maupertuis used the terms "race" and "species" unsystematically and sometimes interchangeably.

9 Mary Terrall has meticulously explored the erotic undertones of Maupertuis's writings on reproduction (Terrall 1996).

10 "In exactly the period when Maupertuis was breeding his dogs and reflecting on hereditary variations, Réaumur was developing techniques to improve poultry breeding, especially through artificial incubation of eggs" (Terrall 2007, 267).

11 Andrew Curran argues that "Maupertuis's use of the albino became the hidden foundation of a white-centred *science de l'homme* for the next decades" (Curran 2011, 22).

12 On Kant's understanding of the "germs" that clearly differed from preformationist understandings and was compatible with his epigenetic position, see Bernasconi 2014.

13 The text has been published as *Worin besteht der Fortschritt zum besseren im Menschengeschlecht. Ein bisher ungedruckter und unbekannter Ausfatz von Kant*. Wiesbaden: Staadt, 1914.

14 Kant also briefly referred to inbreeding, arguing that the reason for the "abhorrence against the mixing of too close relatives" lies in the fact that nature "does not want the old forms to be always reproduced again" (Kant 1788/2007, 202). This resonates with the process of "a re-tabooing of incest" in the late eighteenth century that Christine Lehleiter analyses in her chapter in this volume on the Mignon episode in Goethe's *Wilhelm Meister*.

15 Zöller and Louden translate as "pure phyletic origin."

16 The French word "degeneration" is mostly translated as "Entartung." However, in the German texts of the late eighteenth century, words like

"Verartung," "Abartung," or "Ausartung" were also used to describe the modifications of the "kind" (*Art*) that sometimes but not always were understood as decline. I thus translate "verarten" as "to degenerate" because no systematic distinction between these term exists.

17 In chapter 5 of book 7 he explained that nature has "drawn her boundaries between far away countries not for nothing" (255). The "history of conquests" and the "history of diseases," he argued, reveal that the Europeans who recklessly transgress these boundaries "degenerate" (*entarten*).

18 In 1788, Meiners published the translation of a French article in his journal the *Göttingisches historisches Magazin*, in which an anonymous author celebrated the example of the Georgians who "have remained unmixed" (*unvermischt*) (1788, 410–11, quoted from Figal 2014, 176) and were thus an independent people with powerful leaders that "are regarded as regional protectors" (176). Here, racial purity emerges as a precondition of political power.

19 Meiners referred to Kant in a handwritten note to his *Sketch of the History of Mankind* (*Grundriss der Geschichte der Menschheit*, 1785) and in the essay *On the Nature of African Negroes* (*Über die Natur der afrikanischen Neger*) (Dougherty 1990, 103).

20 Meiners's writings were met with interest among French historians of the early nineteenth century. Many of his writings were translated into French soon after their appearance in German but not his racial philosophy of history. However, close contacts between the university of Göttingen and French scientists like the members of the group Observateurs de l'homme make it likely that these writings, too, circulated among French scholars (Dougherty 1990, 94–6).

REFERENCES

Bernasconi, R. 2002. "Kant as an Unfamiliar Source of Racism." In *Philosophers on Race: Critical Essays*, edited by J.K. Ward and T.L. Lott, 145–66. Oxford: Blackwell. http://dx.doi.org/10.1002/9780470753514.ch8.

Bernasconi, R. 2014. "Heredity and Hybridity in the Natural History of Kant, Girtanner and Schelling during the 1790s." In *Reproduction, Race and Gender in Philosophy and the Early Life Sciences*, edited by S. Lettow, 237–58. Albany, NY: SUNY Press.

Buffon, G.-L. Leclerc, Comte de. 1753. "Le Cheval." In *Histoire naturelle*, vol. 14, edited by P. Corsi and T. Hoquet, 174–257. http://www.buffon.cnrs.fr/, accessed 17 Feb. 2013

Buffon, G.-L. Leclerc, Comte de. 1766. "De la degeneration des animaux." In: *Histoire naturelle*, vol. 14, edited by P. Corsi and T. Hoquet, 311–74. http://www.buffon.cnrs.fr/, accessed 17 Feb. 2013.

Carol, A. 1995. *Histoire de l'eugénisme en France: Les médecins et la procréation XIXe–XXe siècles*. Paris: Seuil.

Condorcet, M.J.A.N. de Caritat, Marquis de. (1793) 1988. *Esquisse d'un tableau historique des progrès de l'esprit humain: Fragment sur l'Atlantide*. Paris: Flammarion.

Curran, A. 2011. *The Anatomy of Blackness: Science and Slavery in the Age of Enlightenment*. Baltimore: Johns Hopkins University Press.

Davidson, J. 2009. *Breeding: A Partial History of the Eighteenth Century*. New York: Columbia University Press.

Diderot, D. (1792) 2007. *Supplément au Voyage de Bougainville*. Paris: Flammarion.

Dougherty, F.W.P. 1990. "Christoph Meiners und Johann Friedrich Blumenbach im Streit um den Begriff der Menschenrasse." In *Die Natur des Menschen: Probleme der Physischen Anthropologie und Rassenkunde (1750–1850)*, edited by G. Mann and F. Dumont, 89–111. Stuttgart: Gustav Fischer Verlag.

Eigen, S. 2006. "Policing the Menschen=Racen." In *The German Invention of Race*, edited by S. Eigen and M. Larrimore, 185–212. SUNY Press.

Eigen, S. 2008. *Heredity and the Birth of the Modern*. London: Routledge.

Figal, S. 2014. "The Caucasian Slave Race: Beautiful Circassians and the Hybrid Origin of European Identity." In *Reproduction, Race and Gender in Philosophy and the Early Life Sciences*, edited by S. Lettow, 163–86. Albany, NY: SUNY Press.

Frank, P.J. 1779–1819. *System einer vollständigen medicinischen Policey*. Mannheim: C.F. Schwan, http://gdz.sub.uni-goettingen.de/dms/load/toc/?PPN=PPN333514955, accessed 26 Feb. 2013.

Frängsmyr, T., J.L. Heilbron, and R.E. Rider, eds. 1990. *The Quantifying Spirit in the 18th Century*. Berkeley: University of California Press.

Gissis, S. 2011. "Visualizing 'race' in the 18th Century." *Historical Studies in the Natural Sciences* 41 (1): 41–103. http://dx.doi.org/10.1525/hsns.2011.41.1.41.

Heilbron, J.L. 1990. Introduction. In *The Quantifying Spirit in the 18th Century*, edited by T. Frängsmyr, J.L. Heilbron, and R.E. Rider, 1–23. Berkeley: University of California Press.

Herder, J.G. (1784–91) 2002. *Ideen zur einer Philosophie der Geschichte der Menschheit*. Munich and Vienna: Carl Hanser.

Hilts, V. 1984. "Enlightenment Views on the Genetic Perfectibility of Man." In *Transformation and Tradition in the Sciences*, edited by Everett Mendelssohn. 255–71. Cambridge: Cambridge University Press.

Kant, I. (1775) 2007. "Of the Different Races of Human Beings." In *Anthropology, History, and Education*, edited by G. Zöller and R. Louden, translated by M. Gregor. The Cambridge Edition of the Works of Immanuel Kant, edited by P. Guyer and A.W. Wood, Vol. 1, AA 02, 82–98. Cambridge: Cambridge University Press.

La Mettrie, J.O. de. (1748) 1996. "Man as Plant." In *Machine Man and Other Writings*, translated by A. Thomson., 75–88. Cambridge: Cambridge University Press. http://dx.doi.org/10.1017/CBO9781139166713.007.

Lettow, S. 2014. "Generation, Genealogy and Time: The Concept of Reproduction from *Histoire naturelle* to German *Naturphilosophie*." In *Reproduction, Race and Gender in Philosophy and the Early Life Sciences*, edited by S. Lettow, 21–44. Albany, NY: SUNY.

Maupertuis, P.-L.M. de. (1745) 1780. *Vénus physique*. Geneva: Jean Samuel Cailler.

Maupertuis, P.-L.M. de. (1752) 1756. "Lettre sur le progrès des sciences." In *Oeuvres* 2:420–1. Lyon: Bruyset.

Mazzolini, R. 2007. "'Las Castas': Interracial Crossing and Social Structure, 1770–1835." In *Heredity Produced: At the Crossroads of Biology, Politics, and Culture, 1500–1870*, edited by S. Müller-Wille and H.-J. Rheinberger, 349–73. Cambridge, MA: Massachusetts Institute of Technology Press.

Meiners, C. 1788. "Über die Völkerschaften des Kaukasus." In *Göttingisches historisches Magazin*, 110–11.

Meiners, C. (1785) 1793. *Grundriss der Geschichte der Menschheit*, 2nd ed. Lemgo: Meyersche Buchhandlung. http://babel.hathitrust.org/cgi/pt?id=nyp.33433082394754;view=1up;seq=7, accessed 26 Feb. 2013.

Meiners, C. (1790) 2000. *Über die Natur der afrikanischen Neger (On the Nature of African Negroes)*. Hannover: Werhahn.

Müller-Wille, S. 2014. "Reproducing Difference – Race and Heredity from a *longue durée* Perspective." In *Reproduction, Race and Gender in Philosophy and the Early Life Sciences*, edited by S. Lettow, 217–36. Albany, NY: SUNY.

Müller-Wille, S., and H.-J. Rheinberger. 2007. "Heredity–The Formation of an Epistemic Space." In *Heredity Produced: At the Crossroads of Biology, Politics, and Culture, 1500–1870*, edited by S. Müller-Wille and H.-J. Rheinberger, 3–34. Cambridge, MA: MIT Press.

Pratt, M.L. 1992. *Imperial Eyes: Travel Writing and Transculturation*. London: Routledge.

Roger, J. 1997. *Buffon: A Life in Natural History*. Ithaca and London: Cornell University Press.

Spallanzani, L. Abbé. 1784. *Dissertations Relative to the Natural History of Animals and Vegetables*. Vol. 2. London: J. Murray.

Spary, E. 1996. "Political, Natural and Bodily Economies." In *Cultures of Natural History*, edited by N. Jardine, J.A. Secord, and E. Spary, 178–95. Cambridge: Cambridge University Press.

Stoler, A.L. 2002. *Carnal Knowledge and Imperial Power*. Berkeley: University of California Press.

Terrall, M. 1996. "Salon, Academy and Boudoir: Generation and Desire in Maupertuis' Science of Life." *Isis* 87 (2): 217–29. http://dx.doi.org/10.1086/357481.

Terrall, M. 2007. "Speculation and Experiment in Enlightenment Life Sciences." In *Hererdity Produced: At the Crossroads of Biology, Politics, and Culture, 1500–1870*, edited by S. Müller-Wille and H.-J. Rheinberger, 253–75. Cambridge, MA.: MIT Press.

de Vandermonde, C.-A. 1756. *Essai sur la manière de perfectionner l'espèce humaine*. Paris: Vincent. http://babel.hathitrust.org/cgi/pt?id=ucm.5323757755;view=1up;seq=7 accessed 26 Feb. 2013.

6 New Attention to Incest and Inbreeding as Ways of Reproduction around 1800: A Case Study of the Mignon Episode in Goethe's *Wilhelm Meister*

CHRISTINE LEHLEITER[1]

In discussions of eighteenth-century German literature, the biological dimension of incest and its effect on reproduction have hardly been touched. The assumption behind this neglect is largely that knowledge about biological laws of inbreeding was not substantial at the time so that any attempt to discuss such laws in the context of literature is anachronistic and, therefore, unjustified. However, as research in the last ten years has demonstrated impressively, documented knowledge on the biological effects of inbreeding predates the advent of genetics by many decades and was widely circulated throughout eighteenth-century Europe. To address the question of how knowledge on reproduction and inbreeding mattered for literature around 1800, this chapter focuses on the incest-child Mignon in Johann Wolfgang Goethe's *Wilhelm Meister* (1795–6). Drawing on work by Daniel Wilson (1984) and Hartmut Nonnenmacher (2002), I explore the ways in which the Mignon episode introduces a radical innovation in the discussion of incest by shifting the attention from the incestuous parent to the incest-child. As Wilson has argued, for Goethe the question concerning incest is not what the parents did and how they dealt with their deed, but rather what consequences does incestuous reproduction have for the child and for genealogy? I suggest that Mignon's inability to reproduce and to enter a heterosexual society is not the result of a trauma, as often claimed, but the consequence of inbreeding leading to – what was called at the time – the "monstrosity" of the hermaphrodite body. By placing Mignon in the context of contemporary discussions on inbreeding, we will also see that Goethe's shift in attention from parent to child is deeply connected to a new understanding of nature as a sphere that follows laws independent from ethical considerations.

Incest and Natural Law

Mignon's death at the end of *Wilhelm Meisters Lehrjahre* has often been explained by the fact that her artistic existence has no place in the economic circle of the Tower Society (Jaumann and Voßkamp 1992; Ammerlahn 1981). This secretive society is defined by an enlightened social utopia that requires the individual to devote her life to practical work to further the common good. The society shapes Wilhelm's biography at crucial points and, at the end of his years of apprenticeship, Wilhelm becomes a useful member as a surgeon. Although Mignon had been one of Wilhelm's closest companions during his formative years within a theatre group, her early death seems to indicate that there is no space for her poetic existence in the rational world of the "Tower."

While the dichotomy of poetry and economy has been discussed frequently, little attention has been paid to the difference between Mignon and Wilhelm in terms of their ability to establish a family or a genealogy. However, I want to revisit the significance of the fact that for Wilhelm the process of formation ends with the foundation of a family, while Mignon's genealogy ends with her death. Wilhelm's process of formation arguably ends in the very moment in which he recognizes Felix as his son:

> [Wilhelm] surveyed the world around him, but not like a bird of passage ... Everything he planned was now to mature for the boy, and everything he built was to last for several generations. His apprenticeship was therefore completed in one sense, for along with the feeling of a father he had acquired the virtues of a solid citizen. (*Apprenticeship*, 307)[2]

Paternity, citizenship, and adult selfhood coincide. For Mignon – whose nomadic existence seems to be evoked in the image of the migratory bird – this inscription in genealogy is impossible because of Mignon's incestuous origin and her inability to reproduce.

As Nonnenmacher has described most comprehensively, Goethe's text stands at a curious point in the history of incest. It was the conviction of Enlightenment authors that the prohibition of incest had no basis in natural law. On one hand, this argument was made with reference to indigenous populations who were thought to live in the natural state and for whom incest was not a taboo (e.g., the "Tahitians"). On the other hand, the argument was supported by the claim that the reproduction of the first people had to be necessarily incestuous, if one assumed with the Bible that there was only one couple in the beginning. Some authors were even convinced that the offspring of incestuous relationships were more perfect than others since they ignored or detested social conventions and combined innate blood inclination with erotic attraction, a phenomenon which was called "voice of the blood." At the end of the eighteenth century, though, there was a re-tabooing of incest. However, following a tradition which Luther contributed to when he pleaded for the continuation of marriages that were postnuptially discovered to be incestuous, there was basically no objection to relationships that developed without knowledge of their incestuous quality. Our question is: how does Goethe fit in this tradition of incest? What are his innovative contributions to it?

Considering Mignon's early death and her parents' tragic fate, Goethe's portrayal could be considered as taking part in the mentioned re-tabooing of incest. However, as Wilson has pointed out, it is remarkable that although Mignon's parents fall in love and conceive without knowing their kinship, this family's case is still depicted as being problematic and tragic. As Wilson states, it is also interesting that where authors before Goethe had focused on the consequences of incest for the incestuous couple and had asked for the causality of incest (be it providence, fate, or voice of the blood), Goethe focuses on the incest child. What are Goethe's motivations for this new emphasis?

Answering this question requires examining the justifications that Mignon's father, Augustin, provides to defend his incestuous relationship. In opposition to his brothers who argue that the incest taboo as historical norm and tradition has reached quasi natural validity, Augustin asks: "Haven't there been noble peoples that have sanctioned marriage with one's sister? Don't talk about your gods, you only refer to them when you want to fool us, lead us away from nature, distort our noblest instincts into crimes by infamous coercion" (*Apprenticeship*, 357).[3] Much like natural law philosophers, Augustin refers to indigenous, "noble" peoples who do not know the incest taboo (cf. Nonnenmacher 2002, 195). In the centre of his apology stands the reference to nature. He exclaims: "Consider the lilies: Do not husband and wife grow on one and the same stem? Does not the blossom they bear unite them? And is not the lily the image of innocence? Is not its sibling union fruitful?" (*Apprenticeship*, 357).

Augustin's lily imagery alludes to Matthew 6:28: "And why take ye thought for raiment? Consider the lilies of the field, how they grow. They toil not, neither do they spin."[4] While in the Gospel of Matthew the lilies are used metaphorically, Augustin uses the comparison between the process of reproduction in flowers and the reproduction in humans in the literal sense (reminiscent of Linnaean taxonomy). He argues that reproductive patterns in plants and humans follow the same natural law which justifies and necessitates incest. Nonnenmacher observes that there is basically no literary work before *Apprenticeship* in which incest is connected to the botanical realm. Despite his consideration of biological questions, Nonnenmacher comes to the conclusion that "the plot line leaves it open whether nature justifies incest or, after all, its prohibition" (2002, 199).[5] While Nonnenmacher acknowledges the differences between the standpoint taken by *Apprenticeship* and natural law philosophy, he also stops short of reading the Mignon episode as an argument against the incest taboo. Considering both the tragic outcome of Augustin's and Sperata's relationship and the problematic condemnation of Augustin and Mignon by the Tower Society, it is understandable that scholars hesitate to read any normative statements into the story. However, I see this uncertainty in the assessment of incest as largely based on the fear that an acknowledgment of Mignon's problematic biology would lead to her parents' moral condemnation. It is exactly the split between nature and morality that is decisive for Goethe's take on the question of incestuous reproduction.

Augustin himself confuses the two. Confronted with the brothers' accusations, Augustin invites them to witness a paradisiacal scene: "Visit us [Augustin and Sperata] at those trellises, where lemons and pomegranates surround us ... and then try to frighten us with your dismal, gray, man-made entrapments!" (*Apprenticeship*, 357).[6] Augustin refers to the garden to underline the natural justification for incest. However, it is remarkable that the fruits that he names are trained on a trellis. Hence, the image is not supporting the dichotomy between nature and culture that Augustin wants to evoke. Furthermore, the end of the story makes clear that Augustin's reference to nature does not support his claim that nature justifies his incestuous relationship. Augustin states, "Nature clearly indicates what it abhors: a creature that should not exist, cannot exist, develops wrongly, or is soon destroyed. The marks of her curse, the signs of her severity are: barrenness, stunted growth, premature decay" (*Apprenticeship*, 357).

Augustin's justification of his relationship with his sister appears in the narrative after Mignon's death so that, in hindsight, this justification turns into his accusation: nature has condemned Mignon, which is why she has problems speaking and dies early. Mignon is described as a child of a "strange nature," who has great musical and acrobatic talents, but is unable to articulate her thoughts. It is important to note that this strangeness – located in Mignon's "nature" – is observed already before Mignon is kidnapped and arguably before she could experience any psychological or educational harm. Hence, the plotline suggests that Goethe follows

Augustin's conviction that nature establishes an unbreakable rule that reigns over man-made laws, but also that he draws a different conclusion: the law of nature does not justify incest; it seems to condemn it.

Girl and Orgasm

Scholarly discussion on the Mignon figure so far can be summarized under two connected topics. First, Mignon's androgyny and, second, her inability to overcome this androgyny as the result of a traumatic childhood – in contrast to other androgynous figures in *Wilhelm Meister*, like Therese and Nathalie who eventually embrace their assigned gender roles. Thomas Kniesche interprets Mignon's problems as a hysterical neurosis connected to the social "coercion to become a girl" (1993, 72). Friedrich Kittler argues that the Tower Society explains Mignon's androgyny as an unfortunate result of her traumatic childhood and lack of proper *Bildung* (1978, 36–43). The Tower Society's intention and inability to fit Mignon into established gender norms has been discussed in numerous articles. Although there is often an implied or explicit criticism of the Tower Society, the assumption in these articles remains that woman's clothes are those that fit Mignon's sex and that Mignon's refusal to wear them is the result of a psychological problem. Hence, in the dominant scholarship Mignon has been read as a female figure and has been listed among the female figures whom Wilhelm encounters along his way to *Bildung*.[7] Astonishing is the fact that scholars have not questioned whether or not Mignon *is* a girl. Despite the abundance of discussions on Mignon's androgyny, critics argue within the framework of biologically differentiated sexes in the very moment in which they claim to question it.

Only a few scholars have tried to turn the tide. Rejecting the dichotomy that the Tower Society establishes and drawing on the fact that the word "mignon" was used in the late eighteenth century to refer to male homosexual prostitutes, Robert Tobin has highlighted the homoerotic quality of Wilhelm's relationship to Mignon and has criticized the Tower Society's "medicinalization" of the figure. However, Tobin's wish to rescue a space for homoerotic desire within a system that considers sex a cultural construct makes it also impossible to (re)consider Mignon's body (Tobin 1993, 47). Furthermore, Tobin's claim of a latent homoerotic desire is confusing because he continues to argue that Mignon is a girl. This confusion is highlighted when Tobin refers to Kurt Robert Eissler's interpretation of Mignon's seizure in Book II of *Apprenticeship*. Eissler reads this seizure as a detailed and realistic description of female orgasm (Eissler 1985, 870).

Drawing on Eissler, Tobin argues that of all erotic scenes in the novel, the scene of Mignon's seizure "portrays most explicitly a woman's feelings, sensations, and sexuality." It is, says Tobin, "the only scene in the novel portraying a woman's orgasm" (Tobin 1993, 49). By declaring the seizure a female orgasm and Mignon a girl, scholars have reinforced the two-sex model that they intended to criticize.

Inbreeding and Infertility

In his 1984 article, Wilson addresses the biology of incest in eighteenth-century German literature with explicit reference to Mignon without, however, exploring it in detail. He concludes that contemporary thinkers "did not have the benefit of Darwin, Mendel, and recent studies ... [W]ithout a 1980s knowledge of genetics, they have nothing on which to base their suspicion, so that suspicion took on the status of superstition" (Wilson 1984, 251). Yet, a close look at the literature shows that documented knowledge about the effects of inbreeding predates Darwin and Mendel by several decades and that Goethe is at the forefront of this consideration.

The cultural rejection of the incest taboo in the context of natural law possibly prepared the openness to the use of inbreeding in a growing field of animal husbandry.[8] One of the best examples for the rapid and revolutionary developments within livestock breeding and its effects on the conceptualization of inbreeding is Robert Bakewell (1725–95) of Dishley in Leicestershire, an exceptionally active and internationally recognized breeder in his time. Noting the importance of parentage for the quality of the offspring, Bakewell used inbreeding as his main approach in the attempt to perfect his animals.[9] His success with inbreeding was well-known throughout Europe. In fact, Christoph Gottlieb Sturm (1781–1826), who led the agricultural institute in Tiefurt (Weimar), and whom Goethe used as a source in the context of new breeding results, refers explicitly to Bakewell (cf. Goethe 1993, 312c). Despite the astonishing national and international success of Bakewell's breeding methods, there was a growing rejection of inbreeding in Germany and elsewhere around 1800. However, this rejection was based not on religious and social conventions, but increasingly on observations from inbreeding experiments. Breeding experts like Parry (1806), Sebright (1809), and Sinclair (1823, 93–5) started to issue warnings about the degenerative effect of inbreeding. These warnings referred in particular to loss of sexual differentiation and increased infertility among the offspring of incestuous breeding in sheep (the guinea pig of the period).

In 1806, Caleb Hillier Parry (1755–1822), member of the Royal College of Physicians of London and honorary member of the Physical Society of Göttingen, contributed a long article on the history of the Merino-Ryeland sheep breed to the British *Communications to the Board of Agriculture.*[10] Among other aspects like wool quality, Parry reflects upon the options for the sheep's improvement by means of fattening (the latter had been one of Bakewell's prime concerns). Operating initially within a framework which stressed the influence of environmental factors, he observed that the fattening of the Merino-Ryeland "may probably be accelerated by early and uniform luxuriance of keep." But he added:

> Perhaps also the same end may be promoted by breeding in and in. This has been suggested to me by Mr. Davis, who thinks the early fattening of the New-Leicester breed to be chiefly owing to this cause. He says, that this constant incestuous intercourse produces, in both sexes, a deficiency of the powers of generation, and that of nursing in the female; reducing them to a state approaching to that of eunuchs. (Parry 1806, 471)

The author drew a close connection between incestuous reproduction and degeneration, in particular the loss of clearly distinguishable sexual features which coincides with infertility. What shapes the above quotation is a strange tension between a rehabilitation of inbreeding as a means to improve certain flock qualities and a rejection of incestuous propagation as a cause for sexual degeneration in the offspring. That both statements are possible at the same time is closely related to the fact that the criteria for the assessment of incestuous propagation are biological and economical. The results are judged according to these criteria and therefore the question of whether the outcomes are desirable depends solely on the market and purpose for which the sheep are bred. Without yet having certainty in terms of biology (in fact, we consider the case today biologically rather complex), he explores what it would mean if biology could constitute a determining factor.[11] This consideration is not only interesting from a history of science perspective, but has also implications for the reading of the Mignon episode.

Hermaphrodite and Surgeon

There are a number of scenes which become readable if Mignon's incestuous origin and the possibility of sexual degeneration are considered. In this context, it is important to note that the narrator does not introduce

Mignon as a girl. Mignon's first introduction is as "a young creature" (*Apprenticeship*, 50). Her declaration as a girl is presented as the result of a rather arbitrary decision process: Wilhelm, says the narrator, "looked at the figure with amazement, uncertain whether it was a boy or a girl. But he finally decided in favor of the latter" (*Apprenticeship*, 50). Despite Wilhelm's decision, doubts about Mignon's sex remain throughout the text. Textual evidence pointing to this ambiguity is abundant and particularly voiced by Mignon herself. When Melina wants Mignon to wear "Weiberkleider" (clothes for women), Mignon clings to Wilhelm and responds with agitation: "I am a boy, I do not want to be a girl" (*Apprenticeship*, 122). Even after Mignon's death and the dissection of her body, the boys' choir switches back and forth between female and male pronouns when referring to Mignon: "Oh! How reluctantly did we bring *him* here! Oh! And *he* ought to stay here! ... when we garlanded *her* head, *she* looked dear and friendly" (*Apprenticeship*, 956, translation and emphasis mine).[12] Mignon herself wishes for a state where the gender question is not asked any longer. In her last song, she states, "For all those glorious heavenly forms, / They do not ask for man or woman" (*Apprenticeship*, 316).[13]

Only by understanding that Mignon's problem is biological does it become clear why the androgyny of other figures like Therese and Natalie is not shown as problematic. In contrast to Mignon, Therese and Natalie derive their masculinity from clothes that they wear. Their double gender is the result of masquerade, not of the body.[14] Since they can replace their androgynous role with clearly defined gender roles, they can become adults. Mignon's body, however, is not replaceable within a system marked by contingency. Therefore, she is neither allowed to reproduce nor to become a member of society, which is based on classificatory systems that her body resists.

In her book on comic androgyny in Jonson and Shakespeare, Grace Tiffany has observed that Renaissance authors used the terms hermaphroditism and androgyny still interchangeably (1995, 11).[15] But, as Laqueur has shown, in the eighteenth century the body obtained a new normative power (1990), which at the same time made it possible to distinguish between body and dress, biology and culture, and to define hermaphroditism as bound to the body, while androgyny as a cultural and psychological phenomenon. Goethe's *Wilhelm Meister* is one of the works that contribute to this reformulation of the definition of hermaphroditism and androgyny in light of a new split between the body and its cultural inscriptions. The textual indecision concerning Mignon's sex, which has irritated commentators, invites thoughts that Jarno's rejection of Mignon as "a silly, hermaphrodite [zwitterhaft] creature" (*Apprenticeship*, 113)[16] is more than an annoyed remark about Wilhelm's company with the theatrical nomads and his hesitation to enter a more productive life. Against the backdrop of contemporary animal husbandry, we can conclude that Mignon is presented as deeply shaped by her incestuous origin displaying a "sexual degeneration" that makes it impossible to assign one sex to her body. Drawing on Jarno's statement, I want to suggest that Mignon is biologically a hermaphrodite (or intersex person as we would say today).[17]

These observations cast the seizure scene in a new light. Drawing on Eissler's perceptive recognition of the erotic potential of the scene, I suggest that its closure has been misread. The narrator describes the end of the seizure with the following words: "[Mignon's] rigid members became gentle, her innermost flowed over" (*Apprenticeship*, 82).[18] It is, of course, possible to read this outpouring of the inner as the flow of those tears that are mentioned shortly before in this scene. However, associations surrounding the transition from stiffness to relaxation accompanied by an outpouring of liquid rather suggest an ejaculation. In fact, when considering the hermaphrodite body, surgeons of the time consider ejaculations one of the main criteria in the assessment of its sex (I will return to this below).

The figure of the surgeon plays an important role in the context of the Mignon episode. Mignon's first encounter with the surgeon happens after the theatrical group has been surprised by a band of robbers. Like Wilhelm, Mignon has been hurt in the violent event: "Mignon had for several days been very quiet, and when asked why, she finally admitted that she had sprained her right arm ... They scolded her for not telling them sooner that she was hurt, but they had noticed that she was afraid of the surgeon who all this time had taken her for a boy" (*Apprenticeship*, 140).[19] Mignon's hesitation can be read as an expression of the fear to disclose her sexuality. The "evil" that is discovered is the scandal of her hermaphrodite body (Mignon's dislocated arm can be read as a metonym for another "dislocated member" of her body). The fact that it is the surgeon who discovers that Mignon's body does not fit in the system of clear-cut gender differences stands in close connection to the re-evaluation of the hermaphrodite around 1800.

The seventeenth and eighteenth centuries, as Maximilian Schochow has described in a recent study on the topic (2009), experienced not only a heightened interest in hermaphroditism but also brought forward a new way of observing the hermaphrodite body.[20] In the search for a sexual classification of this body, seventeenth- and eighteenth-century physicians such as Jacques Duval and surgeons like Georg Arnaud and Jean Jacques Louis Hoin did not read the signs of the body any longer for a divine message (as authors such as Augustine had done). Rather, they tried to find the unseen truth by touching and entering the openings of the body to discover the hidden sexual organ (cf. Schochow 2009, 91–101).[21] Stressing this shift in methodology and discipline, Kathleen Long arrives at the conclusion that the hermaphrodite can be associated "with the rise of empirical science and the valorization of the clinical practice over bookish learning" (2006, 29).

Goethe's physician Christoph Wilhelm Hufeland (1762–1836) operates within this new methodological, empirical framework. In 1801, he described the often discussed body of the hermaphrodite Maria Dorothea Derrier whose unusual sexual organs had been discovered when she visited the Berlin Charité for an unrelated reason:[22]

> The rod is of remarkable size, very well and perfectly formed, freestanding except a small part, equipped with a perfectly formed foreskin, which can be glided back and forth over the glands, she also has from time to time, particularly in the early morning, weak erections ... By the way, the female sexual organs are present in the ... natural constitution. (Hufeland 1801, 170, as quoted in Schochow 2009, 220)

Focusing on the sexual organs, Hufeland's surgical eye and hand discovered both sexes. Like Hufeland, contemporary physicians were confronted with a variety of bodily formations (see figure 6.1 for a depiction of Derrier by Mursinna). However, the urge for deciding for one of the two sexes remained strong. Hufeland ends his report on Maria Dorothea Derrier with the reassuring words: "Since apparently the main parts and features of femininity are present, and the main parts of masculinity, the testicles, are missing, the person is to be considered for nothing else than a female being with a monstrous clitoris" (Hufeland 1801, 171–2, as quoted in Schochow 2009, 220).[23]

Hufeland's contemporary Johann Christian Stark (1753–1811) examines Derrier again, but stresses masculinity: "After I and others have pointed out this phenomenon to her – she has seen more often true ejaculation combined with erections during sleep" (Stark 1801, 551, as quoted in Schochow 2009, 223). His conclusion is similar to Hufeland's in the sense that he also denies real hermaphroditism; for Stark, Derrier is a "degenerated man" (*missgestaltete Mannsperson*) (Stark 1801, 551, as quoted in Schochow 2009, 223). Mignon's seizure has to be read within these parameters.

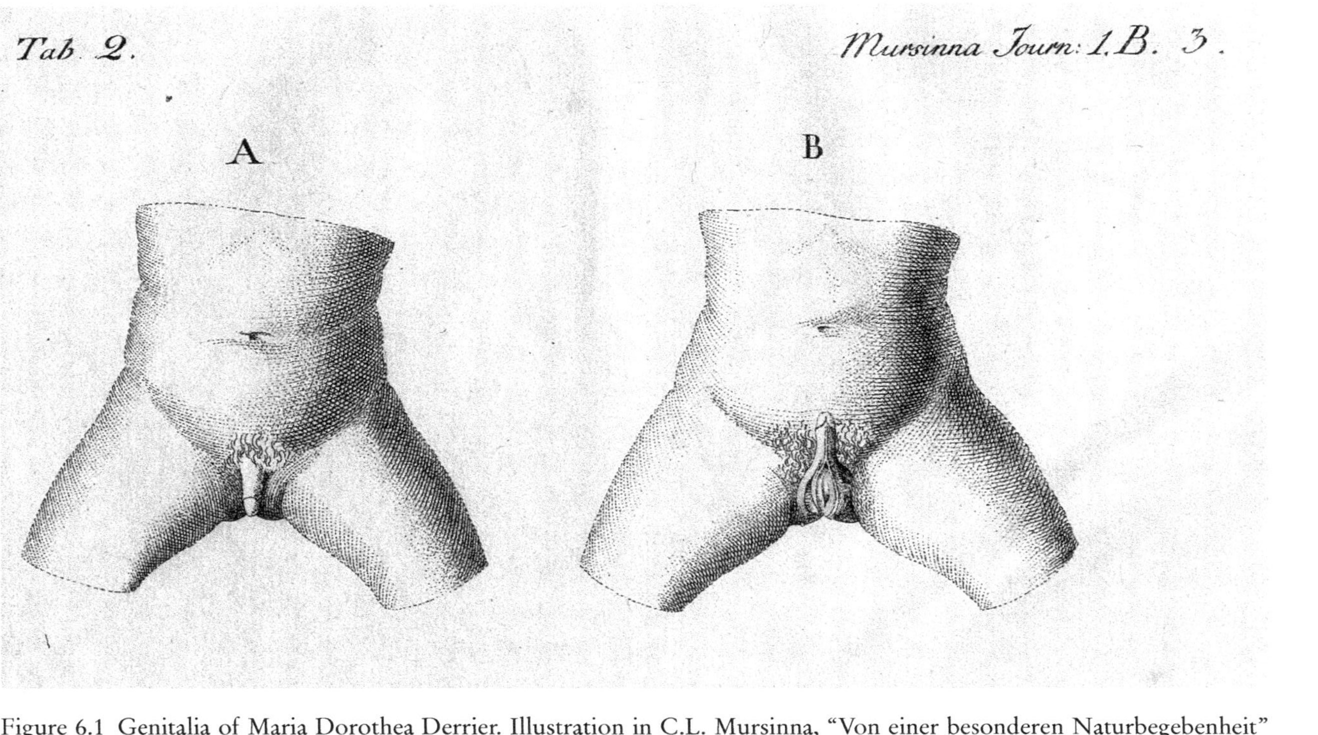

Figure 6.1 Genitalia of Maria Dorothea Derrier. Illustration in C.L. Mursinna, “Von einer besonderen Naturbegebenheit” (Of an Exceptional Event of Nature). *Journal für die Chirurgie, Arzneykunde und Geburtshilfe*. Erster Band, drittes Stück. Berlin: in der Felischischen Buchhandlung, 1801, 555–9. Universitätsbibliothek Leipzig, Allg. med. Lit. 1527-n (1.1801), Abb.

Anatomical Collection and Specimen

While Hufeland seems to have been satisfied with the examination of the living body of the hermaphrodite, Stark exclaims, "However, I have always wished! And still wish it very much, that one dissected a hermaphrodite after death or that one might open the ones which still exist after death, in order to see the correlation of outer and inner parts" (Stark 1801, 540, as quoted in Schochow 2009, 224). It is precisely such a dissection which takes place at the end of *Apprenticeship*. Scholarship so far has claimed that the preparation of Mignon's corpse for the Hall of the Past belongs in the context of mummification practices in reference to Egyptian rituals (Kniesche 1993, 73). It is astonishing that it has not been noticed that this "mummification" is staged as the preparation of a specimen for an anatomical collection. Immediately after Mignon's death, the doctor announces in eerily objectifying language what he and the surgeon have planned all along:

> Stay away from this mournful sight [object], and let me [the doctor] use my art to give some permanence to the remains of this unusual person [strange being]. I will start immediately to employ the delicate art of embalming, and also preserve an appearance of life in this beloved creature. Since I foresaw that she was dying, I have made all preparations, and my assistant [the surgeon] and I will see that we succeed. (*Apprenticeship*, 334)

The uncontained eagerness with which doctor and surgeon seem to have awaited Mignon's death reminds one not only of Stark's wish to dissect a hermaphrodite, but also of the so called "Materialmangel" (lack of material) which in the eighteenth century was felt in the medical sciences regarding the need of corpses for the training of doctors. The resulting lack of respect for the dead and their bereaved families is a topic that occupied Goethe throughout his life (see Baßler 1997 and Egger 2001). In the third book of the *Wilhelm Meisters Wanderjahre* (*Journeyman Years*), but also in a letter written in the last weeks before his own death, Goethe still worked on suggestions to alleviate the need in the medical training by replacing the corpses with wax models.[24]

In *Apprenticeship*, however, wax is employed in a different way. "Embalming," the word that the doctor uses, is a term frequently employed for the description of a preparation method of corpses for the anatomical collection. "Embalmed bodies" form a distinguished group within the systematic of such collections. Caspar Friedrich Jenckel (Neickelio) uses the term when presenting his *Instructions for the Right Definition and Useful Idea of Museums and Anatomic Collections* (1727). According to him, in such collections

> are shown all kinds of dissected or cut, prepared and embalmed bodies and members. The finer the skeletons are positioned ... so that not just the eye but particularly also the mind and memory can draw the most advantage in observation of it, the more beautiful such a cabinet is organized. Particular curiosity in such anatomica consists also in the ability to present monstrous or immense objects. (5)

Not only are the bodies embalmed for display, but this display convinces in particular through its effect on emotions and memory, as it seems intended for the Hall of the Past for which Mignon's corpse is prepared. Jenckel also stresses that the pride of the anatomical collection is its wealth in teratological exhibition pieces, among which Mignon's body could be counted.

Once the connection of Mignon's embalmed body to the anatomical collection and the medical-biological context is established, it becomes clear that the Abbé does not simply describe a mummification process when presenting Mignon's corpse to the mourners, but a modern preservation practice: "[I]f art could not give permanence to her spirit, it could employ every skill to preserve her body and save it from decay. Balsam has been introduced into all her veins and, instead [in place] of blood, this colors those cheeks that faded so early. Come closer, my friends, and see the miracle of art and care!" (*Apprenticeship*, 353).[25] The balsamic mass that fills Mignon's blood vessels is not connected to Egyptian practices (where the body is drained of fluids) as Kniesche would have it, but quotes injection techniques widely used for representation and preservation of blood vessels. These techniques belonged to the highlights of anatomical preparations in the seventeenth and eighteenth century (see figure 6.2). Since the success of the technique depended on size and condition of the vessels, the best results were obtained with corpses of children. The injection technique when used for the bodies of older children, as Mignon was, required the opening of thorax and belly covers. The body was then laid for an hour in water and the blood removed via the vena portae and other vessels. After this work, the (coloured) wax mass was injected in the vessels.

The epistemological questions at the centre of the embalming practice and science are perhaps nowhere clearer than in the work of the Dutch anatomist Frederik Ruysch (1638–1731), one of the most talented and

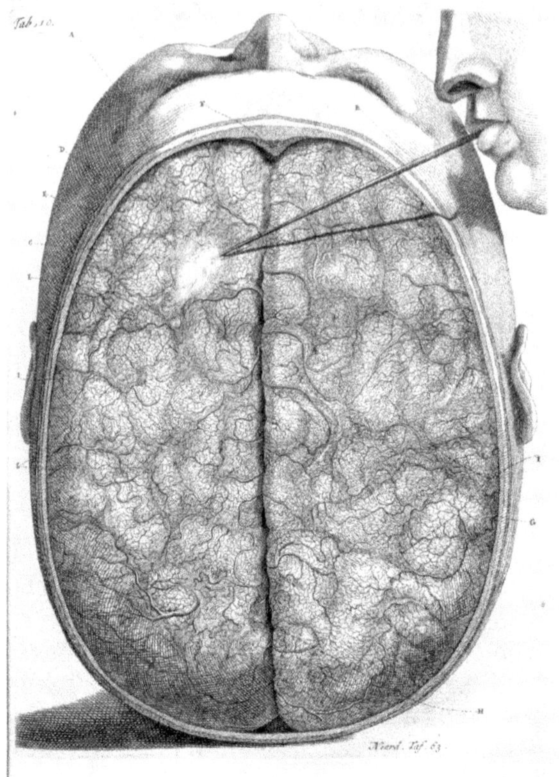

Figure 6.2 Preparation technique in F. Ruysch, *Opera Omnia Anatomico-Medico Chirurgica* (Amsterdam: Janssonio-Waesbergios, 1737), table 10. Courtesy of the Thomas Fisher Rare Book Library, University of Toronto.

famous producers of anatomical preparations in the seventeenth and eighteenth century. Ruysch's preparations were praised for their faithfulness, and his work experienced enormous popularity, which can be estimated from the kind of visitors which his collection attracted. Among the many visitors was Peter the Great from Russia who saw the collection several times and eventually bought significant parts of it. There is a story that Peter the Great kissed one of Ruysch's mummified children because he thought it was alive (cf. Cook 2002, 241, and Hansen 1996, 673). Other segments of the collection were auctioned after Ruysch's death in 1731 by King John Sobieski from Poland and were later bought by the University of Wittenberg (Quigley 2001, 185).[26] Ruysch's publications on his collections were widely distributed and quoted. Margócsy has shown that an important point of Ruysch's publications was that they insisted on a hierarchy between object and text. Ruysch advertised that through his method dead bodies would remain "very beautiful, well-shaped, and full of lively colour" (quoted in Margócsy 2009, 199). This insistency on the actual object obviously had economic motivations – Ruysch charged for the visit to his collection. However, as Margócsy argues convincingly, it also stressed the "epistemological primacy" of the object over the text (2009, 199).[27]

Margócsy's point is well taken and focuses our attention on the conceptualization of the relationship between body and text in the seventeenth and eighteenth centuries. However, it glosses too easily over the fact that the body to which Ruysch's text refers is itself not living nature but its remnant and as such postpones the problem of access to nature and body without ever being able to solve it. The treatment of Mignon's preparation for the Hall of the Past demonstrates that Goethe was acutely aware of the problem. He brings this moment of absence to our attention by highlighting that the preparation and preservation of the body can only take place as a process of replacement. The Abbé's words demonstrate an awareness of the fact that Mignon's embalmed body is representation *not* nature, and that the wax that fills the vessels of her corpse is there *in place* of real blood ("an der Stelle des Bluts").

The complex relationship between the live body and its replacement, nature and its representation, which is brought to our attention by reference to Ruysch, highlights a crucial aspect of the Mignon episode. Mignon's embalmed body can only be a replacement in absence of the living body, which is stressed by the recurrence of a motto from Ruysch's catalogue in Goethe's text. The motto that Ruysch advertised in the foreword to *Opera Omnia* was "venite et videte" (quoted in Margócsy 2009, 199). It is this "come and see" that reappears in the context of the presentation of Mignon's embalmed body. At Mignon's funeral, in the quoted passage, the Abbé invites the friends: "*Come* closer, my friends, *and see* the miracle of art and care!" (*Apprenticeship*, 353, my emphasis). When the Abbé invites the audience to look at the embalmed corpse, the "come and see" promises presence, but the Abbé refers to a body which is only a reference to a living body and, even more, the reference to a text (Ruysch's) which promises life-likeness, but refers to other corpses. The condition of possibility of this circulation of references is a living body, which defies classification and representation and which can only be grasped in its absence. And only in its absence, which is referenced in the embalmed and aestheticized corpse, can the scandal of Mignon's hermaphrodite body be accepted in the culture of the Tower Society.

On the deathbed, Mignon wears the winged garb that she had also worn in the last days before her death. In scholarship so far, this costume has been read as the representation of an angelic figure with focus on the lack of sexuality.[28] This reading seems legitimate in particular since Mignon, in her last song ("For all those glorious heavenly forms, / They do not ask for man or woman") refers to Matthew 22:30: "For in the resurrection they neither marry, nor are given in marriage, but are as the angels of God in heaven."[29] The reference to the biblical verse invites a reading in which Mignon's body transcends gender differences. However, the winged appearance of Mignon's hermaphroditic body also suggests a connection to the antique god Phanes. In Greek mythology, Phanes is described as a winged figure, at times depicted as hermaphrodite, who is invisible but radiates pure light. As the god's name suggests, Phanes (from *phaino*: bringing to light, make appear) makes things visible, but remains invisible him/herself. Benjamin Hederich's *Gründliches mythologisches Lexicon* (*comprehensive Mythological Dictionary*), which was published in Schwaben's revised version in 1770 and which was in Goethe's possession, describes "Phanaeus" as an attribute name of Sol or Apollo, and adds: "Whether he has such attributive name from the mountain range or from an old king, Phanaus ... or just from φάνεϑαι, to appear, because he appears every day anew ... or makes that everything appears and can be seen ... has not been decided yet" (Hederich 1770). Against the backdrop of the Phanes figure, we can read Mignon's last song, which includes the line "lasst mich scheinen" (let me appear, *Apprenticeship*, 895), not as a plea to appear, but as a plea to let her be that source of light that makes the world visible, but remains invisible herself. If an allegorical reading of Mignon's hermaphrodite body is possible, then only as a figure who is the condition of possibility for interpretation to appear, but who has to remain outside the circulation of signs herself. The plea of this figure remains unheard in the dissecting and classifying world of the Tower Society.[30]

In considering the history of incest this chapter has argued that there is a new hesitation concerning incestuous reproduction around 1800. While the incest taboo before the eighteenth century had been understood in an ethical-religious context and the taboo's rejection was closely tied to a rejection of social conventions and laws, the re-tabooing of incest found in Goethe can be understood in the context of new findings in animal husbandry. The hesitations in animal husbandry against inbreeding were connected to the (perceived) loss of sexual differentiation and the failure of inbred animals to produce fertile offspring. Against this background,

Goethe anticipated the discussion on the biological problem of inbreeding in the Mignon figure and by doing so introduced a split between ethical and biological considerations of the incest taboo. Revisiting the Mignon episode, I have argued that Mignon's inability to reproduce and to enter a heterosexual society is not the result of a trauma, as often claimed, but the result of a biological condition. Furthermore, Goethe's use of the figure of the hermaphrodite, in the specific historical moment in which he writes, suggests that he places Mignon's "monstrosity" as a body in opposition to the classificatory world of the Tower Society. Finally, the anatomical collection highlights the epistemological questions raised in the Mignon episode. Only as dead body is Mignon's nature represented and incorporated in the Hall of the Past.

NOTES

1 An expanded version of this material can be found in the chapter "Incest and Inbreeding" in my book *Romanticism, Origins, and the History of Heredity* (Lewisburg, PA: Bucknell University Press, 2014).
2 *Wilhelm Meister* is composed of two volumes, *Wilhelm Meisters Lehrjahre* (Wilhelm Meister's Apprenticeship) and *Wilhelm Meisters Wanderjahre* (Wilhelm Meister's Journeyman Years). In what follows, the abbreviations *Apprenticeship* and *Journeyman Years* will be used. Unless otherwise indicated, I use the Eric A. Blackall/Victor Lange translation (Goethe 1989a). Where I have supplied my own translations I give the page reference to Blackall/ Lange and explain the reasons for my alterations in an endnote.
3 Eric A. Blackall (in cooperation with Victor Lange) translates "edle Völker" as "great nations." This translation overlooks the connection to the discourse around incest in indigenous populations. To make this connection visible, I have modified the translation by replacing "great nations" with "noble peoples."
4 Cf. *Lehrjahre*, 965, note 28. For quotations from the Bible I used the *21st Century King James Version*, http://www.biblegateway.com (accessed 30 November 2014).
5 Unless otherwise indicated, all translations are mine.
6 I have modified Blackall's translation by replacing "in those groves" with "at those trellises" which stays closer to the original German "an jenen Spalieren" (*Lehrjahre* 965).
7 Typical assessments are the following: "From a feminist perspective, the celestial Mignon and the subterranean Melusine ... can be read as *cultural representations of femininity*" (Bäumer 1993, 113, emphasis mine), or

"Particularly, the figures of Mariane and Mignon represent the discussion of the *female body* ..." (Groß 1993, 83, emphasis mine), and "With Mignon in the novels *Wilhelm Meisters Lehrjahre*, Ottilie in *Die Wahlverwandtschaften*, and to some degree with Makarie in *Wilhelm Meisters Wanderjahre*, Goethe created three *female characters*" (Rainer 1993, 101, emphasis mine). Even for readers who have offered comprehensive and careful accounts of androgyny in Goethe's *Meister*, it has remained difficult to accept Mignon's liminal stage. In her detailed study, *Embodying Ambiguity* (1998), Catriona MacLeod assumes that Mignon is a girl. In reference to Natalie's suggestion that Mignon wears female clothes, MacLeod remarks, "It is Natalie who attempts to have Mignon dress in a manner *befitting her sex*" and, in reference to Mignon's preference for the angelic dress, MacLeod continues "[b]ut in keeping the long white dress, she [Mignon] is *not acknowledging her female sex*" (119–22, emphasis mine).

8 In her contribution to this volume, Susanne Lettow shows how important it was still for prominent scholars such as Buffon to insist on giving "foreign males to the native females, and reciprocally to the native males, foreign females" in order to prevent degeneration. Inbreeding was not a desired option for these researchers.

9 For an overview on Bakewell's activities, see Wood and Orel (2001).

10 Parry was a well-known physician who had contact with famous contemporaries like Burke and Jenner. For a short biography of Parry, see Hull (1998).

11 John C. Waller demonstrates in this volume the extent to which biological and non-biological notions of nobility were still undifferentiated around 1800. The crystallization of a biological understanding of hereditary qualities as we can observe it increasingly in animal husbandry and, as I argue, in Goethe marks an innovative step in the understanding of reproduction and heredity.

12 The switch between male and female pronouns is so puzzling that it is ignored in Blackall's translation: "Sadly we brought *her* here, here shall *she* stay ... Her head we crowned with roses, sweet and friendly was her gaze" (*Apprenticeship*, 352, emphasis mine).
In his diary from 22 September 1786, Goethe uses the masculine or neuter article when referring to Mignon: "Ich war lang willens Verona oder Vicenz *dem* Mignon zum Vaterland zu geben" (For a long time, I wanted to make Verona or Vicenz the fatherland of the Mignon, *Lehrjahre* 1139, emphasis mine). Similarly, Lothario refers to Mignon using the masculine article: "*der* arme Mignon scheint sich zu verzehren" (the poor Mignon seems to yearn, *Lehrjahre* 887, emphasis mine).

13 I have modified Blackall's translation by using "woman" instead of "wife" for "Weib" in the German original (*Lehrjahre* 895).

14 Hence, my reading does not confirm earlier claims that Therese's and Natalie's androgyny is a sign of a natural wholeness, as often claimed. See, for example: "The attraction which figures like ... Therese (the 'true Amazone') and Natalie (the 'beautiful Amazone') have for Wilhelm in the novel hints towards the strive for 'harmonious development' of his human nature. The connection of male and female sexual characteristics ... hint towards the ideal of perfection of the human race in the platonic tradition" (*Lehrjahre*, 378, note 6). See also Larrett (1968/9). On the question of androgyny in Goethe, see also Fuhrmann (1995), MacLeod (1993), and Tobin (2000).

15 For a discussion of the distinction between androgyny and hermaphroditism, see also Gilbert (2002, 9–12).

16 Blackall's translation: "a silly androgynous creature."

17 It is also Jarno who has a hermaphrodite aide once he appears as Montan in the *Journeyman Years*. Like Mignon, this aide speaks in a way which is difficult to understand.

18 Blackall translates: "[Mignon's] rigid limbs unfroze her whole inner self poured itself out."

19 In reports on hermaphrodites, the discovery of a person's sexual condition was often connected to a doctor's visit for another reason (cf. Schochow 2009, 220).

20 See also Daston and Park (1995).

21 For a history of the growing tendency to assess hermaphroditism using biological criteria in the nineteenth century, see Dreger (1998) and Mak (2012).

22 Christian Ludwig Mursinna (1744–1823) was professor of surgery in Berlin from the 1780s. Goethe was familiar with his work and when Mursinna died in 1823, Goethe commented on the death with the following words, "May young striving men with the same seriousness and pure strong activity be encouraged ... by such noble model" (8 June 1823) (Goethe 1993, 308).

23 In his 1741 publication on hermaphroditism, James Parsons had already claimed that the hermaphrodite is nothing else than a woman with an enlarged clitoris.

24 Goethe was bothered by the necessity of dissection for medical training. In fact, as Gerhard Müller has pointed out, in *Wilhelm Meisters Wanderjahre* this criticism is included in the third book when Wilhelm starts his training as a surgeon (*Wanderjahre*, 601–8). The problem of mere body as scientific object and the neglect of the feelings of the bereaved because of strong interest in the deceased body occupied Goethe up to the very end of his life. In his essay "Plastische Anatomie" (completed in February 1832, one month before his death) and in the *Wanderjahre* (604), the suggestion is to use wax models instead (cf. Müller 2003).

25 Blackall translates the last sentence of the given quotation as: "Draw near, my friends, and observe the wonders of art, the sum of solicitude!"
26 Among the institutions for which Goethe, together with C. G. Voigt, became responsible for after returning from Italy was an anatomical collection (see Schmid 1998, 39–42).
27 I thank Lucia Dacome from the Institute for the History and Philosophy of Science and Technology (University of Toronto) for pointing me to scholarship on seventeenth- and eighteenth-century techniques of anatomical preservation and display.
28 *Lehrjahre*, 895, note 22.
29 Similarly, Luke 20: 34–6: "And Jesus answering said unto them, "The children of this world marry and are given in marriage. But they which shall be accounted worthy to obtain that World and the resurrection from the dead, neither marry nor are given in marriage, neither can they die any more; for they are equal unto the angels and are the children of God, being the children of the resurrection."
30 The practice of dissecting brings the Tower Society into close connection to Enlightenment paradigms, thereby exposing its latent anachronism. As Barabara Stafford has noted, "Anatomy and its inseparable practice of dissection were the eighteenth-century paradigm for any forced, artful, contrived, and violent study of depths" (Stafford 1997, 47).

REFERENCES

Ammerlahn, H. 1981. "Puppe-Tänzer-Dämon-Genius-Engel: Naturkind, Poesiekind und Kunstwerdung bei Goethe." *German Quarterly* 54 (1): 19–32. http://dx.doi.org/10.2307/405829.

Baßler, M. 1997. "Goethe und die Bodysnatcher." In *Von der Natur zur Kunst zurück*, edited by M. Baßler, C. Brecht, and D. Niefanger, 181–97. Tübingen: Niemeyer. http://dx.doi.org/10.1515/9783110931181.

Bäumer, K. 1993. "Wiederholte Spiegelungen – Goethes 'Mignon' und die 'Neue Melusine." In *Goethes Mignon und ihre Schwestern*, edited by G. Hoffmeister, 113–33. New York: Peter Lang.

Cook, H.J. 2002. "Time's Bodies: Crafting the Preparation and Preservation of Naturalia." In *Merchants and Marvels: Commerce, Science, and Art in Early Modern Europe*, edited by P.H. Smith and P. Findlen, 223–47. London: Routledge.

Daston, L., and K. Park. 1995. "The Hermaphrodite and the Orders of Nature: Sexual Ambiguity in Early Modern France." *GLQ: A Journal of Lesbian and Gay Studies* 1 (4): 419–38.

Dreger, A.D. 1998. *Hermaphrodites and the Medical Invention of Sex.* Cambridge, MA: Harvard University Press.
Egger, I. 2001. "'Verbinden mehr als Trennen': Goethe und die plastische Anatomie." *Germanisch-Romanische Monatsschrift* 51 (1): 45–53.
Eissler, K.R. 1985. *Goethe: eine psychoanalytische Studie 1775–1786.* Vol. 2. Translated by P. Fischer and R. Scholz, edited by R. Scholz, W. Mauser, and J. Cremerius. Basel and Frankfurt a. M.: Stroemfeld/Roter Stern.
Fuhrmann, H. 1995. *Der androgyne Mensch: "Bild"und "Gestalt" der Frau und des Mannes im Werk Goethes.* Würzburg: Königshausen & Neumann.
Gilbert, R. 2002. *Early Modern Hermaphrodites: Sex and Other Stories.* New York: Palgrave. http://dx.doi.org/10.1057/9780230510227.
Goethe, J.W. 1989a. *Wilhelm Meister's Apprenticeship.* Edited and translated by Eric A. Blackall in cooperation with Victor Lange. New York: Suhrkamp.
Goethe, J.W. 1989b. *Wilhelm Meisters Wanderjahre. Sämtliche Werke, Briefe, Tagebücher und Gespräche.* Vol. 10. Edited by G. Neumann and H.-G. Drewitz, 261–774. Frankfurt a. M.: Deutscher Klassiker Verlag.
Goethe, J.W. 1989c. *Sämtliche Werke.* Vol. 12, Zur Naturwissenschaft überhaupt, besonders zur Morphologie. Erfahrung, Betrachtung, Folgerung, durch Lebensereignisse verbunden. Edited by H.J. Becker et al. Munich: Carl Hanser.
Goethe, J.W. 1992. *Wilhelm Meisters Lehrjahre. Sämtliche Werke. Briefe, Tagebücher und Gespräche.* Vol. 9. Edited by H. Jaumann and W. Voßkamp, 357–992. Frankfurt a. M.: Deutscher Klassiker Verlag. (abbreviated *Lehrjahre*)
Goethe, J.W. 1993. *Sämtliche Werke.* Vol. 13.2, *Die Jahre 1820–1826.* Edited by Karl Richter. Munich: Carl Hanser.
Groß, S. 1993. "Diskursregelung und Weiblichkeit: Mignon und ihre Schwestern." In *Goethes Mignon und ihre Schwestern*, edited by G. Hoffmeister, 83–99. New York: Peter Lang.
Hansen, J.V. 1996. "Resurrecting Death: Anatomical Art in the Cabinet of Dr. Frederik Ruysch." *Art Bulletin* 78 (4): 663–79. http://dx.doi.org/10.2307/3046214.
Hederich, Benjamin. (1770) 1968. *Gründliches mythologisches Lexicon: Durchgesehen, ansehnlich vermehrete und verbessert von Johann Joachim Schwaben.* Leipzig: In Gleditschens Handlung.
Hufeland, C.W. 1801. "Beschreibung und Abbildung eines zu Berlin beobachteten weiblichen Hermaphroditen. Vol. 12/3." In *Journal der practischen Arzneykunde und Wundarzneykunst*, by C.W.Hufeland, 170–2. Berlin: Ungers Journalhandlung. (quoted in Schochow 2009)
Hull, G. 1998. "Caleb Hillier Parry 1755–1822: A Notable Provincial Physician." *Journal of the Royal Society of Medicine* 9:335–8.
Jaumann, H., and W. Voßkamp. 1992. "Die Sozialutopie der Turmgesellschaft und ihre Ausgrenzungen." In J. W. Goethe. *Sämtliche Werke. Briefe,*

Tagebücher und Gespräche, edited by H. Jaumann and W. Voßkamp, 9: 1374–8. Frankfurt a. M.: Deutscher Klassiker.

Kittler, F.A. 1978. "Über die Sozialisation Wilhelm Meisters." In *Dichtung als Sozialisationsspiel*, edited by F. Kittler and G. Kaiser. 13–124. Göttingen: Vandenhoeck & Ruprecht.

Kniesche, T.W. 1993. "Die psychoanalytische Rezeption von Mignon." In *Goethes Mignon und ihre Schwestern*, edited by G. Hoffmeister, 61–81. New York: Peter Lang.

Laqueur, T. 1990. *Making Sex: Body and Gender from the Greeks to Freud*. Cambridge, MA: Harvard University Press.

Larrett, W. 1968/9. "Wilhelm Meister and the Amazons: The Quest for Wholeness." *Publications of the English Goethe Society* 39:31–56.

Long, K.P. 2006. *Hermaphrodites in Renaissance Europe*. Aldershot, Hampshire, and Burlington, VT: Ashgate.

MacLeod, C. 1993. "Pedagogy and Androgyny in *Wilhelm Meisters Lehrjahre*." *MLN* 108 (3): 389–426. http://dx.doi.org/10.2307/2904753.

MacLeod, C. 1998. *Embodying Ambiguity: Androgyny and Aesthetics from Winckelmann to Keller*. Detroit: Wayne State University Press.

Mak, G. 2012. *Doubting Sex: Inscriptions, Bodies and Selves in Nineteenth-Century Hermaphrodite Case Histories*. Manchester: Manchester University Press.

Margócsy, D. 2009. "Advertising Cadavers in the Republic of Letters: Anatomical Publications in the Early Modern Netherlands." *British Journal of the History of Science* 42 (2): 187–210. http://dx.doi.org/10.1017/S0007087408001556.

Müller, G.H. 2003. "'Der Künstler setzt sich an die Stelle der Natur': Goethes Alternativen in der Plastischen Anatomie." In *Anatomie: Sektionen einer medizinischen Wissenschaft im 18. Jahrhundert*, edited by J. Helm and K. Stukenbrock, 211–23. Wiesbaden: Franz Steiner Verlag.

Mursinna, C.L. 1801. "Von einer besonderen Naturbegebenheit." *Journal für die Chirurgie, Arzneykunde und Geburtshilfe* 1:555–9.

Neickelio, C.F. [Caspar Friedrich Jenckel]. 1727. *Museographia oder Anleitung zum rechten Begriff und nützlicher Anregung der Museorum oder Raritätenkammern*. Leipzig and Breslau: Michael Hubert.

Nonnenmacher, H. 2002. *Natur und Fatum: Inzest als Motiv und Thema in der französischen und deutschen Literatur des 18. Jahrhunderts*. Frankfurt a. M. Peter Lang.

Parry, C.H. 1806. "Part II. History of the Merino-Ryeland Breed of the Author." *Communications to the Board of Agriculture; on Subjects Relative to the Husbandry, and Internal Improvement of the Country*. Vol. 5, pts 1–2, 433–526. London: Eighteenth Century Collections Online. Gale document number: CW109575029.

Parsons, J. 1741. *A Mechanical and Critical Enquiry into the Nature of Hermaphrodites*. London: Walthoe.
Quigley, C. 2001. *Skulls and Skeletons: Human Bone Collections and Accumulations*. Jefferson, NC: McFarland.
Rainer, U. 1993. "A Question of Silence: Goethe's Speechless Women." In *Goethes Mignon und ihre Schwestern*, edited by G. Hoffmeister, 101–11. New York: Peter Lang.
Ruysch, Frederik. 1737. *Opera Omnia Anatomico-Medico Chirurgica*. Amsterdam: Janssonio-Waesbergios.
Schmid, I. 1998. "Amtliche Tätigkeit." In *Goethe Handbuch in vier Bänden*. Vol. 4/1, *Personen, Sachen, Begriffe A-K*, edited by H.-D. Dahnke and R. Otto, 33–46. Stuttgart and Weimar: Metzler.
Schochow, M. 2009. *Die Ordnung der Hermaphroditen-Geschlechter: Eine Genealogie des Geschlechtsbegriffs*. Berlin: Akademie Verlag. http://dx.doi.org/10.1524/9783050088877.
Sebright, J. 1809. *The Art of Improving the Breeds of Domestic Animals*. London: John Harding.
Sinclair, J. 1823. *Grundsätze des Ackerbaues nebst Bemerkungen über Gartenbau*. Vienna: Obstbaumzucht, Forst-Cultur und Holzpflanzungen.
Stafford, B.M. 1997. *Body Criticism: Imagining the Unseen in Enlightenment Art and Medicine*. Cambridge, MA: Massachusetts Institute of Technology Press.
Stark, D.J.C. 1801. "Kurze Beschreibung eines sogenannten Hermaphroditen oder Zwitters, welcher aber mehr zum männlichen, als weiblichen Geschlechte zu rechnen ist, nebst einer Vorerinnerung von dem Herausgeber." In *Neues Archiv für die Geburtshülfe, Frauenzimmer- und Kinderkrankheiten mit Hinsicht auf die Physiologie, Diätektik und Chirurgie*, edited by D.J.C. Stark, 538–56. Zweyten Bandes, drittes Stück. Jena: Wolfgang Strahl. (quoted in Schochow 2009)
Tiffany, G. 1995. *Erotic Beasts and Social Monsters: Shakespeare, Jonson, and Comic Androgyny*. London: Associated University Press.
Tobin, R. 1993. "The Medicinalization of Mignon." In *Goethes Mignon und ihre Schwestern*, edited by G. Hoffmeister, 42–60. New York: Peter Lang.
Tobin, R. 2000. *Warm Brothers: Queer Theory and the Age of Goethe*. Philadelphia: University of Pennsylvania Press.
Wilson, D. 1984. "Science, Natural Law, and Unwitting Incest in Eighteenth-Century Literature." *Studies in Eighteenth-Century Culture* 13:249–70.
Wood, R.J., and V. Orel. 2001. *Genetic Prehistory in Selective Breeding: A Prelude to Mendel*. Oxford: Oxford University Press.

PART TWO

Fetus, Child, Mother

7 Changing Views on Generation – Images of the Unborn

SEBASTIAN PRANGHOFER

How are the embryo, fetus, and the female body created as an object of knowledge? And what are the identities of the fetal and the female bodies? These are important, historical, and ongoing questions in modern Western culture (Duden 1993; Dubow 2011). These questions have largely been answered through visual representations of the fetal and the female bodies (Petchesky 1987; Newman 1996). The identity of the unborn[1] changed fundamentally from the second half of the seventeenth to the end of the eighteenth century. While preformationist ideas became a challenge to Aristotelian concepts of epigenesis in the late seventeenth century, the eighteenth century saw ongoing debates about the validity of these concepts. Only towards the end of the eighteenth century did neo-epigenetic theories become predominant, based as they were on a secularized account of reproduction.

Within these debates images of embryos and fetuses reflected uncertainties and changes in notions about the unborn. These images were often more than mere illustrations of reproductive processes. Drawing, for example, on Christian iconography or neoclassical aesthetics they expressed more general sociocultural values associated with the unborn. Thus issues of generation not only mattered for the identity of the unborn as a biological entity but also raised questions about both its metaphysical and moral status. This also affected the relationship between the maternal body and the body of the unborn, where traditionally the fate of the unborn and the mother were inextricably linked through the Christian narrative of salvation. Yet Enlightenment science shaped the maternal body and the unborn as separate entities whose identities were not so much determined by their mutual relationship but their individual reproductive capacities.

To discuss such issues this chapter draws on a variety of sources ranging from midwifery manuals to embryological treatises and anatomical prints. It also reviews the literature on the early modern visual representation of the unborn. Beyond their genre-specific function of conveying, for example, practical obstetrical knowledge or anatomical information, images of the unborn always carried surplus meaning. When analysing visual representations of the unborn the focus is on how they mediated, occasionally within the same picture, a variety of ambiguous and contested views of the embryo and the fetus. The first section of the chapter reviews recent research on visual representations and the identity of the unborn since the Renaissance. This shows the difficulties in interpreting early modern images of the unborn as markers of prenatal identity. Subsequently midwifery books and embryological works are used to demonstrate how images of the unborn shaped it as an object of knowledge. While these images were attempts to get a grip on the physical nature of the unborn, they still had to deal with uncertainties about its metaphysical nature. Therefore, the third section of the chapter discusses the construction of fetal identity within the framework of the Christian narrative of salvation, drawing mainly on anatomical and physico-theological literature. The final section shows how images of embryos and fetuses underwent a fundamental change in the second half of the eighteenth century, when Christian iconography was replaced by neoclassical aesthetics to determine the identity of the unborn.

Personhood before Birth?

In *Fetal Positions*, Karen Newman has shown that contemporary images of the unborn are part of a long visual tradition, from late medieval obstetrical illustrations, renaissance anatomy, eighteenth-century obstetrical atlases and anatomical wax models to modern obstetrics (Newman 1996). Her book was the first comprehensive account of the Western visual tradition of representations of the unborn. Newman claimed that common to all these images was that they tended to isolate the fetus from the female body or reduced the female body to its reproductive capacity and inscribed the fetus with individual identity. She assumed that since the Enlightenment the identity of the unborn was modelled on modern subjectivity. Eve Keller argued along similar lines when she claimed with regards to late seventeenth-century embryological illustrations that "competing theories of embryogenesis and the conflicting formulations of the embryo itself take part in the conceptual struggles accompanying the emergence of the early-modern individual" (Keller 2000, 333). Keller also assumed a prenatal individual identity and assigned embryology a crucial role in establishing such an identity for the unborn (Keller 2005). She argued that embryology, especially in its variant as animalculist preformation, provided a mechanist explanation for generation while protecting subjectivity against the threat mechanism posed to itself.

Both Newman and Keller remained rather vague about the specific characteristics of the identity of the unborn before the Enlightenment. They also tended to underestimate the often ambiguous identity of the unborn as a liminal being. As Barbara Duden argued, images of the unborn did not necessarily represent something that was already present, but had to be seen as "emblems of the coming child" (Duden 2002, 27). Only birth could reveal the true appearance and identity of the child. For Duden even microscopic observations revealed more about the theoretical concepts of generation that were imposed on them than what could actually be identified in the specimen (37). However, to determine the identity of the unborn these theories were often deficient and questions about the beginning of human life had strong theological implications. With regards to the Christian narrative of salvation it was crucial to know from what point the immortal soul of the unborn was at stake (31–6).

Although anatomy and embryology were male domains in the early modern period, the ascriptions made to the fetal and the female body in these areas did not remain unchallenged. Male discourses of the fetal and the female body had to consider cultural meanings of the body and concepts of gender. They were also not isolated from predominantly female areas of practice like childbirth and domestic care, and were confronted with genuine female somatic experiences of pregnancy, labour, and childbirth. This led to conflicts especially in the area of midwifery, where male practitioners were in increasing competition with well-established female practitioners from the second half of the seventeenth century (Wilson 2007). Therefore, according to Ludmilla Jordanova, eighteenth-century obstetrical atlases in particular have to be understood as part of a male strategy to establish hegemony over hitherto female dominated areas and experiences (Jordanova 1985). However, Lianne McTavish has recently shown in her work on early modern French midwifery treatises how this process was not a one-sided patriarchal subjection of a previously female domain, but "that men's entry into the lying-in chamber was a complex negotiation involving their adaption to the demands of women" (McTavish 2005, 217). In such a context, gendered inscriptions on the fetal and the female body were complex and contentious as results of power relations in which women were both agents and subjects to male superiority (Fissell 1995).

The illustrations of anatomical handbooks, obstetrical atlases, and embryological works were evidence of the pursuit for the hegemony of male knowledge about generation, and illustrations of the fetal body attributed it with a distinct identity. This identity was framed by early modern natural philosophy, ideas about subjectivity and Christian understanding of human nature. Yet these ideas were not stable and changed fundamentally during the long eighteenth century. While illustrations in midwifery manuals and obstetrical atlases showed the changing relationship between the female and the fetal body, early modern natural philosophers discussed in embryological treatises various concepts of generation, ranging from Aristotelian epigenesis to preformationist theories and early ontogenetic ideas. Meanwhile a moralizing iconography made wide-ranging claims about the status of the unborn within Christian salvation history. Towards the end of the eighteenth century, however, the fetal body became a scientific object in its own right and was gradually disjoined from the female body.

The Unborn as an Object of Knowledge

The most coherent iconography of the unborn in the West was established from the Middle Ages in illustrated midwifery manuals such as the various versions of the *Gynaecia*, a gynaecological text from late antiquity that borrowed heavily from the Greek physician Soranus of Ephesus (first/second century AD). This text circulated widely in medieval Europe and was often illustrated with images representing the situation of the fetus in the womb (Bonnet-Cadilhac 1995). The earliest such illustrations are from the Muscio manuscript (around 900 AD), an abbreviated Latin translation of the *Gynaecia*, dating from around 500 AD. These images were first published in print in the early sixteenth century and remained the iconographical model for the next three centuries (Green 2009). The illustrations depicted the unborn in various poses within the womb and were intended to help midwives understand the different positions of the fetus in utero just before birth and the potential complications during birth, resulting from the abnormal positions of the fetus. The images remained part of the iconographic repertoire of midwifery books throughout the seventeenth and into the eighteenth century (Newman 1996, 26). In frequent reprints the series of images remained in circulation well into the eighteenth century, as in Jane Sharp's *The Midwives Book* (1671) and François Mauriceau's (1637–1709) *Des maladies des femmes grosses et accouchées* (1668).

The illustrations in midwifery books in the tradition of Muscio were primarily concerned with the different positions the fetus might obtain before birth. The importance of the mediation of practical knowledge in illustrations in midwifery books becomes particularly evident with Justina Siegemund's (1636–1705) *Hoff-Wehe-Mutter* (Tatlock 2005).[2] Siegemund was midwife at the court of Brandenburg and published her book in 1690 as a dialogue between an experienced midwife and her pupil (Tatlock 1992). The illustrations in the book included a series of twelve images showing the various positions of the child during birth (figure 7.1). While these illustrations were modelled on older images, which also showed the unborn in a rather abstract uterus with little if any anatomical detail, they were remarkable in how they emphasized the practical aspects of showing the fetal positions. They gave explicit practical advice by showing how the midwife could grab and move the child during difficult births. Simultaneously the way the child had to be held and the particular moves to ensure a successful birth were also explained in the accompanying text.

Yet the interior of the female body often remained obscure in such illustrations, and the unborn appeared as an active individual moving about the womb. This notion of a child trapped inside the uterus conformed to early modern notions of childbirth. Usually the unborn was described as actively pushing itself out of the womb, as if it was captured and contained inside the maternal body, about to liberate itself from its prison during birth (Newman 1996, 33, 126). This view was reflected in the illustrations of midwifery books with the fetus moving independently within a uterus, which was detached from the female body. On one hand, this omission of the female body can be understood as the representation of a notion of the unborn as an autonomous agent and the mother's body its passive host. On the other, the illustrations in midwifery books were situated in a moment of transition when the different poses of the unborn in the womb were usually described as representations of the different positions of the child *at birth*. These illustrations were therefore imaginary representations of the unborn and were characterized by a certain degree of uncertainty about the true appearance of the unborn, which could ultimately only be confirmed after the child was born.

Other obstetrical illustrations also represented the unborn within the womb and provided more anatomical context when they showed the different layers of the womb opening like a flower revealing the fully formed

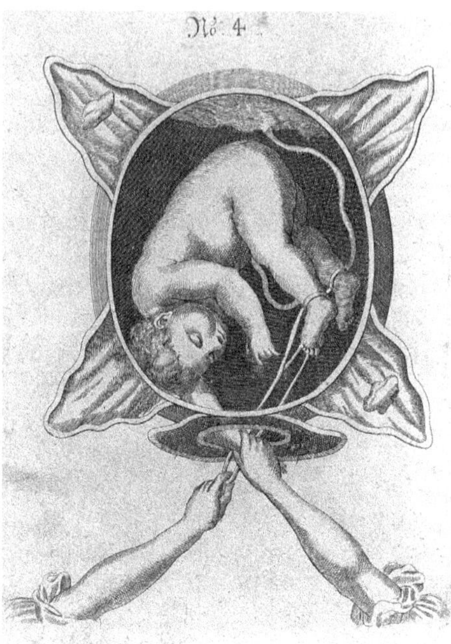

Figure 7.1 Illustration of techniques to move the fetus into a position suitable for birth. Engraving in J. Siegemund, *Die Chur-Brandenburgische Hoff-Wehe-Mutter* (Cölln an der Spree: Liebpert, 1690), plate IV. Courtesy of Wellcome Library, London.

child (McTavish 2005, 199). Such an iconography referred to a discourse in which agricultural metaphors were very common to describe human reproduction (Wagner 2011, 552–7). Illustrations of the positions of the unborn inside the uterus were often supplemented by images showing the unborn in situ. From the sixteenth century, some illustrations from an anatomical context were added to this canon, such as whole-body figures representing the anatomy of the pregnant uterus, some of them showing the unborn crouching inside the womb. These full body figures had their origins in the medieval anatomical manuscript tradition and circulated widely in midwifery manuals and anatomical texts, as well as anatomical fugitive sheets during the sixteenth and seventeenth centuries. These images usually represented a sitting female figure with the legs opened. On the anatomical fugitive sheets, readers would be able to lift the abdominal wall to gaze into the body where they would see the internal organs and frequently the unborn inside the womb.

These anatomical fugitive sheets usually came in pairs of a male and a female figure and frequently made references to biblical history by identifying them as Adam and Eve (Carlino 1999, 74–88). Such biblical references also featured explicitly in midwifery manuals and could still be found, for example, in the 1724 edition of Sharp's book (figure 7.2). Copied from the earlier editions of the book this engraving represents a female figure with her womb opened so that the fetus could be seen curled up in the uterus. A flower covering her pubic area identifies her as Eve after the fall of man. The image is drawing on a series of illustrations from Adriaan van der Spiegel's *De formato foetu* (1626), a book on the anatomy of the fetus and the uterus. In this book a series of four illustrations showed a pregnant female figure with her uterus at different stages of dissection. On the last image the uterus was fully opened and the figure was holding a fruit behind her back while a lily covered her vagina. This reference to Eve not only provided a rationale for the pains of labour as a consequence of original sin, but also held the promise of future redemption. If the flower was seen as a symbol of the annunciation, the image would also refer to the salvation of man through Christ's self-sacrifice (Newman 1996, 82).

Visualizing Preformation

A different kind of knowledge was associated with images of the unborn in embryological texts from the seventeenth to the eighteenth century. In the context of debates about preformation the unborn had become an object of learned curiosity that had far-reaching consequences for its identity. The last few decades of the seventeenth century saw a significant shift in the notion of the unborn when authors such as the Dutch anatomist Theodor Kerckring (1638–93) saw a "child" in the uterus only a few days after conception (Kerckring 1671, 3–4). Keller interpreted such attributions of personhood as a response to the threats posed by mechanist theories of generation and suggested that they were fundamental for the formation of early modern identity (Keller 2005, 125–7).

By the end of the seventeenth century, mechanist theories of generation and the animalculist concept of pre-existence of man in the male semen were widely discussed in natural philosophy (Bowler 1971). Key to this debate were the observations by the Dutch microscopist Anton Leeuwenhoek (1632–1723), published in the *Philosophical Transactions* of the Royal Society, where he had first reported his observations of little animalcula in the male semen (Leeuwenhoek 1677/8). Later he would be credited with the discovery of the spermatozoon as one of the most

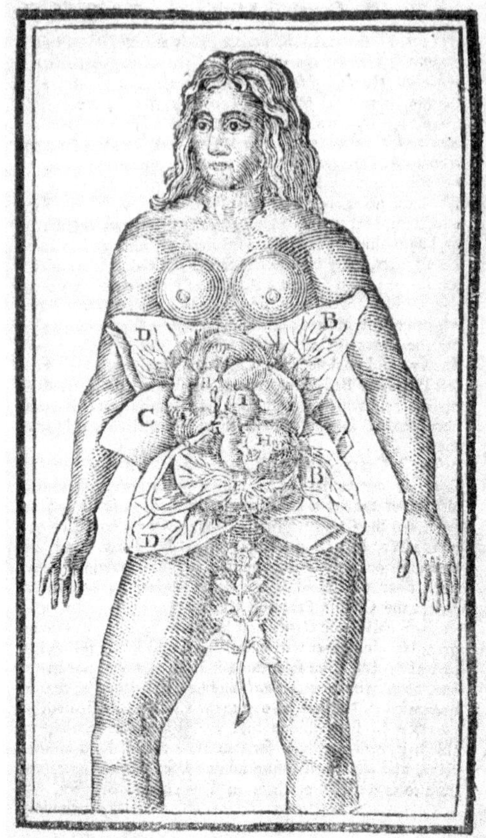

Figure 7.2 Pregnant woman with her womb opened and revealing the unborn. Engraving in J. Sharp, *The Compleat Midwife's Companion; or, the art of midwifery improv'd*. 3rd ed. (London: J. Marshall), 97. Courtesy of Wellcome Library, London.

significant discoveries of the microscope (Ruestow 1983, 190). Leeuwenhoek believed that "the fruits [came] from the male seed, and the females only [contributed] to the nourishment and growth of it" (Leeuwenhoek 1683, 349). However, he stopped short of subscribing to the idea of pre-existence. Although Leeuwenhoek was convinced that the entire human being was in the spermatozoon, he suggested that ultimately the exact appearance of the preformed man would remain unknown (Ruestow 1983, 211).

Accordingly, Leeuwenhoek rejected illustrations of the spermatozoon which had been published under the pen-name Dalenpatius with a letter to the Royal Society in 1699.[3] Leeuwenhoek suggested that because of the limitations of the microscope to make infinitely small objects visible in order to "find such a perfect Human shape ... I am certainly persuaded you will not allow of it" (Leeuwenhoek 1699, 303). Despite Leeuwenhoek's doubts, the idea that a fully formed human being pre-existed in the sperm had already become very convincing. The French naturalist Nicolas Hartsoeker (1656–1725), for example, had an illustration added to his *Essay de dioptrique* (1694), which showed a little human figure crouching in the head of a spermatozoon (figure 7.3). However, what appeared to be icons of pre-existence theories did not establish an iconographic tradition in early modern embryology. While Hartsoeker was only able to claim that his figure represented what we would see if we could look through the skin which hides the little animal in the sperm, Dalenpatius's observations were considered as unreliable by contemporaries because of their high degree of imagination (Leeuwenhoek 1699, 305). As a consequence, visual representations of the spermatozoon and the unborn did not produce strong evidence for animalculist-preformationist theories of generation.

Hitherto the debates about generation during the period between the 1670s and the Haller-Wolff debate of the 1760s and 1770s have often been characterized as dominated by animalculist-preformationist theories (Roe 1981, 9; Pinto-Correia 1997, 3; Cunningham 2010, 168). However, the story appears to be more complex, and rather than being dominated by a particular theory of generation, a variety of often overlapping theories competed in seventeenth- and eighteenth-century debates about generation (Richards 1992, 5–16). The Italian physician and naturalist Antonio Vallisneri (1661–1730) accepted the existence of animalcula in the male semen and duly reproduced illustrations of the observations of other authors in his book on human and animal generation when he discussed the history of the animalcula (Vallisneri 1739, 13; figure 7.4).

But although Vallisneri had accepted the existence of little "semen-worms," he rejected the idea that they were animalcula in which a human being was enclosed (126–7). He thought of them as a kind of worm that could also be found in other parts of the body. According to Vallisneri, the true use of the semen-worms was not reproductive, but was to prevent the semen from coagulating by constantly stirring it with their movement (198–9). Against this background the illustrations of previous authors of their observations of semen-worms became unproblematic and no longer posed a challenge that required an elaborate response within the debates

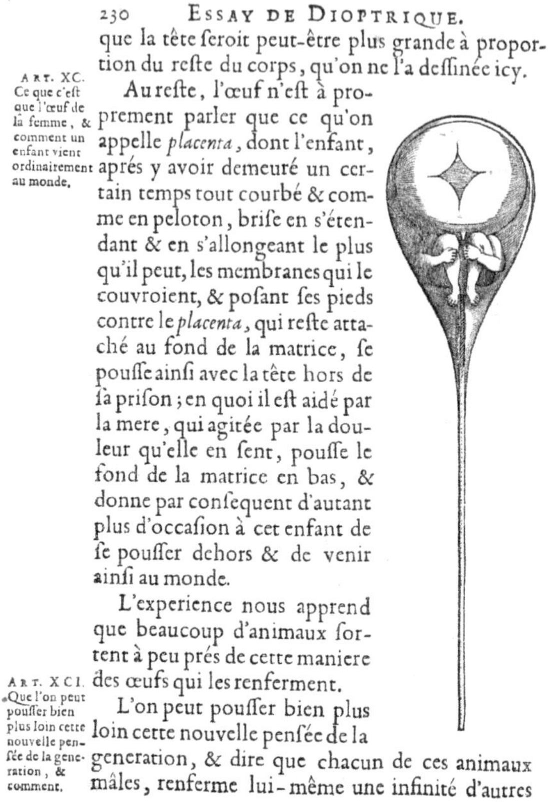

230 ESSAY DE DIOPTRIQUE.

que la tête feroit peut-être plus grande à proportion du refte du corps, qu'on ne l'a deffinée icy.

ART. XC. Ce que c'eft que l'œuf de la femme, & comment un enfant vient ordinairement au monde.

Au refte, l'œuf n'eft à proprement parler que ce qu'on appelle *placenta*, dont l'enfant, aprés y avoir demeuré un certain temps tout courbé & comme en peloton, brife en s'étendant & en s'allongeant le plus qu'il peut, les membranes qui le couvroient, & pofant fes pieds contre le *placenta*, qui refte attaché au fond de la matrice, fe pouffe ainfi avec la tête hors de fa prifon ; en quoi il eft aidé par la mere, qui agitée par la douleur qu'elle en fent, pouffe le fond de la matrice en bas, & donne par confequent d'autant plus d'occafion à cet enfant de fe pouffer dehors & de venir ainfi au monde.

L'experience nous apprend que beaucoup d'animaux fortent à peu prés de cette maniere des œufs qui les renferment.

ART. XCI. Que l'on peut pouffer bien plus loin cette nouvelle penfée de la generation, & comment.

L'on peut pouffer bien plus loin cette nouvelle penfée de la generation, & dire que chacun de ces animaux mâles, renferme lui-même une infinité d'autres

Figure 7.3 The unborn crouching in the head of a sperm. Engraving in N. Hartsoeker, *Essay de dioptrique* (Paris: Jean Anisson), 230. Courtesy of Landesbibliothek Oldenburg (LBO), Nw I 9/51.

about preformation. As a thinning agent the semen-worms could not, unlike the animalcula, enclose a little human being and had lost their significance in debates about generation, while their very existence could still be accommodated. Therefore, Vallisneri did not need to comment on the illustrations in detail, but could simply add them to his book without having to speculate about the implications of the discovery of the "semen worms" on matters of generation.

While Vallisneri adopted the idea of animalcula in the male semen, the works of other authors, who maintained a more traditional view, such as

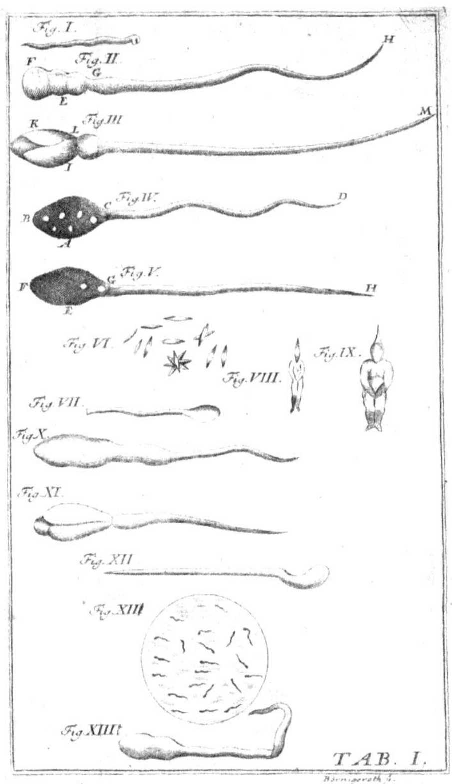

Figure 7.4 Various illustrations of microscopic observations of male semen compiled from different authors. Engraving in A. Vallisneri, *Historie von der Erzeugung der Menschen und Thiere etc.* Translated by C.P. Berger (Lemgo: Johann Heinrich Meyer, 1739), plate I. Courtesy of LBO, Nw III 9b/53.

the French physician Nicolas Venette (1633–98), also circulated well into the eighteenth century (Porter and Hall 1995, 69–82). Venette even dismissed William Harvey's earlier ovist theories, which regarded the human egg as the origin out of which embryonic life grew and developed. Against such theories he still maintained the Galenic view, according to which the fetus was gradually formed out of a mix of male and female semen in the "horns" of the uterus (Venette 1696, 359–63). When it had grown too big for the restricted space of the "horns" the fetus would move into the uterus, a moment Venette was more than happy to illustrate in a crude drawing copied from Reinier de Graaf's (1641–73) *De Mulierum Organis Generationi* (figure 7.5). The image showed how the fetus, which already appeared in a human form, put pressure on the "horns" in order to move into the uterus. From this moment the fetus was attributed with a remarkable degree of subjectivity and had according to Venette the ability to give emotional responses to his mother and express feelings such as joy (399–401).

How divided the opinions on matters of generation had been for about 100 years becomes even more obvious in the reflections of the French physician and male-midwife Joseph Raulin (1708–84) on previous debates. He was keen to emphasize the particular importance of microscopy in these controversies:

> The discovery of the microscope became the source for new systems of generation. Some philosophers abandoned the doctrine of the eggs, in order to come up with others which were even less likely. With it Leuwenhoeck and Hartsoeker believed it was possible to see special bodies in the semen of most males, which appeared to them to be alive, and which they took for embryos, which were solely equipped to reproduce different species of animals over again. (Raulin 1770, 12)

Early modern microscopic images of generation were fundamentally different from the applied knowledge represented in midwifery manuals with their relatively coherent iconographic tradition. Early modern embryological works, however, generally lacked the practical aspects. At the same time a coherent iconography of the unborn did not evolve in embryology, for which the two main reasons were the lack of a dominant theory of generation and the uncertainty created by the lack of or ambiguity of the empirical evidence. Images of the unborn in the context of seventeenth- and early eighteenth-century embryology also struggled with the naturalistic paradigm of visual representations when they tried to create evidence. In the case of the little human beings in the animalcula they failed, since this object could only be imagined.

Salvation and Fetal Identity

Both illustrations in early modern midwifery books and images of generation often portrayed the gendered female body as a dangerous environment for the unborn. In midwifery manuals, focus was usually on the unborn and how it could safely be handled during birth, with the maternal

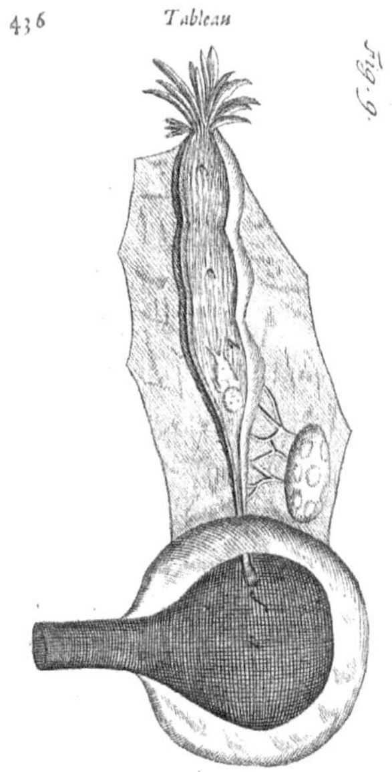

Figure 7.5 Illustration of the unborn (b) on its way through the fallopian tubes to the womb. Engraving in N. Venette, *Tableau de l'amour consideré dans l'estat du marriage*. 7th ed. (Rouen: Frédric Gaillard, 1696), 436. Courtesy of LBO, Nw III 9b/50.

body marginalized (Wagner 2011, 557–8). In embryological works and works on fetal development images of the unborn were generally completely isolated from the female body. Yet this visual emphasis on the unborn did not mean that the female body was not implicitly present or that the unborn was necessarily either an autonomous individual or could be regarded merely as a biological fact. As Kathleen Crowther and others have shown, conception, pregnancy, and childbirth were closely associated with and interpreted through biblical history (Carlino 1999; Crowther-Heyck 2002; Duden 2002). In the debates about preformation this theme featured repeatedly when the question was discussed whether each individual had actually been created by God during Genesis. The creation of Adam and Eve and the fall of man provided a powerful framework for understanding the generation of human life as imperfectly modelled on God's creation of man while the pains and the dangers of labour could be understood as punishment for original sin and the fall from Paradise.

Reflections on the status of the unborn within the Christian narrative of salvation, the sinfulness of man, and self-awareness as integral to human identity were not uncommon in the seventeenth and eighteenth centuries and familiar to a wider learned audience. The famous Amsterdam anatomist Frederik Ruysch (1638–1731), for example, kept several tableaux assemblages which incorporated fetal skeletons in his anatomical collection, a popular destination for young gentlemen on their grand tour (Hansen 1996). Ruysch added prints representing some of these still-lifes to the catalogues of his collection. On the third plate from his *Thesaurus Anatomicus Primus* (1701) Ruysch represented an object where gallstones and vascular trees were piled together with three fetal skeletons on a wooden base (figure 7.6). One of the skeletons held a tiny sickle, while the skeleton to the right was weeping in a handkerchief as if it was mourning. The accompanying text in the catalogue was not just explaining the figures, but contained moralizing biblical and classical quotes such as "Man, who is born of woman, is short-lived and full of turmoil" (Job 14:1–4; Ruysch 1701, 8–9). Such mottos suggested that mortality and sinfulness were inextricably linked with human existence and inescapable for every individual since the beginning of the world, while salvation would only come after death. In Ruysch's *Thesaurus* this insight was emphasized by two further references to the philosophers Heraklit and Demokrit, when the former bemoaned his own mortality, while the latter celebrated the victory over life in death (Ruysch 1701, 9–10; Felfe 2003, 36).

Ruysch published his catalogues during a time when debates about theories of generation were one of the big issues in the European republic of letters. After all, his anatomical collection could be read as a preformationist comment on the inevitable fate of every human being. In these debates Ruysch was a key player when he positioned himself as a supporter of ovist-preformationist views. The sixth catalogue of his collection came with a series of prints showing fetal skeletons and human eggs (Ruysch 1705, tables I–III). On the first of these plates figure 1 represented a fetal skeleton holding a human egg in its right hand and another three eggs tied with hairs to its left hand. The subsequent plates showed further fetal skeletons and dissected eggs containing embryos with rudimentary human features. This arrangement suggested that the fetus not only originated from the egg, but was also inseparable from and identical with it.

A view on human fate and human generation similar to Ruysch's was presented in the *Physica sacra* by the Swiss physician and naturalist Johann Jakob Scheuchzer (1672–1733), which was published between 1731 and 1735 in four folio volumes illustrated with 761 copper engravings. This

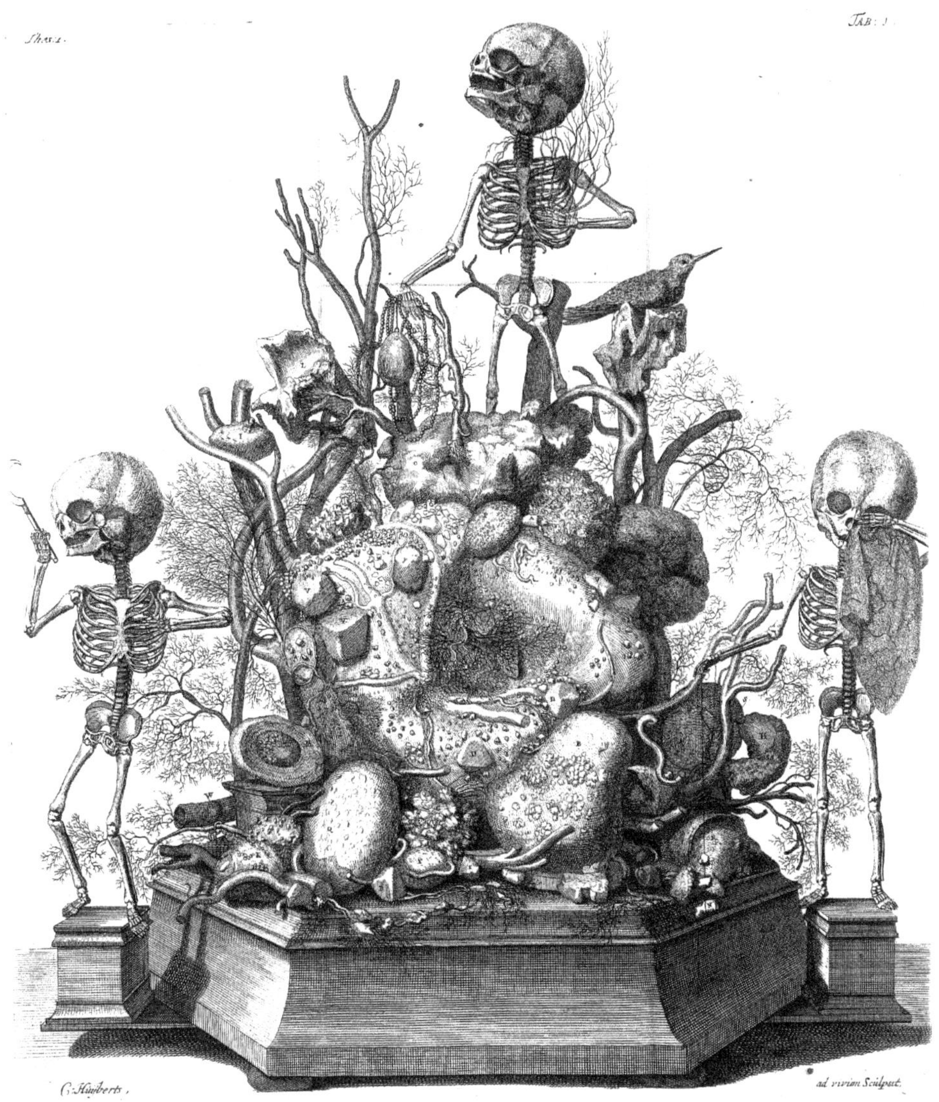

Figure 7.6 Anatomical arrangement featuring fetal skeletons. Engraving in F. Ruysch, *Thesaurus Anatomicus Primus*. (Amsterdam: Jansson-Waesberg, 1701), plate I. Courtesy of LBO, Nw III 3a/98.

biblical natural history had its intellectual background in physico-theology, which held that science would lead to God and functionalized a mechanical world view to prove the existence of God. The twenty-third plate in Scheuchzers's *Physica Sacra* represented Adam in Paradise and was part of a series of illustrations of Genesis (figure 7.7). The scene was framed with female eggs, embryos, and fetal skeletons of different developmental stages. They were copies from Ruysch's *Thesaurus Primus* and *Thesaurus Sextus* and underlined the inevitable fate of human sorrow with a preformationist argument (Felfe 2003, 27–8; van de Roemer 2010, 169–70).

The centrepiece of the plate showed Adam alone in Paradise, sitting under a tree with a rabbit, a symbol of reproductive fertility, at his feet. The background depicted a prosperous landscape with numerous pairs of animals. Adam's gaze was drawn in a mix of fear and admiration to the top left by a divine light from the sky. The picture was framed by the fetal skeletons, embryos, and human eggs. The most prominent of these objects was the mourning skeleton on the right and the skeleton holding the eggs at the top right. Robert Felfe interpreted the composition as a memento mori and prediction that with generation man will become subject to mortality (28). However, the print also allows an alternative reading. The vanitas iconography of the fetal skeletons, together with the depiction of different developmental stages from the beginnings of the human egg, made clear that mortality and sinfulness were not just the future fate of man. They showed that from a preformationist point of view every individual was inherently sinful and had been exposed already before the Fall to the perils of carnal desire, represented by the rabbit at Adam's feet, a traditional symbol of both fertility and sexual exuberance. Scheuchzer was therefore using a preformationist argument to underline the Protestant key doctrine of predestination, which made the individual immediately responsible to God alone, emphasized by the divine light on Adam's face (Stafford 1991, 238–42).

Early modern anatomical images of the fetus were often associated with a moralizing iconography and referred to the inherent sinfulness of self-conscious human beings. Thereby they defined the status of the human as a subject within the Creation. This reflected the ambitions of early modern anatomy as natural philosophy. Instead of merely representing the physical appearance and structure of the human body the aim was to achieve and mediate a superior knowledge of the status and role of mankind within God's creation. While early modern images of the unborn reflected, for example, changing theories of generation, the moralizing and metaphysical iconography remained a key element of the

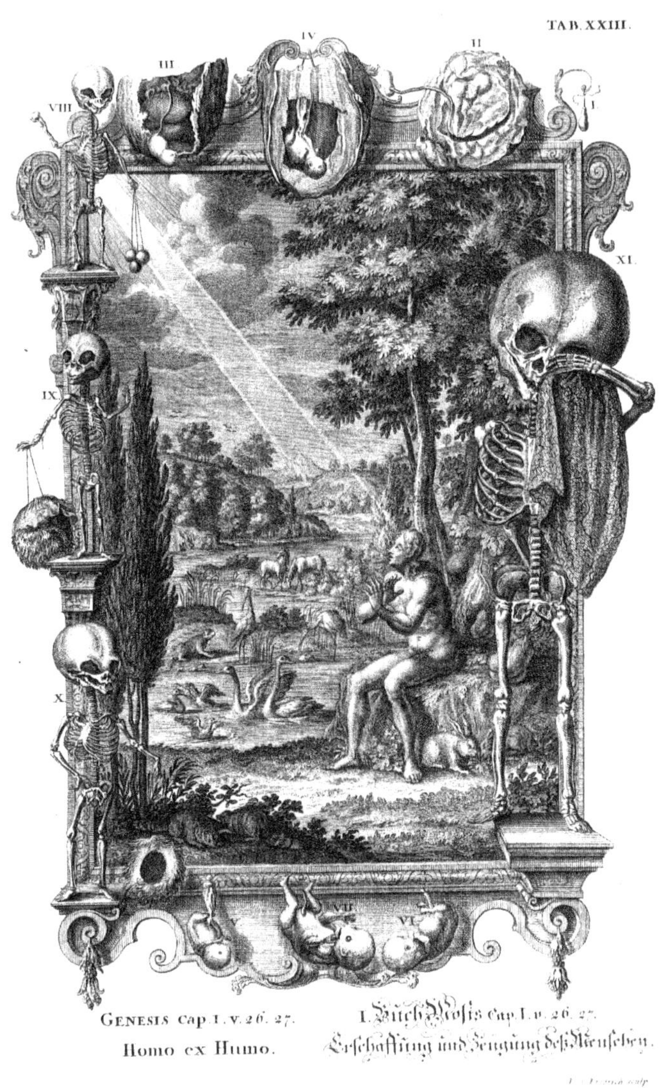

Figure 7.7 Adam in Paradise and the creation of man. Engraving in J. Scheuchzer, *Kupfer-Bibel, In welcher Die Physica Sacra, Oder Geheiligte Natur-Wissenschafft Derer In Heil. Schrifft vorkommenden Natürlichen Sachen, Deutlich erklärt und bewährt*. 4 vols (Augsburg: Johann Andreas Pfeffel, 1731), plate XXIII. Courtesy of LBO, Theol II Ak/27.

visual representation of the fetus into the mid-eighteenth century, which is evident from both Ruysch's *Thesauri* and Scheuchzer's *Physica Sacra*.

Beauty and Truth

While seventeenth- and early eighteenth-century images of the unborn were deeply rooted in Christian cosmology, a very different picture emerged in the second half of the eighteenth century. The most important concern with visual representations of the unborn was now the question how to convey the most truthful images of nature. Based on the ideal of visual truth, these images were framed by Enlightenment aesthetics rather than religious or moral concerns. When William Hunter (1718–83) published his *Anatomy of the Human Gravid Uterus* in 1774, he produced a huge folio set of anatomical plates of the pregnant uterus and the fetus, which were skilfully executed and followed an ideal of truth to nature which was based on accurate delineation of natural objects (figure 7.8; Jordanova 1985, 394–8). They also showed an intimate relationship between the female and the fetal body which made the body of the mother and the child one and subjected them to the gaze of the anatomist (Jordanova 1985, 407–9). Despite their high degree of naturalism these images were still normative images that objectified and standardized the pregnant female body and subjected it to Hunter's authority (Massey 2005, 82–3).

The objectification of the female and the fetal body was emphasized by the lack of applied knowledge in Hunter's plates. Instead they invited a more general interpretation, embracing sociocultural values and notions related to the body of both mother and child (Jordanova 1985, 399–400). Roberta McGrath has argued that Hunter's plates reduced the female body to its reproductive function: "The idea of 'Woman' started and stopped at the womb. In contrast to the fetus, which was granted integrity, the woman was much less than herself" (McGrath 2002, 82). The identity of the unborn became, as Jordanova suggested, shaped by bourgeois subjectivity. She argued that the intimate relationship between the mother's and the child's bodies represented on Hunter's plates "emphasised the intertwining of maternal and child welfare," and indicating that the child had to be cared for in order to create legitimate and healthy offspring (Jordanova 1985, 409).

However, I would suggest an additional interpretation of eighteenth-century naturalistic images of the unborn like those in Hunter's *Anatomy*. Like the authors of the older illustrations from midwifery manuals, Hunter

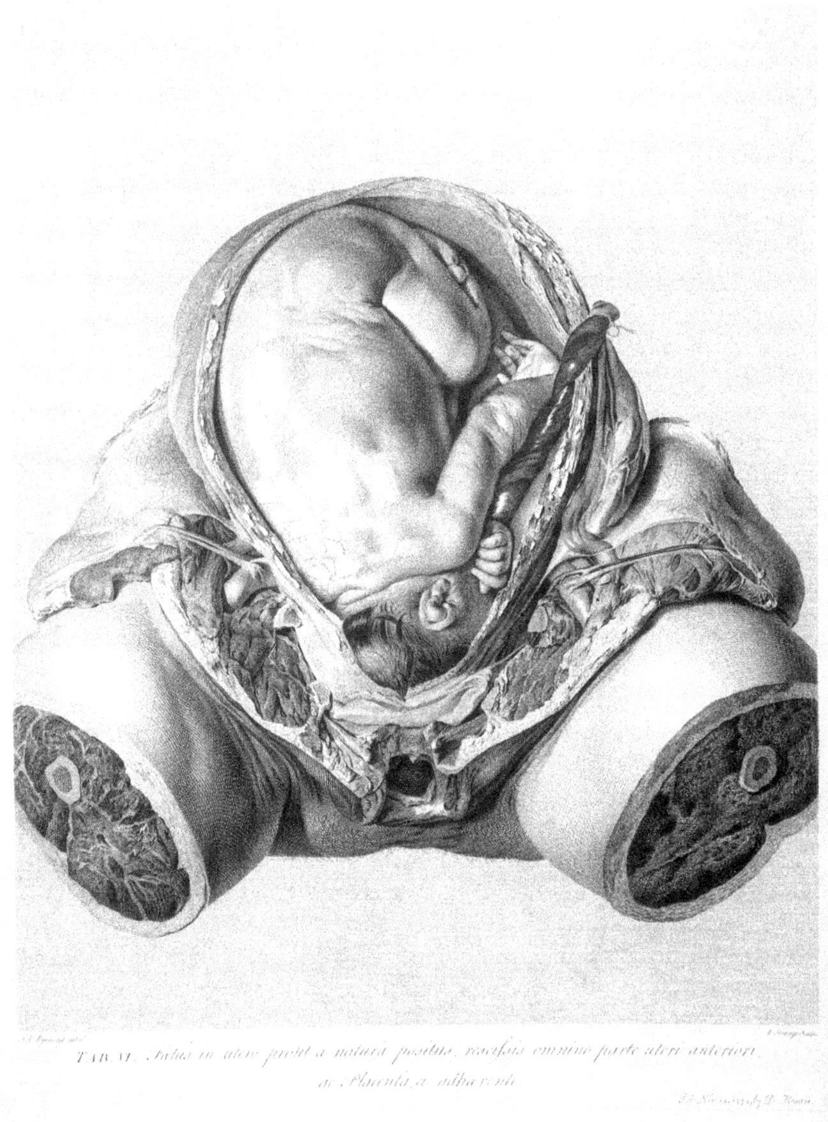

Figure 7.8 A fetus in utero. Engraving in W. Hunter, *Anatomia Uteri Humani Gravidi: Anatomy of the Human Gravid Uterus* (Birmingham and London: J. Baskerville et al., 1774), plate VI. Courtesy of Wellcome Library, London.

was less interested in the representation of fetal development. Although he noted the age of the different fetuses depicted on the plates, the images were not designed to mediate a particular theory of generation. From a pragmatic point of view they were not necessary and ignoring such issues allowed Hunter to avoid the muddy waters of debates about concepts of generation. Instead, by drawing on contemporary aesthetics, the obstetrical images allowed Hunter to raise his professional and social status by representing himself as a skilful anatomist and medical authority in midwifery. Hunter was quite familiar with the aesthetic ideas of the painter and art theorist Joshua Reynolds (1723–92), who was also president of the Royal Academy of Arts, where Hunter lectured on anatomy (Kemp 1992). However, where Reynolds promoted the representation of an idealized natural beauty, Hunter followed in his obstetrical atlas the ideas of his collaborator, the Dutch painter Jan van Rymsdyk (died 1790), who was an advocate of naturalistic imitation of nature (Mount 2006, 86–90). The illustrations in Hunter's obstetrical atlas showed great anatomical detail, were based on dissections of pregnant female bodies, and were characterized by a high degree of naturalism. Focusing on the pregnant female body, Hunter was not particularly interested in the anatomy of the unborn itself, but rather sought to portray the corpses he had dissected as accurately as possible and thereby convey the most truthful image of nature (Daston and Galison 2007, 75–7).

The turn towards the aesthetic values of the Enlightenment was even more obvious in the work of the German anatomist Samuel Thomas Soemmering (1755–1830). In 1799 he published a plate that represented seventeen embryos from about three weeks to four months in his *Icones Embryonum Humanorum* (Soemmering 1799/2000, figure 7.9). This plate was intended as a supplement to Hunter's tables, and together they would represent "a complete series of human fetuses from the first beginnings until complete maturity" (Soemmering 1799/2000, 173). The drawings for the plate had been made from Soemmering's own preparations of miscarried embryos and other specimens from anatomical collections. Unlike earlier images of human generation, these pictures represented a coherent series of embryos undergoing morphological changes, based on empirical observation and could be regarded as early representations of the notion of continuous embryonic development (Hopwood 2000, 33–4).

Soemmering's plate rather offered a comparative view of isolated specimens (Wellmann 2010, 283–91). Although it is difficult to determine whether these illustrations represented a particular view on theories of generation or not, there are some indicators that the series of embryos

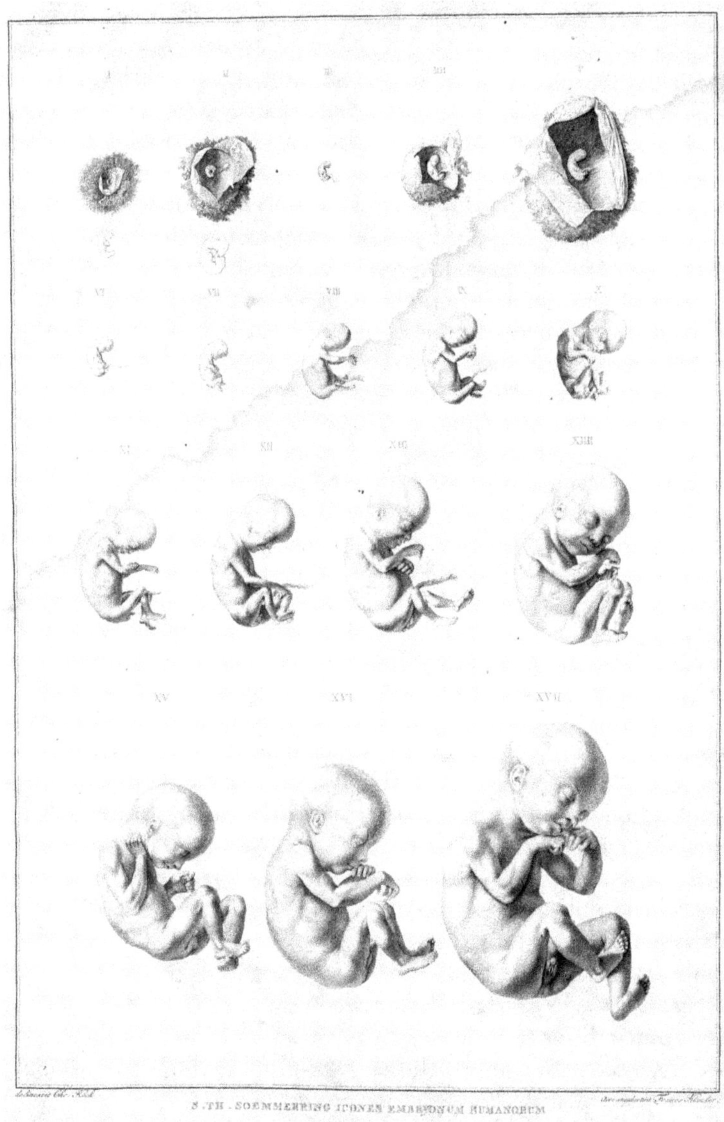

Figure 7.9 Embryos at various developmental stages from between three and four weeks to three and a half months. Engraving in S. Soemmering, *Schriften zur Embryologie und Teratologie*. Edited and translated by U. Enke (Basel: Schwabe Soemmering, 1799). Courtesy of Staatsbibliothek Berlin, gr.2"L 7250.

might be understood as a representation of epigenetic development when Soemmering suggested that his plate should allow the reader to see the "growth and development" of the human body (Soemmering 1799/2000, 172–3). But this development should be regarded as the development of a specific, determined form of a new organism, which would not allow endless variation (Enke 2002, 214–15). Hence the embryonic table represented a restricted idea of the development of the unborn.

Soemmering's reflections on the illustrations used aesthetic categories that were borrowed from neoclassical art theory. Just like Hunter, he was very aware of and involved with contemporary aesthetic debates and art theory. However, where Hunter preferred a naturalistic representation of what could actually be observed during dissections, Soemmering followed the ideal of anatomical perfection (Soemmering 1799/2000, 102). In the introduction to his *Icones* Soemmering marvelled at the beauty of the body of the unborn. Such views were informed by contemporary neoclassical art theory, which linked beauty with truth, for example, in the work of Joshua Reynolds (Reynolds 1798, esp. vol. 1) or the German art historian Johann Joachim Winckelmann (1717–68; Winckelmann 1995). According to Winckelmann beauty and perfection could no longer be found in nature alone. He regarded the study and imitation of ancient art as the appropriate approach to discover ideal beauty and natural perfection (Oehler-Klein 1984, 194). This confronted Soemmering, whose aim was to produce truthful images of the anatomical body, with the problem of how to solve the tensions between the ideal and reality without referring back to ancient works of art. He tried to overcome this problem by generalizing an image of the unborn based on a variety of individual embryonic specimens (Soemmering 1799/2000, 98–104). Together with his artist-collaborator Christian Koeck (1758–1828) (Geus 1985), Soemmering created a truthful image of the unborn that represented perfection and beauty (Oehler-Klein 1984, 207).

Soemmering's images of the embryo were attempts to achieve a truthful representation of the unborn that allowed generalizations about the nature of their subject by identifying them as examples of perfect beauty (Enke 2002, 227). In the caption for the seventeenth illustration he argued that this was a particularly good example to finish the series of embryos because of its perfect proportions and "gracefulness of the very lovely face" of this female embryo (Soemmering 1799/2000, 185). With such judgments Soemmering claimed authority over his subject by deciding categorically the correct arrangement and delineation of embryos (Enke 2002, 226–7). Both Soemmering and Hunter used an aesthetic framework for the visual representation of the unborn, within which it was no longer necessary to understand human generation and the identity of the unborn as part of the Christian salvation narrative, in the context of a greater cosmology, or in relation to the female body. Embryos and fetuses had been turned into mere objects of scientific investigation with their biological sex as the only remaining signifier for their identity.

Conclusions

Early modern images of the unborn represented both practical knowledge and changing embryological theories. These images also made more fundamental statements about the nature of the unborn and life itself, which changed significantly during the long eighteenth century. The question of when human life begins received quite different answers. In midwifery the unborn remained in a liminal state until birth. Only when it entered the world did the child gain its full status as a human being subjected to original sin. Within the debates about preformation as well as in Enlightenment debates about generation, however, both mechanist and vitalist theories of generation suggested that life was always there since the creation of the world, which raised important metaphysical questions. For preformationists this could lead to physico-theological reflections on predestination and whether all beings were actually created at the beginning of the world, as in Scheuchzer's *Physica Sacra*.

Such changing views on the beginnings of life also resulted in changing notions of the unborn as an object of knowledge. From the late seventeenth and into the eighteenth century the identity of this object was more and more shaped by the rationalizing and asexual debates about preformation and epigenesis as well as neoclassical aesthetics. Images of earlier ideas of generation drew on an elaborate iconography that understood the unborn within natural philosophy and Christian cosmology. The aesthetic categories of Enlightenment art theory, however, allowed displaying the unborn as a natural object that was subject to the biological facts of life. Categories such as "beauty," "perfection," or "ideal" provided a secularized language to describe the quality of anatomical specimens and images (Sarafianos 2006, 103–5; Daston and Galison 2007, 69–82). These changing ways of looking at the unborn also had consequences for the identity of the unborn. Before the Enlightenment human identity was inextricably linked to Christian cosmology. The embryonic individuals of Ruysch and Scheuchzer were subjected to predestination and firmly placed within the Christian salvation narrative as inherently sinful human beings. However, these images did not necessarily imply personhood of the unborn, but rather represented the unborn as a liminal being in a precarious position whose future salvation was at stake.

A new and very different way of seeing the embryo and the fetus was introduced by authors such as Hunter and Soemmering, who represented the unborn as an autonomous individual. Now the fetal and the female bodies were created as separate entities, which were determined by their biological sex and reproductive capacities. This natural object was clearly defined, measurable, comparable, and manageable and could potentially be subjected to medical and eugenic interventions. The defining bond of the unborn with the maternal body was cut. By the second half of the eighteenth century the identity of the unborn was no longer defined by its relationship to the female body and the way it was thereby placed in the Christian narrative of salvation. This required a new form of embryonic and fetal identity. As a result the unborn became increasingly an autonomous entity, and as a consequence the question when the unborn had the right to life became key to modern concepts of the identity of the unborn. This notion of the unborn as a (potentially) autonomous individual is still at the heart of contemporary ethical debates.

NOTES

I would like to thank Christine Köhn for her help with the index.

1 My use of the term "unborn" refers generally to what was understood to become a child, such as "seed," "animalcule," "fruit," "embryo," or "child."

2 McTavish made similar observations on French midwifery manuals. She argued that the images in midwifery books "combined iconic and indexical signs to make arguments about the haptic knowledge and gendered medical identity of the practitioner" (McTavish, 2005, 206).

3 For a discussion of the identity of the author, the French naturalist Francois de Plantade (1670–1741) and the fraud allegations against him, see Pinto-Correia 1997, 230–2.

REFERENCES

Bowler, P. 1971. "Preformation and Pre-existence in the Seventeenth Century: A Brief Analysis." *Journal of the History of Biology* 4 (2): 221–44. http://dx.doi.org/10.1007/BF00138311.

Bonnet-Cadilhac, C. 1995. "Les representations du foetus in utero." *Medicina nei secoli* ns 7: 339–50.
Carlino, A. 1999. *Paper Bodies: A Catalogue of Anatomical Fugitive Sheets. Medical History,* Supplement 19. London: Wellcome Institute for the History of Medicine.
Crowther-Heyck, K. 2002. "'Be Fruitful and Multiply': Genesis and Generation in Reformation Germany." *Renaissance Quarterly* 55 (3): 904–35. http://dx.doi.org/10.2307/1261560.
Cunningham, A. 2010. *The Anatomist Anatomise'd: An Experimental Discipline in Enlightenment Europe*. Aldershot: Ashgate.
Daston, L., and P. Galison. 2007. *Objectivity*. New York: Zone Books.
Dubow, S. 2011. *Ourselves Unborn: A History of the Fetus in Modern America*. Oxford: Oxford University Press.
Duden, B. 1993. *Disembodying Women: Perspectives on Pregnancy and the Unborn*. Cambridge, MA: Harvard University Press.
Duden, B. 2002. "Zwischen 'wahrem Wissen' und Prophetie: Konzeptionen des Ungeborenen." In *Geschichte des Ungeborenen: Zur Erfahrungs- und Wissenschaftsgeschichte der Schwangerschaft, 17.-20. Jahrhundert*, edited by B. Duden, 11–48. Göttingen: Vandenhoeck und Ruprecht.
Enke, U. 2002. "Von der Schönheit der Embryonen: Samuel Thomas Soemmerings Werk Icones embryonum humanorum (1799)." In *Geschichte des Ungeborenen: Zur Erfahrungs- und Wissenschaftsgeschichte der Schwangerschaft, 17.-20. Jahrhundert*, edited by B. Duden, 205–35. Göttingen: Vandenhoeck und Ruprecht.
Felfe, R. 2003. *Naturgeschichte als kunstvolle Synthese: Physikotheologie und Bildpraxis bei Johann Jakob Scheuchzer*. Berlin: Akademie Verlag.
Fissell, M. 1995. "Gender and Generation: Representing Reproduction in Early Modern England." *Gender & History* 7 (3): 433–56. http://dx.doi.org/10.1111/j.1468-0424.1995.tb00035.x.
Geus, A. 1985. "Christian Koeck (1758–1818), der Illustrator Samuel Thomas Soemmerrings." In *Samuel Thomas Soemmerring und die Gelehrten der Goethezeit. Beiträge eines Symposions in Mainz vom 19. bis 21. Mai 1983*, edited by G. Mann and F. Dumont, 263–78. Stuttgart: Fischer.
Green, M. 2009. "The Sources of Eucharius Rösslin's 'Rosegarden for Pregnant Women and Midwives' (1513)." *Medical History* 53 (2): 167–92. http://dx.doi.org/10.1017/S0025727300000193.
Hansen, J. 1996. "Resurrecting Death: Anatomical Art in the Cabinet of Dr Frederik Ruysch." *Art Bulletin* 78 (4): 663–79. http://dx.doi.org/10.2307/3046214.
Hartsoeker, N. 1694. *Essay de dioptrique*. Paris: Jean Anisson.

Hopwood, N. 2000. "Producing Development: The Anatomy of Human Embryos and the Norms of Wilhelm His." *Bulletin of the History of Medicine* 74 (1): 29–79. http://dx.doi.org/10.1353/bhm.2000.0020.

Hunter, W. 1774. *Anatomia Uteri Humani Gravidi: Anatomy of the Human Gravid Uterus.* Birmingham and London: J. Baskerville et al.

Jordanova, L. 1985. "Gender, Generation and Science: William Hunter's Obstetrical Atlas." In *William Hunter and the Eighteenth-Century Medical World*, edited by W.F. Bynum and R. Porter, 385–412. Cambridge: Cambridge University Press.

Keller, E. 2000. "Embryonic Individuals: The Rhetoric of Seventeenth-Century Embryology and the Construction of Early-Modern Identity." *Eighteenth-Century Studies* 33 (3): 321–48. http://dx.doi.org/10.1353/ecs.2000.0027.

Keller, E. 2005. *Generating Bodies and Gendered Selves: The Rhetoric of Reproduction in Early Modern England.* Seattle: University of Washington Press.

Kemp, M. 1992. "True to Their Natures: Sir Joshua Reynolds and Dr William Hunter at the Royal Academy of Arts." *Notes and Records of the Royal Society of London* 46 (1): 77–88. http://dx.doi.org/10.1098/rsnr.1992.0004.

Kerckring, T. 1671. *Anthropogeniae Ichnographia, sive conformation foetus ab ovo usque ad ossificationis principa, in supplementum osteogeniae foetum.* Amsterdam: Andreas Frisius.

Leeuwenhoek, A. 1677/8. "De Natis e Semine Genitali Animalculis." *Philosophical Transactions of the Royal Society of London* 12:1040–6. http://dx.doi.org/10.1098/rstl.1677.0068.

Leeuwenhoek, A. 1683. "An Abstract of a Letter from Mr. Anthony Leeuwenhoeck of Delft about Generation by an Animalcule of the Male Seed, etc." *Philosophical Transactions of the Royal Society of London* 13:347–55. http://dx.doi.org/10.1098/rstl.1683.0049.

Leeuwenhoek, A. 1699. "Part of a Letter from Mr. Leuvenhook, Dated June 9th, 1699, Concerning the Animalcula in Semine Humano, etc." *Philosophical Transactionsof the Royal Society of London* 21 (248-59): 301–8. http://dx.doi.org/10.1098/rstl.1699.0054.

Massey, L. 2005. "Pregnancy and Pathology: Picturing Childbirth in Eighteenth-Century Obstetric Atlases." *Art Bulletin* 87 (1): 73–91. http://dx.doi.org/10.1080/00043079.2005.10786229.

Mauriceau, F. 1668. *Des maladies des femmes grosses et accouchées.* Paris: J. Hénault.

McGrath, R. 2002. *Seeing Her Sex: Medical Archives and the Female Body.* Manchester: Manchester University Press.

McTavish, L. 2005. *Childbirth and the Display of Authority in Early Modern France.* Aldershot: Ashgate.

Mount, H. 2006. "Van Rymsdyk and the Nature-Menders: An Early Victim of the Two Cultures Divide." *British Journal for Eighteenth-Century Studies* 29 (1): 79–96. http://dx.doi.org/10.1111/j.1754-0208.2006.tb00636.x.
Newman, K. 1996. *Fetal Positions: Individualism, Science, Visuality*. Stanford: Stanford University Press.
Oehler-Klein, S. 1984. "Anatomie und Kunstgeschichte: Soemmerings Rede Über die Schönheit der antiken Kinderköpfe vor der Société des Antiquités in Kassel (1779)." In *Samuel Thomas Soemmering in Kassel (1779–1784). Beiträge zur Wissenschaftsgeschichte der Goethezeit*, edited by M. Wenzel, 189–239. Stuttgart: Steiner.
Petchesky, R. 1987. "Fetal Images: The Power of Visual Culture in the Politics of Reproduction." *Feminist Studies* 2:263–92. http://dx.doi.org/10.2307/3177802.
Pinto-Correia, C. 1997. *The Ovary of Eve: Egg and Sperm and Preformation*. Chicago: University of Chicago Press. http://dx.doi.org/10.7208/chicago/9780226669502.001.0001.
Porter, R., and L. Hall. 1995. *The Facts of Life: The Creation of Sexual Knowledge in Britain, 1650–1950*. New Haven: Yale University Press.
Raulin, J. 1770. *Von der Erhaltung der Kinder von dem ersten Augenblick ihres Entstehens an bis zu ihrer Mannbarkeit*. 2 vols. Translated by J. Adelung. Leipzig: Siegfried Leberecht Crusius (1st ed., French, 2 vols, 1768–9).
Reynolds, J. 1798. *The Works of Joshua Reynolds*. 2nd ed. 3 vols. London: T. Cadell and W. Davies.
Richards, R. 1992. *The Meaning of Evolution: The Morphological Construction and Ideological Reconstruction of Darwin's Theory*. Chicago: University of Chicago Press. http://dx.doi.org/10.7208/chicago/9780226712055.001.0001.
Roe, S. 1981. *Matter, Life, and Generation: Eighteenth-Century Embryology and the Haller-Wolff Debate*. Cambridge: Cambridge University Press.
Ruestow, E. 1983. "Images and Ideas: Leeuwenhoek's Perception of the Spermatozoa." *Journal of the History of Biology* 16 (2): 185–224. http://dx.doi.org/10.1007/BF00124698.
Ruysch, F. 1701. *Thesaurus Anatomicus Primus*. Amsterdam: Jansson-Waesberg.
Ruysch, F. 1705. *Thesaurus Anatomicus Sextus*. Amsterdam: Johannes Wolters.
Sarafianos, A. 2006. "The Natural History of Man and the Politics of Medical Portraiture in Manchester." *Art Bulletin* 88 (1): 102–18. http://dx.doi.org/10.1080/00043079.2006.10786280.
Scheuchzer, J. 1731–5. *Kupfer-Bibel, In welcher Die Physica Sacra, Oder Geheiligte Natur-Wissenschafft Derer In Heil. Schrifft vorkommenden Natürlichen Sachen, Deutlich erklärt und bewährt*. 4 vols. Augsburg: Johann Andreas Pfeffel.
Sharp, J. (1671) 1999. *The Midwives Book; or, the Whole Art of Midwifry Discovered*. Edited by E. Hobby. Oxford: Oxford University Press.

Soemmering, S. (1799) 2000. *Schriften zur Embryologie und Teratologie*. Edited and translated by U. Enke. Basel: Schwabe.
Stafford, B. 1991. *Body Criticism: Imaging the Unseen in Enlightenment Art and Medicine*. Cambridge, MA: Massachusetts Institute of Technology Press.
Tatlock, L. 1992. "Speculum Feminarum: Gendered Perspectives on Obstetrics and Gynecology." *Signs* (Chicago, Ill.) 17 (4): 725–60. http://dx.doi.org/10.1086/494762.
Tatlock, L. 2005. *Justina Siegemund: The Court Midwife*. Chicago: University of Chicago Press.
Vallisneri, A. 1739. *Historie von der Erzeugung der Menschen und Thiere etc.* Translated by C.P. Berger. Lemgo: Johann Heinrich Meyer (printer) (1st ed., Italian, 1721).
van de Roemer, G. 2010. "From Vanitas to Veneration: The Embellishments in the Anatomical Cabinet of Frederik Ruysch." *Journal of the History of Collections* 22 (2): 169–86. http://dx.doi.org/10.1093/jhc/fhp044.
Venette, N. 1696. *Tableau de l'amour consideré dans l'estat du marriage*. 7th ed. Rouen: Frédric Gaillard (1st ed., French, 1687).
Wagner, D. 2011. "Visualizations of the Womb through Tropes, Dissection, and Illustration, circa 1660–1774." In *Illustration in the Long Eighteenth Century: Reconfiguring the Visual Periphery of the Text*, edited by C. Ionescu, 541–73. Newcastle: Cambridge Scholars Publishing.
Wellmann, J. 2010. *Die Form des Werdens: Eine Kulturgeschichte der Embryologie, 1760–1830*. Göttingen: Wallstein.
Winckelmann, J. 1995. *Gedanken über die Nachahmung der griechischen Werke in der Malerei und Bildhauerkunst. With bibliographic additions*. Stuttgart: Reclam.
Wilson, A. 2007. "Midwifery in the 'Medical Marketplace.'" In *Medicine and the Market in Early Modern England*, edited by M. Jenner and P. Wallis, 153–74. London: Palgrave Macmillan.

8 The Problem of Maternal Violence: Anatomy, Forensic Medicine, and the Mind

CORINNA WAGNER

This chapter explores how late eighteenth- and nineteenth-century investigators of cases of maternal violence – by which I mean child neglect, abuse, abandonment, abortion, but especially infanticide and newborn child murder – used anatomical knowledge to buttress cultural attitudes about motherhood and maternal affection. Scholars have documented the various legal and medical changes in this period, as well as shifting cultural attitudes towards maternal violence, including the increasing reluctance to sentence poor, young, unmarried women to death for crimes of infanticide; the burgeoning faith in the ability of forensic medicine to establish guilt or innocence with more certainty; and the move to identify what we now term psychological reasons for maternal acts of violence.[1] My intention here is not to rehearse these findings, but to focus on the relationship between the rise of anatomy in the eighteenth century and emerging medical and cultural attitudes towards maternal violence in the early decades of the nineteenth. This relationship, I argue, has had a distinctly problematic legacy.

Pioneering work by historians such as Londa Schiebinger (1993), Thomas Laqueur (1990), and Laura Gowing (2003) has established physical contexts for the history of ideas and mentalities. Wider cultural attitudes about maternal emotion, the emphasis on affective motherhood, and beliefs about women's mental and physical capacities grew out of evolving links between anatomical knowledge, changes to the way women's bodies were physically examined, and the print culture surrounding such cases (court records, newspaper accounts, medical treatises). Medical professionals were faced with a dilemma: they had to account for seemingly numerous incidences of maternal violence, which occurred in an era characterized by its celebration of the affective family, domesticity, and motherhood. Forensic knowledge, gathered from the bodies of the deceased and the accused, promised to provide certainty about notoriously opaque crimes like infanticide, which had always been shrouded in secrecy. In addition, medical professionals employed anatomical knowledge to make claims about women's reproductive bodies, and more and more often, their mental capacities and psychological limitations. In the hands of male physicians, forensic examiners, and nascent psychologists, women's bodies were made to *testify materially* to certain legal and biological "truths" about women's "natures," and to shore up the belief in maternal instinct.

Uncertain Bodies, Uncertain Crimes: Forensic Medicine and the Sciences of Mind

If, in terms of sexual practice, masturbation became the subject of a "general neurosis" in the eighteenth century, then maternal violence might be the equivalent in the domain of generation. A vast body of literature describes the real or imagined spectacle of dead babies and the spectre of aberrant mothers who furtively conspired to do away with their offspring. So, for instance, in the late 1730s the philanthropic founder of London's Foundling Hospital, Captain Thomas Coram, "had frequent Occasions of seeing young Children exposed, sometimes alive, sometimes dead, and sometimes dying" in his travels throughout the metropolis (Brocklesby 1751, 12–13). In *The Anatomy of the Gravid Uterus* (1799), the Glasgow surgeon John Burns outlined the five chief means by which abortion may be induced, but assured those who worried about publicizing such information that he was unlikely to attract any but medical readers – readers with whom he shared a worry that purges were being "too frequently employed, by unfortunate and unhappy females" (Burns 1799, 57–8). In addition, eighteenth-century newspapers detailed trials for "the unnatural crime of child-murder" and on any given week of the nineteenth century, columns under headlines proclaiming "Inhuman Atrocity" described how murderous mothers committed "unnatural and unparalleled atrocities" against their defenceless infants.[2] A hundred years after Coram's walks were interrupted by the grievous sight of dead and dying babies, Dr William Burke Ryan described how his own evening walk was similarly troubled by the sight of a "mangled infant" (1862, 45).

Ryan belonged to a medical community that released panic-inspiring statistics, such as the coroner Dr Edwin Lankester's assertion that 12,000 women had committed infanticide in London alone. Lankester's number caused the Reverend Henry Humble to envision dead babies floating in the Thames or left strangled in the streets, one or two of which had "a woman's garter around its throat" (1866, 57). As with the masturbation panic, the language of medicine and morality became entwined in the service of cultural values like domesticity, duty, and familial affection. This hybrid medico-moral discourse infused print culture in the 1850s and 1860s, decades characterized as a time of "maternal panic" in which Britons witnessed "an epidemic of child murder."[3] Of course, masturbation and maternal violence are very different kinds of issues, and to most twenty-first-century minds, the former is a harmless, fairly conventional sexual practice and the latter remains a legitimately grave issue. Yet, it is what they have shared historically that interests me: they both inspired cultural neuroses largely because they were associated with secrecy, uncertainty, and opacity. Maternal violence was also linked with bodily opacity in ways that masturbation was not; but as we will see, developments in anatomy and physiology promised to dispel that bodily uncertainty.

If the fears and anxieties expressed in print culture across a century sound fairly consistent, the legal and medical responses to maternal violence in this same period were not, nor were public attitudes towards punishment. Britons may have been deeply anxious about child murder but they felt sympathy for desperate young mothers; courts were progressively more lenient in cases of infanticide – a fact borne out by steadily declining conviction rates and the repeal of Charles I's punitive 1624 Act to Prevent the Destroying and Murthering of Bastard Children.[4] Under the aegis of the 1624 statutes, many vulnerable and most often unmarried women were executed for delivering in secret or for concealing a stillbirth, rather than for the actual crime of newborn child murder. When the 1624 act was replaced with Lord Ellenborough's 1803 landmark Offenses Against the Person Act (43 Geo 3 c 58), infanticide was brought in line with other crimes, so that the onus was then on the prosecution to obtain conviction through evidentiary proof; in addition, juries could now return a lesser verdict of concealment of birth (punishable by a maximum of two years imprisonment). Yet, for all of the differences between the seventeenth- and nineteenth-century statutes, the anxiety about concealment and the shadowiness of women's bodies remained. Medicine – and specifically, forensic science and the sciences of mind (which would subdivide in the nineteenth century into the related disciplines of psychology and psychiatry) – were two particularly promising weapons in the battle against the inscrutability of intimate bodily crimes like newborn child murder. In turn, the knowledge gained through autopsy promised to reveal anatomical and physiological bases for those crimes.

Medical historians have detailed the professional rise of forensic experts and the increased importance of physical evidence in legal trials.[5] In the third edition of *Principles of Forensic Medicine*, John Gordon Smith (who would become Professor of Medical Jurisprudence at University College London) claimed that "many thousand separate volumes" had been published on the subject of this new science (1821/1827, xvi–xviii). Surgeons with forensic training could tell if and how umbilical cords were cut or torn; they could decide, using the post-mortem hydrostatic test, on the likelihood that a newborn had been born alive or dead (if it breathed outside the womb, its air-inflated lungs would float in water); they could also determine if wounds had been "made upon a living subject" because, as the surgeon William Herring testified in the 29 January 1855 infanticide trial of twenty-year-old Hannah Pipkins, then "the edges are always red, everted, or turned out" (350). Early modern trials in which the opinions of male professionals could conflict with the testimony of female midwives had exposed "the problem of finding clear evidence in the female body" (Gowing 2003, 49). Founded as it was in new anatomical knowledge, forensic medicine did not dispel the problem, and indeed it had its own fallibilities and limits, but it did promise new ways of finding and interpreting bodily evidence. It was a science that countered unreliable testimony and false confession by rendering the body a silent witness, capable of testifying to concealed, secretive acts in newly accurate ways. The obstetrician Michael Ryan expressed this confidence in forensic medicine with a quote by the eighteenth-century anatomist Albrecht von Haller: there were, he wrote, "no secrets in physiology" (1836, 20).

Other historians and critics have traced how, in the eighteenth century, medical witnesses made the mental state of desperate mothers a prime consideration of guilt or innocence. This is reflected in the trial records of cases of infanticide and child murder, which increasingly emphasized links between the accused's state of mind and the physical aspects of the crime. Defendants claimed they were victim of a temporary "phrenzy," "insensibility," or some sort of nervous debility, while the medics who examined them diagnosed a temporary madness that, in the nineteenth century, would be labelled puerperal insanity.[6] So, for example, when the married Mary Dixon's child was found alive at the bottom of a privy, she offered this defence at her 11 September 1735 trial: "I got up from my Husband and went down to the Vault, where my Senses went from me, and I did not recover my self, nor know what I did or said – I was under no Temptation of being so barbarous, for I had a good Husband who was able to maintain the Child" (145). Similarly, at her 8 December 1762 trial for infanticide, Ann Haywood claimed to be "quite insensible" when giving birth over a privy (26). In Hannah Pipkins's trial, her testimony was supported by her examining surgeon, William Herring, who was recorded as saying: "I have no doubt that the pains of unassisted labour are sometimes sufficient to cause an aberration of intellect ... I believe that the pains of unassisted labour may be such as to cause a temporary deprivation of reason" (32). These types of testimonies indicate how infanticide became downgraded from a heinous "crime" (Dixon and Haywood were acquitted, and Pipkins was found guilty of concealment only). In addition, as I will address more fully later, these statements reveal how such crimes began to be described as a regrettable manifestation of the various psychological disorders that plagued childbearing women from the moment of conception to the termination of lactation.

But before doing so, I want to draw connections between forensic science and psychology and to show how both were grounded in anatomy. There has been a tendency to see forensic science and the sciences of mind as developing along perhaps compatible, but separate pathways, and scholars have argued that physical forensic findings were superseded in importance by the new emphasis on psychology. Sheena Sommers points out that "new defences of nonresponsibility" carried more weight than material evidence as to whether a woman had prepared linen in anticipation of birth (2009, 37). According to Dana Rabin, the state of the defendant's mind became so significant in late eighteenth-century infanticide cases, "that evidence about the body no longer determined the outcome of a trial" (2002, 74). Mark Jackson also argues that "testimony as to the mother's state of mind at and after birth" came to dominate medico-legal debates in the nineteenth century, "largely replacing medical evidence derived from the physical examination of the bodies of the mother and child" (2002, 10). Cath Quinn identifies a similar historical trajectory, so that by the last decades of the nineteenth century, "psychiatry increasingly replaced obstetrics as the authoritative medical body" in infanticide cases (2002, 193).

Yet in spite of the distinctions between forensic and psychological approaches to maternal violence, they overlapped in their aims, as is clear in the surgeon William Herring's testimony in the Pipkins case above. Both medical subdisciplines aimed for bodily transparency, and this is part of their shared origin in anatomy. We may commonly think of psychiatry as opening the mind rather than the body, but in its earliest phases of development, it looked for physical, internal origins for diseases like puerperal insanity. Professionalizing forensic scientists and the up-and-coming group of alienists and mind doctors who came to dominate the medico-legal field in the next century aimed to open the body: the former in order to understand the facts of the crime and the latter in order to identify the psychological reasons for this crime. New emphases on the infanticidal mother's state of mind did not lessen the sense that her interior body could dispel secrets.

Opening up a Few Bodies: Anatomy and Visualization

Across the West, the reputation of anatomical study, in spite of ebbs and flows, grew steadily in the eighteenth century. Anatomy evolved from the specialist study of early modern scientific gentlemen to the cornerstone of surgery; it grew in prominence in intellectual centres, from Bologna to Vienna, Paris to Edinburgh, and in North America. In 1800, the American John Collins Warren (who would become Professor of Anatomy and Surgery at Harvard), credited the famous anatomists John and William Hunter for inspiring a "rage" for their discipline in the British Isles (Sappol 2002, 48). The visual cultural element of anatomy cannot be overemphasized: bodies were notoriously hard to come by and they decomposed quickly, so anatomists worked closely with engravers, wax modellers, and other artists to capture their findings. Dissected specimens, preserved pathological samples, lavishly illustrated folio-sized anatomical atlases, and models of wax, wood, plaster, and even terra cotta conserved the structures and textures of veins, arteries, and organs, as well as offering their viewer a chance to see how everything "fit" together.

This visual culture of anatomy has a complex and important relationship to the types of legal, medical, and cultural responses to maternal violence that I am tracing here. In Britain, in the second half of the eighteenth century, anatomists made increasingly fine representational discriminations in their images of the pregnant, parturient, and post-natal female body in particular. Figure 8.1 is an image from one of the many versions of the obstetrician William Smellie's 1754 anatomical atlas.

This image demonstrates how to extract the fetus's head with both hand and tool (a "curved crotchet" in this case). If the body of a dead fetus had come away because of mortification and the remaining head was too large, or if the woman's pelvis was too narrow to allow for its extraction, the obstetrician had to compress and crush the skull before pulling the pieces of the fetal body out. This image illustrates an important obstetrical development, but my interest here is in how medical practitioners increasingly entered, manipulated, and even more to the point, described and visually represented the interior of the vagina and uterus.

Smellie's engraver, the Dutch medical illustrator Jan van Rymsdyk, went on to create the plates for the anatomist William Hunter's enormous and

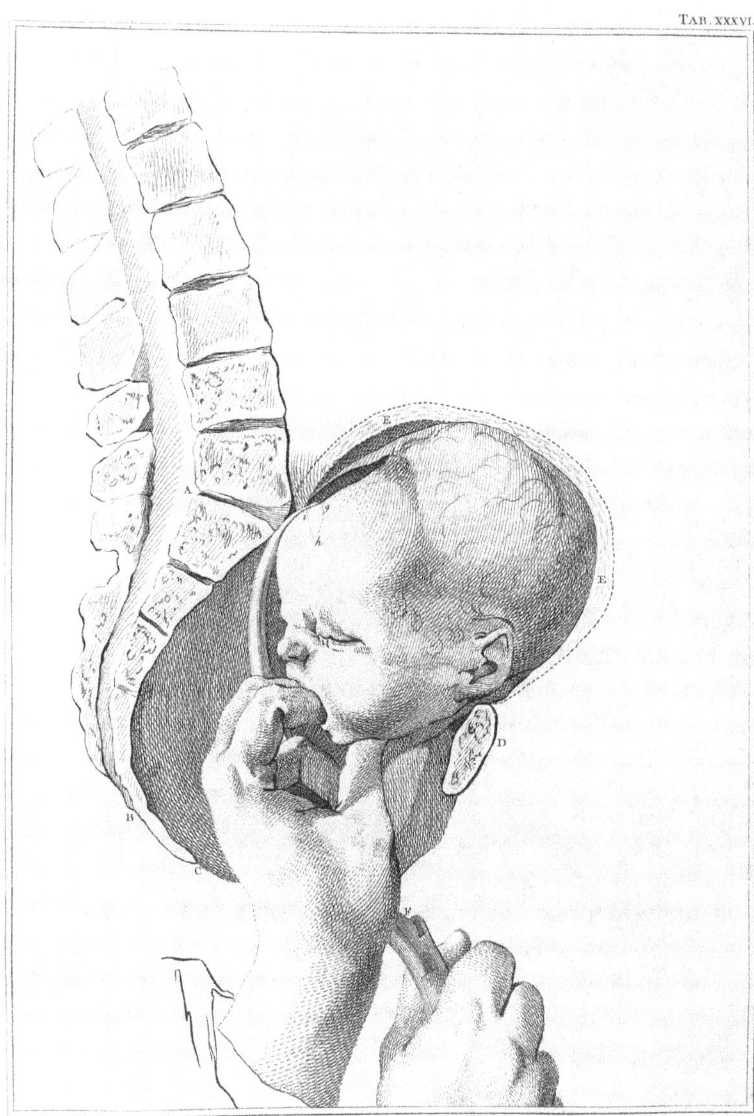

Figure 8.1 Illustration of the lateral view of a woman's pelvis and the method of extracting the head of the foetus. W. Smellie, *A Set of Anatomical Tables with Explanations, and an Abridgement of the Practice of Midwifery* (Edinburgh: William Creech, 1787), plate XXXVI. Courtesy of Wellcome Library, London.

magnificently illustrated *Anatomy of the Gravid Uterus* (1774). Characterized by art historian Martin Kemp as the key figure of the "flesh-and-blood" school of anatomical illustration, Hunter believed that "Representation in the imitative Arts is a Substitute for reality" (Kemp 1993, 85). The principle that medical illustration can and should objectively capture reality informs, for example, Hunter's image opposite (figure 8.2).

It is hard to exaggerate how carefully each anatomical feature is captured in its unrefined materiality. As this image demonstrates, Hunter clung tenaciously to the idea "that the foundation of knowledge must consist in striving for an untainted looking at the raw material" (Kemp 1993, 118). In almost every manual on infanticide, specialists like Hunter claimed that understanding the stages of conception and parturition, and the physiological systems connecting fetus and mother, was the key to recognizing whether a fetus had been voluntarily or involuntarily aborted, or how a full-term infant had died.[7] In such a way, as Roberta McGrath puts it, women's bodies, which had previously "lain beneath the threshold of vision," were now made "tangible" (2002, 30). These anatomical atlases instructed forensic specialists where to look, how to look, and what to look for; in doing so, they also naturalized certain types of looking and touching that dispensed with politeness, privacy, and, as these images indicate, individual identity.

Of course, it was impossible for anatomists, legal experts, forensic specialists, or mind doctors to fully know what a woman's intentions were or what her state of mind was: these were nebulous entities. However, anatomy offered some certitude because it provided visual and physical access to the internal body and knowledge about how to read it. Forensic medicine, as John Gordon Smith explained, "is clearly understood to imply the use made of Medical knowledge in the Courts of Justice" and he singled out anatomy as a particularly important branch of knowledge applied "to clear up doubtful cases of accusation" (1821/1827, x). In his 1821 edition of *A Dissertation on Infanticide in Its Relation to Physiology and Jurisprudence*, William Hutchinson explained that "even though it may be known with moral certainty" that a woman had secretly given birth and killed her child, the medical practitioner was still "generally required to examine the mother" (90). Forensic examiners were instructed, as soon as possible after the suspected birth, to look for stretchmarks, discharge from the nipples, darkened areolas, a dark line on the abdomen, signs of a ruptured perinaeum, dilated uterus, and tumefied labia and vagina (Hutchinson 1821, 91; Simson 1825, 19). In his 1825 *Probationary Essay on Infanticide,* the forensic specialist Dr James Simson encouraged examiners to form a

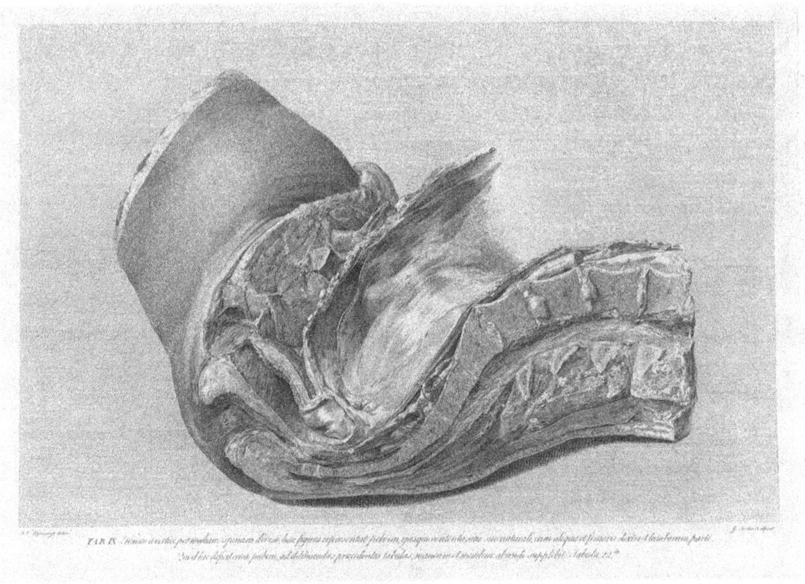

Figure 8.2 Sagittal section of a gravid female pelvis with the fetus removed. W. Hunter, *Anatomy of the Human Gravid Uterus* (Birmingham: J. Baskerville, 1774), plate IX. Courtesy of Wellcome Library, London.

visual and tactile intimacy with the body of the accused, which went below the surface of the body. Like the eye, hands should enter the body: an enlarged uterus may be partially felt through the abdomen, "but still better if we introduce one finger into the vagina" (Simson 1825, 52). Forensic specialists directed readers to the surgeon John Burns's observation that the os uteri of a recently delivered woman "will admit two or more fingers"; a week after delivery, "the womb is as large as two fists"; after three weeks, "the uterus be felt, per vaginum, to resemble its unimpregnated size, but the os uteri rarely, if ever, closes to the same degree as in the virgin state" (1837, 631–3).[8] In addition to such manual examinations, forensic specialists advised students to use their nose: they should check for "a discharge of a bloody sanies or puriform fluid, possessing a very peculiar smell, known to accoucheurs by the name of lociae," variously described as having an "acid odour" or a "sour" tang akin to "fish-oil" (Simson 1825, 5; Montgomery 1857, 482).

Simson also broached the subject of abortion; he cautioned examiners not to miss the underhanded means by which women would seek to rid themselves of their unborn.[9] Professionals should look for hidden evidence of "mechanical means" of abortion, such as punctures or tears along the vaginal walls and "sometimes pieces of wood" and other material concealed inside the uterus (18). Members of "the lower class of society" often attempted abortion by blood-letting, the use of "emetics, cathartics, cantharides, mercury, savine powder [and] oil of juniper," Simson advised, but abortion produced the same signs as a normal delivery, including "a bloody ichorous offensive discharge from the vagina, mixed with clots of blood and mucus – the labia soft, red, and enlarged – the os uteri open, and the vagina relaxed and dilated" (1825, 17). This type of rather graphic medical detail demonstrates how the forensic eye, nose, and hand accessed women's reproductive bodies, as well as reveals how thoroughly male professionals had taken over roles of bodily examination, formerly performed by women.

These treatises also indicate how previously unseen parts of women's bodies entered into a medicalized "ocular economy," to use Lynda Nead's phrase (2000, 66). Like the anatomical illustrations, they raise questions about the social politics and ethics surrounding visual and physical access. Considerations of legitimacy, morality, and professionalism could not be separated from medical advancements, which made new incursions on the female body. The harrowingly graphic physiological detail recounted above may seem far from sexually titillating, but the type of penetrative, no-holds-barred scrutinizing of the female body raises issues about privacy and surveillance, as well as the less objective uses of such evidence gathering. In forensic manuals like those quoted above, there is a struggle between the professionalizing impetus, with its claims to medical objectivity and impartiality; the taint of impropriety and immorality; and rather ironically, an accompanying moralizing, disciplinary discourse about women's character and their appropriate roles.

From Anatomy to Mind

Over the course of the eighteenth century, anatomists who "uncovered" knowledge about the female reproductive body also paved the way for the psychiatric justification of maternal violence in the following century. Many anatomists established a biological foundation for the incommensurability between the sexes and identified a supposedly essential, and physiologically determined, maternal nature. These concepts became the foundation for later prognoses about the mental state of fragile, vulnerable, but violent mothers. Among the influential eighteenth-century texts that linked anatomy and physiology with supposedly inherent gendered traits is Andrew Wilson's 1776 treatise *The Nature and Origin of Hysterics in the Female Constitution*. A fellow of the Royal College of Physicians at Edinburgh and a physician to the London Medical Asylum, Wilson's view of gendered biological difference chimed with the majority of his contemporaries. Compared to men, females were more delicate of frame, their bodily solids and fluids "more yielding and susceptible," their organs more fine and delicate (1776, 40). Notwithstanding his patronizing language about female sensitivity, patience, and moral purity, women were on the losing side of a clear biological line. In addition to female-specific diseases, there were serious "accidents to which the health and constitutions of females are exposed during pregnancy, and how many different kinds, according to the different stages of it!" (66). A great believer in the mother's ability to "mark" or "impress" the fetus, Wilson pinpointed the female "organ of conception" – with its communicative or sympathetic nature – as "the immediate source" of hysteria and potential danger (83). Even if mother and fetus survived the gestational period unscathed, "yet Nature has ordained" that more "uncertain difficulties and dangers" attended childbirth – and "every hour of the mother's recovery from these shocks, *till Nature has repaired them, and re-established the constitution again, in the habits of the Sex*" (66–7).

Wilson shared much with contemporaries who sought biological explanations for women's allegedly impressionable psychologies and their propensity for irrational or violent behaviour. Generation might be inevitable and natural, but it also produced hysteria, temporary insanity, a suspension of reason, and general intellectual instability. In the decades following Wilson's treatise, the nebulous category of hysteria due to childbirth or temporary insanity was subdivided into overlapping categories, among them puerperal insanity, puerperal melancholy or mania, lactational insanity, climacteric insanity, and ovarian mania. In his 1798 collection of case studies, the surgeon and apothecary to Bethlem Hospital, John Haslam, observed a link between insanity and "the natural processes which women undergo, of menstruation, parturition and of preparing nutriment for the infant" (1809, 245). These sentiments were echoed in 1810, by the physician at the Manchester Asylum, John Ferriar, who described the onset of "puerperal mania" – a subcondition of puerperal insanity – as "the application of any exciting cause" such as distressing thoughts or bad news, during gestation or after delivery. The "circulation" is so disturbed when a woman produces breast milk that the disturbing phenomena "may be readily converted to the head, and produce either hysteria or insanity, according to its force and the nature of the occasional cause" (1810, 68). In 1795 the accoucheur at Middlesex Hospital, Thomas Denman, observed that hysterical and maniacal women were in "an altered, but not a morbid state" (1795, 468). In 1810, he used the label *mania lactea* to describe the "aberration of the mental faculties" that can occur during any part of the reproductive process, from conception through pregnancy, from childbirth through months of breastfeeding. This mania was a result of "an uncommon irritation" of the uterus or breasts, which affected the brain, but was not linked to "former disposition or habits" (1810, 37–8). John Burns argued that "all women, at the menstrual period, are more subject than at other times to spasmodic and hysterical complaints" while during pregnancy and/or lactation, they could suffer from "despondency" and could become "much alarmed respecting the issue of their confinement" (1837, 160). These developments in the arena of psychology impacted medical jurisprudence, and were reflected in courtrooms and wider culture. The next section examines the significant dilemma raised by this psychological turn in maternal violence cases.

Medicine, Mind, and the Culture of Sentimentalized Motherhood

Let us consider the cultural context of the medical knowledge described above. The belief that maternal violence had psychological causes, firmly rooted in anatomical and physiological origins, emerged in a culture that celebrated maternity and sentimentalized motherhood. The medical findings of Haslam, Denman, Ferriar, and others, which emphasize the instability and dangers of the pregnant and parturient mind, raised a profound dilemma: if women's biology rendered them as unstable and irrational so as to become violent child killers, how could they be characterized as inherently maternal, nurturing caregivers? Historian of psychiatry and mental health researcher Cath Quinn poses the question this way: how does "a society which held ideals of maternity as synonymous with the role of women, react to the potential rupture in its fabric presented by cases of puerperal insanity and infanticide?" (2002, 194). This dilemma underwrites the testimony of both laypeople and experts, who respond in sometimes surprisingly similar ways.

Crucially, there were prevailing common responses to this dilemma. Laypeople and medical professionals may have used very different vocabularies, but they both employed – whether consciously or not – three key interrelated strategies: they disconnected the violent act from the person committing it; they emphasized the impermanence of the violence; and finally, they grounded that temporary "craziness" in the body – in female anatomy and the processes of generation. What emerges in all of the courtroom testimony is a distinct refusal to relinquish in any way the idea of maternal instinct and a distinctly female, God-given nurturing impulse. So, when Elizabeth Parkins was tried for infanticide on 10 April 1771, her employer John Lang described how "she behaved very well, was a very good servant, and remarkably fond of children" (203). At the 15 September 1779 Old Bailey trial of Elisabeth Gwatkin, one witness declared that he "could not have conceived she could be capable of destroying a child of her own body" (495). In the case of Ann Mountford of Bethnal Green, tried on 24 May 1822 for the murder of her nine-month-old daughter Lucy, her long-term acquaintance Charles Leagow testified that he was "positive she could not be in her right mind" for "she was a kind and humane mother as ever lived, and has nine children now" (331). In similar fashion, Mountford's landlady observed that although physically weakened and likely suffering from milk fever, Mountford was an affectionate mother who was not only "kind to them all," but had even sacrificed her own health by refusing to wean the particularly delicate nine-month-old Lucy (330). These statements are compassionate, personal defences, but they also express profound disbelief that women – whatever their circumstances – could feel ambivalence, resentment, malice, or violence towards their newborns and infants.

The almost absolute faith in maternal instinct as an inherent biological fact is, of course, sorely tested in the light of cold, hard forensic facts, yet that faith underpinned a search for innate biological reasons for violence. This is the case, for example, in the testimony given at the 25 February 1747 infanticide trial of servant Hannah Perfect. The interrogation of Perfect's fellow servant Mary Millet focuses on the defendant's state of mind, as do the witness's answers:

Q. In what Condition was the Prisoner, was she in her Senses?
MILLET. I think she was not in her right Senses.
Q. Was there any Behaviour at that Time that induced you to think she was crazy?
MILLET. I think the Nature of a Woman, except she was out of her Senses, would not make away or destroy her own.
Q. Do you construe by her Behaviour that she was stupified; that she was in her Senses, or was not?
MILLET. I believe she was stupified.

> COURT. You believe she had not the Government of her Understanding?
> MILLET. No, I believe she had not.
> Q. Is she a sensible Woman at other Times?
> MILLET. She is a very sensible young Woman. (83)

Millet's responses to the court's questions disclose much about sensibility and sympathy, but they are also indicative of a struggle to reconcile the fact that otherwise normal, decent girls and women committed secretive violent acts against children with the unequivocal belief that the "Nature of Woman" was to protect and nurture children. Millet's comments, made in 1747, anticipate how, at the end of the century, medical professionals would fashion insanity into a temporary state of mind that was "unrelated to the defendant's true self and sensibility" (Rabin 2002, 92). The true female self could remain sensibly fond of children, while professionals identified the etiologies of an array of temporary psychological conditions – aberrations – that explained maternal violence. Whatever the particular condition, it naturally originated from and inhered in female anatomy and physiology.

Maternal care is, as Sarah LaChance Adams puts it, "one of those rare, mutual assumptions shared by scientists and poets alike" (2014, 2). Indeed, the assumptions underlying the testimony of laypeople like Mary Millet are remarkably alike, and inform the arguments forwarded by medical professionals. Nineteenth-century physicians reconciled the maternal nature/maternal violence paradox by emphasizing the impermanence of the accused's mental state and by casting it as an anomaly, a lapse, a short-term physiological and psychological failure. For example, in the 1805 infanticide trial of Sarah Dixon, the surgeon John Weston was asked if women in labour "are very frequently in so debilitated a state, and the mind so far affected, as to render them incapable" of tying the navel string to prevent their newborn haemorrhaging (422). Weston's affirmative response, and his description of how "a sort of delirium attends labour," clearly contains the episode of maternal violence (422). There is a similar diagnosis, too, in the 1823 case of Lucy Dancer, a thirty-three-year-old mother, charged with the murder of her nine-month-old son William. On 14 March, *The Morning Post* reported the trial testimony of the examining surgeon Downing:

> She said she was sitting upon a chair nursing the child, when a thought suddenly came into her head, that she would kill both her children ... She reached a large knife, she then walked to her chair, sat down, and began to cut the child's throat ... *I believe she was insane in November, and also on the 13th January* [the day of the murder]. (1823; my emphasis)

Tried at the Worcester assizes, Dancer was found not guilty by reason of temporary insanity. What is remarkable here is just how fixed and precise are the dates of the onset and termination of her insanity – an exactness that contrasts remarkably with the lack of specificity or detail about her life.

Downing's insistence that Dancer's insanity was both a direct result of her pregnancy and thereby distinctly transitory is part of a profound struggle to identify medical facts that would explain violence but protect the idea of inherent maternal feeling. Medical professionals used knowledge about psychology, grounded in anatomy and physiology, to reconcile the supposedly instinctual protectiveness of mothers with the reality that across the nation those same mothers were quietly suffocating their children, dropping them down privies, and slitting their throats. We have already seen how Ann Mountford's acquaintances portrayed her as a kind and humane mother of ten children; medicine had developed in ways that squared this maternal kindness with her crimes. Her examining surgeon Joseph Dalton made sense of the bodily evidence he found by pronouncing it a case of *mania lactea*. It was his experience, he testified, that a woman's inability to wean her child could produce "insanity," which was exacerbated by any predisposition to a "melancholy temper":

> I was not at all surprised when I heard she was the subject of insanity. At the time of weaning, the breast remains extremely full of milk, which always produces a degree of irritation. I believe she was an affectionate wife, and had correct parental feelings. (1822, 331)

The juxtaposition here of the physiological and the cultural could not be more marked, but Dalton's testimony draws intimate connections between physiology, psychology, sentiment, and an idealized vision of maternal emotion. Like other filicidal or infanticidal women, Mountford is violently present in the home but psychologically absent. Because these women are wholly in their bodies, they are also periodically out of their minds.

Instinct and Environment

According to historian Kathryn Watson, temporary puerperal insanity was perceived in the medico-legal realm to be "due more to a deplorable personal situation than organic disease" (2011, 108), but it seems to me that there is strong evidence to support precisely the opposite conclusion. Medical men sought an organic source for puerperal insanity, whatever their sympathies for the plight of disadvantaged women. It is true that, as social historians have shown, the public sympathized with defendants who, fearing social shame, the loss of employment, and the withdrawal of poor relief, were driven to commit desperate acts of maternal violence. Still, on the fairly rare occasions when there was sympathetic consideration of circumstances, these are inevitably economic, rather than a consideration of the defendant's desires, motives, frustrations, failed dreams, disappointments, or feelings of powerlessness. Psychological considerations are about general biological categories, that is, about being female, child-bearing, and having anatomical and physiological weaknesses. Certainly, there is a distinct unwillingness to entertain, even briefly, the idea that these acts of violence might stem from maternal ambivalence or a lack of maternal affection.

This is most evident, for instance, in the Mountford trial. What might be the everyday experience of mothering ten children is not considered, nor is that experience seen as a contributing factor to her obviously troubled state of mind. At her trial she simply requested to be returned home, but at the time of her arrest she expressed a rather different desire: "I want to be hung, for I am tired of my life" she stated, and when asked if she "would not sooner go home to her family than be hung" she replied "No" (1822, 331). That being a mother of ten children could lead to feelings other than maternal bliss was never entertained. She would be mad not to want to return to the bosom of her family. Josephine McDonagh's comments on another case, the 1774 Jane Cornforth infanticide trial, applies equally well here: "there is no probing of Cornforth's [read: "Mountford's"] motives, or the circumstances that might have provoked this act … Our gaze jolts back and forth between the wounded corpse of the infant, and the pathetic culprit named in the reiterated refrain: 'poor Jane Cornforth, who loved children'" (2003, 2). Versions of this refrain, which echoed consistently throughout the following decades, is meant to be a reassuring chorus for a society that celebrates motherhood but that also sees itself as beleaguered by maternal violence.

Explanations for maternal violence were almost invariably grounded in the anatomical, the physiological, the biological, even when the issue of the woman's mental state was of prime consideration. Although some professionals did occasionally offer a socio-economic explanation to account for infanticidal violence, this was always a subsidiary explanation. Social pressures were described as mitigating circumstances rather than leading causes in, for example, forensic specialist Charles Severn's *First Lines of the Practice of Midwifery To Which are Added Remarks on the Forensic Evidence Requisite in Cases of Infanticide and Foeticide* (1831). Severn deemed it almost impossible that females who were characterized by the "ardour of the natural affections, could stifle that loud voice of nature" (1831, 136). This view chimes with that of Professor of Forensic Medicine at Paris, Dr P.A.O. Mahon. In *An Essay on the Signs of Murder in New Born Children* (translated from the French in 1813 by Lancaster surgeon Christopher Johnson), Mahon argued that severe public disapproval and social hypocrisy were strong enough to make mothers betray their naturally maternal inclinations, and over time, women could even become "incapable of feeling the loss" of a child (1813, xx, 2).

Critically, though, this allowance for the influence of environmental or cultural factors on the issue of maternal violence is trumped by a belief in the supreme authority of nature. Maternal violence was simply evidence that natural impulses could become "modified by prejudice and education" (Mahon 1813, 9). Ultimately, women were ruled by a common "natural and powerful instinct" that they might criminally resist for a time, yet that did not negate the fact that instinct still determined women's emotions, inclinations, and roles (8). "To judge by actions only" – that is, to interpret abortion, infanticide, and filicide – as proof against the existence of inherent maternal feeling was an unequivocal and dangerous error. We must *not* "disbelieve those natural impulses" Mahon insisted, rather we must acknowledge "the existence of an instinct, so closely allied to [maternal] duty" (9). That the very existence of the infanticidal mother "testifies to the instability of those 'instincts' in the first place" (Kipp 2003, 131) is solved by identifying biological bases for maternal violence and by constructing it as a temporary aberration in the evolutionary plan. Women's "debility" could not "extinguish that pleasure to which the hope of an infant inspires" nor could it override "the instinct which bends her to the new-born," Mahon argued, since that instinct is as "equally involuntary ... as that which united the two sexes" (9). This is an articulation of essentialist efforts to use medical knowledge (or more accurately, assumptions) to confine women to prescribed roles, and to enforce heteronormative relationships. In this respect, Mahon's use of the term "involuntary" could not be more striking.

As I hope to have shown, there is a common thread, which can be followed from atlases of the dissected gravid uterus to guides on forensic medicine, from treatises on mental disorders to court case testimony. This is the search for biological certainty about distinctly uncertain subjects. Eighteenth-century anatomists opened, exposed, and exhibited the female body, and in doing so, provided their successors with the material evidence needed for their claims about women's supposedly delicate yet volatile nervous systems, erratic reproductive organs, and susceptible minds. The words and images of anatomist-obstetricians, notably Smellie and Hunter, can be traced through a succeeding generation of forensic experts and mind doctors who searched for a biological link between reproductive organs and the mind. The construction of motherhood as inherent or essential to woman's nature became so firmly entrenched in the late eighteenth and nineteenth centuries that the idea of maternal ambivalence could not be contemplated. A woman who did not desire children, or a mother who felt resentment or animosity towards her children (or even more frighteningly, felt nothing at all), was a woman who monstrously contravened the biological imperative. According to the dictates of nature, such women could not exist: and so they could only be suffering from a temporary spell of insanity, from which they would return to normality. Arguably, we have much more choice about our bodies today than in previous eras, but we also continue to live with biological destiny dressed up as choice. But of course, that is not *real* choice.

NOTES

1 See Goc, Jackson, Kipp, Marland, Quinn, Rose, and Sommers.
2 *Daily Journal*, London: 1 February, 1729, issue 2518; *Times* 29 October 1822, 3; *The Derby Mercury* (Derby, England), 30 November 1842, issue 5762).
3 See Goc, McDonagh.
4 For statistics about this, see Forbes (1985, 96–9) including the table of Old Bailey Infanticide Trials with Expert Medical Testimony, 1729–1878; but especially, see Clayton (2009, 337–59). Clayton notes that in her study of the trial records, 48 women out of 90 trials (or 53 per cent of women) held between 1674 and 1714 were found guilty, but in the remaining 89 years of the study only 20 women (15 per cent) of 130 were found guilty and none after December 1775. This study was restricted to Old Bailey trials, but it gives a clear sense of attitudinal changes. Rebecca Smith was the last British woman hanged for newborn murder in 1849; see R. Smith (1981, 143).
5 Historians R. Dickinson and J.A. Sharpe chart the increasing importance of medical evidence as the eighteenth century progressed in their study of infanticide cases in the Cheshire court records (2002). Legal scholar Stephen Landsman observes that medical experts became the most frequently called expert witnesses at the Old Bailey, noting that "infanticide cases featured more multiple medical witness presentations than might have been expected"

(1998, 448, 452). Lionel Rose describes the inquest system, which developed in the early nineteenth century, as "a lantern that uncomfortably illuminated the dark recesses of society" (1986, 57).

6 See Marland and Rabin.

7 Hunter's published lecture on infanticide was hugely influential; see Hunter (1783/1836).

8 See also Beck (1823, 137, 144–5); Hutchinson (1821, 92–3).

9 The 1803 Act also clarified the court's position on abortion, which under common law, had been rather ambiguous. According to bioethicist John Keown, in earlier eras, under common law, women were generally left to themselves on this more ambiguous issue, and could legally terminate their pregnancies up until "quickening" or when the fetus became "animated" in the womb (usually in the second trimester) (1988, 20).

REFERENCES

Beck, T. 1823. *Elements of Medical Jurisprudence*. Vol. 1 of 2. Albany: Websters & Skinners.

[Brocklesby, R]. 1751. *Private Virtue and Publick Spirit displayed in a Succinct Essay on the Character of Thomas Coram*, London: J. Roberts.

Burns, J. (1809) 1837. *Principles of Midwifery*. 9th ed. London: Longman et al.

Burns, J. 1799. *The Anatomy of the Gravid Uterus.* Glasgow: Gasgow University Press.

Clayton, M. 2009. "Changes in Old Bailey Trials for the Murder of Newborn Babies, 1674–1803." *Continuity and Change* 24 (2): 337–59. http://dx.doi.org/10.1017/S0268416009007206.

Denman, T. 1795. *An Introduction to the Practice of Midwifery*. Vol. 2 of 2. London: J. Johnson.

Denman, T. 1810. *Observations on the Rupture of the Uterus, on the Snuffles in Infants, and on Mania Lactea*. London: J. Johnson.

Dickinson, R., and J.A. Sharpe. 2002. "Infanticide in Early Modern England: The Court of Great Sessions at Chester, 1650–1800." In *Infanticide: Historical Perspective on Child Murder and Concealment, 1550–2000*, edited by M. Jackson, 35–51. Aldershot: Ashgate.

Ferriar, J. 1810. *Medical Histories and Reflections*. Vol. 1. London: Cadell & Davies.

Forbes, T.R. 1985. *Surgeons at the Bailey: English Forensic Medicine to 1878*. New Haven: Yale University Press.

Goc, N. 2013. *Women, Infanticide and the Press, 1822–1922*. Aldershot: Ashgate.
Gowing, L. 2003. *Common Bodies: Women, Touch and Power in Seventeenth-Century England*. New Haven, CT: Yale University Press.
Haslam, J. 1809. *Observations on Madness and Melancholy*. 2nd ed. London: J. Callow.
"Horrible Case of Infanticide [Lucy Dancer]; Worcester Assizes, March 11." In *The Morning Post* 14 March 1823.
Humble, H. 1866. "Infanticide, Its Cause and Cure." In *The Church and the World: Essays on Questions of the Day*, edited by O. Shipley, 51–69. London: Longmans et al.
Hunter, W. 1774. *The Anatomy of the Human Gravid Uterus*. Birmingham: J. Baskerville et al.
Hunter, W. 1783. "On the Uncertainty of the Signs of Murder in the Case of Bastard Children." Rpt. in W. Cummin. 1836. *The Proofs of Infanticide Considered*. London: Longman et al.
Hutchinson, W.A. 1821. *Dissertation on Infanticide in its Relation to Physiology and Jurisprudence*. London: J. & C. Adlard.
Jackson, M. 2002. "The Trial of Harriet Vooght: Continuity and Change in the History of Infanticide." In *Infanticide: Historical Perspective on Child Murder and Concealment, 1550–2000*, edited by M. Jackson, 1–17. Aldershot: Ashgate.
Kemp, M. 1993. "'The mark of truth': Looking and Learning in Some Anatomical Illustrations from the Renaissance and Eighteenth Century." In *Medicine and the Five Senses*, edited by W.F. Bynum and R. Porter, 85–121. Cambridge: Cambridge University Press.
Keown, J. 1988. *Abortion, Doctors and the Law*. Cambridge: Cambridge University Press. http://dx.doi.org/10.1017/CBO9780511563683.
Kipp, J. 2003. *Romanticism, Maternity, and the Body Politic*. Cambridge: Cambridge University Press. http://dx.doi.org/10.1017/CBO9780511484346.
LaChance Adams, S. 2014. *Mad Mothers, Bad Mothers, & What a "Good" Mother Would Do*. New York: Columbia University Press.
Landsman, S. 1998. "One Hundred Years of Rectitude: Medical Witnesses at the Old Bailey, 1717–1817." *Law and History Review* 16 (3): 445–94. http://dx.doi.org/10.2307/744241.
Laqueur, Thomas. 1990. *Making Sex: Body and Gender from the Greeks to Freud*. Cambridge, MA: Harvard University Press.
Mahon, P.A.O. 1813. *An Essay on the Signs of Murder in New Born Children*. Translated by C. Johnson. Lancaster: C. Clark.
Marland, H. 2002. "Getting away with Murder? Puerperal Insanity, Infanticide and the Defence Plea." In *Infanticide: Historical Perspective on Child Murder and Concealment, 1550–2000*, edited by M. Jackson, 168–92. Aldershot: Ashgate.

McDonagh, J. 2003. *Child Murder & British Culture, 1720–1900*. Cambridge: Cambridge University Press.
McGrath, R. 2002. *Seeing Her Sex: Medical Archives and the Female Body*. Manchester: Manchester University Press.
Montgomery, W.F.H. 1857. *An Exposition of the Signs and Symptoms of Pregnancy*. Philadelphia: Blanchard.
Need, Lynda. 2000. *Victorian Babylon: People, Streets and Images in Nineteenth-Century London. Yale*. Yale University Press.
Quinn, C. 2002. "Images and Impulses: Representations of Puerperal Insanity and Infanticide in Late Victorian England." In *Infanticide: Historical Perspective on Child Murder and Concealment, 1550–2000*, edited by M. Jackson, 193–215. Aldershot: Ashgate.
Rabin, D. 2002. "Bodies of Evidence, States of Mind Infanticide, Emotion and Sensibility in Eighteenth-Century England." In *Infanticide: Historical Perspective on Child Murder and Concealment, 1550–2000*, edited by M. Jackson, 73–92. Aldershot: Ashgate.
Rose, L. 1986. *Massacre of the Innocents: Infanticide in Britain, 1800–1939*. London: Routledge.
Ryan, M. 1836. "Dr Ryan's Lectures on Obstetricy." *London Medical and Surgical Journal* 3 (1): 19–25.
Ryan, W.B. 1862. *Infanticide: Its Law, Prevalence, Prevention and History*. London: J. Churchill.
Sappol, M. 2002. *A Traffic of Dead Bodies: Anatomy and Embodied Social Identity in Nineteenth-Century America*. Princeton: Princeton University Press.
Scheibinger, Londa. 1993. *Nature's Body: Sexual Politics and the Making of Modern Science*. London: HarperCollins.
Severn, C. 1831. *First Lines of the Practice of Midwifery To Which are Added Remarks on the Forensic Evidence Requisite in Cases of Infanticide and Foeticide*. London: S. Highley.
Simson, J. 1825. *A Probationary Essay on Infanticide*. Edinburgh: James Gall.
Smellie, W. (Original work published 1754) 1787. *A Set of Anatomical Tables with Explanations, and an Abridgement of the Practice of Midwifery*. Edinburgh: William Creech.
Smith, J.G. (1821) 1827. *The Principles of Forensic Medicine*. 3rd ed. London: Thomas and George Underwood.
Smith, R. 1981. *Trial by Medicine: Insanity and Responsibility in Victorian Trials*. Edinburgh: Edinburgh University Press.
Sommers, S. 2009. "Remapping Maternity in the Courtroom: Female Defenses and Medical Witnesses in Eighteenth-Century Infanticide Proceedings."

In *The Body in Medical Culture*, edited by E. Klaver, 37–59. Albany: SUNY Press.

Trial of Mary Dixon for Murder. 11 September 1735. *Old Bailey Online.* Reference Number: t17350911–88.

Trial of Hannah Perfect for Infanticide. 25 February 1747. *Old Bailey Onine.* Reference Number: t17470225-1.

Trial of Ann Haywood for Infanticide. 8 December 1762. *Old Bailey Online.* Reference Number: t17621208–26.

Trial of Elizabeth Parkins for Infanticide. 10 April 1771. *Old Bailey Online.* Reference Number: t17710410–35.

Trial of Elisabeth Gwatkin for Infanticide. 15 September 1779. *Old Bailey Online.* Reference Number: t17790915–78.

Trial of Sarah Dixon for Infanticide. 10 July 1805. *Old Bailey Online.* Reference Number: t18050710–37.

Trial of Ann Mountford for Murder. 24 May 1822. *Old Bailey Online.* Reference Number: t18220522–45.

Trial of Hannah Maria Pipkins for Murder. 29 January 1855. *Old Bailey Online.* Reference Number: t18550129–261.

Watson, K. 2011. *Forensic Medicine in Western Society: A History*. Abingdon: Routledge.

Wilson, A. 1776. *Medical Researches: Being an Enquiry into the Nature and Origin of Hysterics in the Female Constitution*. London: S. Hooper.

9 Birth Anomaly and Childhood Disability

DAVID M. TURNER

In December 1748, one "J.D." of Beaminster, Dorset, wrote to the *Gentleman's Magazine* to report a "monstrous child" born to a "poor woman" of that town. The child was remarkable for, besides having "the usual form and parts of a female," she had been born with what appeared to be a "large cyst, or bag, extending itself from the fundament quite down to the toes," being in size "equal to that of a bullock's heart." The membrane covering the "cyst" burst some days after birth and "discovered to view an irregular mass of flesh, perfectly human." Inside were "solid substances, which feel like bones, and on its external surface are visible a distinct hand and foot," with fingers and toes discernible. The correspondent had seen the child, now aged two months, on 20 December, "which feeds heartily." The baby had been visited by "many hundreds" of people, who all seemed to agree that it was "one of the most surprising instances of the kind ever seen or heard of" (J.D. 1748, 535).

J.D.'s careful description of the child's physical traits followed the eighteenth-century pattern of empirical observation of the features of birth anomaly, characterized by the many accounts of such phenomena in the Royal Society's *Philosophical Transactions*. While narratives of monstrous births had long been a significant feature of early modern popular culture, by the eighteenth century it is commonly argued that they were losing their status as signs and wonders of divine or supernatural provenance, and increasingly captured within "rational," "scientific," or "medical" discourses based on firmer anatomical principles. This eventually led to the adoption of the term "teratology" by Geoffrey Saint-Hilaire in 1832 to designate the field of the study of irregular conceptions (Curran and Graille 1997, 2). Yet the author of this account could not resist the opportunity to pass moral judgment. "Such phenomena," he remarked, were "undoubtedly visible proofs of God's displeasure against sin." He further noted that "the parent of the child has been remarkably vile, and her offspring is spurious" (J.D. 1748, 535). Where merited, the recourse to "older" theological interpretations was still compelling.

This chapter examines interpretations of birth anomaly in eighteenth-century England and explores how accounts of "defective" children contributed to broader understandings of physical difference. Eighteenth-century "monstrosity" had a broad definition. As Sally Frampton shows in her chapter in this volume, the spectrum of "monstrosity" extended beyond birth anomalies to include ovarian diseases or the excessive swelling of the body as a result of dropsy. "Monstrous" births were the most visible manifestations of childhood imperfection in early modern England, and have been the most widely studied by modern scholars. Bodies defined as "monstrous" typically included those which were formed of an "excess" of matter, such as conjoined twins, giants, or people with extra fingers or toes, or those whose bodies were characterized by a "deficit," such as missing limbs, hands, or feet, or hindrance of growth (Bates 2005, 113–38). But discussions of "defective" conceptions and imperfect offspring were more wide-ranging. In his *Female Physician* (1724), John Maubray listed alongside various types of "monstrous" births a series of "deformed conceptions," which included children born with a "Scurf-Head, a discolour'd Skin, an Ugly Visage, disagreeable Features, distorted mouth, crooked Nose, Legs, or Arms, maim'd in whole or in Part, Tumours, Pustules, or Bubos against the Groin &c." (373). The definition was thus extended beyond the prodigiously deformed specimens that were the subject of broadside moralizing or empirical observation in learned journals, to include those born with functional impairments, diseases or anomalies of appearance judged by aesthetic standards of what constituted "ugly" or "disagreeable" looks. This broad definition of "deformity" was bound up with anxieties about the breeding of children with "weak" constitutions, more prone to developing intellectual or physical impairments in infancy or childhood, or liable to lack moral fibre in adulthood. Those born without "Nature's gifts and graces," explained Maubray, were particularly liable to become either "Jolt-Heads, Foolish, or Delirious" or else "Lewd Vitious and Licentious Persons," with serious consequences for the nation's strength and its ability to support a population incapable of supporting themselves through honest labour (374).

Congenital birth defects have been of considerable interest to scholars working in a variety of disciplines, including history of medicine, literature, and disability studies. Much work has focused on changing explanations for irregular conceptions, in particular the role of the maternal imagination. Scholars have traced the growing scepticism in learned circles about the power of mothers to influence fetal development or cause harm (Boucé 1987; Huet 1993). Bound up in these changes was a broader set of issues including the increasing "passivity" of women in the reproductive process, professionalization and medical authority, and the growing gap between elite and popular cultures of sexual knowledge (Cody 2005). As "monsters" became subject to increasingly stringent classification, they lost their status as "lusus naturae" – sports of nature – and were increasingly viewed as the product of natural laws that helped to clarify normal embryological development (Hagner 1999, 175). Scientific debates over causation of anomaly thus provided opportunities for advocates of preformationism and epigenesis to set out their claims for authority over the mysteries of generation (Park and Daston 1981, 53). At the same time, the study of "deformity" was central to attempts to map out the "limits of the human" in the age of Enlightenment, both creating and reinforcing models of racial and sexual differentiation (Nussbaum 2003).

Such themes have received a good deal of attention and need little repetition here. However, although the voluminous work on the history of "monstrous" births has usefully shed light on the significance of the anomalous body to understanding broader currents in the social, cultural, and medical history of eighteenth-century England, there has been little attempt to explore the implications of debates about imperfect generation for attitudes towards disability. There was, as Kevin Stagg has observed of the sixteenth and seventeenth centuries, "no simple correspondence between the overlapping discourses of disability and monstrosity," but physical anomaly was at the core of both (21). The central figure in stories of "monstrous" or "deformed" births was a severely impaired child, but the idea of the "monster" as "disabled" was seldom articulated. J.D.'s account of the girl born at Beaminster, for example, dwelt at length on her physical difference, but did not attempt to describe this as "disabling," or pause to think about her future prospects or likelihood of survival. Indeed, the term "disabled" in the eighteenth century was used more narrowly than today, tending to refer to those injured in battle rather than people with congenital deficiencies (Turner 2012, 21). Eighteenth-century representations of "disability" thus tended to focus on "accidental" rather than "natural" deformities, perhaps reflecting the poor survival chances of severely disabled infants in this era. Nevertheless, discussions of the causes of "monstrous" births were an aspect of a broader debate about the nature of "deformity" and raised questions about parental responsibility for the health and well-being of their offspring. Eighteenth-century discussions of hereditary causes of defects and diseases debated whether imperfections might be bred out or avoided by placing restrictions on the sexual conduct and marital opportunities of those deemed most at risk of passing on their own imperfections or illnesses to their children. Discussions of birth anomaly thus raised questions not just about the causes of congenital defects, but also about whether people with certain diseases or impairments should be allowed to procreate and about the value of human life. Such issues take us beyond the well-worked topic of early modern monstrosity, into the less developed field of disability history. This chapter re-assesses these issues and attempts to re-locate the history of birth anomaly within the history of eighteenth-century disability.

I

At the beginning of the period, it was still commonplace to blame "deformed" offspring or sickly children on parental sexual immorality. Although early modern broadsides had sometimes represented the birth of a monstrous child as a warning against extra-marital sex, the emphasis of popular literature on generation was on sexual practices within marriage, focusing on the quality, timing, and frequency of a couple's love making. *Aristotele's Master-Piece* (1684) warned its readers that while birth defects might stem from a variety of causes, "above all, unseasonable copulation, or intemperate Venery, is the cause of so many monsterous shapes" (48). Incorporating Levinus Lemnius's account of "prodigious and monstrous births" from *The Secret Miracles of Nature* (originally published in Latin in 1559 and published in English by John Streater in 1658), *Aristotele's Master-Piece* blamed "unseasonable and unreasonable Venery" for a long list of diseases and disabilities including "scald Heads, bowed and distorted Legs, Arms, and Backs, wry Necks, crumpled Feet, incident to swellings and inherent Diseases, especially swellings in the Groin, Buboes, and Emerods," as well as for producing those whose minds were "dull, stupid, forgetful, foolish, mad and unreasonable" (*Aristotele's Master-Piece* 1684, 51). The principal cause was a couple's refusal to abstain from sex during menstruation, which, according to Maubray, ran not only contrary to the "Express Word of God," but also to the dictates of "right Reason" and "common sense," causing the ejaculated seed to mix with the menstrual blood, corrupting it and running the risk of miscarriage, abortion, or an imperfect conception (1724, 374). The horror of physical or intellectual difference was thus intended to "serve for a memorable Caution to all

Parents, that in their conjugal Duties, they behave themselves orderly and decently," so that their "Families may be preserved, and their Persons succeeded, not by an opprobrious RACE, but by a univocal Generation of hopeful CHILDREN, Men of Probity and Integrity both in BODY and MIND" (Maubray 1724, 377).

Sexual relations needed to be carefully timed, not just to avoid this "menstruous contagion," but also to profit from the most advantageous astrological conditions for conception. Claude Quillet's *Callipaedia: Or, the Art of Getting Beautiful Children*, originally published in 1655 but subject to a series of English translations in the early eighteenth century, blamed "ill-tim'd Pleasure" and ignorance of the "Course of Heaven" for the birth of so many "Shapeless Females, and uncomely Boys" (1733, 45). Children conceived under the sign of Aries, for example, were liable to "disgrace" their parents' bed, being often born with "lank Crane-Neck[s]," pointed heads, legs of disproportionate size and a "stupid leaden look," since the competing planets of Mars and Saturn were both "Foes to Beauty" (46). *Callipaedia* also emphasized the importance of environmental factors such as the heat or cold of the seasons of the year for producing "beauteous Progeny," with the temperate spring climate better for producing the "strongest, sanguine Breed," rather than the excessive heats of summer or "sickly" autumn chills or the "rough raging of a wintry Air" (51–2). Popular guides to generation blamed not just the timing, but also the ardour of a couple's love-making. Nicolas Venette warned his readers that sexual attraction was particularly important in ensuring that the man in particular ejaculated seed that was good in quality and sufficient in quantity. "Forced conjunctions" lacking in sexual chemistry were likely to produce "dull and lumpish" children, living evidence of the "small satisfaction their Father took in the Caressing of their Mother" (Venette 1720, 167).

Drawing on humoral physiology, early modern writers claimed that the various qualities of the seed ejaculated by both partners during conception (though with greater "force" or "violence" by the male), when combined with the mother's blood, determined whether the ensuing child was likely to be hot or cold of constitution and also whether they were liable to suffer birth defects or congenital "weakness" that increased susceptibility to disease or disability in infancy and childhood (Newton, 2012, 36). In the Aristotelian tradition, "defect of seed" was liable to cause the birth of children with "one or more members ... wanting, or more short and decrepit" (Paré 1691, 594), whereas conjoined twins were blamed on an "excess" of seed. As the eighteenth century progressed humoral theory was gradually abandoned by the medical profession, and the notion of each partner contributing "seed" was superseded by the identification of sperma and ova, along with a redefinition of male and female roles in conception. Yet the mother's physical constitution and general health during pregnancy remained crucial in explaining anomaly. For example, James Augustus Blondel regarded it as a universal truth that a child "may suffer by the distempers of the mother, by several accidents, as great falls, and blows she receives" as well as by the "irregularity of her diet, and of her actions by dancing, running, jumping, riding, excess of laughter, frequent sneezing, and all other agitations of the body" (1727, 2).

The risk of birth anomaly or childhood disability was affected not only by a mother's physical health, but also by her emotional well-being. The debate over the role of the maternal imagination in producing defective children was perhaps the biggest controversy surrounding birth anomaly in the eighteenth century, but even the most strident critics of maternal impressions recognized that the mother's passions played an important role in pregnancy and violent emotions might harm the fetus. Blondel noted that miscarriage could be caused by a "sudden surprise, a violent passion of anger, an extraordinary grief, or an apprehension of danger." He also believed it was right to take a pregnant woman's cravings seriously since "the disappointment of what the Mother longs for" might make her "uneasy and pine away" meaning that "the child may be depriv'd of sufficient nourishment, grow feeble and weak, and at last lose its life" (Blondel 1727, 2). Stories of "defective" infants born as a consequence of their mother's passions focused attention on the role of emotion in the production of impairment. Although potentially any strong passion might be used to explain abnormalities, it was "surprizing Fear, or an earnest and longing desire" that were the "most turbulent and impetuous Passions that the Mind is subject to" (N.H. 1697, 477). According to the popular advice book *The Ladies Dictionary* (1697) it was these passions which "exciting the tenuous Humors and Spirits in all parts of the Body, cause both the Infant and Mother remarkable Alterations" (N.H. 1697, 477).

Maternal imagination provided a convenient explanation for more unusual types of deformity that resisted other models of causation. Time and again, "monsters" were attributed to strange sights or to the witnessing of trauma, whether in the form of bodies mutilated in warfare, accidents, or judicial punishment, such as Malebranche's famous story of a woman giving birth to a child with multiple fractures after seeing a criminal broken on the wheel (Turner 1723, 175; Blondel 1727, 16). Stories involving apprehension towards exotic animals were particularly popular. Timothy Sheldrake wrote to the Royal Society in January 1735 about a woman who gave birth to a severely deformed child in Norwich Jail where she was awaiting transportation. It was the "strange Apprehensions that her sentence had put her under, from the uncommon creatures the country to which she was sentenced might bring in sight" that could be the "only thing that had occasioned so great a change from the natural form of the child" (Sheldrake 1739–41, 343). The attribution of monstrous births to fear caused by the sight of unusual creatures gave such stories of birth anomaly an exotic quality and emphasized the liminality of the "monster," placing it on the border between human and animal. Blondel blamed these explanations on credulity: monsters had "sometimes the look and figure of a Monkey" because "the lips and cheeks not being come to perfection, and the Mouth opened from ear to ear, appear frightful to the spectators, and give room to these silly notions" (Blondel 1727, 85).

Fright helped to explain the remarkable physical difference of monstrous births, but it also provided explanations for sensory as well as physical impairments, showing the close connection between the two. In 1668 the Royal Society reported on the case of a young gentleman born deaf who had "continued dumb" until the age of ten or eleven. Hearing loss was occasioned by a "sudden fright" received by his mother during pregnancy by which his "head and face were a little distorted" to such a degree that his left ear was "quite shut up," leading to a "want of due Tension of the Tympanum of his ear" (Holder 1668, 665–6). Maternal imagination was also used by early eighteenth-century physicians and natural philosophers to explain deviation from common pathologies of illnesses. For example, a tumour found on the loins of an infant accompanied by a cloven spine was classed as "praeternatural" by Dr Rutty, a Fellow of the Royal Society and Royal College of Physicians. Since the case did not conform to Frederik Ruysch's observations on the normal causes of spina bifida, it was instead attributed to a fright experienced by the child's mother "occasion'd by her Husband's falling from a Horse and very much bruising his loins," which led to the tumour appearing on the baby's own loins (Rutty 1720–1, 98–101).

Popular advice literature warned pregnant women against the dangers of traumatic events, but also about the effects of day-to-day encounters with "deformed" or disabled people. *Callipaedia* advised mothers to "Guard well your Eyes from Monsters, and beware/ No Aesop or Thersites enter there," referring to the famously "crooked" poet and the bow-legged, lame soldier in the *Iliad* (Quillet 1733, 66). Yet such sights were difficult to avoid, especially in large towns and cities such as London where, as Lady Mary Wortley Montagu described in 1715, the sight of so many "loathsome Cripples" daily "shock'd" the senses (Montagu 1965–7, 1:229). During the early eighteenth century, warnings of the effects of the maternal imagination were harnessed in calls for greater regulation of the disabled poor whose "unsightly" presence was seen as a threat to the progress of commerce and politeness (Turner 2012, 93–4). In *The Trade and Navigation of Great Britain Considered* (1729), the merchant Joshua Gee complained of the attraction of London to beggars "born with any Defect or Deformity, or maimed by Fire or any other Casualty" and urged the authorities to build a hospital for their care and confinement so that honest pedestrians were not subjected to such "obnoxious sights" (Gee 1729, 38–9). "I am of Opinion," he wrote, "that they are by no Means Objects fit to go abroad; and considering the Frights and pernicious Impressions which such horrid Sights have given to pregnant Women (and sometimes even to the disfiguring of Infants in the Womb) should move all tender Husbands to the redress of this Enormity" (42).

Gee's use of the theory of maternal impressions to bolster his calls for the institutionalization of the disabled poor took place against the backdrop of growing controversy over the power of the mother's imagination to affect the development of the unborn child. Both sides in this debate used their support or opposition to the theory of maternal impressions to comment more generally on the problem of the disabled poor in Georgian London. The principal defender of the theory, Daniel Turner, provided examples of cases where the sight of maimed beggars had frightened pregnant women and led to the birth of children with similar defects. There was, he argued, a "sad instance" from London where "a child of Sir J.B. whose Lady frighten'd at the unexpected view of a Beggar's Stump Arm upon her Coach Door, being then with child" was later delivered of a child "wanting one of his hands" (Turner 1723, 176). The story reiterated the common message that pregnant women should avoid frightful sights, but its choice of details reflected a broader range of concerns, including the troubling emotional consequences of encounters between London's wealthier citizens and the disorderly poor and the intrusion of the latter upon the spaces of the elite, marked here by the beggar's stump thrust aggressively at the coach. The way-laying of respectable citizens as they alighted from coaches by beggars imploring assistance was often noted by social commentators. For instance, Edward Ward's *London Spy* (1709) described beggars on crutches "drawing into a body to attack the coach of some charitable Lord" at Lincoln's Inn Fields (Ward 1993, 96), while the anonymous author of *A Trip from St James's to the Royal-Exchange* described being "accosted" in the Strand by "several Beggars, maim'd lame and lazy"

(*Trip from St James's*, 1744, 23). The description of these encounters using the language of violence, and the belief that they were frightening enough to harm an unborn child because of the effects of the "shocking" or "loathsome" display of impaired bodies on the minds of mothers, served to heighten the menace of London's most impoverished citizens and helped to crystallize moral outrage in the media and social commentary.

Turner's opponent, James Augustus Blondel, focused on a different problem related to the disabled poor, using his scepticism of the theory of maternal impressions to denounce the fraudulent presentation of impairments by street beggars. Like Ambroise Paré in the sixteenth century, he included in his discussion of the causes of "monstrosity" artificial productions of physical difference caused by "Abominable Cheats" (Blondel 1727, 11–12; Paré 1691, 606–8). "Some of those deformities attributed to the Strength of Imagination, are often the effects of Imprudence and the most villainous barbarity," he argued, and were used to fraudulently obtain "the charity and benevolence of others," allowing beggars to "live a lazy and indolent life" (Blondel 1727, 11). Blondel had "taken particular notice of several of them in the streets of London," including many who carried children about with them who "have very odd and unusual deformities and mutilations, especially in their hands and feet." The frequency of such aberrations on the children of mendicants fuelled Blondel's doubts, not just about the veracity of the impairments presented, but also about the role of the maternal imagination in causing defects more generally: "If these irregularities were from the birth and occasion'd by strength of imagination why should they appear more on the body of beggars than of any other people? There's certainly a mystery in this" (12). While disagreeing about the power of the maternal imagination, Blondel was no less vocal than his contemporaries in calling for the better regulation of mendacity, reflecting that "many of these vagrants deserve to be tried upon the Coventry Act" – the legislation passed in the reign of Charles II outlawing deliberate disfigurement (Blondel 1727, 12). But whereas defenders of the theory of maternal imagination had drawn upon the example of the frightful effects of viewing a mutilated body in causing birth anomalies to support their argument, Blondel drew upon a different disability metaphor to refute them. Maintaining that the fluid in which the fertilized ovum swims after conception effectively cut it off from the mother and made it impervious to her will, Blondel maintained that "Imagination does command it no more than a man paralitical can move his limbs" (54). Whereas Turner and other supporters of the theory of maternal impressions had attributed a kind of threatening power to people with impairments that threatened the posterity of the social and political elite, Blondel used examples that emphasized the impotence of people with impairments, or ones which associated physical disability with fraud, in order to deny the powers of imagining women over their unborn children.

II

Debates about the power of the maternal imagination focused on the role of fright and other strong passions in harming the unborn child. Yet some writers maintained that if the mother's imagination might cause impairment or deformity, it could also help to reduce the possibility of a child inheriting negative physical traits from its parents, eliminating rather than causing disablement. The *Ladies Dictionary* repeated Galen's advice to a woman married to a "deformed" husband to "gaze earnestly" on a picture of a "lovely person" hanging in her chamber, to bring forth a son with a more "pleasing" physical appearance (N.H. 1697, 476). Stories of adulteresses imagining their husbands when making love to their gallants to avoid the stigma of illegitimacy were also commonplace in early modern popular culture (Maubray 1724, 64).

Such tales formed part of a wider body of literature in seventeenth- and eighteenth-century England offering advice on how to bring forth "beautiful" children. Not just supplying useful counsel on ante-natal care, these publications also held out the possibility of improving the human species by breeding out physical – or moral – imperfections. If procreation had always been a key purpose of marriage, some eighteenth-century texts argued that it was a duty of married couples to strive to generate the most handsome – and by implication the fittest – children possible. The anonymous author of *Procreation Refin'd: A New Method for the Begetting Children with Handsome Faces* (c. 1710) presented a series of "Examples and Experiments applicable and necessary for the commodious Carrying on the Great Work of GENERATION," recommending it as a gift "proper to be given at Marriages instead of Gloves, Rings, etc." (title page). Such texts were also part of a broader eighteenth-century debate about the role of hereditary factors in contributing to birth anomaly and childhood disability which also had significant implications for the reproductive roles of people with notable deformities, disabilities, and diseases. As *Callipaedia* put it:

> Not every Man or Woman was design'd
> To propagate and multiply their kind;
> Forbid we rightly the Deform'd and Foul,
> To clothe with ill-shap'd Limbs the heavenly Soul (Quillet 1733, 21)

Heredity had long been considered important as a cause of congenital malformation (Russell 1986). Stemming from the simple idea that like engenders like, heredity was commonly listed alongside other medical and moral causes of monstrosity in early modern texts. "By injury of hereditary diseases infants grow monstrous," wrote Paré, "for Crook-backed produce Crook-backed ... so Lame produce Lame, Flat-nosed their like, Dwarffs bring forth Dwarffs, Lean bring forth Lean, and Fat produce Fat" (1691, 598). The reason was that "the seed follows the power, nature, temperature, and complexion of he that engendereth it" (Paré 1691, 538). The Hippocratic theory that the seed drew elements from all parts of the body provided a basis for the passing down of impairments such as lameness and physical traits such as baldness through the generations. Orgasm "delighted" the whole body, releasing humours that influenced the seed. Chances of passing on hereditary imperfections were greater in those "that are immoderate in the use of Venus," since increased sexual activity heightened the risks (Crooke 1631, 279). Yet this Hippocratic theory had been challenged by Aristotle who, in the seventeenth and eighteenth chapters of his *De Generatione Animalium*, refuted the idea that the whole body was affected by pleasure during coition. In this way, likeness "proceedeth not so much from the crasse and thicke matters of the seede; as from the formative faculty seated in the particular parts, and communicated to the Testicles, and at length to the seed by the influent spirits which are neare of kinne unto those which have their perpetuall residence in the parts of the body" (Crooke 1631, 280).

The notion that "monsters have in them an hereditary principle" (Hunter 1861, 246) fascinated some enquirers after the secrets of generation in the eighteenth century. Physicians had long identified particular "hereditary diseases" that passed along family lines. Such phenomena tended to be viewed as "curiosities" or as the individual eccentricities of particular families, rather than demonstrating the modern notion that each disease possesses a genetic element (Müller-Wille and Rheinberger 2012, 43). For example, the surgeon John Hunter described a variety of disabilities and deformities that he had observed running in families, including "spina bifidae," "hare lips," and cases such as that of "Sir C.C." who was born with one testicle, a trait passed on to his son (Hunter 1861, 246–7). Hereditary traits might be immediately apparent in the case of some infants "born deformed and sickly," wrote Isaac Bellet in 1765, or might reveal themselves gradually and possibly not until the child reached adulthood (105). "The vessels of the human body are extended, unfolded and dilated successively in our infancy and youth," hence the effects of the "impregnation of the seed" with a hereditary characteristic may be "suspended, and remain concealed so long as the portion of the vessel which it has tainted is of no use, but they will show themselves as soon as the vessels are unraveled, and the defect of its unraveling will give birth to a disease incurable ... a disease which appears without any accidents foretelling it, because its birth is fixed to the intent of the unfolding of these particular vessels" (Bellet 1765, 105–6). The hereditary transmission of a disease or defect could make its effects more virulent in contrast to similar conditions resulting from accidental or environmental factors. John Andree, for example, included in his *Cases of the Epilepsy, Hysteric Fits and St Vitus Dance* (1746), the example of a twenty-three-year-old patient, Mary Lovell, who had been subject to epileptic fits since birth apparently inherited as a result of her mother experiencing similar symptoms during pregnancy. Encompassing a variety of symptoms including pain in her stomach and head, paralysis, a pricking sensation on her skin, and trembling, Andree noted that being "hereditary" it was "so rooted in the Habit" that its effects were particularly "dismal" (Andree 1746, 107).

Nevertheless, the course of heredity was complex and unpredictable. The notion that prevailed until the end of the eighteenth century that each conception was a unique event, an individual act of "generation" rather than "reproduction," meant that the transmission of hereditary characteristics was not as yet seen as following general laws and could be complicated by a variety of factors (Müller-Wille and Rheinberger 2012, 16). Indeed, one reason why theories of maternal imagination causing physical anomaly were slow to disappear in the eighteenth century was that some "monstrous" births patently bore little resemblance to familial traits (Cody 2005, 121). In an account typical of many published in the *Philosophical Transactions*, a description of a "monstrous" boy reported to the Royal Society in 1731 by Dr Andrew Cantwell (published in the *Transactions* in 1739–41) from Montpellier noted that he was the seventh child born to his mother but "all the rest were of the natural shape" (Cantwell 1739–41, 138). In *Orthopaedia* (1743), Nicolas Andry noted the example of a young mother with a "crooked" gait caused by the poor healing of a dislocated thigh who had given birth to "three Boys with each of them a Thigh luxated, and all of them remain Cripples," whereas their three sisters were, on the contrary, "strong and straight." This surprising pattern was, he conceded, "a subject for the Theorists to employ themselves upon" (Andry 1743, 1:148). Medical authorities sometimes noted other unusual characteristics in parents of anomalous offspring as curiosities, although connections with the traits of the "monstrous" birth could be tenuous. Thus the accoucheur William Smellie noted in his account of his delivery of conjoined twins that although their mother had since had "two fine children," it was "remarkable of the father" that "he had no teeth before the age of one or two and twenty, but has now as good a set as I ever saw, and can lift up very great weights with them &c." (Smellie 1764, 401).

Wits made fun of those who might indiscriminately seek hereditary explanations for any kind of medical curiosity. If defects such as absent limbs might be hereditary, then might also artificial appendages used to compensate for their lack be passed on from parent to child? In one joke, a "droll Fellow who has a Wooden Leg" responds to the question posed by his "soft and credulous" friend about how he came to have his prosthetic limb by saying that his "Father had one, and [his] Grandfather before him; it runs in the Blood" (*Complete London Jester* 1764, 70). Jest books speculated on how a pregnant woman who had two lovers, one with a wooden leg, might identify the father of her illegitimate child by seeing whether or not the baby was born with a prosthetic (Turner 2012, 67). When it was reported that a woman at Lynchburg in Virginia had given birth to a baby with a wooden leg in October 1789, fathered upon her by an "invalid out pensioner of Kilmainham Hospital," the prospect that an amputee "with a wooden leg ... has the property of handing down that leg to his posterity" was treated with gleeful derision in the press. One newspaper urged that a Committee of American Literati be "appointed to bleed him, and examine in what proportion the ligneous particles are in his blood – and particularly examine what food he eats, and caution him in future to avoid eating walking sticks, acorns, and bark, or such substances as may propagate trees, for of trees, all wooden legs, we presume, are made" ("Intelligence Extraordinary," 1790).

Despite the uncertainties of heredity, some medical authorities were more forthright in warning against the consequences of unions involving people with disabilities, diseases, or constitutional weakness. The Scottish physician William Buchan, author of the popular family guide to health, *Domestic Medicine*, first published in 1769, was uncompromising in his opposition to marital unions involving people with potentially inheritable medical defects. Providing advice on healthy living and regimen, Buchan was highly critical of the superficialities of eighteenth-century fashionable society that was lacking in responsibility for its own health and future posterity. His work appealed to the anxieties of middling parents concerned about their children's future prospects (Rosenberg 1983, 39). Criticizing a general human tendency to "value things according to their present, not their future usefulness," Buchan emphasized the duty of parents to avoid passing on ill health or bodily defects to their offspring (1772, 8). Drawing on Rousseau's connection between the health of the mother and the future health of her offspring, but not exempting from blame the "irregular lives of fathers," Buchan argued that "no person who labors under any incurable malady ought to marry," for "he thereby not only shortens his own life, but transmits misery to others" (1772, 9). A man who marries a woman "of a sickly constitution, and descended of unhealthy parents," he continued, "cannot be said to act a prudent part" (10). Such warnings complemented medical concerns about the practical problems faced by women with deformed pelvises in giving birth, as highlighted by Pam Lieske in her chapter in this volume. As William Farrer wrote in his 1773 treatise on rickets, it was "prudent to forbid" women from marrying "who were not cured of the Rickets before their fifth year," due to the effects of the disease in making the "cavity of the pelvis very straight" (46). Such texts married a concern about infant health with a belief in the authority of medical men to preside over the processes of generation and childbirth, marked by the rise of the "man-midwife" (Cody 2005).

Eighteenth-century advances in improving livestock by selective animal breeding provided a justification for restricting access to marriage based on physical fitness (Wood and Orel, 2001). "In our matrimonial contracts," noted Buchan, "it is amazing that so little regard is had to the health and form of the object," for "our sportsmen know" that a fine hunting horse could not be bred from a lame one, nor "the sagacious spaniel out of the snarling cur" (1772, 10). According to Buchan the fortune of families was intimately bound up with the body's health: "family constitutions are as capable of improvement as family estates; and the libertine, who impairs the one, does greater injury to his posterity, than the prodigal who squanders among the other" (11). The avoidance of hereditary disease or disability was thus more than a private matter, but one of wider political and economic importance. Buchan praised the Levitical laws that forbade "any manner of commerce with the diseased," and suggested that this was a subject to which "all wise legislators should have a special regard" (10).

Discussions of heredity had a strong moral message, reinforcing familiar themes of parental blame and responsibility. For example, although many cases of eighteenth-century rickets probably resulted from poverty and poor diet, authors of texts on child health sometimes blamed it on parents' poor constitutions, exacerbated by irresponsible behaviour during pregnancy. "One cause of rickets is diseased parents," warned Buchan, who blamed "mothers of a weak and relaxed habit, who neglect exercise, and live upon weak, watery diet" and so "can neither be expected to bring forth strong and healthy children, or be expected to nurse them." Similarly, "children begotten by men in the decline of life, who are subject to the gout, the gravel, or other chronic diseases, or who have been often affected with the venereal disease in their youth, are likewise very liable to rickets" (Buchan 1772, 687). Farrer concurred that the disease was "most incident and fatal to children whose parents are of a lax, and weak constitution, who are addicted to idleness and effeminacy; who live luxuriously," eat badly or were frequent sufferers from venereal infections (Farrer 1773, 3). Contrasting parental vice with a sentimental depiction of the "sorrows" of the disease's young sufferers whom he wished to rescue "from debilities, diseases and an early grave," Farrer sent out a clear warning to those who put their posterity at risk by irresponsible breeding (viii).

At the heart of these warnings about the dangers of children inheriting diseases – or the weak constitutions that made them susceptible to debilitating illness – was the message that parents needed to take more seriously their responsibility for the health and well-being of their progeny. For Buchan, who had witnessed the health problems of the very young first hand as medical officer of the Foundling Hospital at Ackworth, Yorkshire, child welfare was a neglected topic both by medical professionals and by the kind of genteel mother who passed on responsibility for the care of infants to untrained nurses thinking it "below her to take care of her own child, or to be so ignorant as not to know what is proper to be done for it" (Buchan 1772, 2; Rosenberg 1983, 39). Discussion of how diseases might be passed on by the "imprudent" to their offspring, or the responsibilities of the mother to take care of herself during pregnancy for the sake of her child, complemented a more general message about the dangers of poor child-rearing practices in making children more susceptible to diseases and deformities. They should therefore be seen in the context of broader mid-eighteenth-century discussions of child health and the increasing awareness of population strength as a national resource, evidenced elsewhere by medical treatises warning about harmfulness of wet-nursing, the effects on tender infant bones of swaddling, and the development of orthopaedic medical technologies designed to correct the deformities of children (Perry 1991; Andry, 1743).

For some participants in this debate, the blaming of infant weakness or deformity on hereditary factors was an unhelpful distraction from the real problems of poor nursing, inappropriate clothing, lack of cleanliness, and bad diet. Dr William Cadogan argued that "it is not so common for children to inherit the Diseases of their Parents as is generally imagined" and that many defects or illnesses described as "family distempers" were "falsely, and without the least Foundation" blamed on heredity "when the real cause is either in the Complainants themselves, or bad Nursing that has fixed them early in wrong Habits" (Cadogan 1750, 24–5). Yet he also acknowledged that poor infant care might increase the chances of inherited traits becoming harmful as the child developed and argued that with good nursing these illnesses could be avoided (25–6). Eighteenth-century advocates of responsible parenting imposed a more secular morality on the interpretation of childhood disability or deformity based on the welfare of the child and a concern with the future health of the population. This may have been shorn of the language of sin that had characterized earlier discussions of "monstrous" births, but it was no less concerned with the questions of parental guilt and responsibility.

III

This chapter has examined a variety of explanations for birth anomaly and childhood disability found in English medical texts, midwifery manuals, natural philosophy, and popular guides to generation. During this period a diverse range of factors including astrology, emotion, humours and the environment, heredity, and maternal imagination provided explanations for birth anomalies. At first sight, the value of such material for historians interested in attitudes towards disability and bodily difference more generally might appear limited. The literature on monstrosity provides very little evidence of the subjectivity of "deformed" or severely disabled children. The association between disability and devaluation is repeated and unquestioning. For some writers, even infertility might be preferable to giving birth to a "defective" infant. Thus in one of Edward Ward's *Nuptial Dialogues and Debates* (1710) a "tender and religious Husband" listed the possibility for a child to be born with a physical, sensory, or intellectual impairment among the many undesirable traits in a potential offspring as a means of comforting his "barren melancholy lady":

> Had we a son, what Mortal can foresee,
> In spite of Care, how wicked he might be;
> Crooked in Body, or deform'd in Mind,
> Shallow in Intellect, dum, deaf or blind
> Perfidious, cruel, thirsty after Blood,
> Prone to all Mischief, and avers'd to Good (Ward 1710, 1:195)

Such a child might prove a "thorny Bryar" to the couple's "nuptial love" and breed a "variance" in their relationship they might "ne'er survive"

(1:196). The possibility of bearing a "defective" child thus qualified the common assumption that children were a "blessing" to a marriage (Pollock 1983). Furthermore, despite the growing emphasis on child welfare, there was very little either in books of generation or popular medical or midwifery texts on how to care for a physically different child, or any recognition that such children might have different needs to others. The emphasis in these texts, therefore, was on the avoidance of generating "defective" children in the first place.

Nevertheless, discussions about causation had wider implications for the status of people with diseases or disabilities in eighteenth-century society. The debate about maternal impressions intersected with concerns about the unsightly visibility of the disabled poor on the streets of London and other cities in this period. Both sides of the debate drew attention to social problems associated with poverty and disability, such as aggressive begging and fraud. The association of "unsightly" disability with the potential to harm the unborn child, creating further "defective" people, provided moral, political, and economic ammunition for those who wished to banish those deemed to impede the progress of commerce and politeness from the streets. The theory of maternal impressions continued to influence perceptions of "deformed" people. It remained popular in advertisements for human exhibition in the late eighteenth and nineteenth centuries, helping to emphasize the "wondrous" qualities of exhibited humans (McHold 2008, 30; Turner 2012, 46). As late as the 1880s, the deformities of the "Elephant Man" Joseph Merrick were ascribed to his mother's fright at seeing a circus elephant, and women in a "Delicate State of Health" were urged not to attend shows in which he was exhibited (Durbach 2007, 200). Furthermore, developing medical interest in heredity called into question the "prudence" of allowing people with certain medical conditions to marry and bear children, and raised questions about the role of the state in legislating to prevent such unions.

Calls for state intervention to ensure only the healthy should marry ultimately went unheeded by eighteenth-century policy makers. The hereditary passing on of diseases or disabling conditions from parents to children was too uncertain or prone to "vulgar error" (Cadogan 1750, 24) to influence policy, and there was little appetite for legislation that would challenge the religious principle that marriage should be open to all – or at least to those adults deemed mentally capable of entering a matrimonial contract. Nevertheless, the assumption that the "deformed" or diseased made unsuitable partners in the act of generation created a context of suspicion in which relationships involving "defective" partners might be judged.

Jokes about amputees fathering wooden-legged babies might reflect scepticism about heredity, but also served to present sexual unions involving people with physical impairments as ridiculous and transgressive (Turner 2012, 67–8). This suspicion is evident in one of the few eighteenth-century narratives to examine the sexual and marital "rights" of severely disabled people, *Surprising Memoirs of the Meeting, Courtship, and Sundry other Humorous Adventures of the most Renowned of CRIPPLE-BEGGARs, Manupedirus and Stumpanympha* (1734), which described the relationship of two well-known Dublin vagrants Joanna Magennis (alias "Stumpanympha") and Thomas Murphy ("Manupedirus"). The couple was forced to confront public concerns that their match was a "mad and wicked one" being likely to "propagate Objects of Terror and Wretchedness to the World's End." Although ultimately undeterred by these objections, and satisfied that since "Stumpanympha's" mother "had both hands and feet but had no suspicion her child would be born without either," then there was every chance "we may see a comely breed yet" (*Surprising Memoirs* 1734, 9–10), this account highlighted a popular anxiety about breeding that would gain increasing medical authority as the period wore on. Emphasis on judicious choice of marriage partner and a healthy lifestyle in avoiding the risk of disabled children, together with calls for the "unfit" to be denied opportunities to reproduce, is often seen as symptomatic of the eugenics movement of the late nineteenth and early twentieth centuries, but evidence surveyed in this chapter suggests that such themes would repay further attention by historians of generation, disability, and the body in earlier periods.

REFERENCES

Andree, J. 1746. *Cases of the Epilepsy, Hysteric Fits, and St Vitus Dance*. London: W. Meadows and J. Clarke.

Andry, N. 1743. *Orthopaedia: Or, the Art of Correcting and Preventing Deformities in Children*. 2 vols. London: A. Millar.

Aristotele's Master-Piece, or, the Secrets of Generation Displayed in all the Parts Thereof. 1684. London: J. How.

Bates, A.W. 2005. *Emblematic Monsters: Unnatural Conceptions and Deformed Births in Early Modern Europe*. Amsterdam: Rodopi.

Bellet, I. 1765. *Letters on the Force of Imagination in Pregnant Women*. London: Griffin.

Blondel, J.A. 1727. *The Strength of Imagination in Pregnant Women Examin'd: And the Opinions that the Marks and Deformities in Children arise from thence Demonstrated to be a Vulgar Error*. London: J. Watts.
Boucé, P.G. 1987. "Imagination, Pregnant Women, and Monsters in Eighteenth-Century England and France." In *Sexual Underworlds of the Enlightenment*, edited by G.S. Rousseau and R. Porter, 86–100. Manchester: Manchester University Press.
Buchan, W. 1772. *Domestic Medicine: Or, A Treatise on the Prevention and Cure of Diseases by Regimen and Simple Medicines*. London: Strahan.
Cadogan, W. 1750. *An Essay upon Nursing and the Management of Children*. London: J. Roberts.
Cantwell, Andrew. 1739–41. "Extract of a Letter dated at Montpelier, Dec. 21 1731, N.S. from Andrew Cantwell, M.D. Monspel. To T.S. M.D. and by him translated from the French, giving an Account of a Monstrous Boy." *Philosophical Transactions of the Royal Society* 41:137–8.
Cody, L. 2005. *Birthing the Nation: Sex, Science and the Conception of Eighteenth-Century Britons*. Oxford: Oxford University Press.
The Complete London Jester, or Wit's Companion. 1764. London: T. Lownds.
Crooke, H. 1631. *Mikrocosmographia: A Description of the Body of Man*. London: T. and R. Coles.
Curran, A., and P. Graille. 1997. "The Faces of Eighteenth-Century Monstrosity." *Eighteenth Century Life* 21 (2): 1–15.
D., J. 1748. "Of a Monstrous Birth." *Gentleman's Magazine* 18:535.
Durbach, N. 2007. "Monstrosity, Masculinity and Medicine: Re-Examining 'The Elephant Man'." *Cultural and Social History* 4 (2): 193–213. http://dx.doi.org/10.2752/147800307X199047.
"Extraordinary Intelligence." 1790. *The Daily Advertiser*, 18 May.
Farrer, W. 1773. *A Particular Account of the Rickets in Children; and Remarks on the Analogy to the King's Evil*. London: J. Johnson.
Gee, J. 1729. *The Trade and Navigation of Great-Britain Considered*. London: Samuel Buckley.
H., N. 1697. *The Ladies Dictionary*. London: John Dunton.
Hagner, M. 1999. "Enlightened Monsters." In *The Sciences in Enlightenment Europe*, edited by W. Clark, J. Golinski, and S. Schaffer, 175–217. Chicago: University of Chicago Press.
Holder, W. 1668. "An Account of an Experiment, concerning Deafness, communicated to the R. Society" *Philosophical Transactions of the Royal Society* 3, 665–8
Huet, M.-H. 1993. *Monstrous Imagination*. Cambridge, MA: Harvard University Press.

Hunter, J. 1861. *Essays and Observations on Natural History, Anatomy, Physiology and Geology*. Edited by R. Owen. London: J. Van Voorst. http://dx.doi.org/10.5962/bhl.title.61787.

McHold, H. 2008. "'Even as You and I': Freak Shows and Lay Discourse on Spectacular Deformity." In *Victorian Freaks: The Social Context of Freakery in Britain*, edited by M. Tromp, 21–36. Columbus: Ohio State University Press.

Maubray, J. 1724. *The Female Physician, Containing all the Diseases Incident to the Fair Sex*. London: James Holland.

Montagu, Lady M.W. 1965–7. *The Complete Letters of Lady Mary Wortley Montagu*. 3 vols. Edited by R. Halsband. Oxford: Oxford University Press.

Müller-Wille, S., and H.-J. Rheinberger. 2012. *A Cultural History of Heredity*. Chicago: University of Chicago Press. http://dx.doi.org/10.7208/chicago/9780226545721.001.0001.

Newton, H. 2012. *The Sick Child in Early Modern England, 1580–1720*. Oxford: Oxford University Press.

Nussbaum, F.A. 2003. *The Limits of the Human: Fictions of Anomaly, Race and Gender in the Long Eighteenth Century*. Cambridge: Cambridge University Press.

Paré, A. 1691. *The Works of Ambrose Parey, Chyrurgeon to Henry II, Francis II, Charles IX and Henry III Kings of France*. London: J. Hindmarsh.

Park, K., and L. Daston. 1981. "Unnatural Conceptions: The Study of Monsters in Sixteenth- and Seventeenth-Century France and England." *Past & Present* 92 (1): 20–54. http://dx.doi.org/10.1093/past/92.1.20.

Perry, R. 1991. "Colonizing the Breast: Sexuality and Maternity in Eighteenth-Century England." *Journal of the History of Sexuality* 2 (2): 204–34.

Pollock, L. 1983. *Forgotten Children: Parent-Child Relations from 1500 to 1900*. Cambridge: Cambridge University Press.

Procreation Refin'd. A New Method for the Begetting Children with Handsome Faces. c. 1710. London: R. Griffin.

Quillet, C. 1733. *Callipaedia: Or, the Art of Getting Beautiful Children*. Translated by N. Rowe. London: Feales.

Rosenberg, C. 1983. "Medical Text and Social Context: Explaining William Buchan's *Domestic Medicine*." *Bulletin of the History of Medicine* 57 (1): 22–42.

Russell, N. 1986. *Like Engend'ring Like: Heredity and Animal Breeding in Early Modern England*. Cambridge: Cambridge University Press.

Rutty, Dr. 1720–1. "An Account of a Praeternatural Tumour on the Loins of an Infant, attended with a Cloven Spine." *Philosophical Transactions of the Royal Society* 31: 98–102.

Sheldrake, T. 1739–41. "A Letter from Mr Timothy Sheldrake to Sir Hans Sloan, Bart. Pr. R.S. &c. concerning a Monstrous Child born of a Woman under

Sentence of Transportation." *Philosophical Transactions of the Royal Society* 41: 341–3.
Smellie, W. 1764. *A Collection of Preternatural Cases and Observations in Midwifery*. London: D. Wilson and T. Durham
Stagg, K. 2006. "Representing Physical Difference: The Materiality of the Monstrous." In *Social Histories of Disability and Deformity*, edited by D.M. Turner and K. Stagg, 19–38. London: Routledge.
Surprising Memoirs of the Meeting, Courtship, and Sundry other Humorous Adventures of the Most Renowned of Cripple-Beggars, Manupedirus and Stumpanympha. 1734. Dublin: George Faulkner.
A Trip from St James's to the Royal-Exchange. With Remarks Serious and Diverting on the Manners, Customs and Amusements of the Inhabitants of London and Westminster. 1744. London: E. Withers, M. Cooper, and J. Joffe.
Turner, D. 1723. *De Morbis Cutaneis: A Treatise of Diseases Incident to the Skin*. London: R. Bonwicke.
Turner, D.M. 2012. *Disability in Eighteenth-Century England: Imagining Physical Impairment*. New York: Routledge.
Venette, N. 1720. *Conjugal Love Reveal'd; in the Nightly Pleasures of the Marriage Bed, and the Advantages of that Happy State*. 7th ed. London: Thomas Hinton.
Ward, E. 1710. *Nuptial Dialogues and Debates*. 2 vols. London: H. Meere.
Ward, E. 1993. *The London Spy*. Edited by P. Hyland. East Lansing, MI: Colleagues Press.
Wood, R.J., and V. Orel. 2001. *Genetic Prehistory in Selective Breeding: A Prelude to Mendel*. Oxford: Oxford University Press.

10 Motherhood, Hysteria, and the Eighteenth-Century Woman Writer

HEATHER MEEK

The category of "motherhood" as it developed in the mid-eighteenth century incorporated two distinct strands of discourse. On the one hand, we find the emerging elevation of the "natural" mother – one whose maternal feelings were supposedly "instinctual and innate" (Nussbaum 1991–2, 131); writers of conduct and medical manuals typically defined this figure as nurturing, self-sacrificing, domestic, sexless, and committed utterly to her children. Predictably, however, the construct of the "natural" mother required its opposite in order to exist. The *unnatural* mother – the one who "fail[ed] to 'nurture'" (Fasick 1997, 17) and who assumed qualities of bodily excess and emotional changeability more consistent with the figure of the hysteric – ostensibly disappeared in discussions of post-1750 maternity. A close examination of women's writing and medical texts from the period reveals, however, that the hysteric lingered, exerting her influence and reformulating conventional discourses of motherhood. Like the experience of maternity, the mother's hysteria was an ambivalent force, a painful burden that at the same time offered an escape from the strictures of motherhood.

In my discussion of discourses of maternity and hysteria, I focus primarily on the second half of the eighteenth century, drawing upon documents across a range of genres. I look at a selection of women's life-writing, fiction, and poetry that provides varied portrayals of pregnant women and mothers. The generic diversity of these texts is crucial to gaining access to women's voices with regards to maternity and hysteria, states more often described (and usually oversimplified or appropriated) by male professionals, whose views are expressed in a comparatively abundant number of medical and instructional manuals, a selection of which I also examine. For this reason, in addition to exploring mainstream representations of maternity, this chapter considers women's depictions of a range of autobiographical and constructed mother-figures to uncover a more complete, nuanced, and productively fraught model of what it meant to be a mother in the period than that provided by the dominant discourse alone.

Hysteria and Maternity before 1750

In the first half of the eighteenth century, discourses of hysteria and maternity overlapped in several important ways and for a variety of complex reasons. For one, hysteria was (like pregnancy, childbirth, and motherhood), according to medical wisdom, with few exceptions, a female condition. And just as all women possessed reproductive organs, it was believed that all women suffered from hysteria to some degree.[1] Lingering (though ostensibly rejected) archaic notions attributed the condition to wandering or noxious wombs, and the terminology adopted by physicians suggested that they had not yet rejected the womb as cause for the affliction: "hysteria" was a term applied almost exclusively to women, and outdated synonyms, such as "Fits of the Mother," or "Suffocation of the Womb" (Blackmore 1725, 100), were still commonly used. Even Thomas Sydenham, the progressive late seventeenth-century physician whom Lady Mary Wortley Montagu called her "Oracle in Physic" (1708–62/1965–7, 2:442), saw the female sex as constitutionally weaker and claimed that "there is rarely one [woman] who is wholly free from" hysterical complaints (1682/1979, 85). Dr Richard Blackmore's 1725 assertion – that women's nerves were "of a finer and more delicate Thread, and their Spirits more fugitive and apt to lose their Coherence than those of Men" (130) – prevailed in medical treatises, most of which were rife with resonances of female pathology. G.S. Rousseau observes that women of the period were defined through a series of "incontrovertible universals": an "innate propensity to nervousness," a "domestic situation in a private world conducive to hysterical excess," and an "insatiable sexual voracity granted from time immemorial" – all of which were viewed as "God given, inevitable, unchangeable conditions." Consequently, Rousseau contends, the category "woman" "naturally – almost preternaturally – seemed to lend itself to the hysteria diagnosis" (1993, 174).

Woman's propensity towards hysteria and illness was, in the accepted medical view, only aggravated by pregnancy and motherhood. As Linda Pollock observes, "Medical practitioners considered women to be particularly prone to disease." They were, she writes, subject to "fevers," "ill vapours," "hysteria," and "general bad health"; moreover, "to the ailments endured by all their sex," they could add "those induced by reproduction and child care." Many female patients treated for mental illness, she notes, "complained of a gynaecological or obstetrical illness, and the fear, stress, and illness caused by difficult births contributed to [their] mental disorders" (1990, 45). The association of mental illness with pregnancy and childbirth was often articulated in medical texts. In Sydenham's 1689 treatise on hysteria, for instance, he asserts a direct link between hysteria and childbirth, declaring that "[the disease] often occurs immediately after delivery, and with a great loss of blood, being due to either a difficult labour or to some violent mental emotion" (1682/1979, 85–6). Not surprisingly, such declarations of a correspondence between specifically female manifestations of mental illness (especially hysteria) and the experience of maternity exerted an influence on later conceptions of motherhood. As Pollock concludes, "[r]ather than associating childbearing with a sense of well-being and joy, pregnancy … was correlated with physical discomfort and mental unease" (1990, 45).

In fact, doctors into the first half of the century often viewed pregnancy itself as an illness, much like hysteria. The physician William Sermon described it as "the greatest disease that can afflict women" in his 1671 *The Ladies Companion, or the English Midwife* (quoted in Hobby 1999, xxiv). This phenomenon is aptly illustrated in François Mauriceau's late seventeenth-century treatise, *The Diseases of Women with Child, and in Child-bed*, which was translated into English and circulated widely in England into the eighteenth century: "What *Hippocrates* very well notes in his book of *Humane Parts*, (that the Womb … causeth most Diseases in Women) is not to be doubted" (1710, xvii). Because the womb occupied this role, Mauriceau believed, the experience of pregnancy and childbirth was precarious at best. He explains:

> A Woman with Child, in respect of her present Disposition, altho in Good Health, yet ought to be reputed as tho she were sick … (for to be with Child, is also vulgarly called a Sickness of nine Months) because she is then in daily Expectation of many Inconveniences, which Pregnancy usually causes to those that are not well governed. She should in this Case resemble a good Pilot, who being imbarqued on a rough Sea, and full of Rocks, shuns the Danger, if he steers with Prudence; if not, 'tis by chance, if he escapes Shipwrack: so a Woman with Child is often in danger of her Life, if she doth not her best endeavour to shun and prevent many Accidents to which she is then subject. (48)

This passage provides an instance of what Susan C. Greenfield and Carol Barash call the malleability of "maternal images and metaphors" (1999, 26). On the one hand, probably unwittingly, Mauriceau gives the pregnant woman a degree of agency. She is the "good Pilot" who boldly "imbarqu[es] on a rough Sea," "shuns ... Danger," "prevent[s] many Accidents," and "steers with Prudence." On the other hand, the woman and her womb are prone to disease, and pregnancy in particular is a dangerous voyage for which the "great belly'd Woman" (Mauriceau 1710, 119) must be "well governed." Thus the maternal body was perceived as being acutely vulnerable, and the mother, who was thought to be on the verge of hysteria and so risked mismanaging her condition, had to be supervised and directed by the likes of Mauriceau. In fact, the view that is articulated in Mauriceau's treatise anticipates the medical management of maternity so current in the second half of the century.

The "Natural," Good Mother

After about 1750, women were viewed less and less as inferior, inverted versions of men, and the figure of the physically corrupt, emotionally unstable, sexually voracious hysteric began to give way to that of the "natural," good mother. As Felicity Nussbaum observes, "[a]n ideal of motherhood made the uterus, which had been the site of sickness, into the site of maternal health and the location of unquestioned sexual difference" (1989, 205). A new "female domestic ideal," Laura Fasick concurs, framed the mother-child bond as something that was beautiful, sexually pure, and unequivocally blissful (1997, 18). Within this emerging ideal, the mother-figure was self-effacing, nurturing, and intuitive. In her 1797 manual *The Pupil of Nature*, for instance, Martha Mears, "Practitioner in Midwifery," suggests that "the study of nature" and the language "of the heart" allowed mothers to encourage "the vigour, growth, and beauty of their offspring" (2–3). Mears calls pregnancy a state of "perfection" rather than one of "disease," insisting that what some physicians have described as an "irritability" is more aptly called "an increased sensibility of the womb" (2–3). Indeed, though there was, as Nussbaum observes, a lingering belief that women were "prone to hysteria and irritability due to their reproductive organs," many child-rearing books "named women for the first time as 'managers' of their children and of the domestic space" (1989, 205). Knowledge of motherhood in these books was framed as something that could potentially lend women purpose and influence. Thus, in a 1779 treatise, Sarah Brown establishes her authority as a mother by touting her experience of having "suckled and superintended" seven children (iii). In the new spirit of reverence for natural motherhood, Brown, Mears, and others vigorously promoted breastfeeding as a matter of good health. As Sonja Boon argues elsewhere in this collection, "Maternal breastfeeding was understood as a beneficent practice that had a profoundly positive impact on both mother and child" (270). This view is apparent in William Cadogan's *Essay Upon Nursing* (1764), in which he claims that "When a Child sucks its own Mother, which, with very few exceptions, would be best for every Child and every Mother, Nature has provided it with such wholsome [*sic*] and suitable nourishment" (18). He extols the wonders of mother's milk, which is "poured forth from an exuberant, overflowing, urn, by a bountiful hand, that never provides sparingly" (20). Such praise of breastfeeding and women's distinctive skills as nurturers shows, at least to a degree, that the emergence of the good mother as a rhetorical construct meant that women's maternal capabilities were now perceived as both powerful and unique.

Predictably, however, this turn towards a veneration of the good mother – and the consequent disappearance of the hysteric – was not wholly empowering for the female sex. In some respects, the cult of natural motherhood served to imprison women and their bodies more than ever before. Thomas Laqueur suggests that women lost their passion after mid-century (1986, 23), while Ruth Perry holds that they became sexless "paragons of virtue" (1990, 113). Elaborating on what she calls the "colonization of the female body for domestic life" (113), Perry argues that it was commonly believed "that women needed bodily instruction in matters of [childbirth, breastfeeding,] and childrearing," and that, consequently, women's bodies became increasingly appropriated in medical literature after 1750 (127–9). Nussbaum, for her part, notes the insidious influence of medical management: "Though child care would seem to be transferred to mothers directly because of the plethora of books on management addressed to them, it shifts instead to male doctors who then dispense and publish advice to mothers who do their bidding" (1989, 207). Motherhood in the period was, indeed, in many respects oppressive. It was, as Toni Bowers observes, "[an] institution defined according to a limited set of supposedly timeless behaviours and sentiments: all-engrossing tenderness, long-term maternal breastfeeding, personal supervision and education of young children, complete physical restriction to domestic space, absence of sexual desire, [and] withdrawal from productive labor." By mid-century, she suggests, "these criteria ... became ... universally imposed on women of all social positions" (1996, 28). Thus, the emergence of the figure of the "natural" mother was not greeted only with celebration. The transition from a conception of women as emotionally unstable and sexually voracious beings to "natural," sexless, "good" mothers brought with it a new set of restrictions.

In fact, medical and conduct manuals often undercut the authority of mothers, gossips, and female midwives, even as they cast the mother-figure as a manager of domestic space. William Cadogan, for instance, in the opening passages of his *Essay Upon Nursing*, expresses relief at the medicalization of maternity: "It is with great pleasure I see at last the preservation of Children become the care of Men of Sense" (1764, 3). While he supports a "more reasonable and more natural method of nursing," he nonetheless expresses the opinion that "this business has been too long fatally left to the management of Women, who cannot be supposed to have proper knowledge to fit them for such a talk, notwithstanding they look upon it to be their own province" (3). In his *Domestic Medicin[e] or, The Family Physician* (1772), William Buchan similarly blames the "ignorance" or "carelessness" of parents for the fact that many of their offspring "perish in infancy" (1). The increasingly widespread belief in the virtues of breastfeeding that proliferated in these manuals also served to hinder women. Cadogan is both reproachful and condescending in a remark following his detailed (and equally patronizing) instructions on how to nurse infants: "The plain natural plan I have laid down is never followed, because most Mothers, of any condition, either cannot, or will not undertake the troublesome task of suckling their own Children; which is troublesome only for want of proper method" (1764, 28). In fact, as Boon observes in her chapter in this collection, "the vast majority of infants were nursed by women other than their mothers" (263); nor did the figure of wet nurse escape scrutiny, for she, according to Boon, was subject to a "close surveillance of every aspect of her being" before being deemed employable. In many ways, such post-1750 medical wisdom pretended to give mothers control and authority, when in truth it infringed upon a province previously governed by these very women, stripping them of the ability to make decisions about their children and their bodies.

Considering these maternal strictures, it is not surprising, then, that in some of the literature of the period written by women, mother-figures surface who simultaneously embrace a romantic ideal and find themselves restricted or unsatisfied by it. The notion of the "natural" mother as it emerges in many conduct manuals and treatises is not merely reproduced or reiterated; it is, rather, reworked and made more complex so that the very notion of motherhood comes to appear as a condition fraught with contradiction and ambivalence. For instance, Jane Cave's 1786 poem "Written a Few Hours before the Birth of a Child" simultaneously emphasizes an unbreakable bond between mother and child, and addresses a mother's apprehension as childbirth approaches. The speaker asks God to "prepare [her] for [the] hour" of childbirth (line 1) and looks ahead not only to "pain" and "agony," but also to the possible deaths of both her and her babe (lines 15–16). The poem conveys the impression that pregnancy is by no means an idyllic state in which would-be mothers bask.[2] Women writers such as Cave did not, in other words, discard the discourse of hysteria quite so readily.

A more thorough and visibly ambiguous engagement with discourses of motherhood emerges in Hester Thrale Piozzi's "Family Book," a diary that spans the years 1764–78 and that documents, among other things, the births, deaths, illnesses, accomplishments, and tribulations of Piozzi's twelve offspring, only four of whom lived into adulthood. On the one hand, Piozzi presents herself as an effective "manager" of her many children and the domestic space they inhabit. The very title of the book is suggestive of an existence limited to the domestic sphere, and this initial impression is supported by the many entries in the book that speak to her all-consuming dedication to motherhood and her proficiency at breeding, nurturing, educating, and raising children. However, a counter-narrative reveals itself in Piozzi's defiance of some of the expectations of this dominant discourse. For Piozzi, motherhood was in many respects a thankless task filled with sorrow and hardship. She experienced conflict with most of her daughters, particularly her eldest, Queeney, and the feelings she records are nothing short of embittered. In one instance, she says of three-year-old Susanna that she is "peevish," that her "person" is "Displeasing," and that "I do not love to converse with her" (1764–78/1977, 62). Moreover, she repeatedly describes herself as moving beyond the boundaries of her prescribed domestic space. She travels often with her husband, with Samuel Johnson, and with Queeney, leaving the rest of her children to the care of others. The "Family Book" also highlights Piozzi's involvement in the political and financial affairs of her first husband, Henry Thrale. She describes, for instance, her tireless work "getting Votes all day, & Settling Books with the Clerks all Night" (108) as he campaigns to keep his seat in the Borough of Southwark. Piozzi further defies her role as "natural" mother by flouting – even criticizing – medical advice and boldly taking on the medical care of her children within the home. When her children are sick with the measles, she tells us, "I sent for no Drs. Nor 'Pothecaries, but kept diluting all I could with cooling Liquors varied so as to avoid

Disgust" (215). Thus, although Piozzi follows the advice of conduct and medical manuals and assumes the role of dutiful wife and mother, she simultaneously subverts and challenges such advice by boldly exiting the domestic sphere to occupy the distinctly un-motherly roles of traveller, accountant, and doctor.[3]

A similarly complex treatment of the construct of the "natural" mother surfaces in Mary Wollstonecraft's *The Wrongs of Woman; or Maria, a Fragment* (1798). In this short novel, Wollstonecraft offers a conception of motherhood that asserts a powerful connection between mother and child but at the same time challenges the validity of the "natural mother" construct as an accurate or healthy measure of the female state. In Wollstonecraft's descriptions of the mother-child bond, a vivid sense emerges of the discrete nature of domestic space and of how a sense of vulnerability is engendered by the performance of the role of "natural" mother. In the opening chapter, the heroine recalls her communion with her infant daughter, from whom she has been forcibly separated:

> Her infant's image was continually floating on Maria's sight, and the first smile of intelligence remembered, as none but a mother, an unhappy mother, can conceive. She heard her speaking half cooing, and felt her little twinkling fingers on her burning bosom – a bosom bursting with the nutriment for which this cherished child might now be pining in vain. From a stranger she could indeed receive the maternal aliment, Maria was grieved at the thought – but who would watch her with a mother's tenderness, a mother's self-denial? (1788, 1798/2009, 69)

Wollstonecraft echoes here a notion that most physicians and moralists insisted upon – that breastfeeding was, as Amanda Gilroy notes, the "supreme sign of maternal commitment" and the "essentialist bedrock of maternal identity" (2000, 22–3). Maria's belief that a mother's "tenderness" and "self-denial" are singular and irreplaceable qualities further aligns the text with discourses of "natural" motherhood. A key political point is being made here, however, that in effect qualifies the condition of motherhood. For Maria, the beauties and joys of motherhood are deflated by societal cruelty and injustice. Her infant daughter has been torn from her by a tyrannical husband and father, the lecherous George Venables. This reading has some affinity with Jennifer Golightly's interpretation of the novel in another chapter in this collection. Golightly observes that the purity of the relationship between Maria and her daughter "is interrupted by the cruelty and the lack of paternal feeling of the child's father"

(286). "[I]t is the presence of the father," she continues, "that makes the experience of reproduction and maternity miserable" (286). Maria, in fact, sees the mother-child bond as tainted by patriarchal tyranny: "she mourned for her child, lamented she was a daughter, and anticipated the aggravated ills of life that her sex rendered almost inevitable" (1788, 1798/2009, 69). Even as Wollstonecraft elevates the mother figure, she recognizes the material realities of a society that granted men the legal power to arbitrarily strip women of their maternal attachments.

The Lingering Hysterical Mother

Central to the more official, medical discourses of maternity was an attempt to eradicate the figure of the hysteric that was so prevalent in discussions of motherhood before 1750. Indeed, many doctors set an idealized maternity in direct opposition to hysteria. John Aitkin, for instance, in his *Principles of Midwifery* (1784), includes a discussion of hysteria within a section titled "Diseases peculiar to Women, and not connected with Pregnancy." One aspect of his conception of hysteria is the idea that it includes characteristics that are absent in the "good" mother. In Aitkin's view, the female hysteric's body is out of control; it experiences convulsions, "flatulence," "belching," "palpitation," "yawning," "laughing," and "costiveness" (63). The hysteric is governed by emotion and sexuality, and she experiences "violent emotion of the mind, such as results from *disappointed love*" (61). One particular symptom, "Globus hystericus, or a convulsion of the alimentary canal, particularly the gullet" (62), recalls – both in name and description – the outdated and long-rejected manifestation of a condition in which the womb, as it wandered through the body, deprived the victim of air and voice. A similar discussion is found in Edward Foster's *The Principles and Practice of Midwifery* (1781), which includes a section, "Hysterics," listing symptoms and describing cures for a variety of conditions that inhibit "generation." Manifestations are, much like those listed by Aitkin, characterized by bodily excess; among others, Foster lists "propensity to cry and laugh," "vomiting," "strangulation," "difficulty of respiration," "anxiety," "irregular pulse," and "fornication" (59). Certainly, some of Aitkin's and Foster's symptoms – major gastro-intestinal or respiratory difficulties – are pathological and could genuinely have inhibited a woman's ability to conceive. However, most of the symptoms – such as flatulence, constipation, fatigue, emotional excess, or sexual fervour – are merely innocuous, or they are simply antithetical to the restrictive characteristics of the good mother. Even though most of these symptoms would have had no effect on the reproductive process, Foster and Aitkin insisted nonetheless that they needed to be overcome in women hoping to conceive. For this reason, such physicians listed "indications of cure," which included, among other so-called remedies, "warm, stimulating purges, the warm bath, antispasmodics, and nervous medicines" (Foster 1781, 59). In the context of this opposition between hysteria and motherhood, breastfeeding was, not surprisingly, thought to curb hysteria. Cadogan declares that "the mother would ... in most hysterical nervous cases, establish her own health by [giving suck to her Child], though she were weak and sickly before" (1764, 18). In their attempts to separate hysteria from reproduction and motherhood, therefore, some doctors imposed an ideal of motherhood in which there was no place for the desiring, emotional, "impure" body of the female hysteric.

Like discourses of motherhood, discourses of hysteria tended to offer restrictive prescriptions that aimed to do away with the female hysteric, and these prescriptions were largely ideological. Perry argues that the expectation of maternal purity as it developed in the second half of the century was "[a] cultural construction" that "served in its own way the male appropriation of female sexual and reproductive services" (1990, 112). Treatments for hysteria were similarly oppressive; like the tenets of motherhood, they promoted notions of female selflessness and sexlessness, and they often involved the patient's relegation to the domestic sphere. Katharine Rogers refers to the "needlework and amateurish painting with which women were supposed to divert their spleen" (1989, 24). And John Mullan observes that the "most popular prescription" for hysteria was marriage (1984, 161). According to Guenter Risse, treatments were often nothing more than "blueprint[s] for matrimonial living" (1988, 16). Moreover, once married, there was an expectation that women become mothers. In his 1771 medical treatise, John Ball writes, "if the patient be single and of a proper age, the advice of Hippocrates should be followed, who wisely says, that *a woman's best remedy is to marry, and bear children*" (quoted in Mullan 1984, 161). Such prescriptions often served as attempts to reinstate – sometimes rather aggressively – established gender roles. We see this taken to an extreme by the physician Patrick Blair's early administration of shock therapy. In his 1725 treatise, he describes stripping and blindfolding one of his hysterical patients, only to dump several tons of water upon her until she agrees not only to "become a Loving obedient and dutifull wife," but also to "go to bed with her husband that night" (1725/1998, 75) – with the implied aim of eventually making of her a "good" mother.[4] Blair's treatment is especially punitive; in most cases, however, both hysterics and mothers were at the very least instructed to suppress their rebellious natures and assume their proper domestic roles.

The attempts of some medical men to stifle the hysterical woman were not entirely successful though, and the unruly hysteric, the frightening opposite of the mother who is "rational, tender, [and] non-coercive" (Gilroy 2000, 20), continued to linger, and exert her will, in a variety of texts in the latter half of the eighteenth century. As the above examples show, the figure of the hysterical woman appeared in medical and conduct manuals on the subject of motherhood. Despite their best efforts, these (mostly) male writers ultimately failed to imprison the hysteric, whose laughing, uncontrolled crying, flatulence, vomiting, and sexual voraciousness surfaced in their treatises. Many women writers of the period also contributed to the emergence of the repressed hysteric, but with the key difference that, in their works, she found voice. More than mere bodily excess and passion, hysteria becomes in some of the literature produced by women a form of potential resistance – a revolt against the constraints and limitations of motherhood. Understood thus, the figure of the hysteric comes to reflect a phenomenon Toni Bowers describes with regards to the idealization of eighteenth-century motherhood: "Though silenced, mothers remain authoritative; though complicit, resistant; though co-opted, outside" (1996, 25).

In poetry that features pregnant women – by Jane Cave, Isabella Kelly, Anna Laetitia Barbauld, and others – the maternal ideal is often embraced, but so too is the figure of the hysterical mother. Just as the poet elevates and aestheticizes the experience of maternity, the hysteric appears as part of a process in which the mother-to-be grapples with her tortured mental state and insists upon the power, mystery, and general unruliness of the gestating body. The pregnant body becomes, in effect, the hysterical body. Such a process is evident in Kelly's "To an Unborn Infant" (1794), where the speaker, a pregnant woman, describes both an idyllic physical connection with her child, and her own profound anxiety at the prospect of childbirth and motherhood. Certainly, a romantic attachment between mother and child is apparent as the maternal body "safely guard[s]" the babe's "yet unfinished form" from the "bleak" and "beating storm" of the outside world (lines 2–4). But this visceral connection is tied directly to the mother's hardships, which become the speaker's primary focus. The bodily experience of pregnancy allows the mother to unload her "rising anguish" (line 15) onto her unborn babe. Though she expects that the infant, like her, will "taste of sorrow," she is hopeful that she will fare better "[t]hrough a world of varied woe" (line 27). Because this speaker, like

Cave's, assumes that she will "give being" to her babe and then "retir[e] to endless rest" (lines 39–40), she hopes that the child will carry on with her legacy, asking her to remember her "mournful story" (line 30) and "supply [her] vacant place" (line 36). Kelly's injection of the body into verse results in a tension. Consistent with discourses of "natural" motherhood, the "mother's frame" (line 3) provides a form of protection for the child, who is snuggled within the womb (line 3). But the "mother's frame" is also powerfully linked to the pregnant woman's hysterical tendencies – to her "sorrow" and "suffering," and to her fear of death. Kelly aligns good and hysterical mothers by exalting the maternal body both as idyllic entity and as raw, hysterical force.

Barbauld's "To a Little Invisible Being Who is Expected Soon to Become Visible" (c. 1795) similarly illustrates a process by which good and hysterical mothers come together, but, more so than Kelly's, this poem makes central the power of the female poet both to reformulate discourses of maternity and to ease the mother's suffering. As in Kelly's poem, the mother-child bond is elevated and idealized. The "powers" of the unborn babe "[expand]" in the mother's womb, waiting for "full perfection" (1795/2010, lines 1–2), and the mother-figure "longs to fold to her maternal breast / Part of herself, yet to herself unknown" (lines 21–2). Also like Kelly, Barbauld injects into this mother's experience a foreboding which is suggestive of an incarnation of hysteria. The pregnant woman is "anxious" (line 15) as she awaits, through "many a tedious moon" (line 24), her babe's arrival. Uniquely, however, Barbauld presents a poet who takes it upon herself to alleviate the mother's pain, a process made easier by the speaker's alignment not with the mother-figure (from whom she is made explicitly distinct) but with the poet herself. This speaker/poet urges the "little captive" babe to "burst thy prison doors" (line 29) and to make "haste" (line 12). She expresses a wish that her "charmed verse" could "speed thee on thy way .../ Till thy wished smile thy mother's pangs o'erpay" (lines, 33–4, 36). Ironically, this wish has already been realized through the very "verse" here referenced. The poet has liberated the mother of her troubles; through verse, she has granted the mother the ability to lay a kiss "on [a] soft cheek" (line 16), fold the child "to her maternal breast" (line 21), "see and salute the stranger guest" (line 23), and hear "the first accents of [a] feeble cry" (line 28). Barbauld, therefore, like Kelly, describes an experience of maternity that reflects a productive tension between the good mother, the hysteric, and the poet.

Kelly and Barbauld, along with Piozzi, Wollstonecraft, and Cave are representative of a group of eighteenth-century women whose writing expresses an ambivalence towards the cult of natural motherhood. On the one hand, they embrace its ideals, but on the other, they show that mothers are not merely sexless, obedient, domestic figures. Rather, the mothers featured in their texts sometimes experience anxiety and unhappiness in the face of maternal strictures. At times, these mothers also take on traits of the bodily driven hysteric, thus defying the tenets imposed upon them. The figure of the hysteric does not simply disappear, then, after 1750. Rather, she sometimes emerges in women's writing (and to a degree, in medical texts) as a figure who is both a product of and challenge to the construct of the natural mother.

The Hysterical Mother-Writer as Healer

Inherent in this convergence of motherhood and hysteria was an obvious paradox. Prescriptions for both demanded that mothers fulfil domestic duties, embrace the role of natural mother, and suppress a hysterical nature, but these prescriptions (as some women writers detected) led to the sort of despair that conventional treatments for hysteria were meant to suppress and control. Central to this paradox is the fact that, like remedies for hysteria, eighteenth-century discourses of motherhood tended to encourage the suppression of extreme emotion. According to Amanda Gilroy, Martha Mears's conduct manual outlines "rules for the management of the temper and passions" that are intended to enable women "to acquire a habit of serenity" (quoted in Gilroy 2000, 20), and while she refers specifically to pregnant women, Mears's "rules" extend to "management" within the "new-style sentimental family," where women are defined by their "sweet manners, and mild address" (Gilroy 2000, 20). Expectations of sweetness and compassion were imposed upon hysterical women and mothers alike as a means of containing their rebellious natures, but attempts to fulfil these expectations and repress so-called negative emotion could lead women to assume the very "hysterical" traits – such as anger, passion, and bitterness – that natural mothers were expected to stifle.

Piozzi's "Family Book" offers an apt illustration of this paradox. The work as a whole ostensibly offers a selfless narration of Piozzi's children's early lives, and yet, particularly as the journal progresses, it becomes more of a personal confession of Piozzi's own troubles as she struggles, mostly in vain, to reconcile her conflicting roles as both benevolent, morally pure mother, and introspective, and oftentimes depressed, woman. Indeed, Piozzi's attempts to embrace a maternal nature and follow the demanding expectations of Mears and others ultimately led to frustration, misery, passion, paranoia, and neurosis – symptoms of hysteria. She succumbs to her role as mother, but she also displays a passionate resistance to this very role. For instance, after exhibiting an expected "all-engrossing tenderness" towards her children, and educating them diligently over the course of years, Piozzi begins to feel frustration and resentment. In a July 1776 entry, she notes, "I have really listened to Babies Learning till I am half stupefied – & all my pains have answered so poorly" – which is a reference to the many children (seven of ten) who had died by this point. She looks back on her education of Henry and Lucy in particular, and asks: "The Instructions I labor'd to give them – what did they end in? The Grave – & every recollection brings only new Regret." "[A]t Present I can not begin battling with Babies," she continues, "I have already spent my whole Youth at it & lost my Reward at last" (1764–78/1977, 163). Piozzi's tangible despair shows her as a "stupefied" and "Regret[ful]" mother. Her role as selfless educator has brought her to a state that has much in common with contemporary diagnoses of hysteria. Indeed, as a whole, the "Family Book" emerges as a record of experiences and emotions that Piozzi, as a mother, was expected to contain. She "performs" the role of "natural" mother, but tells us in her journal that there is a sad, passionate, and angry woman lurking beneath.

At the same time, however, we find in Piozzi's journal an alternative to medical approaches that essentially aggravated or incited hysteria. Piozzi experiences many of the hysterical symptoms enumerated by certain doctors (such as what late seventeenth-century doctor Thomas Sydenham calls, quite simply, "an incurable despair" [1682/1979, 88–9]), but she manages these symptoms in her own, unique way. She provides reasons for her despair in the journal, which effectively becomes a therapeutic outlet for her pain. Doctors such as Sydenham, Richard Blackmore, and Robert Whytt listed groundless fears, "ridiculous fancies" (Whytt 1765, 74), frightful dreams, and "melancholy forebodings" (Sydenham 1682/1979, 88–9) as hysterical symptoms, all of which Piozzi complains of at various points. In one 1777 passage, for instance, written four months into her twelfth pregnancy, Piozzi worries that the child she carries has died: "I felt [today] none of the usual Motion of the Foetus," she writes, "which I fear never was endued with Life nor now ever will be." She goes on to describe a rather horrific dream in which she "deliver'd of a Boy – all bathed in blood." "Last Night," she writes, "I dreamt there was a Mourning Coach at the Door to carry my dead Son to the Grave" (1764–78/1977, 198). In the next entry, Piozzi feels the foetus move inside of her, which reinforces her fears of having indulged in "ridiculous fanc[y]." Her indulgence in some sense confirms her as one of Sydenham's neurotic hysterics, who, "see in their dreams ... funerals and the shadows of departed friends" (1682/1979, 88–9). However, to frame Piozzi's "fancies" and "forebodings" as strictly pathological would be a mistake, for her experience of watching children die (she had lost seven children by this time, five of them in the previous five years), as well as the incredible pressure she felt to produce a boy are revealed as legitimate causes for her mental ills. Moreover, her writing makes sense of her supposedly "unruly" emotions and thoughts.

Maria, of *The Wrongs of Woman*, similarly displays signs of hysteria, and, as in Piozzi's journal, the mother-figure explores possible causes of her hysterical attacks, resulting in a form of self-therapy. Wollstonecraft, moreover, adds a political dimension to this exploration. Maria shows symptoms of hysteria as she contemplates her particular circumstances as a wife terrorized by her husband and as a mother forcibly separated from her daughter. She sits in a "mansion of despair" and "endeavour[s] to recal [*sic*] her scattered thoughts." She also experiences "[s]urprise [and] astonishment that [border] on distraction" (1788, 1798/2009, 69). Rather than merely inhabiting the role of oppressed, silenced, and hysterical mother, however, Maria attempts to uncover the reasons for her despair. She "wak[es] by degrees to a keen sense of anguish, a whirlwind of rage and indignation," but then goes on to acknowledge the social and psychological causes for her confused and tormented mental state (69). Later, when Maria describes her fear of being caught by her husband, from whom she is fleeing, she further underscores a socio-political facet to the condition of hysteria. She is anxious, paranoid, and plagued by insomnia, and she has nightmares, fits of trembling, and delusions – all common symptoms of hysteria – but it is clear that her behaviour is justified by her circumstances. Far from being controlled by a wandering womb, Maria's anxiety and paranoia appear as sane responses to an oppressive situation:

> [S]o accustomed was I to pursuit and alarm, that I seldom closed my eyes without being haunted by Mr. Venables' image, who seemed to assume terrific or hateful forms to torment me, wherever I turned. – Sometimes a wild cat, or a roaring bull, or a hideous assassin, whom I vainly attempted to fly; at others he was a demon, hurrying me to the brink of a precipice, plunging me into dark waves, or horrid gulfs; and I woke, in violent fits of trembling anxiety, to assure myself that it was all a dream. (1788, 1798/2009, 158)

Maria might here be diagnosed with hysteria, but this hysteria is tied directly to her domestic role. Her delusions – the "wild cat[s]," "roaring bull[s]," "hideous assassin[s]," and "demon[s]" – are all manifestations of Mr Venables within her psyche. Her symptoms are therefore traceable to a terrifying husband, an intolerable marriage, and a dreadful experience of motherhood. Venables, a symbol of an oppressive patriarchy that imposes limiting maternal strictures, is portrayed as the cause of Maria's hysteria.

The literary text and the process of writing could be central to the woman writer's recognition of the potential shortcomings of medical diagnosis and management. In the case of Piozzi, an indulgence, through writing, of her so-called hysterical emotions seems to have had therapeutic effects, which suggests that conventional treatments for hysteria and guidelines for motherhood – which promoted a suppression of hysteric tendencies – were at the very least misguided. Although she claims to keep her troubles to herself, repeatedly lamenting that she has no one to "tell the little Foibles of my heart" (1764–78/1977, 65), or, as she puts it elsewhere, that she has "nobody to tell my Uneasinesses to, no Mother, no Female Friend – no Nothing: so I must eat up my own Heart & be quiet" (198), the journal itself becomes her confidante. Piozzi does not, as many doctors would have suggested, suppress her pain merely through needlework or caring for her children; rather, she soothes herself by releasing and exploring her passions in writing, which, incidentally, was a creative pursuit considered by most physicians to be too taxing for the weak female constitution to bear. Similarly, Maria's narration of her struggles offers solace. Writing becomes an obvious outlet for the heroine, who otherwise has few political, legal, or social freedoms. "The events of her past life pressing on her," the narrator observes, "[Maria] resolved circumstantially to relate them, with the sentiments that experience, and more matured reason, would naturally suggest" (1788, 1798/2009, 75). Writing promises to free her of "tears of maternal tenderness," "various phantoms of misery," "cruel remembrances," "gloomy reveries," and "the dark horizon of futurity" (74), and she begins composing "some rhapsodies descriptive of the state of her mind" (75). As with Piozzi, writing serves both as an expression of and a release from the pains of motherhood and hysteria. Wollstonecraft's heroine is, in contrast, comforted by writing in another sense, for her "rhapsodies" are intended to "instruct her daughter, and shield her from misery, the tyranny her mother knew not how to avoid" (75). And, by extension, the text operates as counsel for Wollstonecraft's female readers, specifically mothers. *The Wrongs of Woman* thus serves many purposes. It points to the comforts of literature and creativity; it alleviates hysteria's "phantoms" and "maternal tears"; and it becomes a manifesto of sorts, warning both Wollstonecraft's contemporaries and subsequent generations of mothers of the "wrongs of woman." In this regard, hysteria, though to a degree a debilitating condition, becomes a source of strength. It provides a medium and a language through which Maria – and Wollstonecraft herself – can challenge and reformulate restrictive maternal strictures.

Thus, in a range of ways, these women writers transcend medical management by producing literary works that incorporate and rework circulating notions of maternity and hysteria. They reveal the ways maternal discourses can oppress and restrict; they challenge the notion of the mother as sexless and pure and insist upon the lingering presence of the hysteric; and they boldly highlight the difficulties of motherhood. They also show how writing can relieve the mother of such difficulties. Isabella Kelly and Anna Laetitia Barbauld present an emotionally driven, bodily mother, whose pains are relieved by a more reserved, incorporeal female poet. Hester Thrale Piozzi's writing is therapeutic in the sense that it allows her to articulate a version of herself that incorporates both her role as devoted, selfless mother, and as private, passionate, embittered hysteric. In Mary Wollstonecraft's novel, Maria finds solace as she produces a letter of instruction to her absent daughter. In their various depictions of mother-figures, these women writers foreground the hysterical body as a raw, emotional, and oftentimes positive force, and they elevate and alleviate – through the creative process – the experience of motherhood. They both rework medical ideas to provide a constructively nuanced model of maternity and – to return to Barbauld's words – "[o'erpay]" the "mother's pangs."

NOTES

1 Because eighteenth-century hysteria was an elusive condition with myriad incarnations, it was – and is – difficult to define. Nonetheless, the affliction shared many characteristics with what we know as psychosis or depression; frightful dreams, drowsiness, nightmares, peevishness, wandering thoughts, impaired memory, groundless fears, and disturbances of the imagination were some common manifestations. Physical symptoms were the central diagnostic criteria, however. These symptoms ranged from headaches, salivation, and trembling, to paralysis, choking, and epileptic-like fits. The root cause of hysteria, physicians insisted, was woman's weak constitution and her consequent susceptibility to disorder.

2 As Linda Pollock notes, though maternal death in childbirth was relatively uncommon – about 1 or 2 per cent – childbirth was often "imbued with dread. [It] was a very conspicuous *single* cause of mortality and a fate which a prospective mother had several long months to contemplate" (1990, 47– 8).

She also refutes the notion that parents were "unconcerned when a child was ill and unmoved at a child's death" and offers many examples of parents' extreme anxiety over such occurrences (1983, 124–30).

3 Felicity Nussbaum takes a similar position in her essay on the "Family Book." According to her, Piozzi "define[s] herself as the prototypical bourgeois mother" even as "she counters [that role] by asserting her authority against doctors" and by positioning herself variously as "wife, mother, intellectual, writer, tradeswoman, and election campaigner" (1989, 204). She is, in Nussbaum's estimation, "a woman who manages and is managed" by discourses of motherhood (222).

4 In this instance, Allan Ingram notes, "[i]nterest in the mind is subordinated by a preoccupation with the body and with ways of reducing it to submission." The account "exposes a therapy as a species of rape performed on behalf of an estranged husband by a male medical practitioner on a female patient" (1998, 73).

REFERENCES

Aitkin, J. 1784. *Principles of Midwifery, or Puerperal Medicine*. Edinburgh. Eighteenth Century Collections Online. Gale document number: CW3307613960.

Barbauld, A.L. (1795) 2010. "To a Little Invisible Being Who is Expected Soon to Become Visible." In *The Broadview Anthology of Literature of the Revolutionary Period, 1770–1832*, edited by D.L. Macdonald and A. McWhir, 113. Peterborough, ON: Broadview.

Blackmore, R. 1725. *A Treatise of the Spleen and Vapours: or, Hypochondriacal and Hysterical Affections. With Three Discourses on the Nature and Cure of the Cholick, Melancholy, and Palsies*. London. Eighteenth Century Collections Online. Gale document number: CW107181454.

Blair, P. (1725) 1998. "Some Observations on the Cure of Mad Persons by the Fall of Water." In *Patterns of Madness in the Eighteenth Century: A Reader*, edited by A. Ingram, 73–5. Liverpool: Liverpool University Press.

Bowers, T. 1996. *The Politics of Motherhood. British Writing and Culture, 1680–1760*. Cambridge: Cambridge University Press.

Brown, S. 1779. *A Letter to a Lady on the Management of the Infant*. London. Eighteenth Century Collections Online. Gale document number: CW3307196593.

Buchan, W. 1772. *Domestic Medicin[e] or, The Family Physician*. Philadelphia. Eighteenth Century Collections Online. Gale document number: CB127917488.

Cadogan, W. 1764. *An Essay Upon Nursing and the Management of Children, From their Birth to Three Years of Age.* London. Eighteenth Century Collections Online. Gale document number: CB3326576475.

Cave, J. (1786) 1989. "Written a Few Hours before the Birth of a Child." In *Eighteenth-Century Women Poets: An Oxford Anthology*, edited by R. Lonsdale, 376–7. Oxford: Oxford University Press.

Fasick, L. 1997. *Vessels of Meaning: Women's Bodies, Gender Norms, and Class Bias from Richardson to Lawrence*. DeKalb: Northern Illinois University Press.

Foster, E. 1781. *The Principles and Practice of Midwifery*. London. Eighteenth Century Collections Online. Gale document number: CW3308886436.

Gilroy, A. 2000. "'Candid advice to the fair sex': or, the Politics of Maternity in Late Eighteenth-Century Britain." In *Body Matters: Feminism, Textuality, Corporeality*, edited by A. Horner and A. Keane, 17–28. Manchester: Manchester University Press.

Greenfield, S.C., and C. Barash. 1999. *Inventing Maternity: Politics, Science, and Literature, 1650–1865*. Lexington: University of Kentucky Press.

Hobby, E. 1999. Introduction. In *The Midwives Book, Or the Whole Art of Midwifry Discovered*, written by Jane Sharp, edited by E. Hobby, xi–xxxi. Women Writers in English 1350–1850. New York: Oxford University Press.

Ingram, A. 1998. *Patterns of Madness in the Eighteenth Century: A Reader*. Liverpool: Liverpool University Press.

Kelly, I. (1794) 1989. "To an Unborn Infant." In *Eighteenth-Century Women Poets: An Oxford Anthology*, edited by R. Lonsdale, 482–3. Oxford: Oxford University Press.

Laqueur, T. 1986. "Orgasm, Generation, and the Politics of Reproductive Biology." *Representations* (Berkeley, Calif.) 14 (1): 1–41. http://dx.doi.org/10.1525/rep.1986.14.1.99p0120h.

Mauriceau, F. 1710. *The Diseases of Women with Child, and in Child-Bed*. London. Eighteenth Century Collections Online. Gale document number: CW109817161.

Mears, M. 1797. *The Pupil of Nature; or Candid Advice to the Fair Sex*. London. Eighteenth Century Collections Online. Gale document number: CW3307242294.

Montagu, M.W. (1708–62) 1965–7. *The Complete Letters of Lady Mary Wortley Montagu*. Edited and introduced by Robert Halsband. 3 vols. Oxford: Clarendon.

Mullan, J. 1984. "Hypochondria and Hysteria: Sensibility and the Physicians." *Eighteenth Century Theory and Interpretation* 25 (2): 141–74.

Nussbaum, F. 1989. *The Autobiographical Subject: Gender and Ideology in Eighteenth-Century England*. Baltimore: Johns Hopkins University Press.

Nussbaum, F. 1991–2. "'Savage' Mothers: Narratives of Maternity in the Mid-Eighteenth Century." *Cultural Critique* 20 (winter): 123–51. http://dx.doi.org/10.2307/1354225.

Perry, R. 1990. "Colonizing the Breast: Sexuality and Maternity in Eighteenth-Century England." In *Forbidden History: The State, Society, and the Regulation of Sexuality in Modern Europe*, edited by J.C. Fout, 107–37. Chicago: University of Chicago Press.

Piozzi, H.T. (1764–78) 1977. "The Family Book, 1764–1778." In *The Thrales of Streatham Park*, edited by M. Hyde, 21–218. Cambridge, MA: Harvard University Press.

Pollock, L.A. 1983. *Forgotten Children: Parent-Child Relations from 1500 to 1900*. Cambridge: Cambridge University Press.

Pollock, L.A. 1990. "Embarking on a Rough Passage: The Experience of Pregnancy in Early-Modern Society." In *Women as Mothers in Pre-Industrial England*, edited by V.A. Fildes, 39–67. The Wellcome Institute Series in the History of Medicine. London: Routledge.

Risse, G.B. 1988. "Hysteria at the Edinburgh Infirmary: The Construction and Treatment of a Disease, 1770–1800." *Medical History* 32 (1): 1–22. http://dx.doi.org/10.1017/S0025727300047578.

Rogers, K.M. 1989. "Finch's 'Candid Account' vs. Eighteenth-Century Theories of the Spleen." *Mosaic* 22 (1): 17–26.

Rousseau, G.S. 1993. "'A Strange Pathology': Hysteria in the Early Modern World, 1500–1800." In *Hysteria Beyond Freud*, edited by S.L. Gilman, H. King, R. Porter, G.S. Rousseau, and E. Showalter, 91–221. Berkeley: University of California Press.

Sydenham, T. (1682) 1979. "Epistolary Dissertation to Dr. Cole." In *The Works of Thomas Sydenham, M.D.* Vol. 1, introduction by R.G. Latham, 53–118. Birmingham, AL: Classics of Medicine Library.

Whytt, R. 1765. *Observations on the Nature, Causes, and Cure of Those Disorders Which Are Commonly Called Nervous, Hypochondriac, or Hysteric*. Edinburgh. Eighteenth Century Collections Online. Gale document number: CW107623706.

Wollstonecraft, M. (1788, 1798) 2009. *Mary* and *the Wrongs of Woman*. Revised edition. Edited by G. Kelly. Oxford: Oxford University Press.

11 Mothers and Others: The Politics of Lactation in Medical Consultation Letters Addressed to Samuel-Auguste Tissot

SONJA BOON

Breastfeeding and wet-nursing have been the focus of extensive research in the humanities and social sciences. This includes scholarship on the conceptual role of the wet nurse in social life, to histories of motherhood (Badinter 1981; Fildes 1988 Yalom 1997), histories of wet-nursing as a social practice (Apple 1987; Hedenborg 2001; Klimaszewski 2006; Roberts 1976; Rollet 1982; Sherwood 2010), studies on the relationship between maternal milk and public health (Senior 1983; Nathoo and Ostry 2009), breastfeeding in literature (Bowers 1996, 1999), the organization and economics of the wet-nursing industry (Sussman 1982; Klimaszewski 2006; Wolf 1999), breastfeeding in public and political discourse (Bartlett 2005; Giles 2003; Hausman 2004, 2006; Lindemann 2007; Shaw and Bartlett 2010), and theoretical and methodological work on breastfeeding and lactation (Bartlett 2000, 2005; Cixous 1975; Giles 2002, 2005; Irigaray 1991; Kristeva 2000).

Scholarship in the broad area of eighteenth-century studies has been particularly rich, offering insight into lactation, nursing, and public health as it manifested itself in literature, visual art, social policy, health, and morals (Badinter 1981; Boon 2009; Bowers 1996, Brouard-Arends 1991, 1998; Gutwirth 2004; Jacobus 1992; Lastinger 1996, 1997; Ohayon 1986; Perry 1991; Richter 1996; Senior 1983; Sherwood 1995, 2010; Sussman 1982). This work reveals that, during the second half of the eighteenth century in particular, human lactation was a subject of intense political debate, not only in the broad area of public health – which acknowledged the general health benefits of the practice – but also in the areas of public policy and moral reform. Medicine and morality constructed the maternal nurse as the ultimate balm for social woes, offering the selfless benevolence of the lactating mother as a cure for the myriad ills that plagued eighteenth-century society. In the words of Jean-Jacques Rousseau: "When mothers deign to nurse their children, then will be a reform in morals" (1974, 13). Wet-nursing, by contrast, the practice of putting one's infants and children into the care of a woman who would be responsible for their nutrition and development for an extended period of time, was frowned upon by the medical and philosophical establishment, who saw in the practice the problematic transmission of both physical disease and moral corruption. The eighteenth-century's antipathy towards wet-nursing is well documented. Doctors, midwives, philosophers, and others lined up to condemn the practice, instead urging women to take up their "natural" nursing duties. Nevertheless, it was a very common practice during the Enlightenment, a period during which it is thought that some 90 per cent of children of all social classes were sent out to nurse (Senior 1983, 368; for more on the British politics of lactation, see the chapter by Golightly in this volume).

According to proponents of maternal nursing such as Marie-Angélique Anel Le Rebours, a midwife and author of the bestselling *Avis aux mères qui veulent nourrir leurs enfans,* the overreliance on wet-nursing contributed, among other things, to depopulation (Le Rebours 1767). A return to the natural beneficence of maternal nursing, she argued, could contribute to reversing this trend. Others, among them Roze de l'Epinoy, Regent of the Faculty of Medicine in Paris and author of the 1785 *Avis aux meres qui veulent allaiter*, made no clear distinction between the maternal nurse and her mercenary other. Developing their arguments with broad strokes that encompassed both maternal and mercenary, they asserted that the "nurse" was a conduit for morality. Roze de l'Epinoy insisted on the moral fortitude of the nurse in question:

> As for moral qualities, they are no less essential: it is to be desired that the soul of the wet nurse be as beautiful as her body; that she be sweet, bright, and lively; that her comportment project candour; her face, modesty; and her eyes, the calm of her soul; that she be neither angry nor fearful in nature; nor given to wine; and that she abstains from the pleasures of coitus without regret. This last quality is of utmost importance, because if she finds it too difficult, then the violence of her desires will most certainly have a negative effect on her milk. Finally, if she is to be a good nurse, she must avoid all violent passions. (1785, 8–9)[1]

As the anonymous author of the *Encyclopédie* entry on the wet nurse explains, an immoral wet nurse could do much harm: "We have seen entire villages infected with venereal disease that a few sick wet nurses have communicated by giving their children to other women to nurse" ("Wet-Nurse" 2006). While such concerns, which entangle medical with moral, may seem curious to the contemporary reader, they were very real in an era that understood "health" to be defined by the proper flowing of the humours through the body, and located social salvation in maternal lactation. What they also demonstrate, particularly in the slippage between maternal and mercenary, is the abject position of the lactating body. At once a beneficent entity whose corporeal generosity could nurture and nourish the health of the population as a whole, the lactating body was also a troubling, potentially unruly body whose actions could disrupt the presumed "naturalness" of the social order.

In medical and philosophical thought, the word "nourrice," or nurse, properly refers to the lactating woman who uses her milk to feed and nourish her infant or child. However, during the eighteenth century, this term was qualified by two very different adjectives: there were "nourrices naturelles," or biological mothers whose selfless generosity ensured the quality of their milk and the health of their child; and "nourrices mercénaires," quite literally mercenary mothers who sold their bodies – and their milk – for financial gain. While some eighteenth-century thinkers and writers were very clear in their terminology, others – like Roze de l'Epinoy and Samuel-Auguste Tissot – were far less so, resulting in a slippage between the beneficence of one and the potential danger of the other. Contemporaneous correspondence, memoirs, and literature provide evidence that such slippages did occur; that is, that virtuous maternal bodies were subject to the same kinds of censure ostensibly reserved for their mercenary surrogates. The heroine of Louise-Florence-Pétronille Tardieu d'Esclavelles, Marquise d'Epinay's *Histoire de Madame de Montbrillant*, for example, details the difficulties she had in convincing her husband to allow her to nurse her child (Epinay 2000), echoes of which are found in Isabelle de Charrière's *Lettres de Mistriss Henley*. Charrière's heroine, the thoughtful "Mistriss Henley," finds her lactational ambitions thwarted by a husband worried that his wife's over-imaginative mind and agitated temperament might be dangerous for the health of his child (Charrière 1993, 40). The prospect of maternal breastfeeding is also a point of strife in Samuel Richardson's *Pamela* (Bowers 1999; for more on literary representations of reproductive politics, see the chapter by Golightly in this volume).

This slippage between maternal and mercenary is the focus of this chapter. In it, I am interested in considering the roles that lactation – and more specifically, the tensions between so-called natural and mercenary nursing – played in the ways that eighteenth-century individuals understood and navigated their bodily selves. How was breast milk – maternal or mercenary – imagined in the body politics of maternal autobiography during the eighteenth century? To consider this question, I draw on letters from a rich corpus of some 1300 medical consultation letters addressed to the Swiss physician, Samuel-Auguste Tissot, during the second half of the eighteenth century. These letters, concerning the health of over 800 patients, were written by doctors, laypeople, patients, and family members. Both wet-nursing and maternal breastfeeding figure in these life narratives.

For the correspondents that wrote to Tissot, it is clear that bodies stored memories, and that, in their sufferings, bodies also revealed stories. Bodies, in this sense, were sites of somatic autobiography, spaces upon and through which individuals could craft narratives of self, but also, and importantly, agentive spaces that could, of their own accord, *tell* stories of self. Bodies revealed selves, selves that were sometimes in contradiction with the narratives constructed by those who inhabited them. Considering such themes as bodily memory, maternal performance, bodily resistance, and epistolary silence, I suggest that these letters demonstrate that individuals engaged with dominant medical and moral ideologies in myriad ways, in the process complicating – and sometimes challenging – often highly normative and essentialized medical and moral discourses around infant feeding, population concerns, and moral regeneration. Furthermore, the letters offer insight into the lived experience of the often-fraught relationship between the "good mother," on the one hand, and her mercenary Other, on the other.

Bruce Redford has observed that performance is an integral aspect of letter writing (Redford 1986, 2). Letters, a fundamentally dialogic genre, required the careful fashioning of the self in and through the eyes of the intended recipient. By the same token, letters also inevitably *produced* identities; that is to say, it was through letters that individuals came to understand themselves and their world. As "instrument[s] of politeness," in the words of Clare Brant, letters facilitated social interactions and smoothed over any potential rough edges (Brant 2006, 3). But letters were much more than this. Indeed, letters served vital social, cultural, and political functions in eighteenth-century Europe. Caroline Bland and Máire Cross argue that letters, as a genre, are "crucial to politics" (Bland and Cross 2004, 5). Letters are not, as might be superficially assumed, transparent and easily decodable documents. While they may, in their content, reflect an immediacy of lived experience, they are also marked by the conscious choices of their authors: the silences of conscious omission, for example, stand in stark contrast to what is actually written. The vagaries of correspondence, from content to form to materiality, require us to consider letters in a much more complex way.

These insights are vitally important for understanding the impulses that directed patients to correspond with Tissot. In content, style, and form, all of their letters are shaped by these very elements. These correspondents, too, were navigating the complexities of identity within a highly stratified society. As self-consciously aware individuals, they wanted to elicit a response from the good doctor. Fashioning an appealing self was, therefore, of utmost importance. But they were also doing something more. Their letters required them to articulate their bodily experiences in written form; to put the body into text – to, quite literally, *write the body* so that another individual, in this case the most famous physician in Enlightenment Europe, might understand.

Samuel-Auguste Tissot, a Swiss-born physician trained in Montpellier, spent the majority of his professional life in Lausanne, Switzerland. His international celebrity derives largely from a series of profoundly influential books published, reprinted, and translated throughout Europe and beyond for over a century. The *Avis au people sur sa santé*, for example, a veritable bible of public health, appeared originally in 1761 (Tissot 1761; 1765).[2] Over the next century, it appeared in 16 languages and over 140 editions. This book's international influence can also be confirmed by the extant correspondence; many correspondents reference the *Avis* in relation to their ailments and sufferings.

Tissot's approach to breastfeeding can be read through his understanding of women's health more generally speaking. To a large extent, Tissot's medical philosophy paralleled that of his contemporaries. Women's bodies, he noted, were fundamentally shaped and influenced by their reproductive functions. Accordingly, these functions – dictated by an all-powerful and agentive "Nature, who intended Women for the Increase, and the Nourishment of the human Race" (Tissot 1765, 352), needed to be safeguarded at all costs. Within Tissot's medical philosophy, women served specific social roles as wives and mothers, performing civic duties directly linked to these roles. Any deviation from these roles could have disastrous consequences. A girl who read too many novels at the age of ten, for example, would grow up to be a poor nurse to her children (Tissot 1758, 183–4); a woman who chose not to breastfeed, meanwhile, could suffer "a species of palsy in the uterus, which follows the loss of the milk and renders them insensible to the pleasure, and unfit for the purposes of generation" (Tissot 1771, 144). By contrast, conformity to naturalized social roles was understood to be beneficial to women's health: according to Tissot, single women or widows could find a happy cure in marriage, matrimony being "the most universally acknowledged Specific against so manifold a Disease" (Tissot 1766, 22–3).[3]

At a medical level, Tissot believed that lactation was nothing more than an extension of the reproductive process initiated at conception: the nurturing female body, whose blood and fluids had nursed the fetus in utero, now continued to nurse the newborn infant. Those fluids once directed towards the womb now flowed towards the breast where they emerged in the form of breast milk (Tissot 1766, 4). Like Roze de l'Epinoy, Tissot placed a high premium on the physical and moral behaviours of the nurse. In the *Avis*, for example, he observed that convulsions could come about as a result of the quality of the milk:

> Whether it be that the Nurse has fallen into a violent Passion, some considerable Disgusts, great Fright or frequent Fear: whether she has eat unwholesome Food, drank too much wine, spirituous Liquors, or any strong Drink: whether she is seized with a Descent of her monthly Discharges, and that has greatly disordered her Health; or finally whether she prove really sick: In all these Cases the Milk is vitiated, and exposes the Infant to violent Symptoms, which sometimes speedily destroy it. (Tissot 1765, 392)

For Tissot, "corrupted Milk," which emanated from the psychic or somatic corruption of the nurse, could undermine the physical and moral health of the child in her care.

While Tissot was, in his published works, generally vague in his delineation of the boundaries between the natural and mercenary nurse, he made this distinction much more explicit in chapter 13 of his unpublished "Traité des maladies des femmes" (BCUL, Fonds Tissot, IS3784/I/47.1). Here, Tissot outlined a detailed method for assessing the suitability of a potential wet nurse. His method was founded on three basic principles: the suitability of the wet nurse herself; the constitution and quality of her milk; and finally, the quality of her breasts and their suitability for the job at hand (BCUL, Fonds Tissot, IS3784/I/47.1, 446). In this recitation of qualities, the wet nurse is imagined not as a lactating mother, but rather, as an instrument of medical technology (Sherwood 2010), whose efficacy can be measured through close surveillance of every aspect of her being.

Tissot asked prospective employers to consider age, health, constitution, and habits, all of which could be assessed by looking not only at her weight, teeth, breath, skin, and genital area, but also her reproductive history. Other indicators of her fitness to nurse could be gleaned by examining the health of her husband and child. In addition to this, the potential wet nurse's physical features – her hair colour, complexion, and gender presentation – could provide insight: drawing on the work of Mauriceau, Tissot observed, for example, that women with pale skin and dark hair would have hot, sour, and smelly milk (BCUL, Fonds Tissot, IS3784/I/47.1, 456). The size, shape, texture, nipples, and lactational capacity of the breasts were also points of consideration, as were the quantity, consistency, texture, taste, and smell of the breast milk itself (BCUL, Fonds Tissot, IS3784/I/47.1, 456; 450; 449).

This attention to detail, mirrored in other treatises of the period and also in the *Encyclopédie* article on the wet nurse, suggests a deep desire to control every aspect of the wet nurse's body; a desire that recognized the inherent volatility of the lactating body within the contours of medical technology. Unlike the forceps, another new instrument that emerged during this period (see also Peakman and Watkins in this volume), lactating bodies were not inanimate, material objects whose actions could be controlled and determined by medical professionals. Rather, as Joan Sherwood and Melissa Klimaszewski have observed, wet nurses were living, breathing entities who ultimately existed outside of medical scrutiny (Sherwood 2010; Klimaszewski 2006). While wet-nursing bodies could be assessed and their milk examined, their thoughts and actions were harder to control: the moral imperative was almost impossible to police.

Many doctors, including Tissot, argued that a wet nurse's morals were more important than her physical characteristics. Tissot stressed that employers needed to consider not only the physical health and well-being of the prospective wet nurse, but also her emotional, psychological, and moral suitability to the task at hand. According to Tissot, a good wet nurse had to be hard working, chaste, gracious, serious, clean, happy, and laughing; she would not be fearful (BCUL, Fonds Tissot, IS3784/I/47.1, 448). She would be well spoken but not argumentative nor haughty, as such qualities would lead to continual disagreements which, in turn, could poison the milk (BCUL, Fonds Tissot, IS3784/I/47.1, 459). Finally, the ideal wet nurse would come from a healthy family with no history of epilepsy or insanity. These kinds of details were important for it was believed that moral qualities could travel through breast milk thus having a direct impact on the health and well-being of the infant or child (BCUL, Fonds Tissot, IS3784/I/47.1, 459).

All of this suggests that lactation was, at both conceptual and concrete levels, a messy business. This unruly potential of lactation has been of great interest to feminist theorists, who have engaged actively with the conceptual potential of breast milk and breastfeeding. Of particular relevance has been a focus on fluidity and permeability; that is, on the ways that breast milk, like other fluids that emanate from within the body and are expelled from it, can challenge normative understandings about the taken-for-granted stability – indeed, fixity – of the body. In this formulation, bodily fluidity is imagined as inherently threatening: unruly and volatile, fluidity fundamentally challenges a philosophical imaginary that has invested heavily in the presumed autonomy and self-containment of the bounded "man of reason" (Grosz 1994, 194). But such "threat" has also been interpreted otherwise. Most famous, perhaps, is the response of Hélène Cixous, who aligns "mother's milk" with creativity, writing, and pleasure (Cixous 1975). Breast milk is, for Cixous, the ultimate gift; by extension, Cixous imagines the maternal body as a site of knowledge and of generosity, a corporeal generosity that nourishes not only children, but creativity – that source of the self – itself. As a gift – the embodied manifestation of maternal generosity – breastfeeding must also be understood, as Alison Bartlett suggests, as inherently performative in nature. Bartlett observes that breastfeeding is integral to the successful performance of motherhood; it is a conscious and repeated act that gives the illusion of a stable, beneficent maternal identity. Such a framing is highly productive in the case of breastfeeding, an act which has in both the eighteenth-century and contemporary period, been associated not only with public health, but also with the moral health of the nation-state (Boon 2009; Edgren 2010; Nathoo and Ostry 2009. See also Golightly in this volume).

Breastfeeding as performance fundamentally destabilizes the presumed naturalism of breastfeeding, in the process suggesting possibilities for transgression and subversion. As Bartlett observes:

> What happens when breastfeeding is considered an act? It can be an act of defiance, or an act of conformity; an act of love and an act of duty; an act of necessity, of pleasure or pain, of theatricality, or all of these things and others. The limitations of such acts are much less finite than the limits placed on speaking of breastfeeding as natural. (Bartlett 2005, 22)

These insights are useful in the context of eighteenth-century lactational politics and practice. Thus, while advocates for maternal breastfeeding situated their arguments within the Enlightenment's veneration of "the natural," the lived experience of breastfeeding was often much more complex. In the letters addressed to Tissot, breastfeeding – both maternal and mercenary – takes on numerous meanings, meanings that are as unique and diverse as the people who wrote them. Considering the performative nature of breastfeeding allows for a deeper engagement with the politics of lactation as they manifested themselves in both eighteenth-century rhetoric and embodied experience. In the letters I examine below, breastfeeding – both maternal and mercenary – is an act. In some instances it is an act of defiance. In other instances, it is an ideological act. In some instances, it is both. Finally, it is an act that fundamentally shapes how individuals – both women-as-mothers and their children – understood themselves and their bodily experiences and identities.

Breastfeeding – maternal or mercenary – usually appears within the first few sentences of the letter. It is included as part of the longer medical history, and thus, linked to questions of heredity and temperament. This, in itself, is interesting, as it gestures towards the idea of bodily legacies: the nurse, through her milk, left a mark on the child, imprinting not only her physical health, but also her moral core. In the following pages, I analyse a selection of letters that consider not only bodily experiences of mercenary nursing (as related by those who suckled at the breasts of wet nurses), but also bodily experiences of maternal nursing, as related by mothers writing on behalf of their children. These letters would appear to conform to the dominant medical and moral paradigms of the period. I then consider a selection of letters that complicate normative understandings, before moving towards a conceptual engagement with silence and its role in the lived experience of lactational politics.

Bodily Memories of Wet-Nursing

A correspondent writing in 1792 introduced the case of a three-year-old child. Born of a "delicate" but attentive mother, she appeared to have a healthy constitution at birth but suffered numerous ailments since that time: pneumonia, then smallpox and, in the period immediately preceding the date of the letter, various other vague stomach and bowel problems. While the child's mother admitted that her most recent illness might have been caused, in part, by teething, the prime cause of illness was imputed to the corruptions of the wet nurse:

> The child was sent to nurse with a very healthy woman, and we have reason to believe that her too rich milk could have produced all the sufferings that

> have clouded the first three years of this young girl's life, leaving her without a moment of health. (BCUL, Fonds Tissot, IS3784/II/144.05.04.32)

The anonymous correspondent opened her letter by suggesting that the parents in question had obviously chosen their wet nurse with care, for there is no question about the nurse's health: she was, as the author points out, a "very healthy woman." But even this fact could not guard against the problems that could arise as a result of sending one's child out to nurse: in this case, the milk was "too rich." Mercenary milk had compromised this child's health, leaving a legacy that had now affected the whole of her still short life.

Another letter details the continued sufferings of a thirty-eight-year-old priest. Health problems seem to have begun after he left the seminary: mild fevers and hemorrhoids gave way to a more curious ailment that began with numbness in one arm that soon progressed to other parts of his body. Doctors had tried a whole range of options to no avail. A look at the priest's long term medical history offers some insights. While the patient passed a relatively uneventful childhood, "without serious illness," he was, nevertheless "born with a weak complexion and poorly nursed by several wet nurses, one of whom died of consumption" (BCUL, Fonds Tissot, IS3784/II/144.03.04.22). This statement, in the very first sentence of the letter, points to two possible primary causes of the priest's sufferings: inherent physical weakness, possibly hereditary, and corrupt milk. Central to this framing is an understanding that suffering emanates not from the priest himself, but from some form of external corruption. Alongside his "weak complexion," it is the milk of mercenary mothers – women whose actions were not the result of a natural love of mothers for their children, but rather, from a desire for monetary recompense – that has fundamentally affected this man's bodily experience and identity.

Bodily memories of wet-nursing also manifested themselves in other ways. One anonymous doctor recounted the tale of a four-year-old child who was sent out to nurse for twenty-one months (BCUL, Fonds Tissot, IS3784/II/146.01.05.09). She appeared healthy upon her return, but then began to suffer numerous problems, among them something he labelled "dementia": she was unable to fix her eyes on anything, she ground her teeth, and her limbs were constantly in motion. Most interesting, however, was that she had worms. According to the child's parents, the source of contamination was clear: the wet nurse's children had also suffered from worms, as had a "foreign child" that she had nursed. Worms, in this sense, appear to corporeally manifest the contagion inherent in the body of the wet nurse herself. In this instance, the life of an otherwise innocent child had been irrevocably changed; wet-nursing, read through the presence of worms and in the seemingly "irrational" behaviours of the child, had permanently branded her body.

This pattern – an explication of sufferings, combined with sometimes oblique references to problematic encounters with wet nurses – is common to many of the letters that make mention of wet nurses. These letters, then, would appear to confirm the suspicions of doctors and moralists. Wet nurses were imagined as harmful and potentially life-threatening elements, dangerous contagion that could – and would – adversely affect not only individual health, but also had the potential to affect the health of the populace as a whole. Maternal milk – liquid gold in the parlance of some contemporary lactivists – was here, in its mercenary incarnation, reconceived as a pathological entity that invaded and undermined the body, leaving permanent physical effects.

Maternal Performance and the *nourrice naturelle*

In comparison, it may be worth examining a few of the letters that make express reference to natural breastfeeding. Madame de Bombelles, Marquise de Louvois, writing in the 1780s, observed that she owed the life of her son to Tissot's wise counsel. Born at seven months' gestation, her son thrived despite the dire predictions of her local doctors. This she attributed to following Tissot's guidance, as laid out in his *Avis*:

> It was your method, Sir, that saved the life of a child born in a most terrible state at seven months' gestation. All the doctors in Paris assured me that I would be unable to raise him. [But] I nursed him with my milk [and] I bathed him in cold water, despite the rigour of the depth of winter. He will [soon] be one year old. He is a superb child, both in terms of strength and weight ... he is able to roll on a carpet, crawls, and within a month, he will walk on his own. But I don't want to force him. I am waiting until nature commands him to support his own weight. I have just weaned him ... (BCUL, Fonds Tissot, IS3784/II/144.03.04.18)

A close reading of this excerpt reveals a few things: first and foremost, we note the Marquise's commitment to maternal breastfeeding and her understanding of maternal nursing as integral to a health-giving maternal regimen. The results of her commitment are clear: her son is strong, vital, and healthy. He is rolling, crawling, and close to walking. Maternal breastfeeding played a strong role in this; after all, according to her narrative, most of the doctors in Paris foresaw a very different outcome. But there is more at play. The final sentence links all of this activity with the idea of "Nature" – for this correspondent, nature is not a passive force; rather, it is an active agent that demands – orders – certain behaviours. Maternal breastfeeding fits this ethos – it is a physical representation of nature in practice.

As the following case of a mute six-year-old boy suggests, "Nature" – in the form of maternal breastfeeding – was understood to be integral to the performance of beneficent motherhood. This child appeared to develop according to established expectations until the age of three, when he suddenly began to have difficulties expressing himself. According to his mother, Madame Possel, he found it hard to find words and started making faces and strange, convulsive movements. But while the letter catalogues her son's various sufferings, it is, as a whole, not so much about the child as it is about his mother, the letter's author. The letter offers a maternal performance par excellence: Madame Possel indicates that she nursed her son for fourteen months before weaning. Very attentive to his development, she engaged directly with her child to find out more about his changed behaviours. She also attempted numerous remedies herself. Indeed, Madame Possel presents herself throughout the letter as a caring, loving, and conscientious mother, and it is from this position, rather than from that of the child, that she requests Tissot's assistance:

> You will agree, sir, that this is not a natural state; my affections were alarmed and, if I didn't attempt something, could not indulge in the hope of seeing the changes about which we flattered ourselves; please, sir, help me with your counsel; you love children, you've proven this many times through your various publications; have pity on mine, and even more, have pity on this unfortunate mother who will owe you more than a new existence if you tell her how she can relieve her anxieties; I am so sorry, sir, that distance and my position prevent me from travelling to see you in person; I would have done so already, but I have faith in your knowledge. (BCUL, Fonds Tissot, IS3784/II/144.04.06.18)

In this letter, it is tender motherhood – Possel's "alarmed affections" and her concern – that gave her the authority to request an audience with the doctor. And it is maternal breastfeeding – for fourteen months – that serves as material proof of her maternal virtue. In this instance, the corporeal generosity of maternal breastfeeding imprinted itself on Madame

Possel's moral performance of beneficent motherhood (for more on ideologies of motherhood, see Meek and Nichols, in this volume).

What can we take from these letters? The tone of the vast majority of letters that deal with maternal or mercenary breastfeeding suggests that most writers would support at least some of the insights of medical professionals and moralists. Maternal breastfeeding was understood as a beneficent practice that had a profoundly positive impact on both mother and child, and in the process, could pave the way for a revolution in social morals. Wet-nursing, by contrast, was understood as a practice that undermined both infant and maternal health, in the process compromising lived experience. In both instances, the politics of lactation powerfully shaped questions of bodily identity. In this sense, the somatic autobiographies and the dominant medico-moral prescriptions would appear not only to sustain, but further, to reinforce one another.

Other Mothers

There are, however, disruptive narratives; that is, there are letters that complicate and even challenge dominant paradigms. Thus, while dominant paradigms venerated the corporeal beneficence of the natural nurse, these letters ask us to consider alternative maternal performances; bodily narratives of self constructed by mothers who, for a variety of reasons, did not breastfeed some or all of their children. These letters suggest that maternal performance, an integral element of many letters written by mothers on behalf of their ailing children, does not always rest on the corporeal generosity of the lactating mother. Indeed, some mothers take great pains to assert a beneficent maternal identity even as they also engage the services of wet nurses.

The majority of these letters concern problems with milk production. The 1769 case of an anonymous mother of two can serve as a useful example (BCUL, Fonds Tissot, IS3784/II/144.01.03.12). This woman's medical history details numerous reproductive problems, including challenging pregnancies and births, a stillbirth, and issues with lactation. She was finally able to nurse her third child, but was obliged to stop after three and a half months when her milk dried up. Since that time she experienced pain throughout her body, and her head in particular. In this instance, maternal performance appears to rest not on life-giving milk offered freely by a beneficent reproductive body; rather, it emerges through her physical pain; it is her suffering – the suffering of a mother who tried but was unable to nurse her child – that functions as proof of her maternal generosity.

There is certainly some ambivalence here. Even as this narrative challenges normative understandings, it also confirms them; that is, this mother's illness could also be read as a sign of fundamental bodily disorder, her sufferings proof that "Nature," in the form of maternal breastfeeding, knows best. Nevertheless, it is also equally clear in this case that "Nature" has not been generous to this mother. Her experiences suggest bodily resistance to and refusal of dominant paradigms (Boon 2012). Pregnancy, birth, and lactation were fraught and through no apparent fault of her own, she was unable to take up her reproductive responsibilities. For this particular mother, corporeal suffering was the only way that she could engage with dominant maternal ideologies. In the absence of maternal breastfeeding, bodily suffering manifested her care and concern for her children, in the process, enabling her to articulate and assert her maternal identity.

Similar tensions are at play in the case of Madame Moreau de la Ville Gille, who wrote Tissot a pair of letters in 1785. On the surface these letters seem relatively straightforward. But in other ways, this narrative – like the previous one – challenges and resists normative assumptions. Madame Moreau de la Ville Gille's letters introduce her troubled reproductive history. At the time of writing, she was pregnant with her sixth child. Four of her children were strong and healthy. The fifth had died of an apparent case of smallpox at the age of two years and eight months. Like the majority of her contemporaries, Madame sent the first four of her children out to nurse. But, like the heroines portrayed by Madame d'Epinay, Samuel Richardson, and Isabelle de Charrière, she had also expressed a strong desire to breastfeed. However, she was actively discouraged from the practice by others. As she explained:

> I nursed only the child that I lost; I wanted to nurse the others, but with my first, I had no milk during the first days; I had no experience [and] nobody told me that it could still come in. My child was sent to nurse and this hurt me considerably. My birth was complicated, I had rheumatic fever: first in my bowels, then in my chest and finally, throughout my limbs. I was in this state for two and a half months. As for the others, I was reminded about how ill I'd been and was discouraged from fulfilling my responsibility. Finally, I took it upon myself to try to nurse my fifth child and despite everything I had been told and in spite of the fact that the child did not want to nurse for eight days, I kept at it. I followed the advice for mothers in the *Avis*. I did not swaddle my son and washed him in cold water. I was in good health and my son was very strong and very big. (BCUL, Fonds Tissot, IS3784/II/144.02.03.24)

According to dominant medical ideologies, this decision to take up her maternal "responsibility" should have set her son up for a healthy future; it should have assured his well-being. But this was not to be. In an inversion of dominant logic, it was her son – the child she nursed with the life-giving milk from her own maternal body – who perished while the other four – all of whom she had sent out to nurse – thrived.

This experience put Madame Moreau de la Ville Gille into an impossible bind. Torn between a resistant body that challenged essentialized understandings of women's "natural" propensity for reproduction, and a family framework that discouraged attempts, on her part, to rewrite her maternal narrative on her own terms, and struggling to recover from a loss that should not, according to dominant ideologies, have occurred, Madame Moreau de la Ville Gille had nowhere to turn. She put her faith – and her maternal identity – in Tissot's hands and in his method, only to see it fail. And yet, it is in this very promise of maternal transformation through breastfeeding that she sought healing. Haunted by the death of a son who was healthy and strong and whose death occurred almost before she had had a chance to process the fact of his illness, Madame Moreau de la Ville Gille hoped that breastfeeding her sixth child would help her recovery:

> [The death of my son] is always present and fills my days with bitterness; I am also melancholy and serious. [Nevertheless] I confront with pleasure that which hurts me; I would like to nurse the child that I am carrying [and] I am convinced that this will be the best way to distract me from what I have lost. I do not dissimulate; if I do not nurse this child, I will experience true sorrow. (BCUL, Fonds Tissot, IS3784/II/144.02.03.24)

For Madame Moreau de la Ville Gille, maternal breastfeeding was about much more than infant health; in her case, it offered the promise of maternal redemption.

The politics of lactation thus manifest themselves in a range of ways, from narratives that confirm and sustain dominant ideologies to those that challenge and complicate them. But there is also something further to consider. A rereading of the archival materials as a whole suggests the necessity of considering an area well-recognized by life-writing scholars: silence. Only a very small percentage of the letters mention wet-nursing at all, a surprising fact given that the vast majority of infants born during this period were nursed by women other than their mothers and that a whole host of ills were imputed to wet-nursed milk. What this suggests is that although most of those who contacted Tissot likely engaged the services of a mercenary nurse or suckled at the breast of one, they did not associate these experiences with later bodily disorders; unlike doctors, midwives, and moralists, all of whom stressed the dangerous threats posed by mercenary wet nurses, those patients who contacted Tissot did not engage actively with this rhetoric. Rather, they attributed their sufferings to a range of other causes, among them heredity and physical environment. These letters, then, do not support dominant medical and moral ideologies of the period. For most of the correspondents, nursing – maternal or mercenary – left no bodily traces at all. Silence, in this sense, speaks louder than words.

Silence, as a conceptual lens, may also help us to better assess the letters of those individuals who *did* make reference to wet-nursing. Again, a turn to the performative and dialogic quality of eighteenth-century epistolary practice can be useful. By invoking the spectre of the wet nurse, the correspondents could deflect any potential moral blame that might otherwise be directed towards them. In other words, the wet nurse, already publicly identified as a source of contagion, enabled the patient to perform moral and bodily virtue, even in the face of profound corporeal suffering. "It isn't my fault," these letters proclaim. "I may be corporeally weak. But it isn't my fault. My bodily weaknesses are not the result of any inappropriate behaviours or bodily indiscretions. The blame lies somewhere else." In these instances, bodily memories of mercenary wet-nursing enabled the articulation of unmarked bodily identities and untainted autobiographical selves. As a performative gesture, engaging with the figure of the wet nurse could be powerful indeed.

Conclusion

Breastfeeding, as Alison Bartlett has observed "has always been political" (2005, 18). Nowhere was this more the case than during the second half of the eighteenth century, a period populated by doctors, midwives, moralists, philosophers, and others who saw in the corporeal generosity of the *nourrice naturelle* the promise of medical, moral, social, and political salvation. This natural nurse was, however, always haunted – indeed, threatened – by her mercenary other, a corrupt mother who undermined the natural order and, in so doing, could offer only tainted milk. But as the letters in the Fonds Tissot demonstrate, individuals engaged with the politics of lactation in a variety of ways. For all of these individuals, bodily experience was the frame upon which they wove the narratives of their lives. For some individuals, bodies stored memories, acting as repositories for past nursing experiences. For others, lactating bodies were stages upon and through which they could perform their maternal identities. For others still, bodily experience was much more complex – a tangled web that simultaneously confirmed and resisted normative understandings. Finally, many correspondents appear not to have engaged with these debates at all, ascribing altogether different meanings to their bodily experiences. In all of these letters, mothers and their others weave in, through, and around these texts, leaving traces of their presence in the stories that remain.

NOTES

I thank the Social Sciences and Humanities Research Council of Canada for their generous support of this research.

1 Unless otherwise indicated, all translations are my own.
2 I reference the 1765 English version for the sake of clarity and contextualization in relation to translation.
3 The authorial attribution might be spurious in this instance; however, it is worth including because the reading public would likely have taken the attribution at face value and understood the work as Tissot's.

REFERENCES

Apple, R.D. 1987. *Mothers and Medicine: A Social History of Infant Feeding, 1890–1950*. Madison: University of Wisconsin Press.

Badinter, E. 1981. *The Myth of Motherhood: An Historical View of the Maternal Instinct*. Translated by Roger De Garis. London: Souvenir Press.

Bartlett, A. 2000. "Thinking through Breasts: Writing Maternity." *Feminist Theory* 1 (2): 173–88. http://dx.doi.org/10.1177/14647000022229146.

Bartlett, A. 2005. *Breastwork: Rethinking Breastfeeding*. Sydney: University of New South Wales Press.

Bibliothèque cantonale et universitaire de Lausanne (BCUL). Fonds Tissot, IS3784/I/47.1: Traité des maladies des femmes.

Bibliothèque cantonale et universitaire de Lausanne (BCUL). Fonds Tissot, IS3784/II/144: Dossiers de consultation.

Bibliothèque cantonale et universitaire de Lausanne (BCUL). Fonds Tissot, IS3784/II/146: Dossiers de consultation.

Bland, C., and M. Cross, eds. 2004. *Gender and Politics in the Age of Letter Writing, 1750–2000*. Aldershot: Ashgate.

Boon, S. 2009. "Maternalising the (Female) Breast: A Comparison of Marie-Angélique Anel Le Rebours' *Avis aux mères qui veulent nourrir leurs enfans* (1767) and La Leche League International's *The Womanly Art of Breastfeeding* (1963)." *Limina: A Journal of Historical and Cultural Studies* 15: 1–16.

Boon, S. 2012. "Autobiography by Numbers; or, Embodying Maternal Grief." *Life Writing* 9 (2): 191–202. http://dx.doi.org/10.1080/14484528.2012.667362.
Bowers, T. 1996. *The Politics of Motherhood: British Writing and Culture, 1680–1760*. Cambridge and New York: Cambridge University Press.
Bowers, T. 1999. "'A Point of Conscience': Breastfeeding and Maternal Authority in *Pamela*, Part 2." In *Inventing Maternity: Politics, Science, and Literature, 1650–1865*, edited by S.C. Greenfield and Carol Barash, 138–58. Lexington: University Press of Kentucky.
Brant, C. 2006. *Eighteenth-Century Letters and British Culture*. Basingstoke, England, and New York: Palgrave Macmillan.
Brouard-Arends, I. 1991. *Vies et images maternelles dans la littérature française du dix-huitième siècle*. Oxford: Voltaire Foundation.
Brouard-Arends, I. 1998. "Entre nature et histoire: dire la maternité au siècle des Lumières." In *Sexualité, mariage et famille au XVIIIe siècle*, edited by O.B. Cragg and R. Davison, 233–9. Montréal: Les presses de l'université Laval.
Charrière, I. de. 1993. *Lettres de Mistriss Henley, publiées par son amie*. New York: Modern Language Association.
Cixous, H. 1975. "Rire de la méduse." *L'Arc* 61:39–54.
Edgren, M. 2010. "Colonizing Women's Bodies: Population Policies and Nationhood in Eighteenth-Century Sweden." *Journal of Women's History* 22 (2): 108–32. http://dx.doi.org/10.1353/jowh.0.0146.
Epinay, L.-F.-P. Tardieu d'Esclavelles, Marquise d'. 2000. *Les contre-confessions: Histoire de Madame de Montbrillant*. Edited by E. Badinter. Paris: Mercure de France.
Epinoy, R. de l'. 1785. *Avis aux meres qui veulent allaiter leurs enfans*. Paris: P.F. Didot.
Fildes, V. 1988. *Wet-Nursing: A History from Antiquity to the Present*. New York: Basil Blackwell.
Giles, F. 2002. "Fountains of Love and Loveliness: In Praise of the Dripping Wet Breast." *Journal of the Association for Research on Mothering* 4 (1): 7–18.
Giles, F. 2003. *Fresh Milk: The Secret Life of Breasts*. New York: Simon & Schuster.
Giles, F. 2005. "The Well-Tempered Breast: Fostering Fluidity in Breastly Meaning and Function." *Women's Studies* 34 (3–4): 310–26.
Grosz, E. 1994. *Volatile Bodies: Towards a Corporeal Feminism*. Bloomington: Indiana University Press.
Gutwirth, M. 2004. "Suzanne Necker's Legacy: Breastfeeding as Metonym in Germaine De Staël's *Delphine*." *Eighteenth Century Life* 28 (2): 17–40. http://dx.doi.org/10.1215/00982601-28-2-17.
Hausman, B. 2004. "The Feminist Politics of Breastfeeding." *Australian Feminist Studies* 19 (45): 273–85. http://dx.doi.org/10.1080/0816464042000278963.

Hausman, B. 2006. "Contamination and Contagion: Environmental Toxins, HIV/AIDS, and the Problem of the Maternal Body." *Hypatia* 21 (1): 137–56. http://dx.doi.org/10.1111/j.1527-2001.2006.tb00969.x.

Hedenborg, S. 2001. "To Breastfeed Another Woman's Child: Wet-Nursing in Stockholm, 1777–1937." *Continuity and Change* 16 (3): 399–422.

Irigaray, L. 1991. "The Bodily Encounter with the Mother." In *The Irigaray Reader*, edited by Margaret Whitford, translated by David Macey, 34–46. Oxford, UK, and Cambridge, MA: Basil Blackwell.

Jacobus, M. 1992. "Incorruptible Milk: Breast-Feeding and the French Revolution." In *Rebel Daughters: Women and the French Revolution*, edited by Sara E. Melzer and Leslie W. Rabine, 54–75. New York: Oxford University Press.

Klimaszewski, M. 2006. "Examining the Wet Nurse: Breasts, Power, and Penetration in Victorian England." *Women's Studies* 35 (4): 323–46. http://dx.doi.org/10.1080/00497870600669077.

Kristeva, J. 2000. "Motherhood [according to Giovanni Bellini]." In *French Feminism Reader*, edited by Kelly Oliver, 176–80. Lanham, MD, and Oxford, UK: Rowman & Littlefield.

Lastinger, V. 1996. "Re-Defining Motherhood: Breast-Feeding and the French Enlightenment." *Women's Studies* 25 (6): 603–17. http://dx.doi.org/10.1080/00497878.1996.9979141.

Lastinger, V. 1997. "To Nurse and to Die: Rousseau and the Test of Fiction." *European Journal of Women's Studies* 4 (4): 421–33. http://dx.doi.org/10.1177/135050689700400402.

Le Rebours, M.A. 1767. *Avis aux mères qui veulent nourrir leurs enfans*. Utrecht and Paris: Chez Lacombe.

Lindemann, H. 2007. "Breasts, Wombs, and the Body Politic." *Hastings Center Report* 37 (2): 43–4. http://dx.doi.org/10.1353/hcr.2007.0028.

Nathoo, T., and A.S. Ostry. 2009. *The One Best Way? Breastfeeding History, Politics, and Policy in Canada*. Studies in Childhood and Family in Canada. Waterloo, ON: Wilfrid Laurier University Press.

Ohayon, R. 1986. "Rousseau's Julie; or, The Maternal Odyssey." *CLA Journal* 30 (1): 69–82.

Perry, R. 1991. "Colonizing the Breast: Sexuality and Maternity in Eighteenth-Century England." *Journal of the History of Sexuality* 2 (2): 204–34.

Redford, B. 1986. *The Converse of the Pen: Acts of Intimacy in the Eighteenth-Century Letter*. Chicago: University of Chicago Press.

Richter, S. 1996. "Wet-Nursing, Onanism, and the Breast in Eighteenth-Century Germany." *Journal of the History of Sexuality* 7 (1): 1–22.

Roberts, A. 1976. "Mothers and Babies: The Wetnurse and Her Employer in Mid-Nineteenth Century." *Women's Studies* 3 (3): 279–93. http://dx.doi.org/10.1080/00497878.1976.9978396.

Rollet, C. 1982. "Nourrices et nourrissons dans le département de la Seine et en France de 1880 à 1940." *Population* (French Edition) 37 (3): 573–604. http://dx.doi.org/10.2307/1532172.

Rousseau. J.J. (1762) 1974. *Émile*. Translated by Barbara Foxley. London: J.M. Dent & Sons; Rutland: Charles E. Tuttle.

Senior, N. 1983. "Aspects of Infant Feeding in Eighteenth-Century France." *Eighteenth-Century Studies* 16 (4): 367–88. http://dx.doi.org/10.2307/2738104.

Shaw, R., and A. Bartlett. 2010. *Giving Breastmilk: Body Ethics and Contemporary Breastfeeding Practice*. Toronto: Demeter Press.

Sherwood, J. 1995. "Treating Syphilis: The Wetnurse as Technology in an Eighteenth-Century Parisian Hospital." *Journal of the History of Medicine and Allied Sciences* 50 (3): 315–39. http://dx.doi.org/10.1093/jhmas/50.3.315.

Sherwood, J. 2010. *Infection of the Innocents: Wet Nurses, Infants and Syphilis in France, 1780–1900*. Montreal: McGill-Queen's University Press.

Sussman, G.D. 1982. *Selling Mothers' Milk: The Wet-Nursing Business in France, 1715–1914*. Urbana: University of Illinois Press.

Tissot, S. 1758. *De la santé des gens de lettres*. Lausanne: François Grasset; Lyon: Benoit Duplain.

Tissot, S. 1761. *Avis au peuple sur sa santé*. Lausanne: Zimmerli; Lausanne: François Grasset.

Tissot, S. 1765. *Advice to the People in General, with Regard to Their Health*. Translated by J. Kirkpatrick. London. Eighteenth Century Collections Online. Gale document number: CW107351460.

Tissot, S. 1766. *The Lady's Physician*. London: J. Pridden. Eighteenth Century Collections Online. Gale document number: CW106833282.

Tissot, S. [1771 ?]. *An Essay on the Disorders of People of Fashion*. Translated by Francis Bacon Lee. London: Richardson and Urquhart; S. Bladon; and J. Roson. Eighteenth Century Collections Online. Gale document number: CW106599157.

Wet-Nurse. 2006. *The Encyclopedia of Diderot & d'Alembert Collaborative Translation Project*. Translated by Sonja Boon. Ann Arbor: MPublishing, University of Michigan Library. http://hdl.handle.net/2027/spo.did2222.0000.596 (accessed 14 December 2012). Originally published as "Nourrice," in *Encyclopédie ou Dictionnaire raisonné des sciences, des arts et des métiers*, 11:260–1. Paris, 1765.

Wolf, J.H. 1999. "'Mercenary Hirelings' Or 'A Great Blessing'? Doctors' and Mothers' Conflicted Perceptions of Wet Nurses and the Ramifications for Infant Feeding in Chicago, 1871–1961." *Journal of Social History* 33 (1): 97–120. http://dx.doi.org/10.1353/jsh.1999.0012.

Yalom, M. 1997. *A History of the Breast*. New York: Ballantine Books.

12 Reproduction in British Women's Novels of the 1790s

JENNIFER GOLIGHTLY

At the end of Mary Wollstonecraft's fragmentary novel *Maria, or the Wrongs of Woman* (1798), among several "scattered heads" for the continuation of the narrative, the longest of the plans for the novel's conclusion found by William Godwin after Wollstonecraft's death was appended. This passage, consisting of five or six full paragraphs, is remarkable for the range of reproductive images it includes. In the first paragraph, the heroine swallows laudanum and considers the fact that, while she is ending her own life, she is also ending the life of her unborn child; she imagines her "murdered child," one conceived and born during her disastrous marriage, appearing to her again, "mourning the babe of which she was the tomb" (Wollstonecraft 1798, 136). By the last paragraph of the short passage, Maria resolves to live after having her first child restored to her by her companion, Jemima, who enters the room to find Maria faint and near death only to revive her by exhorting her to think of her child: "I snatched her from misery – and (now she is alive again) would you leave her alone in the world, to endure what I have endured?" (137).

Such a juxtaposition is in fact highly characteristic of literature written in Britain by women during the French Revolution: abortions, miscarriages, stillbirths, and child deaths occur frequently, particularly in the radical novels written by women such as Wollstonecraft, Mary Hays, and Eliza Fenwick. However, such images of stifled reproduction very often coexist with images of other, more successful types of reproduction, frequently within the same text. Biological reproduction, for example, is an important part of Wollstonecraft's novel. She dwells at length upon the strength of her radical heroine's attachment to the daughter that results from her disastrous marriage. Images of the heroine remembering her infant daughter's tiny fingers upon her breast, of her baby being snatched from her even as she was engaged in "discharging the tenderest maternal office," fill the novel and form the basis for the construction of the narrative: the bulk of the text is supposed to be a memoir written by Maria for the benefit of this child who, as a female, will need guidance to survive in late eighteenth-century British society (Wollstonecraft 1798, 12). Adoptive reproduction features in Mary Hays's *Memoirs of Emma Courtney* (1796) and in fact provides a means of value transmission where biological reproduction fails: Emma Courtney's biological daughter dies at age fourteen, but her adopted son lives, and it is for him that Emma Courtney's memoirs are written. Reproduction is an important issue for female radical novelists such as Wollstonecraft, Fenwick, and Hays, whose novels frequently include heroines who marry early in the narrative and which are focused to a large degree on the problems facing women after they marry, including the dangers of childbirth.

Novels written by less explicitly radical novelists, such as Amelia Opie, Charlotte Smith, and Mary Robinson, deal differently with the problems of reproduction for women. Unlike their more radical counterparts, novelists such as Robinson and Smith often concluded their narratives with the marriage of the heroine and thus avoid examination of the heroine's experience with reproduction and maternity as a consequence of marriage. Transmission of values through reproduction as a means of widespread social reformation is also less of a concern. Reproduction in these novels is frequently experienced by secondary characters, and images of miscarriage, abortion, or stillbirth are relatively scarce, though not wholly absent (Robinson's heroine, Martha, is horrified by her sister's participation in the murder of that sister's illegitimate baby). Like more radical novels, these novels include an exploration of the problems for women that result from reproduction, including the vulnerability of both mother and child in a society that accords no legal protection to either. Smith's novels, for example, describe the struggles that women who have "fallen" experience in trying to regain their footing in society through the depiction of Adelina in *Emmeline* (1788) and Josephine in *Desmond* (1792). In novels such as Elizabeth Inchbald's *Nature and Art* (1796), Robinson's *The Natural Daughter* (1800) or Opie's *The Father and Daughter* (1801), such illegitimate reproduction becomes a crisis that precipitates the primary heroine's alienation from society and thus the origination of the novel's exploration of social problems and prejudice facing women.

In the novels written during the 1790s, regardless of the political orientation of the text or its writer, images of reproduction serve as a kind of indicator of the novel's attitudes towards society and the possibility of reforming that society. In both radical and more mainstream novels, reproduction serves as a means of illustrating the depth of society's prejudice against women as well as the carelessness with which both women and their offspring were treated. Problems inherent in reproduction, including the dangers it posed to the health of women, as well as the difficulties women faced in ensuring the survival of themselves and their children, are common themes in women's novels of the 1790s. Interestingly, novels of the period that are most frequently identified by scholars as bleakest in their treatment of reproduction and maternity are often those that include the most optimistic elements: the formation of a family unit, frequently one comprised entirely of women and children, and the education of children, especially daughters, offer hope for the future in novels by writers such as Wollstonecraft, Hays, and, to a lesser extent, Smith. Novels by writers such as Inchbald and Opie, on the other hand, are much more pessimistic about the possibility that reproduction and maternity can offer as a means for reforming society. In Inchbald's and Opie's novels, the heroine who has erred must die, along with her children. Other novels of the period offer complications that resist classification: Fenwick's novel *Secresy* (1795), one of the most radical of the period politically, concludes with the heroine dying after giving birth to a dead child. Charlotte Smith's novels, which span the period, offer a range of reproductive and maternal possibilities. Smith's early novels, such as *Emmeline* and *Desmond*, feature secondary characters who become pregnant outside of wedlock; her later novels, such as *The Banished Man* (1794) and *The Young Philosopher* (1799), conclude (as does Inchbald's *Nature and Art* [1796]) with the depiction of communities of adults and their grown children, usually married but not reproducing.

This chapter explores the varieties of reproduction depicted in the literature written by Wollstonecraft, Hays, and Fenwick during the last decade of the eighteenth century and focuses on the seemingly paradoxical nature of these images. Analysis of novels written by these three authors too often ignores the complexity of the depictions of maternity and reproduction presented in the texts. Many scholarly studies of reproduction in the literature of the 1790s, particularly of the politically radical novels written during the period, emphasize the "impossibility" of reproduction and show a high number of depictions of "failed" reproduction. Many of these readings focus upon Wollstonecraft's novel *Maria, or the Wrongs of Woman*, though Eliza Fenwick's *Secresy* and Mary Hays's *Victim of Prejudice* (1799) and *Memoirs of Emma Courtney* have also received similar attention. Tilottama Rajan, for example, has argued in her essay "Dis-Figuring Reproduction: Natural History, Community, and the 1790s Novel" that the radical novels of the 1790s by Hays and Wollstonecraft point to the failure of reproduction as a means of transmitting values from one generation to the next and suggests that community is shown to be nearly impossible to achieve in these novels. In her book *Romanticism, Maternity, and the Body Politic*, Julie Kipp argues that in Wollstonecraft's novel, "pregnancy is described as a state of imprisonment within one's own flesh" and states that "motherhood is depicted in the novel as a condition pregnant with possibilities which will subsequently be aborted because they are conceived in violence, poisoned by dissimulation, and thwarted by greed" (Kipp 2003, 85). Physical reproduction, as well as the social and legal consequences women faced as a result of reproduction, is a primary (and often negative) focus in the novels of the 1790s. At the same time, however, it is important to recognize, as these writers themselves do, the metaphoric potential of reproduction for depicting the regeneration and reformation of society. If, as most scholars of the novels of the 1790s agree, the ultimate aim of radical novels such as those written by Wollstonecraft, Hays, and Fenwick was to point to problems in British society at the time and to encourage readers to work to reform them, it is often through reproduction that these aims are achieved within the scope of the novels.

Contexts

Scholarship on the literature written during the French Revolution is virtually unanimous in agreeing that the end of the eighteenth century witnessed the solidification of idealized maternity in Britain, France, and America. From mid-century on, as Susan Greenfield and Carol Barash argue in *Inventing Maternity: Politics, Science, and Literature 1650–1865*, the role of the mother was inscribed in these cultures as inherently natural, a function that came to women as a result of their sympathetic and feeling natures, though, as Kipp has observed, it was a role that apparently still required a great deal of oversight and instruction. Greenfield and Barash state that prior to 1750, maternal breastfeeding in Britain was unpopular and uncommon; after 1750, it was common and widely encouraged. As Sonja Boon writes, both medical writers and philosophers increasingly viewed maternal breastfeeding as a "cure for the myriad ills that plagued eighteenth-century society" (see Boon's chapter in this volume, p. 258). By the end of the century, the failure of mothers to breastfeed their own children was pointed to by writers such as Wollstonecraft and Maria

Edgeworth as the catalyst for the corruption of families, lack of harmony between husbands and wives, and even physical illness in "unnatural" mothers such as Edgeworth's Lady Delacour in *Belinda* (1801). In addition to becoming essentially feminine qualities, maternity and motherhood, by the end of the eighteenth century, were supposed to provide women with a clear role in society, one that ostensibly offered them greater independence and importance – they were the mothers of the future citizens of the state, and as such, women were critically important in ensuring the success of the British nation and, as Linda Colley and Kipp argue, its imperialistic mission.

With the start of the French Revolution in 1789, French rhetoric about the importance of mothers to the new republic was heightened. Women in revolutionary France could not be considered citizens except through their status as mothers; women without children were not citizens of France (Kipp 2003, 24). Women's contribution to the revolution and the formation of a new republic in France was therefore limited to their ability to reproduce and swell the population with a new generation of properly patriotic citizens. Likewise, the contribution British women could make to the state as reproductive agents was a trope that applied to a variety of political situations. Gary Kelly, Anne Mellor, and Claudia Johnson, to name a few, have all illustrated the ways in which British writers from Hannah More and Maria Edgeworth to Mary Wollstonecraft and Charlotte Smith urged women to take seriously their duties as mothers to the future citizens of the British state. More, for example, in her *Strictures on the Modern System of Female Education* (1800), impressed upon all women the significance of their influence in the lives of children, both for the sake of their families and their nation.

Such an emphasis upon maternity as a civic duty in the face of national crisis, coming as it did at the end of a period that witnessed an increasing fixation upon women as reproductive agents first and foremost, makes it unsurprising to find women writers of different political shades focusing in their work upon what exactly reproduction and maternity meant, in practical terms, for women. Perhaps more than in any other period of British women's writing, the literature written by women in the 1790s examines closely the experiences and implications of reproduction for ordinary women. Also unsurprising is the fact that many of these literary depictions of generation as a physical act are negative. No woman in late eighteenth-century Britain could escape noticing that pregnancy and childbirth were risky business, from the most basic point of view: lots of women and babies died as a result of both pregnancy and childbirth. Miscarriages and stillbirths, as research by Roy Porter and Lisa Forman Cody has shown, were not uncommon because of the lack of reliable prenatal healthcare, because of inadequate nutrition, and because of unknown complications and health factors. Despite the introduction in the seventeenth century of forceps to ease complications during birth and the use of Caesarean sections (used very rarely but occasionally successfully, as Cody documents), there was no intervention for relatively common problems that occur in utero, such as breech births, placenta previa, or pre-eclampsia. Even those women who had given birth successfully once or even five times were still at risk of dying during subsequent deliveries – the risk of infection was extremely high, and, as now, previous successful deliveries were no guarantee of future ones. These problems are central in novels such as Wollstonecraft's *Maria, or the Wrongs of Woman.* Wollstonecraft's novel is highly characteristic of radical women's writing of the 1790s in its examination of the physical experience of reproduction, depicted largely negatively, as well as in its much more positive evocation of maternity as a means for social reformation in Britain.

Mary Wollstonecraft's *Maria, or the Wrongs of Woman*

Wollstonecraft's novel is painfully clear about the problems of reproduction and motherhood for women. The novel's opening lines describe the pain the heroine feels, both emotionally and physically, as a result of her forcible separation from her infant daughter. Emotionally, Maria is frantic over her daughter's fate and worried that her daughter may be ill, hungry, mistreated, or even dead. Physically, Maria is in agony because her breasts are engorged with milk, for which, she despairingly thinks, her daughter "might now be pining in vain" (Wollstonecraft 1798, 7). From the outset of the novel, then, Wollstonecraft introduces the binary existence in which mothers in the novel live: love felt for their children, and vulnerability as a result of this love. The novel is startlingly graphic about the physical experience of reproduction: in addition to referring several times to Maria's desire to breastfeed her daughter and her physical and emotional pain at being unable to do so, Wollstonecraft is unflinchingly honest about Maria's repugnance for the sex she has with her husband. Maria describes in her memoir her feeling of absolute disgust towards her husband, whose personal habits – he drinks heavily, does not wash, and is generally slovenly – are no more appealing than his personality. She tells her daughter that she is ashamed to confess that she again "allowed" her husband to be "familiar with her person"; yet she cannot wholly regret the act, no matter how much she hates him, because permitting it produced her daughter. In addition, the novel includes the stories of women whose children die, women who kill themselves and their unborn babies, women who take "potions" to abort unwanted babies, women left to provide for children alone, and women who give birth and then die, leaving their children without protection. Each of these stories links in some way to another, so that the reader's perception is one of repetition, accretion, and the universality of women's experience. One of the earliest of these stories is of course Jemima's narrative, in which she details her mother's despair on learning of her pregnancy, a despair that Jemima experiences when she learns of her own pregnancy. Jemima's experience is replicated when she urges the man with whom she will live as mistress to expel another young woman whom he has impregnated. Turned out into the street at Jemima's insistence, the young woman drowns herself.

As Kipp has pointed out, the novel is no less graphic about the emotional toll reproduction takes on women. The asylum in which Maria has been incarcerated by her husband has as one of its inmates a woman who is young like Maria but who, the narrator states, is suffering from a delirium induced by her first childbirth, or, as Heather Meeks argues elsewhere in this volume, what would have in the period been considered a hysterical condition that medical writers often associated with pregnancy and childbirth. Wollstonecraft probably had familiarity with this phenomenon, and not just as a result of her own experience after the birth of her oldest daughter, Fanny Imlay; Janet Todd has suggested that Wollstonecraft's sister Eliza may also have been suffering from "acute post-natal depression" when she, with Wollstonecraft's help, abandoned her husband and newborn daughter in 1783 (Todd 2000, 45). The woman imprisoned with Maria in Wollstonecraft's novel is described as having "been married, against her inclination, to a rich old man ... and in consequence of his treatment, or something which hung on her mind, she had, during her first lying-in, lost her senses" (Wollstonecraft 1798, 21). Such a scenario invites the reader to align this inmate's circumstances with those of Maria, whose marriage is clearly an unhappy one and who wishes, after seeing Darnford from her window for the first time, that her daughter "had a father whom her mother could respect and love" (23).

Maria's jailor, Jemima, who has received a great deal of critical attention, is a lower-class woman who, from the beginning of her life, has been neglected and abused as a result of her gender and the status of her birth. Jemima's mother and father were not married; Jemima's mother, embittered by her seducer's indifference to her plight, dies nine days after

Jemima's birth. Jemima's mother dies as a result of her attempts to "famish" herself as a means to hide or possibly terminate her pregnancy so she will not be dismissed from her position as a servant. Once Jemima is born, her mother's physical strength is exhausted, which leads to her death as well as to the first cause of Jemima's miserable life. As she recounts her life story to Maria and Darnford, Jemima links her misfortunes to her lack of a mother, whose love and protection could have changed the course of her life: "I cannot help attributing the greater part of my misery, to the misfortune of having been thrown into the world without the grand support of life – a mother's affection. I had no one to love me; or to make me respected, to enable me to acquire respect. I was an egg dropped on the sand" (40). As Jemima is "hunted from family to family," she begins work as a servant, only to be raped by her master (40). When she learns of her pregnancy, Jemima is filled with "a mixed sensation of despair and tenderness" (41). Her ambivalence manifests itself in her reluctance to use the abortifacient her master has procured for her: "I burst into tears, I thought it was killing myself" – a phrase which, given Jemima's identification of her own plight as a "bastard" with that of her unborn baby, is richly ambiguous.

However, despite the narrative's focus on these negative experiences with reproduction, the novel also shows that Maria's relationship with Jemima is cemented by their mutual sympathy for Maria's daughter. After hearing Jemima's narrative, Maria realizes the severity of the prejudices facing women at the time and pleads with Jemima to help her regain her infant, and, in so doing, prepare the child for the problems it will face as a female in British society: "With your heart, and such dreadful experience, can you lend your aid to deprive my babe of a mother's tenderness, a mother's care? In the name of God, assist me to snatch her from destruction! Let me but give her an education – let me but prepare her body and mind to encounter the ills which wait her sex, and I will teach her to consider you as her second mother, and herself as the prop of your age" (Wollstonecraft 1798, 55). In portraying Jemima, a woman who is not a mother, as prompted to allow Maria her freedom because Maria promises to teach her daughter to consider Jemima "as a second mother," Wollstonecraft demonstrated the strength that reproduction and maternity have to create lasting bonds between women (Johnson 1999, 169) and the work all women – mothers or no – must do together to educate the nation's young women. Contrasted with the portrayal of Darnford as an example of the failures of republican masculinity, Maria's relationship with Jemima, as Johnson has argued, provides the basis for a social reformation that will transcend relationships between men and women, which many politically radical novels of the decade depict as hopeless. Instead, the social reformation to which the novel looks forward in the longest of the fragments appended to the narrative by Godwin was to be based upon maternity and communities of women drawn together by children. Despite the difficulties of reproduction as depicted in the novel, maternity itself – the result of reproduction – is depicted positively, particularly once this maternity has been disconnected from biological paternity. It is significant that Maria's daughter has been snatched from her breast at the instigation of Maria's husband. The relationship between Maria and her daughter, portrayed briefly but strongly throughout the novel and particularly in the opening description of Maria feeling the baby's "twinkling fingers" on her breast, is a pure one that is interrupted by the cruelty and the lack of paternal feeling of the child's father. Indeed, as in much radical literature of the 1790s, we might say that in Wollstonecraft's novel, it is the presence of the father that makes the experience of reproduction and maternity miserable. The politically radical novel can only offer a portrait of reformed society by excluding him from the new community that forms around the child.

Mary Hays's *Memoirs of Emma Courtney*

The same is true in Mary Hays's 1796 novel *Memoirs of Emma Courtney*. After a tumultuous passion for a man who apparently does not return her affection, Emma Courtney marries another man, Montague, simply because she has no other viable options – she is alone in the world, and, as a woman, has few avenues for maintaining herself by honourable occupation. Montague, who has been in love with Emma throughout the whole of the narrative, offers again to marry her, and after some reluctance, she consents. Her marriage is initially a success. Emma relates her interest in her husband's profession (he is a physician) and describes her marriage to him as a partnership in more ways than one – she works alongside him, but they also have, as Emma relates, a companionate marriage, one that is strengthened by the birth of their daughter. Emma's respect and esteem for Montague is enhanced by her love for their child, and, in a description reminiscent of ones included in Wollstonecraft's earlier *Vindication of the Rights of Woman*, Emma feels a "chaste, an ineffable pleasure" in watching Montague "caress his infant" (198). Montague occasionally manifests jealousy over the coolness of Emma's regard for him, which she counts as one of the advantages of their union. As she tells Montague, "I feel for you all the affection that a reasonable and virtuous mind ought to feel – that affection which is compatible with the fulfilling of other duties" (197). Ostensibly, the portrait of this marriage is intended to alleviate the reader's fears that Emma Courtney is encouraging young ladies to offer themselves freely to any man with whom they imagine they have a mental and emotional compatibility in the way that Emma has offered herself to Augustus Harley, the man whom she imagines, early in the novel, is her soul-mate. Emma is at great pains to renounce her previous passion for Augustus Harley as one created by excessive sensibility, the very danger against which her narrative is supposed to serve as a warning. She tells her husband that her "first attachment was the morbid excess of a distempered imagination. Liberty, reason, virtue, usefulness were the offerings I carried to its shrine," and urges him to be glad that she is "restored to reason" (197). Yet Emma is not quite successful in conveying this moral purpose of her memoir. The reader cannot help noticing that though her marriage to Montague begins well and is based upon rational esteem and mutual respect, something goes spectacularly wrong: the marriage ends when Montague commits suicide after killing the baby he has fathered with Emma's maid.

As in Wollstonecraft's novel, there are a variety of different types of reproduction depicted in Hays's novel. Biological reproduction, while important, is ultimately (and unambiguously) unsuccessful. Emma Courtney's daughter dies at the age of fourteen, and the only other birth that takes place in the novel is that of the illegitimate child born to Emma's maid, Rachel, after Montague seduces her. We hear first of the death of this infant from Rachel. Frenzied by the loss of her baby, she insists repeatedly that she did not murder it and pleads with Emma not to send her to prison. Rachel's fear of being imprisoned reminds readers that unmarried women whose infants died after birth or who were born dead could be tried and hung for murder. Under the strictures of a 1624 law that remained on the books until 1803, "if an unmarried woman were to have a child, and if that child were to die, and if she had concealed the birth and failed to inform anyone of her pregnancy, then she would be considered guilty of murdering the baby, the penalty for which was death by hanging" (McDonagh 1999, 217). Rachel is unmarried, and at Montague's instigation, she has concealed her pregnancy. The fact of its death is, as Rachel seems to know, enough to convict her of its murder – for, as McDonagh states, the 1624 law was exceptional for its immediate presumption of guilt in such cases.

As Rachel claims and he himself confesses, Montague has murdered the baby. Montague is a physician with easy access to abortifacients; he tells

Emma that he repeatedly doses Rachel in an attempt to effect an abortion but is thwarted by Rachel's youth and health. He does, however, succeed in weakening the health of the fetus such that it is born prematurely. In his confession to Emma, Montague writes:

> Six weeks before the allotted period, the infant saw the light – for a moment – to close its eyes on it for ever! I, only, was with the unhappy mother. I had formed no deliberate purpose – I had not yet arrived at the acme of guilt – but, perceiving, from the babe's premature birth, and the consequences of the pernicious potions which had been administered to the mother, that the vital flame played but feebly – that life was but as a quivering, uncertain, spark – a sudden and horrible thought darted through my mind. I know not whether my emotion betrayed me to the ear of Rachel – but, suddenly throwing back the curtain of the bed, she beheld me grasp – with savage ferocity – *with murderous hands*! (Hays 1796, 217)

Unlike Wollstonecraft's *Maria*, where men are so removed from the narrative as to be only indirectly involved in reproduction and attempts to stifle it, in Hays's novel, men are directly responsible for both attempted abortion and infanticide. Rachel, the mother of the child, is merely a passive receptor of potions – she receives doses from Montague, is delivered by him of the child, and only recovers any agency she might possess when she sees Montague (presumably) strangling the baby, though she remains ultimately powerless to stop him. In both Wollstonecraft's and Hays's novels, however, men disrupt and destroy the relationships between women and their children as well as the relationship between women and other women.

Despite the failure of biological reproduction in Hays's novel, adoptive reproduction is entirely successful. On his deathbed, Augustus Harley implores Emma to accept the care of his only living son (he has had two other children, both of whom, his brother informs Emma, died as a result of smallpox). Emma swears that she will raise the young Augustus with the tenderness of a mother, a promise she keeps. The strength of Emma's love for the young Augustus Harley is only equalled by the strength of her love for her own daughter. Emma's love for her children is evidenced throughout the end of the novel: there are numerous references to Emma breastfeeding her infant daughter, of fearing to "give it a pernicious substance" in the midst of her anxiety for Augustus Harley's life, of Emma's division of time between her nursery and Augustus Harley's sickbed, and of her visiting the wet nurse to whose care her infant is given while Emma is ill.

By the end of the narrative, Emma tells her adopted son that she finds happiness only in her role as mother to him and to her (now dead) daughter. She states that after moving to a new part of the country, she lives in retirement, dividing her "heart and her attentions" between her children (Hays 1796, 218).

The relationship between Rachel and Emma is not as equitable as that between Jemima and Maria, but it is nevertheless an important one in the novel. Emma works to prevent Rachel's ruin before her pregnancy, telling Montague that, should he "corrupt the innocence of this girl, she is emphatically *ruined*" because she lacks the mental resources to recover in the face of the world's opprobrium. Emma recognizes the danger that her husband poses to Rachel's future security and happiness, and, rather than blaming Rachel, as most ladies in the literature of the period are depicted as doing, Emma very rationally decides she must release Rachel from her service in the hopes of thereby sheltering her from Montague's attention. It is a strategy that does not work – Montague continues to visit Rachel at her new place of employment – but it is significant that Emma makes the attempt at all. Even before Montague implores Emma in his confession letter to shelter Rachel from the consequences of his actions, Emma has reassured Rachel that she will care for her. At the end of the novel, Emma tells her adopted son, Augustus, who is now a young man, that she nursed Rachel back to health and Rachel has served her faithfully until the present. The novel thus concludes with a depiction of an independent woman, living with only her maid and two children.

The termination of *Memoirs of Emma Courtney* also provides a clear focus on the education of the two children whom Emma raises alone. As Emma tells Augustus, whom she addresses as "my more than son," her primary occupation as a mother has been to educate her children according to principles of "active virtue" and "generous sentiments." The two children, a boy and a girl, receive the same education "from the same masters" until Augustus is twelve; Emma points out that her daughter "emulated, and sometimes outstripped" Augustus's progress, making clear that ability is not gendered in her perception (and, by extension, preventing any such notions from taking hold in the young Augustus's mind). Emma puts a great deal of thought into Augustus's education and future occupation; she hopes to prepare Augustus for a "commercial line of life," thereby indicating that she harbours no aristocratic pretences for him. She frets about his inclination to science and literature because she worries that the study of either will render him "unfit" for any career in trade. A university education is rejected because Emma fears that Augustus's morals will be degraded as a result, and he is finally settled as apprentice to a surveyor, a profession that Emma approves because of Augustus's aptitude for "drawing and architecture." Emma's plans for Augustus's education, then, demonstrate a great deal of careful planning and sensitivity to the natural strengths of his mind, but they also reveal an egalitarian and anti-aristocratic foundation. Emma wishes Augustus to be a practical, industrious, honest man without pretence to upper-class tastes and absolutely without aristocratic vices and corruption, which might be the effect of a university education. Emma's plans for her daughter's education are not as detailed as those for Augustus – her daughter dies when she is fourteen – but after Augustus's apprenticeship has begun, Emma tells him that her daughter "learned from you to draw plans, and to study the laws of proportion" (Hays 1796, 219). Had she lived, little Emma, like her mother before her, would have learned from her mate to work in a male profession. The education that Emma bestows on her children is clearly designed to prepare them for a society much different from the one in which Emma grew up; it is a society in which Emma's daughter will have the opportunity to work in a field reserved for men, one in which Augustus will be valued for his contributions to society, or his merit, rather than his birth.

Eliza Fenwick's *Secresy, or the Ruin on the Rock*

Eliza Fenwick's 1795 novel *Secresy* differs in marked ways from both Hays's and Wollstonecraft's. The primary difference is that in Fenwick's, there is little exploration of the heroine as mother and thus no real emphasis upon breastfeeding or the pleasures of maternity such as may be found in *Maria* or *Memoirs of Emma Courtney*. The pregnant heroine, Sibella, dies shortly after giving birth to a dead baby at the end of the novel. However, the fact of Sibella's pregnancy, which occupies a significant portion of the novel, provides Fenwick with a means to examine the figure of woman as a reproducing body and thus to investigate both the ways in which women's status as reproductive agents changes their role in society as well as the potential that reproduction and maternity hold for effecting social change. The conclusion that Fenwick comes to about the latter is, at least on the surface, much more pessimistic than ones drawn by Wollstonecraft or Hays. As Meghan L. Burke argues, while illegitimate pregnancies occur frequently in eighteenth-century novels, "Sibella's pregnancy is vastly different in that her growing gravid body is not an emblem of female weakness and helplessness or 'the result of women's bodily subjection,' but provides visual, irrefutable evidence of her assertion of agency" (Burke 2009, 379). Combined with Sibella's friendship with Caroline Ashburn, one that parallels Sibella's relationships with Clement Montgomery and Arthur Murden, the novel offers an examination of reproduction and the ability of a female community to support women against patriarchal oppression and exploitation.

Fenwick's Sibella Valmont becomes pregnant as a result of a secret "union," or marriage, as she believes, with her childhood companion, Clement Montgomery. Sibella believes fervently that her union with Clement is pure and holy, but Clement knows that his "marriage" to Sibella is not valid and that she thus has no legal claim upon him. In one sense, then, this episode can be read as evidence of Sibella's oppression and exploitation by patriarchal legal structures and villainous men. In such a reading, Clement uses his worldly knowledge to dupe Sibella, allowing him to have sex with her and then abandon her completely. In another reading, however, Sibella's pregnancy can be seen as evidence of her rejection of the claims her uncle, Lord Valmont, makes upon her obedience and passivity to his wishes. As Clement insists and as Sibella herself tells Caroline Ashburn, the union between Clement and Sibella is one of Sibella's own creation. She proposes the union to Clement; she insists that they consummate the union as a pledge of their "fervent unspotted faith" (Fenwick 1795, 131). As Burke states, "Sibella is literally pregnant with her own power and volition" (2009, 379). Strikingly, the reality of Sibella's pregnancy leads to the decline and death of the man upon whom Caroline and Sibella are relying to be her saviour: Arthur Murden, who has fancied himself in love with Sibella based on Clement's descriptions of her. Murden cannot cope with the fact of Sibella's pregnancy when he comes to rescue her from Castle Valmont. His conduct and speech change as soon as he sees Sibella's pregnant body; as Burke states, Sibella's "pregnancy presents visual, and therefore undeniable, evidence that she is not the ethereal idol of his creation but an active being who possesses a sexual, corporeal body with its creative power" (2009, 380). The various male characters' responses to the physical evidence of Sibella's pregnancy encompass a range of attitudes towards women's reproductive agency, sexual activity, and physicality. Murden is "unmanned" by the sight of Sibella's pregnant body; Lord Valmont is infuriated because he reads it correctly as a sign of Sibella's rebellion against his rule; and Clement Montgomery proclaims that, by becoming pregnant, Sibella has "ruined" him.

After her pregnancy is revealed, rather than responding as female characters in the literature of the period typically respond, Sibella acts with resolution and vigour. She refuses, even with the evidence of her "ruin" visible on her body, to accede to Valmont's demands for obedience, instead attempting to swim across the moat at Valmont Castle to achieve her freedom. As Burke notes, this "wild action ... apes the stock situation of many unwed mothers in sentimental novels, while at the same time carrying a drastically different meaning; rather than wishing to drown and die with the evidence of her sin, as so many 'fallen' literary heroines do, Sibella jumps in the water in order to actively swim away and assert her – and her unborn baby's – right to a continued independent existence" (2009, 379). However, Sibella's resolve to live independently with her child is thwarted by her recognition of the reality of society in Britain at the time. Lord Valmont has educated Sibella in absolute seclusion; following Rousseau's principles for a natural education for boys, Valmont has attempted to make an Emile of Clement Montgomery and Sibella his Sophy. Raised in perfect rural seclusion, Sibella's only friends are Clement, who soon departs to experience society at Valmont's instigation; Caroline Ashburn, with whom she has an epistolary friendship; and a fawn. The fawn is both a representation of Sibella's simplicity and purity and of her proximity to the natural world, a world that is uncorrupted by civilization. Sibella is thus not fitted for society – she has not received the practical education that Wollstonecraft's Maria has realized is essential for her young daughter if she is to survive as a female in Britain at the time. Sibella cannot live in the real world; she is, as she realizes at the end of the novel, "a shadow! A dream ... Am I not dead already?" (Fenwick 1795, 356). Upon finally securing her release from Valmont Castle, a release orchestrated by Caroline Ashburn and effected by Arthur Murden, Sibella is confronted with the truth of Clement Montgomery's behaviour to her. She learns that he has secretly married Caroline's mother, a mercenary marriage contracted from motives of greed on one side and vanity on the other. The truth of Clement's nature and her own credulity are too much for Sibella to bear, though she does so without any of the weeping or fainting typically assigned to women in novels of the period. The shock brings on Sibella's labour, and she gives birth to a dead child. Caroline's attempts to urge Sibella to focus on her – to listen only to her, rather than to the callous Mrs Ashburn or to Clement – cannot prevent the death of either Sibella's child or Sibella herself.

The question, then, is which is more important in Fenwick's novel – the fact that Sibella, confronted with "things as they are," cannot survive, or the novel's earlier depictions of reproduction as an act of agency and female bonds as a source of resistance against patriarchal oppression. The answer is neither. Fenwick's novel is part of a tradition of radical writing during the 1790s that depicts characters as too pure, too unworldly and uncorrupt, to be able to survive in British society at the end of the eighteenth century. While the beginning of *Secresy* has much in common with novels such as Wollstonecraft's *Maria* and Hays's *Memoirs of Emma Courtney*, the ending of the novel aligns it with others such as Amelia Opie's later *Adeline Mowbray* (1804), in which the heroine dies as a result of her commitment to unrealistic ideals. Sibella's Godwinian notion that she and Clement need only pledge their faith to one another to be married in a truer sense than any legal ceremony could make them is echoed in Adeline Mowbray's determination to transcend the problems inherent in marriage as an institution by living openly with Glenmurray. Like Sibella, Adeline is too idealistic and thus cannot survive – she, like Sibella, is lacking an education that would equip her to live in the real world. Adeline, like Sibella, dies at the end of Opie's novel.

Still, reproduction and the bonds between women are shown in Fenwick's narrative to have power, and this power is not totally negated by the novel's ending. Caroline Ashburn, the novel's moral voice and the orchestrator of so much of its action, lives on after both Murden and Sibella have died. The novel concludes with the reformation of Lord Filmar, the aristocratic rake of the novel. Filmar is a Lovelace-like character who plots to abduct and marry Sibella for her fortune; it is also worth noting that he shares a name with the author of the seventeenth-century political tract *Patriarcha, or the Natural Power of Kings* (Filmer 1680), and thus likely represents patriarchy generally. Filmar's infatuation with Sibella begins when he falls in love with her portrait, which he sees on a visit to Valmont Castle with his father, who is Sibella's other guardian. He, like Murden and Clement, objectifies her on the basis of her physical beauty. However, unlike Murden, whose death is hastened by the sight of Sibella's reproductive body, Filmar's reformation is prompted when he sees Sibella's pregnancy. He is moved to sympathy by Sibella's plight, and after listening to her story, he, like the reader should, can see that "Miss Ashburn is an angel, Mr. Murden a fine fellow, Mr. Valmont an ideot, Sibella a saint, and Montgomery – a scoundrel" (Fenwick 1795, 339). The last letter of the novel is written to Filmar by Caroline Ashburn, and it details the ways in which Sibella's death has achieved what she herself could not: Clarissa-like, Sibella's death has created agonizing remorse in the implacable Lord Valmont, the repentance of Clement Montgomery, and the humiliation of Mrs Ashburn. Though she cannot live to see it,

Sibella's actions have prompted a reformation of the segment of society in which she lives. Through Filmar and Caroline Ashburn, who live on, the novel implies that the reformation will spread.

Reproduction and Maternity in the Novels of the 1790s

In the literature of the 1790s, reproduction was a trope that carried a wide and sometimes conflicting range of meanings. In the most basic sense, reproduction as a physical act was something that concerned women writers such as Wollstonecraft, Hays, and Fenwick enormously; pregnancy and childbirth were conditions that were not only physically dangerous for women at the time but also carried with them long-lasting responsibilities. These responsibilities had the potential to provide women with a great deal of autonomy and, as writers of the period such as Hannah More emphasized, power, but they also made women vulnerable. In addition to being subject to legal and social prejudice as a result of their status as mothers or mothers-to-be, women with children had equipped their oppressors with an easy means of tormenting them, a means that was legally sanctioned since fathers, not mothers, by law had custody of their children in the event of marital estrangement or dissolution. Indeed, recognition of the fact that their children, especially their daughters, would have to be prepared to live in a society such as that in Britain at the end of the eighteenth century was cause for both anxiety and grief. Despite these problems of reproduction, however, many radical novels of the period recognize the potential in maternity for reforming society and making it more congenial to women and their children, an aspect frequently overlooked in analyses of the problems of reproduction in the novels of the 1790s. Novels such as those by Wollstonecraft, Hays, and Fenwick depict the power of maternity and reproduction, biological or adoptive, to produce real social change in which women had a critical role to play. If women had "acknowledged power," as More described it, when it came to the education of their children, and if mothers had almost exclusive control of their children's lives during their early years, then maternity, with its consequent responsibilities of educating children, offered women a chance to instil values that would, in time, effect social change. Motherhood offered a means for women's participation as citizens in the future of the nation. In addition, if reproduction and maternity were essentially feminine occupations, they then had the power to draw women, even women of different social classes, together. In many of the most radical novels of the 1790s, communities of women working together to educate children provide hope for social reformation and thus the successful transmission of values where reproduction alone cannot.

REFERENCES

Burke, M.L. 2009. "Making Mother Obsolete: Eliza Fenwick's *Secresy* and the Masculine Appropriation of Maternity." *Eighteenth-Century Fiction* 21 (3): 357–84.

Cody, L.F. 2005. *Birthing the Nation: Sex, Science, and the Conception of Eighteenth-Century Britons*. Oxford: Oxford University Press.

Colley, L. 2009. *Britons: Forging the Nation 1707–1837*. New Haven: Yale University Press.

Edgeworth, M. (1801) 1994. *Belinda*. Edited by K.J. Kirkpatrick. Oxford: Oxford University Press.

Fenwick, E. (1795) 1998. *Secresy: or, the Ruin on the Rock*. 2nd ed. Edited by I. Grundy. Peterborough, ON: Broadview Press.

Filmer, R. 1680. *Patriarcha, or the Natural Power of Kings*. Early English Books Online. Gale document number: BL3025067389.

Godwin, W. (1798) 2001. *Memoirs of the Author of a Vindication of the Rights of Woman*. Edited by P. Clemit and G.L. Walker. Peterborough, ON: Broadview Press.

Greenfield, S.C., and C. Barash. 1999. *Inventing Maternity: Politics, Science, and Literature 1650–1865*. Lexington: University Press of Kentucky.

Hays, M. (1796) 2000. *Memoirs of Emma Courtney*. Edited by M.L. Brooks. Peterborough, ON: Broadview Press.

Hays, M. (1799) 1998. *Victim of Prejudice*. Edited by E. Ty. Peterborough, ON: Broadview Press.

Inchbald, E. (1796) 2005. *Nature and Art*. Edited by S.L. Maurer. Peterborough, ON: Broadview Press.

Johnson, C. 1999. "Mary Wollstonecraft: Styles of Radical Maternity." In *Inventing Maternity: Politics, Science, and Literature 1650–1865*, edited by S.C. Greenfield and C. Barash, 159–72. Lexington: University Press of Kentucky.

Kelly, G. 1993. *Women, Writing, and Revolution 1790–1827*. Oxford: Clarendon Press.

Kelly, G. 1996. *Revolutionary Feminism: The Mind and Career of Mary Wollstonecraft*. New York: St Martin's Press.

Kipp, J. 2003. *Romanticism, Maternity, and the Body Politic*. Cambridge: Cambridge University Press. http://dx.doi.org/10.1017/CBO9780511484346.
McDonagh, J. 1999. "Infanticide and the Boundaries of Culture from Hume to Arnold." In *Inventing Maternity: Politics, Science, and Literature 1650–1865*, edited by S.C. Greenfield and C. Barash, 215–37. Lexington: University Press of Kentucky.
Mellor, A. 2000. *Mothers of the Nation: Women's Political Writing in England, 1780–1830*. Bloomington: Indiana University Press.
More, H. (1799) 1800. *Strictures on the Modern System of Female Education*. 8th ed. Eighteenth Century Collections Online. Gale document number: CW109368188.
Opie, A. (1801) 2003. *The Father and Daughter*. Edited by S. King and J.B. Pierce. Peterborough, ON: Broadview Press.
Opie, A. (1804) 1999. *Adeline Mowbray; or, The Mother and Daughter*. Edited by S. King and J.B. Pierce. Oxford: Oxford University Press.
Porter, R., and L. Hall. 1995. *The Facts of Life: The Creation of Sexual Knowledge in Britain, 1650–1950*. New Haven: Yale University Press.
Rajan, T. 2002. "Dis-figuring Reproduction: Natural History, Community, and the 1790s Novel." *The New Centennial Review* (East Lansing, MI) 2 (3): 211–52. http://dx.doi.org/10.1353/ncr.2002.0056.
Robinson, M. (1800) 2003. "The Natural Daughter." In *A Letter to the Women of England and The Natural Daughter*, edited by S.M. Setzer, 89–296. Peterborough, ON: Broadview Press.
Smith, C. (1788) 2003. *Emmeline*. Edited by L. Fletcher. Peterborough, ON: Broadview Press.
Smith, C. (1792) 2001. *Desmond*. Edited by A. Blank and J. Todd. Peterborough, ON: Broadview Press.
Smith, C. (1794) 2006. "The Banished Man." In *The Works of Charlotte Smith*, edited by M.O. Grenby, 103–480. London: Pickering & Chatto.
Smith, C. (1799) 1999. *The Young Philosopher*. Edited by E. Kraft. Lexington: University Press of Kentucky.
Todd, J. 2000. *Mary Wollstonecraft: A Revolutionary Life*. New York: Columbia University Press.
Wollstonecraft, M. (1791) 1982. *Vindication of the Rights of Woman*. Edited by M. Brody. New York: Penguin.
Wollstonecraft, M. (1798) 1994. *Maria, or the Wrongs of Woman*. Edited by. A.K. Mellor. New York: W.W. Norton.

PART THREE

Pathologies, Body Parts, Display

13 "Unfit for Generation": Body Size and Reproduction

SARAH TOULALAN

In discussions of barrenness and sterility – infertility in modern terms – bodies considered too fat or thin were understood as reproductively dysfunctional. These ideas were not simply repeated as unquestioned truths from classical medical literature, although authors often cited Galen, Hippocrates, and Aristotle or recycled the same words, phrases, sentences, and paragraphs from earlier sixteenth- and seventeenth-century books. Rather, they found a receptive audience in a society and culture where successful reproduction was highly valued, and where remedies for those concerned about their fertility were widely available. There was considerable continuity from the early sixteenth century to the late eighteenth century in how fat was understood and how its over-abundance or paucity in the body was thought to affect reproduction. Authors invariably paired fat and thin bodies when explaining causes of infertility to their readers. Some shifts in thinking can be identified in the later eighteenth century, mostly reflecting newer knowledge and theories about conception, such as that women contributed eggs from ovaries, as Sally Frampton discusses in more detail in this volume, and that men's seed contained "animalcules." There was also one significant change in relation to ideas about miscarriage, where it was recognized that a starving or emaciated woman's body did not seem to starve her infant of nourishment in the womb leading to its premature demise, as was previously believed to happen. There were also more ways in which a fat body was thought to be inimical to reproduction than one that was too thin, as a large amount of flesh itself was thought to present an obstacle to both sexual intercourse and to conception. Increasingly, then, into the later eighteenth century the pairing of fat and thin bodies was uncoupled, and fatness or "Obesity" began to be listed alone, or received much greater attention as a cause of impaired fertility, including miscarriage. While ideas about very thin bodies were to some extent modified, longer-lasting perceptions of fat bodies as unreproductive may have contributed to the more general continued stigmatizing of fat bodies.

More than simply received wisdom, discussions about body size and fertility reflected eighteenth-century anxieties about population and the health of the nation, social stability through the patriarchal family model, and concepts of manhood, womanhood, and parenthood. Concerns about fertility and social, economic, political, and religious stability related to inheritance. Men and women were expected to conform to their allotted social, gender, and familial roles, at a time when procreation was the primary aim of marriage and a measure of a successful marital union. Bodies that did not reproduce to ensure continuity were disruptive bodies, resisting conformity to these expectations. However, while fat bodies were continually subjected to moral judgment for impairing fertility through unrestrained appetites, there was much less condemnation of bodies that were infertile because too lean. Being very slender was often beyond personal control, caused by disease, poverty, and starvation. Exceptions included those who became emaciated, hence infertile, through overindulgence of sexual appetite, either in debauchery that also brought the risk of venereal disease, or through masturbation, which became of increasing concern in publications in the eighteenth century. Ruth Perry has identified a "growing demographic consciousness on the part of a nation in the process of industrializing and building an empire" as an imperative driving an eighteenth-century valorization of motherhood (1991, 206–9). A few years later Roy Porter and Lesley Hall suggested that "pro-natalist" books such as *Aristotle's Masterpiece*, first published in 1684, resonated with contemporary anxieties "that the nation was being weakened by underpopulation" (1995, 52–3). Demographic historians had demonstrated that steady population growth ended in the mid-seventeenth century, and explained its subsequent fall as a combination of several factors: late age of marriage; high mortality (especially infant), caused by endemic disease and wars both national and international; and emigration to the West Indies and the North American colonies (Wrigley and Schofield 1981, 161–2). Early eighteenth-century population growth that became noticeable from mid-century was caused by couples marrying at an earlier age, so extending their active fertile period and increasing the birth rate (Hitchcock 1997, 26). Yet concerns about fertility persisted. In a world where life continued to be precarious due to endemic and epidemic fatal diseases, recurrent conflicts, accidents, crime, and poverty, there was a continuing perception of the need to enhance and preserve reproductive health, to ensure more healthy pregnancies leading to more surviving children, and hence sufficient bodies for economic and military strength (Harvey 2004, 141–5). Church teachings and prescriptive literature also promoted procreation as the primary aim of marriage, binding couples together in mutual support to nurture their offspring and ensure social, economic, and political stability through clear lines of inheritance (Berry and Foyster 2007, 166–9; Cody 2005, 6–7; Toulalan 2007, 62–91). Successful generation was therefore of enormous importance throughout this period, but also highly desired by childless couples, as the plethora of advertised fertility remedies available to them strongly suggests.

Awareness of these concerns has led historians in recent years to pay much greater attention to contemporary knowledge about sexual practices and fertility. Scholars have investigated barriers to fertility, especially the use of contraception and abortion, and considered the impact of unwanted pregnancy and illegitimacy (McLaren 1984; Ingram 1987). Laura Gowing has noted the importance of pregnancy and childbearing to women's lives as a signifier of womanhood and communal status, while Helen Berry and Elizabeth Foyster have argued for the importance of fatherhood to perceptions of male status and reputation (Gowing 2003, 114; Berry and Foyster 2007, 164–74). Jennifer Evans has also noted that knowledge of and demand for remedies for barrenness and impotence were widespread (2012, 7–15). However, while some historians have noted that fat was regarded as one cause of infertility, including impotence, it has only very recently been investigated in any detail (Berry and Foyster 2007, 170; McLaren 2007, 80; Stolberg 2012, 372, 376–7; Toulalan 2014). Christopher E. Forth has identified the late eighteenth and early nineteenth centuries as "a pivotal period for the acceleration of anti-fat sentiment," and it may be that this increasing concern was linked to concerns about population and impediments to successful reproduction, although such anxieties were clearly not new to the eighteenth century (2012, 217). Its opposite body type, extreme leanness or emaciation, has not been considered in scholarship as an eighteenth-century reproductive problem. This chapter aims to go some way towards rectifying these omissions. Pam Lieske's discussion of the malformed pelvis elsewhere in this volume points to further concerns about body size and the final reproductive hurdle for women: childbirth. Concerns about extremely lean bodies and birth included that the pelvis might be too narrow for the infant to pass through (Baudelocque 1775, 86–99; Spence 1784, 452–5).

Early modern people did not generally tend to quantify fat by weight or size, although, as Michael Stolberg has shown, some authors did use specific weights when referring to particular examples of extremely fat persons (Rogers 2010, 23–4, 37 note 16; Stolberg 2012, 372). Eighteenth-century physician George Cheyne was acutely aware of his weight, and a vogue developed among the upper classes at the end of the century for weighing oneself, but how widespread this practice may have been is unknown (Guerrini 2000, 136; Schwartz 1986, 17). Although listed by the *OED* as occurring respectively from 1611 and 1651, the words "obesity" and "obese" were infrequently used in English medical texts. The terms most used for overly fleshy bodies were "fat," "corpulent," or "gross." Eighteenth-century authors also spoke of "fulness of habit." These terms were used interchangeably, and often together, to indicate a generally greater degree of flesh or fat, without specifying how much was too much. Authors referred to bodies that were considered too thin as "very spare and lean," or as having "too much Leanness," or "extream leanness of the whol body" (*Of the Crime of Onan* 1724, 91; Salmon 1700, 131; Riverius 1655, 513). Whatever the variation in size or weight of these bodies, they were understood as suffering from reproductive dysfunction that was rectifiable by modifications to diet: either to eat more sparely to reduce fat, or to eat more, and more nourishingly, to increase it. However, those who were too thin through wasting diseases such as consumption could only achieve a healthy "plumpness" on recovery, so were not perceived to have the same agency in improving their fertility as those who were too fat.

Conception and Seed

Despite medical historians' assertions that there was a shift away from humoral theory in the eighteenth century, medical books continued to describe and explain fat within this model, and repeated the same ideas about its nature and purpose in the body. Thus bodies regarded as too fat or thin were generally understood to be so as a result of their humoral constitution. Bodies were understood as composed of four humours: blood, yellow bile, black bile, and phlegm, associated with four qualities – hot, dry, cold, and wet. The constitution of a body was related to the particular balance of humours in the body, with men more hot and dry, women more cold and moist. There was some debate about whether fat should be understood as hot or cold in nature, as its composition might change from solid to liquid depending on whether it was cold or hot, but ultimately it was widely accepted that it was cold, as fat was congealed by cold. Bodies that were fat were therefore understood to be constitutionally cold and moist, those that were thin were hot and dry, as heat melted fat; women naturally thus had more fat than men. Fat was understood as made from blood: "Fat is the matter of blood: and although it be made of the cream of blood, yet notwithstanding it is cold, and without blood, degenerating into fat by the want of heat, and frigidity of the membrane" (Browne 1669, 180). James Drake in the early eighteenth century described it as "the *Oyly* part of the *Aliment*, separated from the *Arterial* Blood by the *Adipose Glands*," a description repeated over sixty years later when it was described as "the oily part of the blood or *fat*" (Drake 1717, 1:19; *Elements of Anatomy* 1781, 125). Fat served several necessary functions in the body, including cushioning the parts for comfort, oiling the joints to ease movement, keeping the body warm, providing nourishment in times of famine, and improving appearance by filling up the empty spaces of the body. Although constitution affected how much fat there was in the body, it was also observed that behaviour modified its quantity: "This substance increases in quantity by rest and good living; and, on the contrary, diminishes by hard labour and a spare diet" (*System of Anatomy* 1791, 474).

In the humoral model of the body a satisfactory balance of humours was essential for conception to take place. Authors advised that too much hot, cold, dryness, or moisture in the generative parts, particularly in the womb for women or the seed in men, could prevent conception. Thus bodies with an excess of cold and moist humours, and hence fat, would suffer reproductive problems from insufficient heat, including lack of desire and defective generative matter. Heat was crucial to both sexual pleasure and successful conception – desire was inflamed by heat, and heat was increased by the friction of intercourse and, for a woman, the special properties of semen itself, which had vital heat in three elements (Toulalan 2007, 74–7). Heating foods, herbs, and wines might arouse lust in both sexes, as could applying oils and ointments with heating properties to the genitals (Evans 2012, 7–9). But too much heat was equally problematic: it destroyed generative matter and impaired sexual function, paradoxically, through over-indulgence of an inflamed sexual appetite. Those with an excess of heat – therefore extremely thin – were also regarded as reproductively impaired, and remedies recommended for infertility contained the opposing properties of coolness and moisture.

In too fat and too thin bodies impaired or insufficient generative matter – seed and menstrual blood – were understood to cause infertility. In men this meant defective or insufficient seed (sperm). In the Aristotelian model of reproduction where only men contributed seed, women had insufficient menstrual blood; in the Galenic-Hippocratic two-seed model in which women also contributed seed (albeit weaker, thinner, and less perfect) it included both seed and menstrual blood. In both models male seed was the principal generative material that acted upon the female matter to form and shape the fetus. Texts citing these classical models of reproduction circulated alongside newer works that incorporated seventeenth-century theories about egg-producing ovaries in women and the observation of animalcules in sperm, revealed through investigations by Harvey, de Graaf, Malpighi, Leeuwenhoek, and others (Cobb 2007, 243–6). However, these newer works on generation did not yet have any substantial impact on ideas about bodies that were perceived as too fat or too thin and their fertility.

The amount of fat in the body, either too much or too little, was understood to have an effect upon fertility because both fat and seed were made from blood. John Marten reiterated the idea that "in Fat People, part of that Blood which should go to the making of *Seed*, turns into Fat, whereby the *Genital Parts* are depriv'd of that quantity, and of that Spirit and Strength which is requir'd to quicken the *Seed* and make it fertile" (1709, 23). Stolberg has noted that some renaissance authors even thought that obese people had little blood at all because it was converted into fat (2012, 374). William Salmon, in editions of midwifery books attributed to Culpeper and Aristotle published into the later eighteenth century, thus concluded that in those who were fat the seed was "vitious, or unfit for Generation ... the Matter of it being defective." He further observed that seed was destroyed in those who suffered from "too much Leanness, or continual Wasting or Consumption of the Body ... Nature turning all the Matter and Substance thereof into Nutriment of the Body" (1700, 131). Excessively fat or thin bodies were thus understood as inherently infertile because they both diverted resources for generative matter to the body's own use. As the theory that women produced eggs gained ground, so discussion of production of little or defective seed increasingly referred only to men. Earlier concerns about women's seed do not seem to have been transferred to their production of eggs. However, the earlier humoral ideas about heat and cold and their effect on both body fat and seed continued to be held in relation to women's bodies into the late eighteenth century, as the too hot or cold womb was still thought to be inimical to male seed ejaculated into a woman's body during intercourse. Robert Barret had written at the end of the seventeenth century that a woman would be barren "if their Womb be cold, and the Seed be not receiv'd with some wellcome war[m]th ... Or if the Womb be moist, by reason of the Seed's being choak'd and extinguish'd in the prevailing moisture, which is commonly accompany'd with a cold temperature" (1699, 62). Just over seventy years later John Ball succinctly concluded that "the most frequent cause of all, is a cold and moist indisposition of the whole body and womb" (1770, 71). While eighteenth-century authors did not always further explain why fatness caused infertility, readers would undoubtedly have understood that it was because fat bodies were constitutionally very cold and moist bodies and therefore suffered from the reproductive disorders associated with this constitution. Late eighteenth-century authors continued to identify "too much fatness," "excessive fatness," or "Obesity" as a cause of barrenness (Ball 1770, 70; Baudelocque 1790, 213; Aitken 1786b, 137). Women who were, in contrast, constitutionally very hot and dry and therefore extremely slender as fat was melted by heat, were also understood as barren, heat and dryness being as inhospitable to the seed as cold and moisture. Barret explained that "if the Womb be too dry and hot, for then the Seed is burnt up and exhal'd" (1699, 62). Nearly fifty years later in the mid-eighteenth century Jean Astruc also listed as another cause of sterility, "Obstructions of the Body of the *Uterus*; such as proceed from an over-hot or otherwise vicious Temperament" (1743, 342).

These older humoral understandings of conception were thus not discarded as changing knowledge about conception from the late seventeenth century became more widely accepted, but were adapted to encompass newer ideas. This shift is explicit in discussions of barrenness caused by the destruction of male seed in the too hot or cold womb. Previously general discussions of seed now incorporated Leeuwenhoek's observation of animalcules in sperm, and some authors modified their explanations to state that the climate of the womb destroyed these animalcules. Astruc identified as a cause of barrenness, "The excessive Heat of the *Uterus*, whereby the *Animalcula* are destroyed before the *Ovum* descends into the *Matrix* to be impregnated by one of them." Remedies, as in preceding centuries, therefore consisted in countering heat with the opposing qualities of cold and wet, such as "cooling Broths of Veal and Pullet ... Asses Milk, cold or acidulous mineral Waters" (Astruc 1743, 346, 349).

Menstruation

Body size had a further effect on women's fertility through the impact it had upon the other matter of generation: menstrual blood. In both Aristotelian and Galenic-Hippocratic models of generation the menstrual blood played a role in conception and gestation, and so a regular and sufficient menstrual flow was understood as important to a woman's reproductive health (van de Walle 1997, 189–90, 196–8). Menstrual blood contributed matter both to the fetus and to its subsequent nourishment within the womb. Although by 1703 John Freind, in his influential treatise on menstruation, *Emmenologia*, translated from Latin in 1729, had noted that menstrual blood was "not altogether *necessary* to conception," he nevertheless allowed that it helped "Women *Conceive the more easily*" because it "opens the uterine Passages, that the *Semen* has a freer entrance into the Blood" (1729, 52). Ball in 1770 still referred to the menses as that "supply of blood which women ought to collect for the use and aliment of their offspring" (17). But by 1786 John Aitken, in *Principles of Anatomy and Physiology*, set out the three theories of fetal nutrition as from the amniotic fluid, from the mother's blood "through continuous vessels," or fluids from the mother "absorbed through the placenta," and concluded that it was the third of these (1786a, 148). The importance of menstruation to reproduction thus continued to be recognized even if the exact nature of its contribution was debatable.

At the end of the sixteenth century Philip Barrough in his popular (seven editions) *The Methode of Phisicke* repeated the idea that menstruation would be disrupted "against nature, either through ouer much grossenes, or slendernes" because in "fat folke" the blood turned to fat and their veins were more narrow, while "they that are leane and slender which be wasted with some continuall sicknes" had no superfluous blood for evacuation. As well as sickness that caused wasting, suppression of the menses was caused by "aboundaunce or scarcitie of foode" bringing either too much fat which obstructed the passages preventing the evacuation of the blood, or too little, so that blood was immediately consumed by the body leaving none to accumulate requiring regular evacuation (1583, 145). These ideas were reiterated into the eighteenth century. Freind, too, maintained the long-held understanding that the menstrual period "is terminated sooner in those of a grosser Habit, and in those that use a slender Diet, or much Exercise" (1729, 3). Menopause would also occur earlier in fat women, around the age of thirty-five, thereby further reducing their potentially fertile years. This idea was perpetuated into the late eighteenth century by William Smellie and John Ball, among others (Freind 1729, 51–3; Smellie 1790, 197; Ball 1770, 18–19). That women themselves believed that body fat had an impact on menstruation was suggested by Smellie in one of his childbirth case studies, where a woman of thirty, "inclining to be corpulent," whose menses were stopped, and who had previously borne three children, did not believe that she was again pregnant, but rather "imagined it was the consequence of her growing fat" (1790, 187).

Women themselves, then, as well as physicians, understood that a regular and sufficient menstrual flow was essential for reproduction, and women clearly consulted physicians or self-treated for menstrual disorders (Evans 2012, 9–14). Cathy McClive has noted that establishing a regular menstrual flow was important for a girl's transition to womanhood and reproductive success in marriage, while Susan Broomhall identified it as key to deciding whether a girl was ready to begin sexual relations as it indicated she was able to conceive (McClive 2007, 177–82; Broomhall 2002, 3). By the end of the eighteenth century, however, some writers were less concerned about the quantity or regularity of the menses in relation to fertility. David Spence, for example, noted that regularity had no impact on ability to conceive (1784, 49–5). Nevertheless, the idea that too much or too little fat had a negative effect on menstruation, and hence on women's fertility, still circulated throughout the century. The fertility of both fat and very slender women was understood to be impaired because, lacking enough blood, a regular and sufficient menstrual flow could not be established.

Male Sexual Dysfunction

Both fat and emaciated men were believed to suffer from sexual difficulties that diminished their fertility. Fat men's virility was understood as diminished in two specific ways: first, because of erectile difficulties; second, because body fat prevented the close conjunction of genitals during sex so that seed was not ejaculated deeply enough into the vagina. This meant that the seed became too cold to spark a conception, losing its vigour or "vital spirits" before it could enter the womb. Like fat, seed was understood as made from blood. In a complicated process of concoction it became "*a frothy Liquor*," characterized by a saltiness that gave the seed "its fruitfulness and balsamic Power," and giving rise to the term "salacity" for lust. So, "in drier Bodies, where salt Humours predominate, much Seed is generated, which makes 'em more able for the Sports of *Venus* ... Because the increasing of that in quantity excites an itching Titillation, and provoke to Lasciviousness." Therefore, thin, dry bodies had more sexual desire than fat ones which had fewer salt humours, so less seed and reduced desire for sex, minimizing their generative potential: "Because in fat Bodies, where fat and sulphurous Humours predominate, there is little Seed generated, and hence they have little proclivity to Venus" (De Diemerbroeck, 1689, 190–1). This explanation was perpetuated into the eighteenth century by other authors such as William Salmon, who translated De/Van Diemerbroeck and repeated it in his own anatomy, *Ars Anatomica*

(1714, 360). Lack of sexual desire caused by little and poor-quality seed meant that fat men were likely to have fewer and less sustainable erections, further impairing their generative ability. Marten thus noted that a fat man, having seed that lacked vigour, would have weak erections that "are not so frequent, nor altogether so potent as before he arriv'd to that fatness," so that even if he managed coitus "it is seldom found that the *Seed* is prolifick, or any thing comes on that conjunction" (1709, 23). By describing a fat man's seed as rarely "prolifick," meaning "full of blood," Marten alluded to the understanding that in fat people blood was diverted from seed-production to fat-production, diminishing its quality and quantity so that intercourse was unproductive. The poor quality of a fat man's seed meant that it lacked the "vitall spirit" necessary to spark conception, whether in women's "imperfect" seed or her "ova," but its diminished strength and quantity also decreased desire for sex and erectile function. These generative defects suggest that fat men were regarded as lacking in virility and hence inherently less sexual. Such perceptions were likely to have undermined a man's social standing, as it might be suspected that he was unable to father children, intimating a loss of manhood (Fletcher 1995, ch. 5; Foyster 1999, 67–72; Shepard 2005, 281–95; Toulalan 2014).

Wasting of the body leading to lack of sexual energy was paradoxically attributed to the over-indulgence of an over-heated sexual appetite: the effect of a life of debauchery was loss of flesh and hence loss of health, including sexual and procreative ability. The physician John Floyer told his readers at the beginning of the eighteenth century about "A *Gentleman* with a decay'd Stomach, a wan and pale Look, staggering under a load of nothing but Skin and Bone, his Cat-stick-leggs not being able to support his Cat-like *Carkass*. From a strong young Man, as he told me, Wine, Women and Watching, had reduc'd him to a meer *Skeleton*." This life of debauchery resulted in his wasting away and also had consequences for his sexual abilities, causing "a decay in *Virility*, tho' he was a young Man not above 27 or 28 Years of Age" (1706, 182–4). This decayed virility comprised both lack of sexual energy and impaired seed quality, and hence sterility. As in other discussions of male seed, the discovery of the existence of animalcules in semen was now incorporated into the idea that over-heated, excessively lascivious, and hence emaciated, bodies destroyed seed: "It has been observ'd, that they [animalcules] are not found in those that are much addicted to Venery. This agrees with Experience, which teaches us, that those who are given to Women are barren" (*Physical Essays* 1734, 137). Loss of virility from excessive leanness was, though, like that from too much fat, a temporary condition that could be restored through diet – and if the debauched behaviour that led to it ceased. Floyer's cure for the young man he treated restored him to health so that, significantly, "his Flesh came on" and he lost his former emaciation along with his sexual debility (1706, 184).

Masturbation also affected virility. This deleterious effect was reiterated in the anti-masturbation works that began to appear from the early eighteenth century. A correspondent with the anonymous author of the *Supplement to the Onania, Or the Heinous Sin of Self-Pollution* wrote that "this abominable Practice caused me to look lean and thin" (1724, 140). The same consequences were repeated in Samuel Tissot's hugely popular work on masturbation, *L'Onanisme*, published in English in 1766 as *A Treatise On The Crime of Onan*, where a correspondent wrote, "I have a devouring appetite, and yet I grow very lean, and never but look extremely ill" (1766, 31). This effect applied to both sexes, as the anonymous author of *Of the Crime of Onan* pointed out, and led to families becoming "frequently extinct for want of Heirs." It brought "Impotency in one Sex, and Barrenness in the other" so that "very few" could "boast of the Fruits of a married State." Furthermore, any children that were, against these odds, conceived and born, were "most commonly weak puny little sickly things" that would either soon die or grow up to be "tender Sickly Persons." Such impaired fertility came from having "enervated, consumed, drained, wasted, and worn out" their bodies "by this detestable Habit of Self-Defilement" (1724, 14–15). McLaren identified anxieties over masturbation and its dangers for sexual health and reproductive ability as driven by the "belief that Europe's population was declining" (2007, 84). Attention to male impotence, especially as a cause of marital infidelity and cuckolding of a husband, corresponded to later eighteenth-century concerns about sexual and reproductive success, where failure undermined social stability as well as contemporary notions of manhood (Toulalan 2007, 213–17; Turner 2002, 85–94).

Sexual Impediments

The flesh of the fat body was itself identified as an impediment to successful intercourse and hence conception: "by greatness of the Belly, hinders the right and fit Conjunction of the man with the woman" (Riverius 1655, 503). Excessive flesh in one or both partners presented a physical obstruction to fully penetrative sex preventing ejaculation sufficiently far into the vagina to enable seed to reach the womb without losing its heat and procreative vitality. *The Problemes* of *Aristotle* included a question asking why fat women seldom conceived and answered that it was "because the mouth of their matrix is very strait, that the seed cannot enter in: or if it doe goe in, it goeth in very slowly, for that the seed doth wan cold in the meane time, and so is unfit for generation" (1634, E6v). Male seed again became defective and "unfit" for generation because a fat woman's body obstructed and retarded its passage into the womb. Fat bodies were inherently non-sexual and non-reproductive bodies as they were also unsuited to the act of intercourse. However, by the end of the eighteenth century at least one author had noted that conception was still possible "when the semen has been deposited barely within the labia," suggesting that belief in this particular impediment to conception may have weakened by this time (Couper 1797, 40).

As remarked in *The Problemes of Aristotle*, fat offered a further obstacle to conception by narrowing the entrance to the womb, preventing the male seed from passing through it. From the sixteenth century medical authors had repeated Hippocrates's observation that in fat women the omentum (also termed the cawl or epiploon – tissue connecting the stomach with the liver, spleen, and colon) compressed the womb, preventing the seed from entering it, so causing barrenness. Anatomists identified this as a part of the body that was by nature fatty, so it grew even fatter in those who were corpulent (Heister 1721, 95; Aitken 1786a, 2:37; see also Bracken 1737, 20; Maubray 1724, 387). Some authors now also referred to fat compressing the Fallopian tubes and preventing conception, reflecting acceptance of the idea that women contributed eggs from their ovaries rather than seed. William Cheselden did not mention the potential obstruction to conception caused by the omentum in fat women in the first edition of his anatomy, but in the third edition he speculated that fat might obstruct the Fallopian tubes to prevent conception: "perhaps the fat in the membrane that connects the Ovaria to the tubes, may in very fat women, so keep these tubes from the Ovaria as to interrupt impregnations" (Cheselden 1713, 168–9; 1726, 303–4).

In addition to the usual recommendations to reduce fat through diet to restore fertility, some authors also suggested changing sexual position from the prescribed missionary position. Nicholas Venette's *Tableau de l'Amour Conjugal* was translated into English in 1703 as *Conjugal Love Reveal'd* and reprinted in different versions during the eighteenth century, finally reaching, questionably, twenty editions, suggesting that it was a highly popular book of sexual advice (Porter and Hall 1995, 81–3). Although Porter and Hall claimed that "Venette had few remedies to offer" for infertility, he had an explicit recommendation when too much fat prevented intercourse: penetration should be from behind, so that "no Suffocations or Miscarriages ever happen thereupon" (Porter and Hall 1995, 78; Venette 1720, 126–9). Although not specifying exactly how, Bracken also advised that the woman be put "in a proper Posture" for sex when fat presented an obstacle to coitus (1737, 20). Such advice, which conflicted with contemporary prescriptions for acceptable sexual behaviour, suggests that promoting fertility trumped upholding sexual propriety, further supporting the idea that eighteenth-century society was pro-natalist. It also suggests that the preservation of marital intercourse itself was thought to be important because sexual debility, particularly male impotence, might be a cause of marital infidelity that had the potential to disrupt bloodlines and inheritance, threatening the foundations of patriarchal society (Berry and Foyster 2007, 166–7).

By contrast, authors were not as concerned with counselling against excessive slenderness. While advising against sexual debauchery and masturbation that wasted vital spirits, there seems to have been little concern with self-imposed starvation. Emaciation through starvation was mainly a problem for those who were too poor to afford adequate nourishment, and authors of medical and midwifery books did not exhibit particular concern about this except in the context of childbirth, where starving, emaciated poor women suffered hard labours, lacking the strength to cope with prolonged labour and hence requiring assistance (Smellie 1790, 2:263, 265–6, 297–9, 302–3). The fasting and consequent emaciation of extreme religious piety, sainthood, and prophecy encountered in earlier centuries, particularly in women, does not seem to have been of concern to those who wrote about extreme slenderness and fertility in the eighteenth century (Bell 1985; Vandereycken and van Deth 1994). Similarly, references in earlier medical texts to wasting caused by witchcraft, where sufferers were "tortured with lingring consumptions," disappear from eighteenth-century works, reflecting the decline in witchcraft belief (Roberts 1616, 17; Tourney 1992, 296).

Miscarriage

Despite these impediments to conception, fat and lean women did become pregnant. However, these pregnancies were perceived as more precarious with a high risk of miscarriage. Maubray also noted that miscarriage carried more danger for these women: "LEAN and *tender Women* are much endanger'd in *ABORTION*, by Reason of their *Debility* and *Infirmity*: As Women too fat are, on the other Hand; because of the great *Astriction* and

Narrowness of the PASAGES" (1724, 127). Obesity continued to be listed as a cause of miscarriage throughout the eighteenth century. The multiple miscarriages of Queen Anne in the later seventeenth century, as well as the absence of further conceptions after 1700, may have been understood in this context – as an inevitable result of her increasing corpulence. Anne's first three pregnancies (one stillbirth, two live births, both dying in infancy) were followed by three miscarriages; the birth of her son William in 1689 was followed by two live births neither of which survived a day, then by another eight miscarriages. Emson notes that Anne was obese by the age of thirty and had no more pregnancies after 1700, aged thirty-five (1992, 1365).

Just as blood was diverted, in fat bodies, from the production of generative materials to further increasing the body's store of fat, reducing its generative potential, so, too, nourishment was diverted from the fetus to the fat, starving the infant to death in utero. Maubray wrote that "A *nimious* and too great an *Obesity* or *Fatness* ... converts the *CHILD*'s *Nourishment* to itself" (1724, 119). Furthermore, the fetus could be suffocated by a woman's consumption of too much or too rich, poorly digested food, preventing its growth to full term (122). At the end of the century Martha Mears continued to warn against over-indulgence or "luxury," causing "the juices, retarded in their circulation, [to] stagnate and grow foul" so that "the powers of the womb in particular are enfeebled or perverted" (1797, 70). Similarly, those who suffered from "extream leanness of the whol body, wherein there is not Blood enough to nourish the Infant" were more likely to miscarry because they too were unable to provide it with adequate nourishment for growth: "too great a *Gracility* or *Leanness* of the *Woman's* Body ... starves the *INFANT* for want of its *natural Requisites*" (Riverius 1655, 513; Maubray 1724, 119). Whether from sickness or starvation, "a want of food" caused miscarriage as it "hinders the Infant from acquiring its perfection" (Baudelocque 1790, 466; Mauriceau 1672, 132).

Authors were therefore concerned with the question of proper nourishment in the womb for the growing fetus in both types of body, and advised on diet and other remedies to regulate and bring them back to a better "habit" of body. Maubray in the early eighteenth century repeated the same advice as Röesslin had given two centuries earlier: "IF it proceeds from too much FATNESS, her *Body* is to be reduced; if it comes from too much LEANNESS, a convenient *Diet* and good *Regimen*, &c. will help to restore her" (Röesslin 1540, Mii[v]; Maubray 1724, 130). Fat women were thus advised to eat more sparely, and sometimes to take gentle purgatives – although "strong Purgatives" were to be avoided because they might themselves provoke miscarriage (Astruc 1743, 362; Mears 1797, 76). Those who were too thin, whether through sickness or poverty, were also to eat sparingly, but often, of highly nourishing foods (Astruc 1743, 369). But some practitioners perceived those who were fat as not always amenable to treatment: Bracken commented that "Fat People are unwillingly perswaded to live so sparingly, as may bring them to Leanness" (1737, 24). Fat bodies might thus be resistant to social expectations and control, resonating with Sally Frampton's evocation in this volume of the disturbing pregnant and dropsical female body as "beyond the control of both medicine and nature."

By the later eighteenth century, however, these earlier understandings about very thin bodies were being rejected, particularly in relation to the wasting caused by consumption. John Stedman wrote that rather than the mother's body taking nourishment from the fetus, it appeared to be the other way around: "After impregnation the foetus seems to be supplied with nourishment preferable to any part of the mother's body. Women, labouring under wasting diseases, particularly pulmonary consumptions, are frequently delivered of children, whose full and healthy appearance bears no proportion to the emaciated state of the mothers" (1769, 90). Although Denman also listed insufficient or improper nourishment as a cause of fetal death in utero, he also noted that those with "very weak and reduced states of the body, particularly in consumptions" were no more likely to miscarry than others, "yet a state more feeble and more irritable could with difficulty be pointed out" (1794, 2:191, 319). Nevertheless, those who advised women on ante-natal care, like Mears, continued to advise regulating diet to promote fetal survival.

Authors had also repeated throughout the previous two centuries, often without further explanation, the idea that "Fat Women are subject to Miscarry by reason of the slipperiness of their Wombs," and presented it also as a cause of barrenness where the seed slipped out of the womb before conception could occur (Culpeper 1651, 146). In the humoral model, it was obvious that the fat body's excess of cold, moist humours made the womb "so slyppery that the feture slyppeth and slydeth forth" (Röesslin 1540, fol. XLI); furthermore, as fat was an oily, slippery substance, the wombs of fat women would naturally be slippery. Although works such as those on midwifery by Culpeper and *The Problemes of Aristotle* continued to circulate this notion, towards the end of the century it was rejected. Denman referred to it as "the opinion originally entertained and still pursued" that the womb "failed to perform its office on account of its excessive lubricity, as if the *ovum* slipt out of the *uterus*" and concluded: "but this idea will not bear examination" (1794, 2:320). Denman did not explain why he rejected this idea, but it was unlikely to have been a consequence of the abandonment of the humoral ideas which had prompted it, as these clearly persisted.

Conclusion

Men and women perceived to be too fat or lean were categorized as reproductively impaired. Authors repeated old stereotypes – usually accompanied by moral comment – about the superior fertility and childbearing capacity of labouring women, particularly those dwelling in the country rather than in cities (e.g., Sharp 1671, 178). Fertility problems were often attributed to self-indulgence, with Denman telling his readers unequivocally that "these evils are not to be attributed to physical infirmities, but to moral errors" (1794, 2:13). Although clearly repetitions of common stereotypical representations, the ubiquity of these strictures about lifestyle and fertility nevertheless imply a contemporary anxiety about wealth and social class and their relationship with unsuccessful reproduction (Ganev 2007, 42). Elizabeth A. Williams has noted that by the seventeenth century medical advice was characterized by "antagonism toward gastronomic indulgence," and such hostility clearly featured in these stereotypes of indolent, self-indulgent women and their reproductive dysfunction that resisted contemporary expectations of maternity (2012, 392). But it was not only women whose reproductive abilities were affected by body size. Fat men were regarded as likely to be impotent and infertile, potentially affecting their social standing: sexual and reproductive incompetence diminished manhood, hinting at lack of patriarchal authority. Fat bodies, signalling possible reproductive impairment, generated anxieties about inheritance and the smooth transfer of lands, titles, and wealth down through the generations in those classes for whom such issues were of paramount importance. Authors thus tended to be more condemnatory about fat bodies and their consequent reproductive difficulties than they were of thin bodies, whose emaciation was usually a result of poverty or disease, factors beyond individual control – although some emaciated men might be suspected of debauchery that caused wasting and reduced virility. Both types of body disrupted gendered social expectations for maternity and paternity. The medical narratives that linked body size to infertility and miscarriage thus also had a regulatory and disciplinary function. They contributed to a pro-natalist culture in which it was important to ensure bodies were fit and suitable for reproduction assuring economic, political, and social stability.

REFERENCES

Aitken, J. 1786a. *Principles of Anatomy and Physiology*. 2 vols. London: J. Murray.
Aitken, J. 1786b. *Principles of Midwifery, Or Puerperal Medicine*. 3rd ed. London: J. Murray.
Astruc, J. 1743. *A Treatise on All the Diseases Incident to Women*. London.
Ball, J. 1770. *The Female Physician: Or, Every Woman Her Own Doctress*. London: L. Davis.
Barret, R. 1699. *A Companion for Midwives, Child-Bearing Women and Nurses*. London: Tho. Ax.
Barrough, P. 1583. *The Methode of Phisicke*. London: Thomas Vaurroullier.
Baudelocque, J.-L. (1775) 1790. *A System of Midwifery*. 3 vols. Translated by J. Heath. London.
Bell, R.M. 1985. *Holy Anorexia*. Chicago: Chicago University Press.
Berry, H., and E. Foyster, eds. 2007. *The Family in Early Modern England*. Cambridge: Cambridge University Press. http://dx.doi.org/10.1017/CBO9780511495694.
Bracken, H. 1737. *The Midwife's Companion; Or A Treatise of Midwifery*. London: J. Clarke, J. Shuckburgh.
Broomhall, S. 2002. "'Women's Little Secrets': Defining the Boundaries of Reproductive Knowledge in Sixteenth-Century France." *Social History of Medicine* 15 (1): 1–15. http://dx.doi.org/10.1093/shm/15.1.1.
Browne, T. 1669. *Nature's Cabinet Unlock'd*. London: Edward Farnham.
Cheselden, W. (1713) 1726. *The Anatomy of the Humane Body*. 3rd ed. London: N. Cliff, D. Jackson, and W. Innys.
Cobb, M. (2006) 2007. *The Egg & Sperm Race: The Seventeenth-Century Scientists Who Unravelled the Secrets of Sex, Life and Growth*. London: Pocket Books.
Cody, L.F. 2005. *Birthing the Nation: Sex, Science, and the Conception of Eighteenth-Century Britons*. Oxford: Oxford University Press.
Couper, R. 1797. *Speculations on the Mode and Appearances of Impregnation in the Human Female*. 2nd ed. Edinburgh: Peter Hill; London: T. Cadell Junior & W. Davies.
Culpeper, N. 1651. *A Directory for Midwives*. London: Peter Cole.
Denman, T. (1762) 1794. *An Introduction to the Practice of Midwifery*. 2 vols. London: J. Johnson.

De Diemerbroeck, I. 1689. *The Anatomy of Human Bodies*. Translated by W. Salmon. London: Edward Brewster.
Drake, J. 1717. *Anthropologia Nova: Or, A New System of Anatomy*. 2nd ed. 2 vols. London: Judith Drake.
Elements of Anatomy and the Animal Oeconomy. 2nd ed. 1781. London: J. Walker.
Emson, H.E. 1992. "For the Want of an Heir: The Obstetrical History of Queen Anne." *British Medical Journal* 304 (6838): 1365–6. http://dx.doi.org/10.1136/bmj.304.6838.1365.
Evans, J. 2012. "'Gentle Purges corrected with hot Spices, whether they work or not, do vehemently provoke Venery': Menstrual Provocation and Procreation in Early Modern England." *Social History of Medicine* 25 (1): 2–19. http://dx.doi.org/10.1093/shm/hkr021.
Fletcher, A. 1995. *Gender, Sex & Subordination in England 1500–1800*. New Haven and London: Yale University Press.
Floyer, J. 1706. *Ψυχρολουσια:Or, The History Of Cold Bathing*. 2nd ed. London: S. Smith and B. Walford.
Forth, C.E. 2012. "Fat, Desire and Disgust in the Colonial Imagination." *History Workshop Journal* 73 (1): 211–39. http://dx.doi.org/10.1093/hwj/dbr016.
Foyster, E.A. 1999. *Manhood in Early Modern England: Honour, Sex and Marriage*. London: Longman.
Freind, J. (1703) 1729. *Emmenologia*. Translated by T. Dale. London: T. Cox.
Ganev, R. 2007. "Milkmaids, Ploughmen, and Sex in Eighteenth-Century Britain." *Journal of the History of Sexuality* 16 (1): 40–67. http://dx.doi.org/10.1353/sex.2007.0037.
Gowing, L. 2003. *Common Bodies: Women, Touch and Power in Seventeenth-Century England*. New Haven and London: Yale University Press.
Guerrini, A. 2000. *Obesity & Depression in the Enlightenment: The Life and Times of George Cheyne*. Norman: Oklahoma University Press.
Harvey, K. 2004. *Reading Sex in the Eighteenth Century: Bodies and Gender in English Erotic Culture*. Cambridge: Cambridge University Press.
Heister, L. (1717) 1721. *A Compendium of Anatomy*. London: Tho. Combes and James Lacy.
Hitchcock, T. 1997. *English Sexualities: 1700–1900*. Basingstoke: Palgrave Macmillan.
Ingram, M. 1987. *Church Courts, Sex and Marriage in England*. Cambridge: Cambridge University Press.
Marten, J. 1709. *Gonosologium Novum*. London: N. Crouch.
Maubray, J. 1724. *The Female Physician, Containing all the Diseases Incident to that Sex, in Virgins, Wives, and Widows; Etc.* London: James Holland.

Mauriceau, F. (1668) 1672. *The Diseases of Women with Child, and in Child-bed*. London: John Darby.
McClive, C. 2007. “L’âge des fleurs: le passage de l’enfance à l’adolescence dans l’imaginaire médical du XVIIe siècle.” *Biblio* 17:171–85.
McLaren, A. 1984. *Reproductive Rituals: The Perception of Fertility in England from the Sixteenth Century to the Nineteenth Century*. London: Methuen.
McLaren, A. 2007. *Impotence: A Cultural History*. Chicago: Chicago University Press. http://dx.doi.org/10.7208/chicago/9780226500935.001.0001.
Mears, M. 1797. *The Pupil of Nature; or Candid Advice to the Fair Sex, on the Subjects of Pregnancy; Childbirth; the Diseases Incident to Both Etc.* London.
Of the Crime of Onan Or, The Hainous Vice of Self-Defilement with all its Dismal Consequences etc. 1724. London: H. Parker.
Perry, R. 1991. “Colonizing the Breast: Sexuality and Maternity in Eighteenth-Century England.” *Journal of the History of Sexuality* 2 (2): 204–34.
Physical Essays on the Parts of the Human Body and Animal Oeconomy. 1734. London: John Clarke.
Porter, R., and L. Hall. 1995. *The Facts of Life: The Creation of Sexual Knowledge in Britain, 1650–1950*. New Haven: Yale University Press.
The Problemes Of Aristotle. 1623. London: A.G. for Godfrey Emondson.
Riverius, L. (1640) 1655. *The Practice of Physick, Etc.* Translated by N. Culpeper, A. Cole, and W. Rowland. London: Peter Cole.
Roberts, A. 1616. *A Treatise of Witchcraft*. London: N. O. for S. Man.
Röesslin, E. 1540. *The Byrth of Mankynde newly translated out of Laten into Englysshe, etc.* Translated by R. Jonas. London: T.R.
Rogers, P. 2010. “Fat Is a Fictional Issue: The Novel and the Rise of Weight-Watching.” In *Historicizing Fat in Anglo-American Culture*, edited by E. Levy-Navarro, 19–39. Columbus: Ohio State University Press.
Salmon, W. 1700. *Aristotle’s Compleat and Experience’d Midwife*. London.
Salmon, W. 1714. *Ars Anatomica: Or, The Anatomy Of Humane Bodies.* London: I. Dawes for D. Browne; W. Taylor; and J. Browne.
Sharp, J. 1671. *The Midwives Book, or the Whole Art of Midwifry Discovered*. London: Simon Miller.
Shepard, A. 2005. “From Anxious Patriarchs to Refined Gentlemen? Manhood in Britain, circa 1500–1700.” *Journal of British Studies* 44 (2): 281–95. http://dx.doi.org/10.1086/427128.
Schwartz, H. 1986. *Never Satisfied: A Cultural History of Diets, Fantasies and Fat*. New York: The Free Press.
Smellie, W. 1790. *The Theory and Practice of Midwifery*, 1752–1764. London: Alexander Cleugh.

Spence, D. 1784. *A System of Midwifery, Theoretical and Practical.* Edinburgh: William Creech.

Stedman, J. 1769. *Physiological Essays and Observations.* Edinburgh: A. Kincaid & J. Bell; London: T. Cadell.

Stolberg, M. 2012. "'Abhorreas pinguedinem': Fat and Obesity in Early Modern Medicine (c. 1500–1750)." *Studies in History and Philosophy of Biological and Biomedical Sciences* 43 (2): 370–8. http://dx.doi.org/10.1016/j.shpsc.2011.10.029.

A Supplement to the Onania, Or the Heinous Sin of Self-Pollution, And all its Frightful Consequences, &c. 1724. London.

A System of Anatomy and Physiology, with the Comparative Anatomy of Animals. 3 vols. 1791. Edinburgh: William Creech.

Tissot, S. 1766. *A Treatise on The Crime of Onan.* Translated from 3rd ed. London.

Toulalan, S. 2007. *Imagining Sex: Pornography and Bodies in Seventeenth-Century England.* Oxford: Oxford University Press.

Toulalan, S. 2014. "'To[o] much eating stifles the child': Fat Bodies and Reproduction in Early Modern England." *Historical Research* 87 (235): 65–93. http://dx.doi.org/10.1111/1468-2281.12031.

Tourney, G. 1992. "The Physician and Witchcraft in Restoration England." In *Articles on Witchcraft, Magic and Demonology: Witchcraft in England.* Vol. 6 of 12, edited by B.P. Levack, 285–97. New York and London: Garland.

Turner, D.M. 2002. *Fashioning Adultery: Gender, Sex and Civility in England, 1660–1740.* Cambridge: Cambridge University Press. http://dx.doi.org/10.1017/CBO9780511496103.

Vandereycken, W., and R. van Deth. (1988) 1994. *From Fasting Saints to Anorexic Girls: The History of Self-Starvation.* New York: New York University Press.

van de Walle, Etienne. 1997. "Flowers and Fruits: Two Thousand Years of Menstrual Regulation." *The Journal of Interdisciplinary History* 28 (2):183–203.

Venette, N. (1686) 1720. *Conjugal Love Reveal'd.* London.

Williams, E.A. 2012. "Sciences of Appetite in the Enlightenment, 1750–1800." *Studies in History and Philosophy of Biological and Biomedical Sciences* 43 (2): 392–404. http://dx.doi.org/10.1016/j.shpsc.2011.10.031.

Wrigley, E.A., and R.S. Schofield. 1981. *The Population History of England 1541–1871: A Reconstruction.* London: Edward Arnold.

14 Deformity of the Maternal Pelvis in Late Eighteenth-Century Britain

PAM LIESKE

In June of 1799, Elizabeth Thompson, a dwarf with a contracted pelvis, was transported by litter to the Manchester Lying-Hospital for emergency delivery (Wood 1799, 464). Eight hours after admission, she gave birth to a healthy male child by Caesarean. The child flourished and was named Julius Caesar (*Medical* 1799, 473). Thompson was not so fortunate. She died seventy-six hours after surgery (Wood 1799, 470). Interest in her case, however, did not fade with her death as she became a household name among select obstetricians. Her reproductive organs were meticulously dissected, measured, and weighed, and the surgeon who performed Thompson's surgery provided seventeen detailed measurements of her pelvis and lower spine in a report he submitted to the Medical Society of London (473–6). Additional reports as well as models and engravings of Thompson's pelvis began to appear. Plaster of Paris replicas were available for sale in Manchester and London while an engraving of Thompson's pelvis appeared in works by two practitioners closely associated with the case (Wood 1799; Hull 1799, plate VII).

This chapter examines written and visual rhetoric about the eighteenth-century female pelvis to understand the importance of Elizabeth Thompson, and women like her, whose fame rests on their difficulty to give birth due to pelvic deformity. A related objective is to understand when and how interest in contorted pelvic bones came about and what this interest suggests about the nature of emergency obstetrical practice at the end of the eighteenth century. That era's medical practice, of course, was always keen to establish parameters between what is normal and what is not. Elsewhere in this collection, Sally Frampton explains medical practitioners' attempts to distinguish between ovaries of normal size and function and those that are abnormally large, or swollen, with attendant interiors of bone, hair, and teeth reminiscent of monstrous births. Elsewhere, Sarah Toulalan examines the relationship between body size and infertility, discovering that corpulent or emaciated bodies were linked to infertility and miscarriage and thus served as negative, or cautionary, examples of what body size and habits mothers (and fathers) should strive to maintain.

This chapter follows suit. It illustrates how study of distorted maternal pelvises, both when the mother was alive and after her death, prompted practitioners to make distinctions between normal and abnormal pelvises, and by extension, normal and abnormal births. Since many practitioners would not encounter extreme pelvic deformities in their pregnant patients on a regular basis, being able to see and touch pelvic models, study pelvic engravings, and read case histories about emergency births of mothers with distorted and small pelvises served an important pedagogical function. Such activities allowed practitioners to formulate methods of assessment and treatment, debate them with peers, or if they worked alone, to decide on which surgical or nonsurgical interventions to implement should they encounter an expectant mother with pelvic distortion that made vaginal birth difficult, if not impossible.

This chapter will not argue that the era of deformed maternal pelvises led to an important breakthrough in obstetrical knowledge or technique. Texts and case histories discussed here do not reflect such a change. What archival material studied does show is that pelvic contraction in expectant mothers was an area of intense interest among certain late eighteenth-century obstetrical specialists, particularly those at specialized facilities like the Manchester Lying-in Hospital. By treating women like Elizabeth Thompson and then studying and writing about emergency births and abnormal pelvises, these practitioners not only provided immediate assistance to their medical peers by preparing them for possible emergencies in their own clinical practice, but they also added to a growing body of written, visual, and physical evidence of distorted maternal pelvises. Though it appears knowledge of pelvic malformations was not known beyond select networks of medical men and did not uniformly advance the clarification and treatment of maternal pelvic deformity in this time period, this little-known pocket of medical history still deserves its rightful place within the larger narratives of eighteenth-century science and medicine as well as emergency midwifery.

Discourse on the Pelvis in Early British Midwifery Texts

Before we can understand the late eighteenth century's heightened interest in distorted pelvises, it is useful to understand how little attention was given to the pelvis in early midwifery texts. Prior to the 1730s midwifery texts published in Britain contained little original content. A number of important French writers were translated into English, and seventeenth-century midwives Jane Sharp and Percival Willughby provided original content, but Willughby's midwifery treatise, though written between 1730 and 1760, was not published until 1863, and its 200 case histories contain scant mention of pelvises. In contrast, Jane Sharp's *The Midwives Book* (1671) largely ignored labour and delivery to focus on maternal duties related to pregnancy and motherhood. Sharp's work does contain two illustrations: one shows the womb, dissected like a rose petal, within a standing female figure, while the second shows eight images of single or twin fetuses in standing and sitting postures within egg-shaped wombs with each womb's covering peeled away to reveal the figure or figures within. Both illustrations are crudely rendered, lack anatomical detail, and provide only a broad idea of the womb and delivery positions.

Edmund Chapman's *An Essay towards the Improvement of Midwifery* [1733?], a collection of fifty case studies and "the first account in print of the midwifery forceps," ushered in a number of British-authored midwifery works with original content to appear in print in the 1730s (Wilson 1995, 6). Chapman, though, only briefly mentions pelvic bones, and not one of the other midwifery treatises or pamphlets published in the next decade, including one by the female midwife Sarah Stone, and a new edition by Chapman, discusses pelvic bones in a substantive way and certainly none treats its relationship to the mechanics of labour and delivery (Giffard 1734; Chapman 1735; Douglas [1736?]; Bracken 1737; Stone 1737; Ould 1742). For instance, the opening of Henry Bracken's *The Midwife's Companion* (1737) begins in this way:

> The Womb is situated in the lower Part of the *Hypogastrium*, or lower Belly, between the Bladder and straight Gut; the *Os pubis*, commonly called the Sheer bone, is a Fence to it before, the *Sacrum* behind, and the *Ilium* on each Side: These form as it were a Bason for it [the womb], but because it must swell whilst Women are with Child, therefore these Bones are larger than in Men, and is the Reason why Women are bigger in the Haunches. (1)

For Bracken, as for all British midwifery writers of the 1730s, the uterus is the focus. Bones may be named individually, but all midwives need to know about the female pelvis is that it is broad and capacious and, as a boney cage, it houses and protects the uterus. Three of the seven midwifery texts from the 1730s include illustrations, but none are of pelvic bones. William Giffard's work contains five engravings: two of extractors, an early forceps, and three crude dissections of the uterus and related tissues and organs (1734, n.p.) while Fielding Ould's treatise includes images of the "Terebra Occulta," an ice pick-like instrument used to lessen the child's head in cases of intractable labours (1743, 167). Finally, in keeping with growing interest in obstetrical instruments, Alexander Butter's 1735 essay includes what is likely the first engraving of a forceps to appear in a British authored text (Cutter and Viets 1964, 60).

To be fair, scattered remarks on maternal pelvic rigidity and softening during labour were made by seventeenth-century British authors like Percival Willughby and William Harvey; the former suggested that the maternal pelvis was unduly rigid while Harvey felt its joints softened during labour (Allotey, 2:97–102). Moreover, early eighteenth-century audiences could see anatomical waxwork collections in London that included maternal and fetal figures, and by the 1740s students in London and large urban centres could obtain instruction in surgery, midwifery, and dissection in private anatomy and midwifery schools (Lieske 2011, 69–70; Bates 2008, 2–3; Mitchell et al. 2011, 96). For instance, London's *Daily Advertiser* for 8 Nov. 1742 announces that J. Parsons MD will soon be giving "lectures on the structure of the pelvic and uterus" at his residence, while a second advertisement announces William Smellie's lecture course on midwifery for men and for women "illustrated with proper Machines so contriv'd as to represent real Woman and Children."

More attention to the importance of the pelvis during labour and delivery took shape once the Dutch physician Hendrik van Deventer's ideas became established in Britain. Translated into English in 1716, Deventer's 1701 midwifery treatise contains "the first account of the size, shape and obstetric significance of the female pelvis" and a written description of the effects of rickets on the maternal pelvis (Wilson 1995, 79). Deventer had a life-long interest in pelvic anatomy and its deformities. He also practiced midwifery with his wife, who may have helped him recognize what became the cornerstone of his practice and the foundation of the anti-forceps movement in Britain: realization that compression on the vaginal wall to move the mother's coccyx and sacrum backward could create additional space for delivery (Wilson 1995, 80). Deventer includes two images of pelvises in his treatise: one from an anterior and one from a cross-sectional view. Both show "a heavy-boned, compact pelvis" more typically seen in men than in women (Allotey 2007, 1:123) (figures 14.1 and 14.2).

Curiously, in his treatise Deventer only speaks generally about normal and rachitic pelvises: how midwives need to see and touch them, how pelvic bones of men and women differ, and how it is difficult to illustrate the

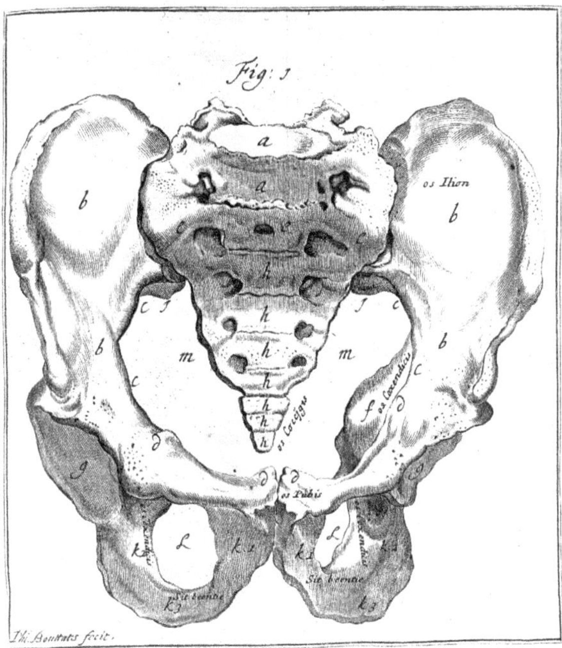

Figure 14.1 Anterior view of the female pelvis. H. van Deventer, *Operationes Chirurgicae Novum Lumen Exhibentes Obstetricantibus* (Leiden: A. Dyckhusien, 1701), figure 1, facing page 16. Courtesy of Wellcome Library, London.

pelvis because "the one Part being in view, easily obstructs the Sight of the other" (1716, 18). He does name individual bones and speaks of angles, but he does not provide exact measurements. That task is left to the British man-midwife William Smellie who delivered women in London for twenty years and applied scientific principles to the theory and the teaching of midwifery. In the first volume of his 1752 midwifery treatise, Smellie minutely details the shape, proportion, and measurements of the pelvis, stating:

> The extent of the brim from the back to the fore-part, commonly amounts to four inches and one quarter; and from one side to the other, the distance is five inches and a quarter: So that this difference of an inch in the different axes, ought to be carefully attended to in the practice of Midwifery. (1762, 4th ed. 1:78)

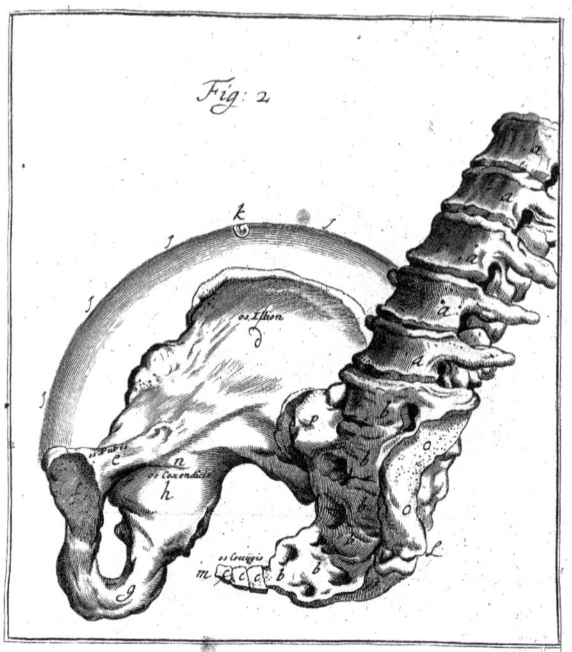

Figure 14.2 Cross-sectional view of the female pelvis, H. van Deventer, Operationes Chirurgicae *Novum Lumen Exhibentes Obstetricantibus* (Leiden: A. Dyckhusien,1701, figure 2, facing page 20. Courtesy of Wellcome Library, London.

This meticulous description of pelvic bones contrasts sharply with more general comments made by earlier British midwifery writers like Bracken.

In 1754, Smellie published an atlas of thirty-nine obstetrical images that correspond to select discussions in his treatise's first volume as well as to 531 individual case histories. The atlas opens with three images of the female pelvis. Two of them mirror Deventer: a frontal view followed by a lateral view of a normal pelvis. The third image represents what Deventer discussed but did not show: a pelvis distorted by rickets (figure 14.3). Including this illustration of a rachitic pelvis is an important milestone in British obstetrical history as it provided lasting visual evidence of pelvic abnormality, far beyond the more fleeting impression that rachitic pelvises seen in lectures or demonstrations could provide.

In the preface to his 1796 collection of eighteen obstetrical plates, the Scottish surgeon and man-midwife James Hamilton provides insight into

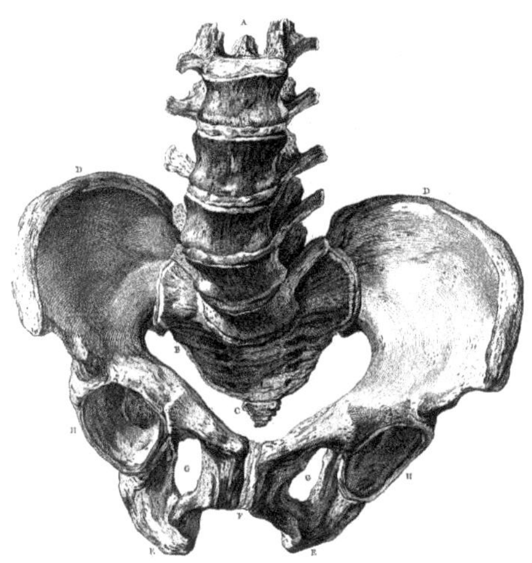

Figure 14.3 A distorted female pelvis. W. Smellie, *A Sett of Anatomical Tables, with Explanations and An Abridgement of the Practice of Midwifery* (London, 1754), plate III. Courtesy of Wellcome Library, London.

how visual and written discourse about the maternal pelvis had become so familiar over the course of the century that some practitioners, Hamilton included, did not hesitate to alter and "improve" images and discussions about pelvises as they saw fit. Hamilton explains that life-sized anatomical plates, including those made by Smellie, are not practical: they cost too much to make, not enough people buy them, and even already published miniatures of Smellie's plates are not attractive to audiences (ix–x). This is why Hamilton has revised Smellie's smaller images, reduced and refigured certain obstetrical plates of William Hunter and Phillipp-Adolphe Boehmer, and included "two or three drawings from preparations" of his father, Alexander Hamilton (x). None of the resulting images is aesthetically pleasing; none is original to Hamilton, and given their crude renditions, none would be useful in clinical practice. Still, they do indicate that pelvises were familiar terrain to some practitioners.

Only two of Hamilton's eighteen obstetrical plates show pelvises, and each of these two plates contains two images. Image 1 of plate I is a vertical section of half of a female pelvis, with the sacrum and coccyx (Hamilton 1796, 2). The second image is an anterior view of the pelvis with attached femurs (2–3) (figure 14.4). Plate II presents two more views: the first depicts a pelvis from a superior viewpoint as if someone were looking down into the boney cavity from above. The second image reverses this perspective and shows the pelvis from an inferior stance, as if someone were peering up into it from below (figure 14.5). Together, these four images show the pelvis from four angles – side, front, above, below. The first image in plate one even cuts the pelvis in half so readers can overcome Deventer's objection that, when viewing the pelvis, "the one Part being in view, easily obstructs the Sight of the other" (1716, 18).

Hamilton also synthesizes ideas and insights of established authorities while he elaborates on specific bones and anatomical features identified by letters in each engraving. He informs readers that the pelvis "lies in a slanting direction from the spine towards the horizon, for the posterior part is situated about three inches higher than the anterior. –The consequence of this is, that the line of the axis of the pelvis is different from that of the body" (3). This passage is easy to understand. Other passages are more obtuse, such as when Hamilton, building on Deventer's idea of the moving coccyx, describes how a fused coccyx that typically moves backward one inch shortens the position of "the longest diameter at the outlet," or the longest distance from the bottom of the pelvis to its brim, or top (6). Hamilton's book of engravings, then, does not just present revised pelvic images, it also presents elaborate and meticulous discussions about what knowledge related to childbirth these images are meant to convey.

Starting in the 1750s, British authors discussed pelvic bones more complexly, mentioning angles, surfaces, depths, and diameters as well as the relationship between the fetal head and the pelvis, and how force and resistance come into play during the birthing process. In 1755 Giles Watts claimed that "the Membranes of the *Fœtus* in *Utero*, with their contained Water, form a spheroidal Figure: now it is very notorious, that the nearer any Form approaches to a perfect Sphere, so much the more capacious such Form is" (11). Indeed, understanding limits of pelvic capacity, force of uterine contractions, and positioning of the fetus during labour and delivery remained central concerns in mid-century texts. As knowledge of the forceps and vectis, or lever, became more entrenched, even more complex data was formulated about the specific angle at which practitioners should insert instruments, and where and how to apply instruments on the

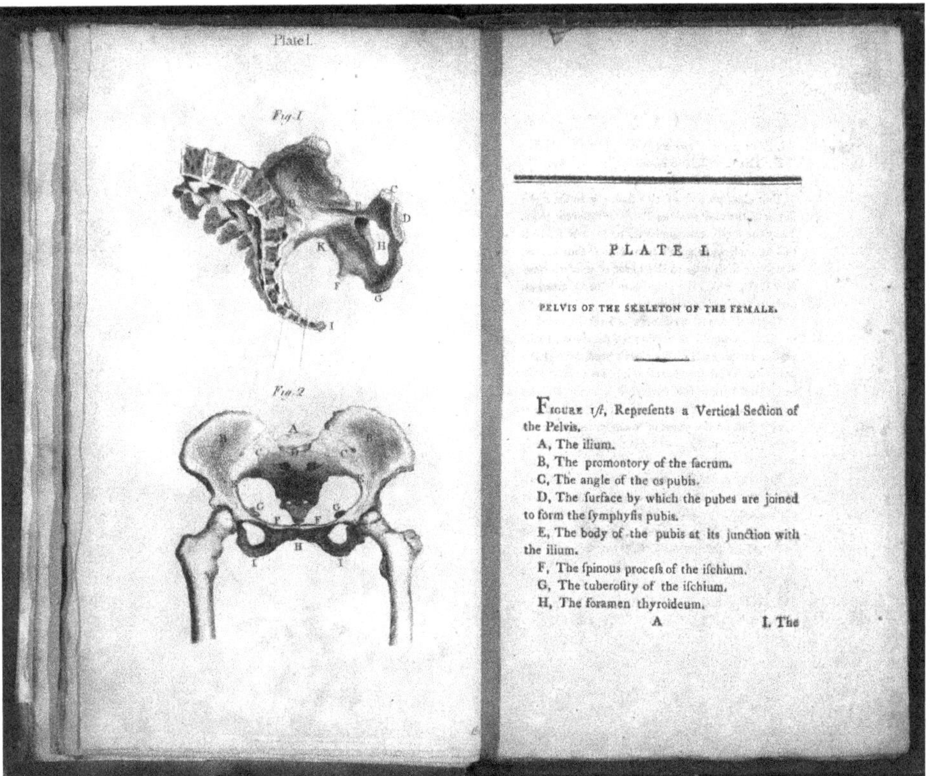

PLATE I.

PELVIS OF THE SKELETON OF THE FEMALE.

FIGURE 1ſt, Repreſents a Vertical Section of the Pelvis.

A, The ilium.

B, The promontory of the ſacrum.

C, The angle of the os pubis.

D, The ſurface by which the pubes are joined to form the ſymphyſis pubis.

E, The body of the pubis at its junction with the ilium.

F, The ſpinous proceſs of the iſchium.

G, The tuberoſity of the iſchium.

H, The foramen thyroideum.

A I. The

Figure 14.4 Cross-sectional view of the female pelvis and anterior view of the female pelvis with attached femurs. J. Hamilton, *A Collection of Engravings, designed to facilitate the Study of Midwifery* (London: G.G. & J. Robinson, 1796), plate I, figures 1 and 2. Courtesy of Wellcome Library, London.

fetal skull, or elsewhere, so that maximum pelvic space and optimal angles for delivery could be obtained.

The Scotsman John Aitken added to empirical work on pelvises when he tried to determine exact measurements of the "average" female pelvis. He apparently did this without internal pelvimeters, whose use, though championed by some French practitioners, never caught on in Britain (Hibbard 2000, 265; Kerr, Johnstone, and Phillips 1954, 22–3). Aitken begins by providing pelvic measurements from three established practitioners – Smellie, Stein, and Baudelocque ([1784?], 9). He follows this with

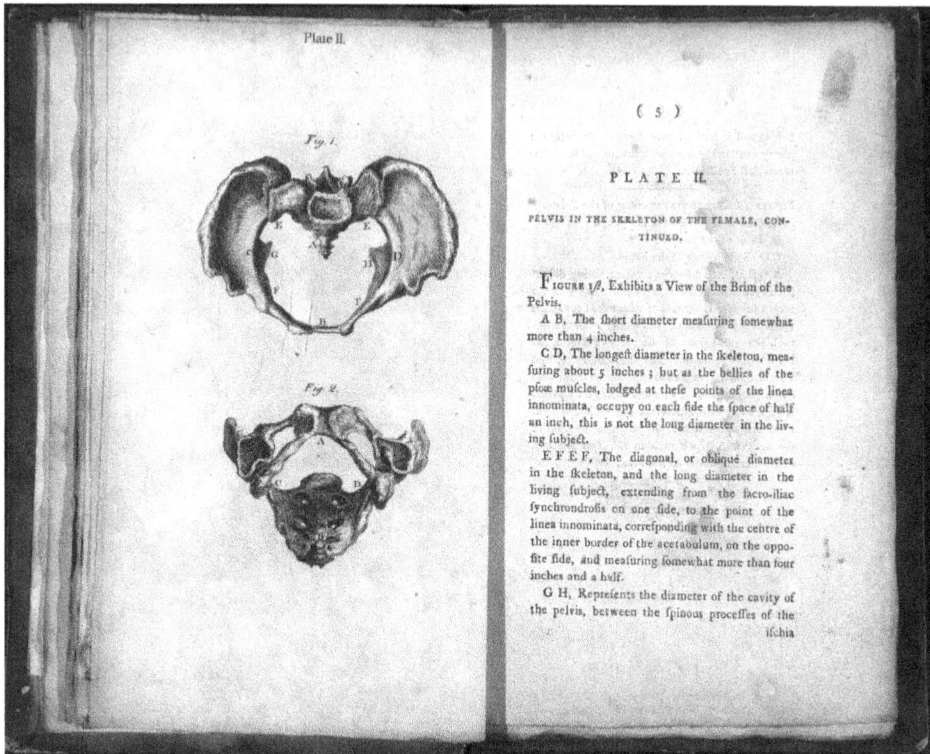

(5)

PLATE II.

PELVIS IN THE SKELETON OF THE FEMALE, CONTINUED.

FIGURE 1ſt, Exhibits a View of the Brim of the Pelvis.

A B, The ſhort diameter meaſuring ſomewhat more than 4 inches.

C D, The longeſt diameter in the ſkeleton, meaſuring about 5 inches; but as the bellies of the pſoæ muſcles, lodged at theſe points of the linea innominata, occupy on each ſide the ſpace of half an inch, this is not the long diameter in the living ſubject.

E F E F, The diagonal, or oblique diameter in the ſkeleton, and the long diameter in the living ſubject, extending from the ſacro-iliac ſynchrondroſis on one ſide, to the point of the linea innominata, correſponding with the centre of the inner border of the acetabulum, on the oppoſite ſide, and meaſuring ſomewhat more than four inches and a half.

G H, Repreſents the diameter of the cavity of the pelvis, between the ſpinous proceſſes of the

iſchia

Figure 14.5 Superior view of the female pelvis and inferior view of the female pelvis. J. Hamilton, *A Collection of Engravings, designed to facilitate the Study of Midwifery* (London: G.G. and J.Robinson, 1796), plate II, figures 1 and 2. Courtesy of Wellcome Library, London.

his own set of four distinct pelvic measurements – from the brim, bottom, angle or arch, and the depth – and claims that his resulting calculations, which he seemingly compared to those of the three authorities, are based on "the mean dimensions of four Pelvises" that he studied (10). Aitken not only wanted to determine the average size, shape, and dimension of the "average" female pelvis, he sought to understand how the position of the mother affected the position of the pelvis and advised that when a hand or surgical instrument is inserted into the pelvis, the angle of insertion should be as close to the axis of the pelvis as possible, or about 23 degrees (7–8).

Like other earnest practitioners of his time, Aitken was an advocate of "a just and scientific practice of midwifery" based on "precise mensuration" of "the form and dimensions of the Pelvis" (8).

While practitioners like Aitken were focused on measurements of the normal female pelvis, others set their sights on measuring distorted pelvises. This was fuelled by news of an innovative procedure to deliver women with impossibly small pelvises: division of the symphysis pubis. First performed in France in 1777, this operation involved cutting the anterior pubic bones to increase pelvic width (Sigault 1778). Like the use of internal pelvimeters on living women, the procedure never gained currency in Britain, but discourse about it sparked further discussions about emergency deliveries of mothers with contracted pelvises. These discussions always circled back to two key questions: What is the smallest possible pelvic diameter a woman can have and still hope for vaginal delivery of a healthy child? And, what procedure(s) should be implemented if a woman's pelvic outlet fell below this mark?

William Simmons, one of two surgeons who saw Elizabeth Thompson before her transport to the lying-in hospital in Manchester, claimed he knew the answers to these questions. He argued that the Caesarean operation "can never be justifiable" when the mother is alive, but when the pelvis is "no more than one inch in diameter" and the mother cannot be delivered by the crotchet, a two-part operative procedure should occur: division of the anterior public bone to create enough space and then vaginal insertion of the hook-like crotchet so the child could be removed piece-meal (1798, 68, 65). Another Manchester surgeon involved in the Thompson case, John Hull, was incensed that Simmons would embrace this dangerous, dual procedure and not endorse what he felt was growing evidence of the efficacy of the Caesarean operation.

Two other physicians, Alexander Hamilton and William Osborn, also differed over how to treat emergency deliveries when the mother's pelvis was small and distorted. Hamilton felt that when the "short diameter of the pelvis at the brim shall admit three fingers" or more, then the mother should be left to deliver the child on her own, as long as the head descends and no urgent symptoms occur (1792, 121). If the pelvis could only admit two average-sized fingers and no more, according to Hamilton, vaginal delivery of a living child was not possible and the child's head should be reduced with the crotchet "as soon as the os uteri [cervix] is nearly or completely dilated" (122). With even smaller pelvic openings, when just one finger, or less, could pass through the short diameter of the pelvis, than "terminating the delivery" through the Caesarean operation was the only option (122).

Osborn felt differently. In his opinion, the smallest pelvic diameter a woman can have and still hope for normal vaginal delivery is "*two inches and three quarters from pubis to sacrum*" (1783, 251). Mothers with smaller pelvic outlets would have to be delivered of a dead child with the crotchet. On this point he disagreed with his long-time teaching partner, Thomas Denman, who felt that the vectis, or lever, should be used. An unwavering fan of the crotchet, Osborn argued that the smallest pelvic space where a child "may be safely extracted by the crotchet ... is a space equal to *one inch and a half from pubis to sacrum*, dimensions much less, than what have invariably been supposed to require the Caesarian operation" (251–2).

To support his claims, Osborn tells the story of Elizabeth Sherwood, a dwarf like Elizabeth Thompson. At only three feet six inches tall, and with extreme pelvic deformity, it is amazing that Sherwood even carried a child to full term. Not surprisingly, she could not deliver vaginally. In a three-hour procedure detailed in his writing, Osborn says he applied the crotchet to lessen the child's head. He then left Sherwood for thirty-six hours believing the delay would result in "putrefaction" of the child followed by its descent in the birth canal (Osborn 1783, 82, 88). Examined by midwives, including William Hunter and Thomas Denman, as well as some thirty students, Sherwood survived the procedure and reportedly "suffered much less than might reasonably have been expected, whether from the length of the labor, or the extreme violence in the delivery" (Osborn 1783, 90, 88–9).

Osborn's meticulous description of the destructive surgery he performed on Sherwood irritated Alexander Hamilton, who believed that application of the crotchet before the cervix was fully dilated, was "highly dangerous and improper" (1792, 121). According to Hamilton, only in cases "where immediate delivery is absolutely necessary" should lessening of the child's head occur (120). Osborn seemingly viewed labour and delivery as potential problems best resolved as quickly as possible. This is suggested in his opinion that four-legged creatures, with horizontal pelvises, have an easier time in childbirth than human mothers with their upright pelvises (1783, 251). Debate over which pelvic outlet size equates with which kind of delivery, and in cases of impossibly small pelvises, which type of instrument to use, were common topics of debate among this network of medical men. Such discussions can make readers squeamish, especially when certain details emerge, such as Sherwood being left with a dead and decomposing fetus inside of her for thirty-six hours, or having thirty students lined up to perform vaginal examinations on her.

Before we level charges of cruelty and callousness on eighteenth-century surgeons and men-midwives, we might consider that today's large teaching hospitals routinely encourage interns and medical students to examine patients with unusual maladies, and that in a reversal of the Elizabeth Sherwood case, brain-dead pregnant women have been kept alive in order to give the living fetus a chance at life.

Moreover, today and in the eighteenth century, practitioners disagree over clinical intervention. Alexander Hamilton's views about childbirth, particularly in cases of contracted pelvises, are measured and less interventionist. He rightly claims that not every man-midwife would have the skill and good luck to deliver Elizabeth Sherwood's child with a crotchet without also killing her. He goes on to relate the story of a mother with a small rachitic pelvis whose three pregnancies resulted in three different outcomes. The mother's first labour ended with lessening of the child's head through application of the crotchet. In the second labour, with the mother's cervix fully dilated, Hamilton unsuccessfully tried a forceps delivery, and then resolved to perform the Caesarean operation; however, while he was preparing for the procedure, the mother felt sudden, sharp pains and within a half hour delivered "a living female child who grew up to be a mother herself" (Hamilton [1792?], 99–100). The third labour ended in a double tragedy. The mother endured a forceps' delivery "of a dead child, in a putrid state," never recovered, and died three weeks later (100–1).

Hamilton relates these three births to inform readers that labour and delivery of all mothers, particularly those with contorted pelvises, is unpredictable. To reinforce this point, he discusses the case of Nelly Sanderson, age forty, who was in labour for three days and eventually gave birth "by the powers of nature alone," to a child with a "flattened and bruised" head (Hamilton [1792?], 118). The child lived for eight days, but died (118). In contrast to this outcome, Hamilton tells of other mothers in labour for two or three days who deliver healthy children. Never knowing what will happen and having faith in the mother's ability to safely deliver without intervention are the hallmarks of Hamilton's unique ideology.

Other midwives besides Hamilton believed that mothers should be left alone to deliver on their own. The foe of William Smellie, Elizabeth Nihell opposed the use of any instruments and felt that female midwives did not require in-depth anatomical knowledge. She would have been appalled by the meticulous measurements of pelvic bones and fetal skulls that became common at the end of the century. Like midwifery writers of the 1730s who favoured the uterus, Nihell felt that the pelvis was merely "a container" for the child; she would not have cared that Nelly Sanderson's pelvic outlet measured less than three inches while her child's head was decidedly larger (1760, 33; Hamilton [1792?], 115–19). Later in the century, the female midwife Margaret Stephen also felt that labour should proceed without practitioner interference. She believed that a mother could safely undergo two or three days of labour before medical intervention was needed (1795, 66–8). Charles White, who attended Elizabeth Thompson's 1799 Caesarean operation, also felt this way as did Sir Richard Croft, the physician and man-midwife who attended the labour of Princess Charlotte in November 1817. Charlotte spent three days in labour; the child's head was lodged in the birth canal for one full day. Results were grim: the child was stillborn. Charlotte died a short time after, and Croft committed suicide out of guilt and shame at what happened (Shingleton 2005). I mention these varying opinions about childbirth to emphasize that concurrent with the late eighteenth-century fad for pelvic measurements and sophisticated methods to deliver women with mangled pelvises, some practitioners held firm to the belief that most mothers, if given the chance, could deliver on their own without practitioner intervention.

Even today there is no definitive answer on when vaginal birth compared to surgical intervention should occur. Two twentieth-century scholars, who spent more than eleven years studying the relationship between pelvic diameters and the outcomes of nearly 4000 labours, "believe that successful vaginal birth in doubtful situations depends largely upon the driving force of the uterus" and not so much on pelvic deformity (Mengert and Korkmas 1957, 154). A more recent study used maternal X-ray pelvimetry and ultrasound to measure fetal head size and the maternal pelvis, but the resulting calculation – the "fetal pelvic index" – did not predict with complete accuracy the method of delivery each woman required (Morgan, Thurnau, and Fishburne 1986). Results of follow-up investigations on the reliability of the fetal-pelvic index to predict the route of delivery appear mixed (Ferguson et al. 1998). Such studies appear to support the views of non-interventionist eighteenth-century midwives like Hamilton, Nihell, and Stephens who felt that uterine contractions could expel a child from the uterus if no obvious sign of danger was present.

Since even modern medicine, with its sophisticated imaging techniques, cannot predict with 100 per cent accuracy the delivery method for women with certain-sized pelvises and fetal skulls, it should come as no surprise that late eighteenth-century midwives held differing views of how to assess and treat pregnant women with impossibly small pelvises. Practitioners like Osborn, Hamilton, Simmons, and Hull tried their best to establish standards of medical care for obstructed delivery caused by extreme pelvic deformity and sway their colleagues to their views. Each arrived at precise pelvic measurements meant to establish definitive surgical (or non-surgical) treatment, and each felt that elaborate, even obsessive, measurements of pelvises and fetal skulls would help them reach decisive knowledge of pelvic anatomy, its relation to the mechanics of childbirth, and which surgical techniques to employ, or avoid.

This is why obtaining contracted pelvises for empirical study was an objective shared by all the practitioners interested in emergency obstetrics. Alexander Hamilton obtained the pelvis of the woman who experienced three different delivery outcomes, and reported that "the short diameter of [her] pelvis at the brim ... was sensibly under three inches" and that the specimen "was shown in our class for several years, but at last was accidently lost" (1792, 101). Hamilton mentioned other unique pelvises that became part of man-midwives' collections, including one from a woman that Thomas Young operated on, which Hamilton then owned, as well as the pelvis of a patient that Dr Cooper treated that belonged to William Hunter (Hamilton [1792?], 63–4).

Cooper also sold Osborn and Denman a teaching apparatus, or obstetrical machine, used in the hands-on teaching of midwifery (see Moscucci). Widely used in Britain, these devices contained a real or artificial pelvis. William Smellie's medical collection, sold after his death, contained a number of obstetrical artefacts, including four obstetrical machines. One of these machines contained a contracted pelvis so students could gain practical knowledge in deliveries of this kind (Paterson 1770, 6–7). Outside of London, the man-midwife William Cockell used a female pelvis, likely of normal shape, in conjunction with William Smellie's obstetrical atlas, to assist him in determining how to treat retroversion of the uterus, while Thomas Pole informed his London midwifery students that he has around 1000 "paintings, drawings, models, and castes in plaster of Paris" that he utilized in his classes (Cockell 1785, 20; Pole 1797, ix). These are just a few of the many practitioners who collected female pelvises – normal, abnormal, real, or artificial. They wanted them so they could teach themselves, or their midwifery students and peers, how best to assess and treat conditions of childbirth.

Elizabeth Thompson

Disputes about contracted pelvises were in full swing when Elizabeth Thompson was delivered by Caesarean operation at the Manchester Lying-in Hospital. Reminiscent of the frenzy caused by the rabbit breeder Mary

Toft in 1726, medical personnel flocked to her side. Two surgeons – James Ogden and William Simmons – examined Thompson before she journeyed to Manchester "in a cart, placed on a feather bed … slung with cords"; four more examined her at the hospital (White et al. 1799, 7). Eight hours after her arrival, William Wood, a surgeon and man-midwife at the facility, performed the Caesarean operation in the presence of eight individuals, mostly men-midwives, but also a female midwife and an apothecary (1799, 4). After Thompson died, eleven men – the hospital's entire medical committee – attended the dissection while eight men inspected her uterus and pelvis that were removed for further study (White et al. 5). Moreover, an unknown number of plaster casts of Thompson's pelvis went on sale in London and in Manchester, and an engraving of her pelvis appeared in two different publications – one by Wood and one by a practitioner previously mentioned, John Hull.

The Thompson case also lived on in various records. For instance, Wood's essay meticulously details how the operation was performed, how the wound was dressed, and the full extent of Thompson's post-operative care – five enemas, a suppository of soap, rectal infusion of tobacco, and a blistering plaster – all standard treatments for the rapid heart rate, abdominal pain, and emesis from which she suffered (Wood 1799, 467–70). Wood stated that he had no choice but to perform the operation since he could only insert two fingers into Thompson's pelvic opening from front to back and only one finger from side-to-side (464). He also related that Thompson had two previous pregnancies. In 1790 she had an easy vaginal delivery of a living child; two years later, she delivered a (dead) child by the crotchet (472). He claimed that gangrene of Thompson's cervix, caused by the cervix and the child's head pressing against the right side of the pelvis, caused her death, and "she would have stood a great chance of recovering" if the Caesarean operation was done earlier at the patient's residence (473). The seventeen detailed pelvic measurements taken by Wood appear excessive to modern-day readers, but they are consistent with measurements of the time and demonstrate clinical interest in her case.

The report of the eminent man-midwife Charles White, written in conjunction with three colleagues, reads like a legal brief as it records the time line of events. It records the names of individuals who attended the surgery, as well as the dissection, and the inspection of the pelvis and uterus. Also included is a copy of the note Ogden wrote to the Manchester Lying-in Hospital asking that Thompson be transferred there, White's reply to Ogden reporting on the outcome of the operation, and White's claim that all the men-midwives present unanimously agreed that delivery by

Caesarean operation was the only humane course of action to take. According to White, crotchet delivery was impossible, and without removal of her child, Thompson would die an agonizing death. White also asserted that Thompson should have been transported to Manchester in a sling carried by two men, stated that the lying-in hospital has such a device, and insinuated that Thompson was jostled too much in the cart that was used (White et al. 1799, 7).

James Ogden's rebuttal, republished with White's remarks, is openly hostile towards the Manchester practitioners. Ogden said that he agreed with William Simmons's opinion after examining Thompson that the "case was one of Dr. Osborne's (*sic*) crotchet cases" (*Medical* 1799, 477). He asserted that Thompson should have been operated on as soon as she arrived at the lying-in hospital and that her bowels should have been evacuated prior to surgery. He ended by declaring that he will never endorse the Caesarean "during the life of the mother" (479). Not surprisingly, Simmons also found fault with the Manchester group. He claimed that Wood unjustly insinuated that he (Simmons) and Ogden caused Thompson's death when it was the Manchester group that did not notice ominous signs of inflammation and deliver Thompson right away. Tellingly, Simmons did not explain why he and Ogden did not deliver the patient themselves. Simmons voiced further disagreement over the clinical findings at autopsy and the after-treatment that Thompson received. He ended by claiming that Thompson died because the Caesarean operation was performed on her and that this surgery should never be done because it is always fatal to the mother (Simmons [1799?]).

Further remarks by George Tomlinson bring the sharp divide between the pro-Caesarean camp at Manchester and the crotchet advocates of Ogden and Simmons into focus. According to Tomlinson, Thompson's only chance at life was the Caesarean, and he was adamant that Simmons's dual procedure of division of the symphysis pubis followed by application of the crotchet would have failed (1799, 7). He said that two maternal pelvises in his possession from previous crotchet cases, joined with his clinical examination of Thompson, assured him that her pelvis was too small for crotchet delivery. Tellingly, he asked the one question about the case that remains unanswered: If Ogden and Simmons felt crotchet delivery was so necessary, why didn't they perform this procedure themselves?

As seen, the Thompson case served as a site for intense debate about standards of medical and surgical care for labouring mothers with severely contracted pelvises. While no agreement between the Caesarean and the crotchet camps was reached, the fact that opinions were aired in print allowed dialogue about contracted pelvises to grow and circulate. This dialogue, it can be argued, reached its full significance in the writings of John Hull. In 1798, a year before the Thompson case, Hull published a work that argued for the Caesarean operation in cases of extreme pelvic contraction and against "either the combination of Embryulcia with the Section of the Symphysis Pubis, or a reliance on the powers of nature" (Hull 1798, 229). Included in the text are charts of seventeen Caesarean operations that allegedly occurred in Great Britain. Each case is discussed at length, and Hull spent extra time on the Caesarean operations he performed on Isabel Redman in 1794 and Ann Lee in 1798. Just over four feet tall with a rachitic pelvis, Lee and her child both died. Hull was more successful delivering Redman. Like Thompson, Redman had already delivered a living child and, like Thompson, she suffered from a softening and degeneration of her pelvic bones. Hull relayed the results of Redman's dissection in full, and then stated that two drawings were made of her pelvis and "that 500 of the best Impressions of each Plate are reserved for another publication" (182). At the end of Hull's text are seven plates (n.p). The first two plates are the engravings of Redman's pelvis that Hull had hoped to have published elsewhere, but apparently never did. Showing the "Superior and Inferior [pelvic] Apertures" or openings, the two plates are elaborately rendered with letters to denote certain pelvic distances that are discussed at length earlier in the text (183–8; figure 14.6, shows Plate I, an anterior view of the Superior Aperture).

Hull's 1798 work also includes an engraving of the base of an average-sized fetal skull preceded by an outline of the pelvis of Ann Lee, the other mother Hull delivered by Caesarean (plates III and IV, not shown here). Hull was so eager to have his readers understand the difficulty in delivering women like Lee that he presented images, or sketches, that juxtapose the base of this fetal skull with Lee's pelvis (plate V, figure 14.7). In another sketch, an average-sized fetal skull is juxtaposed with the deformed pelvis of another mother delivered by Caesarean section – Elizabeth Hutchinson (plate VII, not shown here). There is even a sketch of a crotchet applied to Ann Lee's pelvis to illustrate that crotchet delivery would prove impossible (plate VI, not shown here).

Though these sketches may seem primitive, there is no denying that Hull felt the various sketches of pelvises, alone or with the fetal skull, conveyed important ideas about emergency deliveries. In particular, he wanted readers to realize that the pelvises of the women he mentioned were simply too small and deformed for vaginal delivery. Hull even asked readers to envision scenarios that his seven plates do not show and to compare the different deformed pelvises he has presented. He stated at one point:

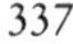

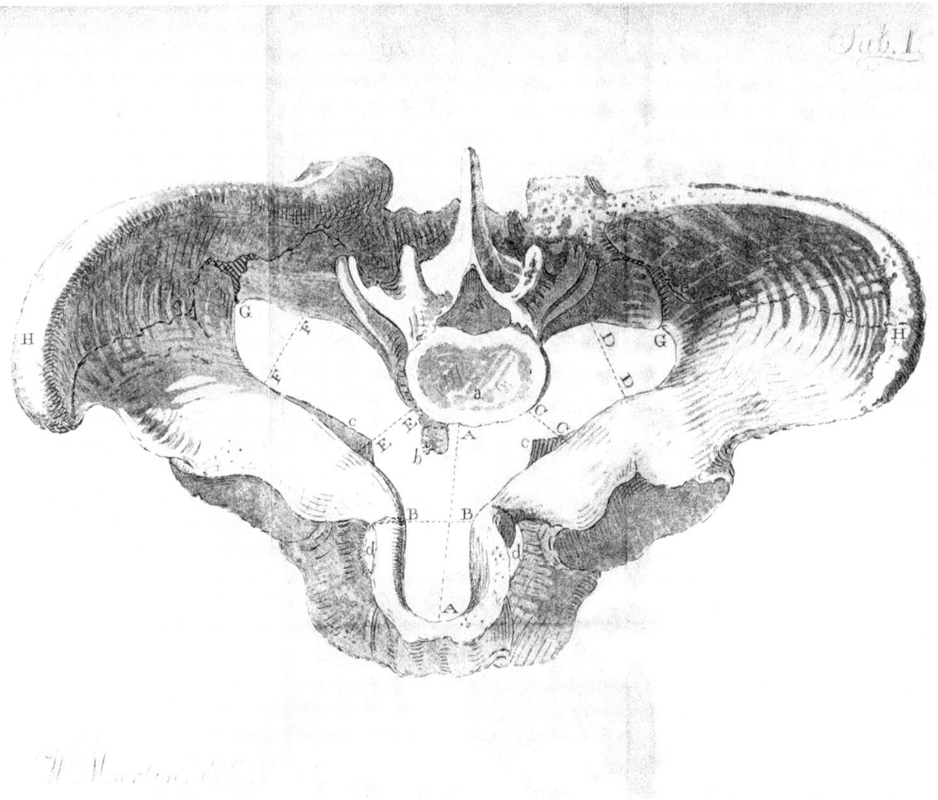

Figure 14.6 Anterior view of the pelvis of Isabel Redman. J. Hull, *A Defence of the Cesarean Operation, with Explanations and An Abridgement of the Practice of Midwifery* (Manchester: R. and W. Dean,1798), plate I. Reproduced by permission of the National Library of Medicine, shelfmark WZ260H917d.

"On applying this cranium, [the average-sized one, Plate IV] in the same manner, to the pelvis of Isabel Redman (Plate I), although its transverse and conjugate diameters are considerably greater than those of the pelvis of Ann Lee [Plate III], we shall find it equally impracticable to accomplish the delivery by *cepthalotomia* [dissection of the fetal head]" (Hull 1798, 202). The full impact of Hull's written and visual discourse on distorted pelvises may be hard for modern readers to fathom, but eighteenth-century practitioners versed in difficult deliveries due to contracted pelvises

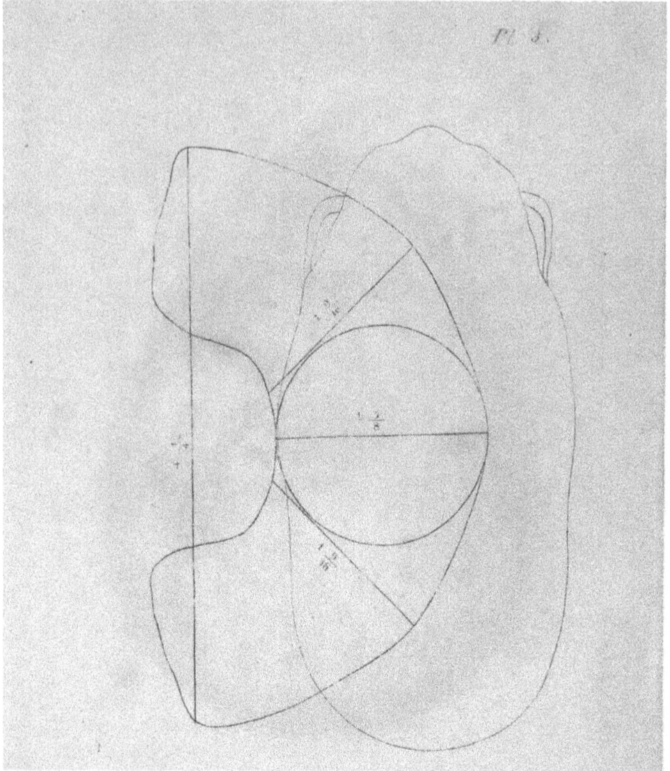

Figure 14.7 Sketch of the pelvis of Ann Lee seen with the base of an average-sized fetal skull, turned sideways. J. Hull, *A Defence of the Cesarean Operation, with Explanations and An Abridgement of the Practice of Midwifery* (Manchester: R. and W. Dean, 1798), plate V. Reproduced by permission of the National Library of Medicine, shelfmark WZ260H917d.

would have understood Hull's argument and been aware of each of the cases discussed.

The year of Thompson's delivery, Hull published another work in favour of the Caesarean operation that opposed the views of William Simmons, the staunch advocate of the crotchet. More than double the length of his 1798 work, Hull included fourteen pages of charts detailing 110 "successful" and 27 "unsuccessful" Caesarean operations performed in Great Britain and Europe from 1500 to the present (277–91). He also included two charts of "forty four cases of the Section of the Symphysis pubis, from which we find, that 30 women have survived the operation, and 11 have died" (n.p., between 94 and 95). He pointed out that most of the women whose pubic bones were severed were permanently injured and that the procedure has fallen out of favour as no new cases have been published since 1787 (Hull 1799, 94).

In Hull's desire to show the usefulness of Caesarean operations, the Thompson case is discussed at some length, and the same engraving of Thompson's pelvis that appeared in Wood's essay appears here (Hull 1799, 109–18, 292, 469–70, Table 7) (figure 14.8). In addition, the twelve plates of images at the end of Hull's 1799 text mix the normal and the abnormal, the universal and the individual. Seen together these images say more about the variability of late eighteenth-century obstetrical practice, including difficult deliveries due to contracted pelvises, than anything that Hull, or other writers, could explain in their writing. The images open with four plates that echo the images produced by James Hamilton. They are largely reprints, without revision, of pelvic engravings from established authorities, like Baudelocque. A few are of abnormally shaped pelvises; many are not. Plate V shows a sketch, or outline, of a superior perspective of the pelvis of Elizabeth Sherwood, as described by Osborn, and drawn by Hull. This is followed by another sketch, from the same perspective, of a cast of a distorted pelvis said to belong to White (468). Near the end of the work are four plates depicting "monstrous children" of various kinds that harken back to the era of Ambroise Paré (Plates VIII–XI). The final plate references present-day obstetrical practice. It shows two images: the head of a child reduced by a perforator and crotchet to show the smallest opening that the head can be brought through the pelvis, and a second image of "a well formed pelvis, with two Pelvimeters applied to it" (Hull 1799, 472).

Tucked in the middle of these images is the engraving of Elizabeth Thompson's pelvis that William Wood first presented. The individuality of this image both competes with, and comments on, attempts by Hull and other practitioners to define normal and abnormal female pelvic anatomy and then link assessments of deformed pelvises to definitive surgical or non-surgical methods of treatment and delivery. While the field of obstetrics at the end of the eighteenth-century never arrived at any uniform consensus about how to evaluate and care for labouring mothers with malformed pelvises, there is no doubt that Elizabeth Thompson, Isabel Redman, Ann Lee, Eliza Sherwood, and other expectant mothers with deformed pelvises were iconic figures in late eighteenth-century specialized obstetrics. While most of these women died during, or shortly after childbirth, their legacy lives on in their written case histories and most importantly in the discussions, images, and models of their uniquely shaped pelvises.

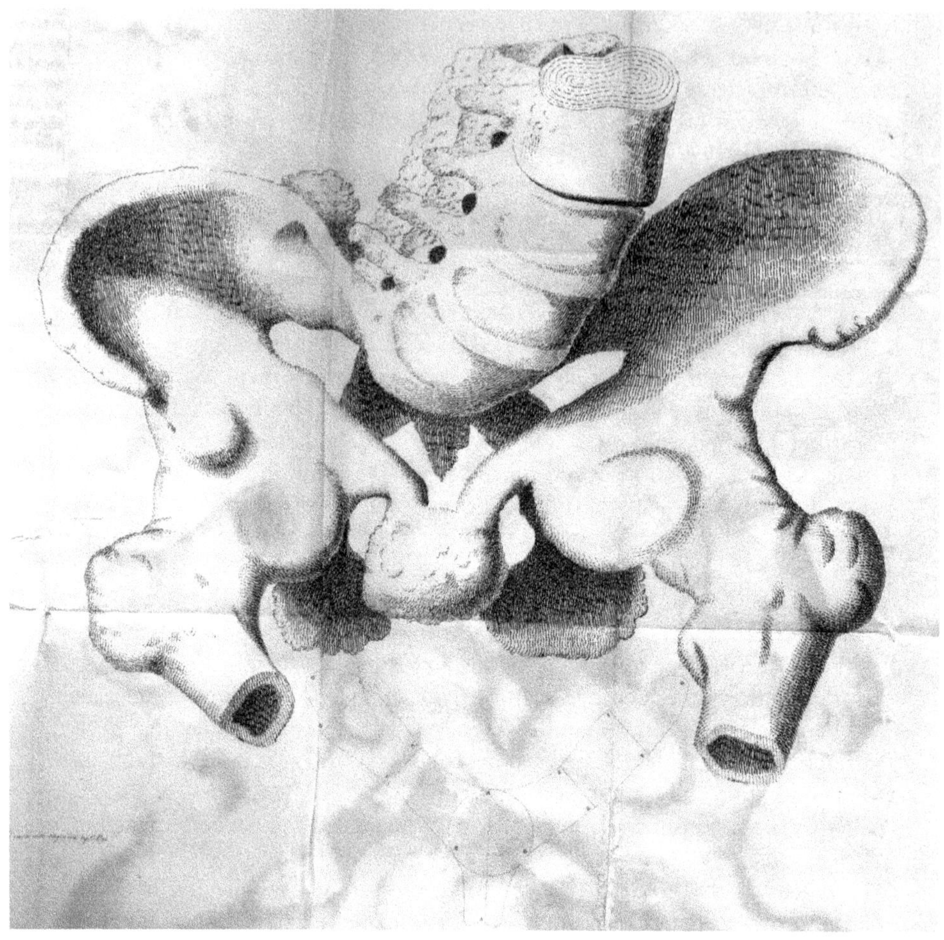

Figure 14.8 Anterior view of the pelvis of Elizabeth Thompson with partial spine and femurs. W. Wood, "Case of Cæsarean Section," In *Memoirs of the Medical Society of London, Instituted in the year 1773* (London: J. Johnson, 1799), final engraving, n.p. Reproduced by permission of the Literary and Philosophical Society of Newcastle upon Tyne.

REFERENCES

Aitken, J. [1784?] *Principles of Midwifery, or Puerperal Medicine*. Edinburgh.
Allotey, J.C. 2007. "Discourses on the Function of the Pelvis." PhD diss. University of Sheffield.
Bates, A.W. 2008. "'Indecent and Demoralising Representations': Public Anatomy Museums in Mid-Victorian England." *Medical History* 52 (1): 1–22. http://dx.doi.org/10.1017/S0025727300002039.
Bracken, H. 1737. *The Midwife's Companion*. London: J. Clarke and J. Suckburgh.
Chapman, E. [1733?]. *An Essay on the Improvement of Midwifery, Chiefly with Regard to the Operation. To which are added Fifty Cases, selected from upwards of Twenty-five Years Practice.* London: A. Blackwell.
Chapman, E. 1735. *A Treatise on the Improvement of Midwifery, Chiefy with regard to the Operation. To which are added Fifty-seven Cases, selected from upward of Twenty-seven years practice. The second edition, with large additions and improvement.* London: John Brindley.
Cockell, W. 1785. *An Essay on the Retroversion of the Uterus*. London: Logographic Press.
Cutter, I.S., and H.R. Viets. 1964. *A Short History of Midwifery*. Philadelphia: Saunders.
Daily Advertiser. 8 Nov. 1742. Issue 3733. London.
Deventer, H. van. 1701. *Operationes Chirurgicae Novum Lumen Exhibentes Obstetricantibus*. Leiden: A. Dyckhusien.
Deventer, H. van. 1716. *The Art of Midwifery Improv'd:* London: E. Curll, J. Pemerton, and W. Taylor.
Douglas, J. [1736?]. *A Short Account of the State of Midwifery in London, Westminster, &c.* London.
Ferguson, J.E., II, Y.G. Newberry, G.A. DeAngleis, J.J. Finnerty, S. Agarwal, and E. Turkheimer. 1998. "The Fetal-Pelvic Index Has Minimal Utility in Predicting Fetal-Pelvic Disproportion." *American Journal of Obstetrics and Gynecology* 179 (5): 1186–92. http://dx.doi.org/10.1016/S0002-9378(98)70129-2.
Giffard, W. 1734. *Cases in Midwifery*. London: B. Motte, T. Wotten, L. Gilliver, and J. Nourse.
Hamilton, A. [1792?]. *Letters to Dr. William Osborn ... on Certain Doctrines Contained in His Essays on the Practice of Midwifery.* Edinburgh: printed for Peter Hill and J. Murray London.
Hamilton, J. 1796. *A Collection of Engravings, Designed to Facilitate the Study of Midwifery*. London: G.G. & J. Robinson.
Hibbard, B. 2000. *The Obstetrician's Armamentarium: Historical Obstetrical Instruments and Their Inventors*. San Anselmo, CA: Norman Publishing.

Hull, J. 1798. *A Defence of the Cesarean Operation, with Observations on Embryulcia, and the Section of the Symphysis Pubis*. Manchester: R. and W. Dean.
Hull, J. 1799. *Observations on Mr. Simmons's Detection, &C. &C.: With a Defence of the Cesarean Operation*. Manchester: R. and W. Dean.
Kerr, J.M. Munro, R.W. Johnstone, and M.H. Phillips, eds. 1954. *Historical Review of British Obstetrics and Gynaecology: 1800–1950*. Edinburgh and London: E. & S. Livingstone.
Lieske, P. 2011. "'Made in Imitation of Real Women and Children': Obstetrical Machines in Eighteenth-Century Britain." In *The Female Body in Medicine and Literature*, edited by Andrew Mangham and Greta Depledge, 69–88. Liverpool: Liverpool University Press.
Medical and Physical Journal. 1799. "A Further Statement of the Case of Elizabeth Thompson" with James Ogden's Letter to the Editors of the Journal. 1:473–9.
Mengert, W.F., and M.V. Korkmas. 1957. "3772 Labors Following Radiographic Mensuration." *American Journal of Obstetrics and Gynecology* 74 (1): 151–8.
Mitchell, P.D., C. Boston, A.T. Chamberlain, S. Chaplin, V. Chauhan, J. Evans, L. Fowler, N. Powers, D. Walker, H. Webb, et al. 2011. "The Study of Anatomy in England from 1700 to the Early 20th Century." *Journal of Anatomy* 219 (2): 91–9. http://dx.doi.org/10.1111/j.1469-7580.2011.01381.x.
Morgan, M.S., G.R. Thurnau, and J.I. Fishburne, Jr. 1986. "The Fetal-Pelvic Index as an Indicator of Felt-Pelvic Disproportion: A Preliminary Report." *American Journal of Obstetrics and Gynecology* 155 (3): 608–13. http://dx.doi.org/10.1016/0002-9378(86)90288-7.
Moscucci, O. (2004) 2007. "Denman, Thomas (1733–1815)." *Oxford Dictionary of National Biography*, edited by H.C.G. Matthew and Brian Harrison. Oxford: Oxford University Press, 2004. Online ed. L. Goldman (accessed 31 Dec. 2012).
Nihell, E. 1760. *A Treatise on the Art of Midwifery*. London: A. Morley.
Osborn, W. 1783. *An Essay on Laborious Parturition: in which the Division of Symphysis Pubis is Particularly Considered*. London: T. Cadell.
Ould, F. 1742. *A Treatise of Midwifery in Three Parts*. Dublin: Oli. Nelson and Charles Connor.
Paterson, S. 1770. *A Catalogue of the Entire and Inestimable Apparatus for Lectures in Midwifery ... by the Late Ingenious Dr. William Smellie, Deceased*. London.
Pole, T. 1797. *A Syllabus of a Course of Lectures on the Theory and Practice of Midwifery*. London: Stephen Couchman.

Sharp, Jane. 1671. *The Midwives Book, or, The Whole Art of Midwifery Discovered, Directing Childbearing Women How to Behave Themselves in their Conception, Bearing, and Nursing of Children*. London: Simon Miller.

Shingleton, H. 2005. "A Famous Triple Obstetrical Tragedy." *American Congress of Obstetricians and Gynecologists Clinical Review* 10 (4):14–16.

Sigault, J.R. 1778. *Discours sur les advantages de la section de la simphyse*. Paris: Quillau.

Simmons, W. 1798. *Reflections on the Propriety of Performing the Cæsarean Operation*. [Manchester]: R. and W. Dean.

Simmons, W. 1799. "It was my Original Intention." In *Discussing the Subject, Not to Advert to Any Particular Instance of the Caesarian Operation*, 1–4. Manchester: Sowler & Russell Deansgate.

Simmons, W. [1799?]. *A Detection of the Fallacy of Dr. Hull's Defence of the Cesarean Operation*. Manchester: Sowler and Russell.

Smellie, W. 1754. *A Sett of Anatomical Tables with Explanations and An Abridgement of the Practice of Midwifery*. London.

Smellie, W. 1762. *A Treatise on the Theory and Practice of Midwifery*. 4th ed., corrected. Vol. I. London: D. Wilson and T. Durham.

Stephen, M. 1795. *Domestic Midwife, or, The Best Means of Preventing Danger in Child-Birth Considered*. London: S.W. Fores.

Stone, S. 1737. *A Complete Practice of Midwifery. Consisting of Upwards of Forty Cases or Observations in that Valuable Art*. London: T. Cooper.

Tomlinson, G. 1799. *A Letter to Mr. Ogden … Pointing out Some of the Misrepresentations of Himself and His Coadjutor, Mr. Simmons, Relative to the Case of Elizabeth Thompson*. Manchester: W. Shelmerdine and Co.

Watts, G. 1755. *Reflection on Slow and Painful Labours and Other Subjects in Midwifery*. London: G. Keith.

White, C., R. Hall, G. Tomlinson, and J. Thorp. 1799. *A Further Statement of the Case of Elizabeth Thompson*. Manchester: Wm. Shelmerdine.

Willughby, P. 1863. *Observations in Midwifery: as also The Country Midwifes opusculum or vade mecum … Edited from the Original MS by Henry Blenkinsop*. Warwick: H.T. Cooke and Son.

Wilson, A. 1995. *The Making of Man-Midwifery: Childbirth in England, 1660–1770*. Cambridge, MA: Harvard University Press.

Wood, W. 1799. "Case of Cæsarean Section." In *Memoirs of the Medical Society of London, Instituted in the year 1773*. 5: 463–76, final engraving, n.p. London: J. Johnson.

15 The Debris of Life: Diseased Ovaries in Eighteenth-Century Medicine

SALLY FRAMPTON

Towards the end of the seventeenth century the "testicles" of females, previously little distinguished from their male counterpart, began to be understood in a fundamentally different way. The middle of the century had seen William Harvey (1578–1657) assert his doctrine of *ex ovo omnia* – everything from an egg – and in the 1660s and 1670s Regnier de Graaf (1641–73), Niels Stensen (1638–86), and Jan Swammerdam (1637–80), among others, began to affirm experimentally that the female testes were egg producing organs. As a consequence, the more congruous terms "ovary" and "ovarium" were seen fit to describe them (de Graaf 1672/1972, 135). This shift from testicle to ovary formed a more secure ground for theories of ovist preformation, which in characterizing the egg (or ovum) as the container of all future pre-formed life, put the ovary at the centre of procreation (Pinto-Correia 1997, 42–4). Yet it did nothing to quell either the rise of spermist preformation, which shone briefly but powerfully during the early part of the eighteenth century, or the concept of epigenesis, which had begun to dominate understandings of generation once more by the end of the century. In fact understanding the ovary as the seat of egg production converged almost as easily with epigenetic theories as it did with ovism. The ovary may have continued to be a locus of research into generation, but its "discovery" neither resolved the question of how life was created, nor fully explained how the organ functioned.

Indeed throughout the eighteenth century much about the ovary remained mysterious; Matthew Baillie (1761–1823), Britain's foremost morbid anatomist and nephew of the Hunter brothers, described it in 1789 as "a part of the animal oeconomy which seems to have been hitherto involved in a considerable degree of obscurity" (Baillie and Hunter 1789, 2). Elaboration as to how and why this was so is markedly lacking in historical accounts of medicine and science in the eighteenth century. In part this is because scholarly work has focused on the organ almost wholly in terms of the investigations into generation that were occurring, such as in Clara Pinto-Correia's monograph *The Ovary of Eve* (1997). Yet there were other ways in which the ovary was perceived as a subject of inquiry, especially if, like Baillie, one was not only an anatomist of some repute but a practising physician too. The "obscurity" he referred to reflected not only a regard of the organ's physiology but also its diseases.

It is the significance ascribed to ovarian pathology in eighteenth-century medicine that I wish to stress in this chapter. The dramatic and controversial rise of gynaecological surgery in the nineteenth century has acted as a byway for historians to examine ideas of ovarian disease during that period (Moscucci 1993). The reasons for doing so have perhaps been less obvious in relation to the eighteenth century. Yet the diseased ovary was an object of intrigue at this time, through which questions regarding the generative powers of women overlapped with the commonplace experiences of medical practitioners. Drawing predominantly on British and French sources, this chapter first examines how diseased ovaries were broadly understood within Enlightenment medicine and their prominent role in pathological discussions. It then goes on to consider the specific ways ovarian pathology interwove with understandings of generation. The first was the not infrequently recorded cases where ovaries affected by dropsy swelled to such a size that a visual imitation of pregnancy was produced, engendering confusion in both practitioners and patients as to whether the growth within was caused by a fetus or disease. The apparent power of ovaries to grow enormously prevented an easy distinction being made between the physiology and pathology of the organ and raised questions about what should be considered normal growth inside the female body. This is further played out in the final part of the chapter where I turn to enlarged ovaries that, upon dissection, were found to contain tissues supposedly foreign to the organ, such as teeth, hair, and bone. These remarkably transformed ovaries seemed to hover somewhere between a firm identity of organ, diseased swelling, or fetus, and practitioners pondered whether the contents of these monstrous growths represented some form of embryonic development – the debris of a life that had ended before it began – or something altogether different. The location of diseased ovaries at boundaries of this kind makes them ideal for historical examination. Through them we gain new insights into how generation, monstrosity, and the uneasy bifurcation of normal and pathological growth were perceived in the eighteenth century. We can also observe the crystallization of familiar characteristics of the ovary that resonate today.

"Her Appearance Was Truly Deplorable": Locating Diseased Ovaries in Enlightenment Medicine

Andrew Cunningham has characterized the long eighteenth century as a time when "the generation of humans – or certain aspects of it – became more important for the medical or surgical practitioner than ever before" (2010, 170). Certainly, as he suggests, the encroachment of male medical practitioners upon the realm of childbirth gave added impetus to anatomical investigations into the female reproductive system. Most famously this was borne out in the works of William Smellie (1697–1763) and William Hunter (1718–83), both of whom made their names and fortunes as man-midwives. Hunter's *Anatomia Uteri Humani Gravidi Tabulis Illustrata* (1774) in particular, provided novel knowledge about embryonic development (Cunningham 2010, 182; "The Anatomy" 1774, 412). However, obstetrical texts were not usually written with an eye to explicitly supporting one theory of generation or another. As Carin Berkowitz has argued, knowledge in Enlightenment anatomy was "produced and disseminated in a pedagogical setting" (360), and certainly prominent man-midwives like Smellie were primarily concerned with producing pedagogical texts and atlases for fellow man-midwives (Jordanova 1985, 399). As such, it was childbirth and its complications that tended to be their focus.

At first glance the ovary, with its more ambiguous role in relation to childbirth, is harder to locate in this discourse. By the early decades of the century, it was generally understood that the egg played a key role in generation, and by the later decades the Edinburgh anatomist John Aitken (1747–1822) was advising that the ovaries be considered "the only organs, on the part of the female, which are truly seminal and genital" (1784, 27). But notions of how exactly the ovary functioned in relation to pregnancy remained decidedly vague; "how the Ovum is impregnated, how it breaks through the Integuments of the Ovaria, and how it gets into the Womb, is not yet sufficiently demonstrated," wrote the physician John Burton (1710–71) (1751, 35). The female generative process as a whole remained abstruse, but the ovaries were more inscrutable than the womb, the latter continuing to dominate vernacular as well as medical understandings of women's bodies, and its diseases a common site of medical intervention (Wagner 2011, 542).

The ovary, unlike the womb, was largely absent from traditional constructions of female pathology. Buried deep within the peritoneum, the organ was quite literally inaccessible, and the slow, painless progression thought to characterize ovarian disease in its early stages made it difficult to diagnose until it was advanced. Because of this, most medical authors took a rather pessimistic view as to what could be done to treat diseased ovaries; some pondered whether it was even necessary for practitioners to fully comprehend the nature of the organ when they could do so little for it. When the physician Henry Manning (dates unknown) published his extensive *Treatise on the Diseases of Women* in 1771, he claimed to do so because female diseases had been neglected by other medical authors (Manning 1771, iii–iv). Yet Manning devoted little more than a page to discussing the diseases of the ovaries, stating that "it is generally extremely difficult to ascertain when these parts are particularly affected; and the diseases to which they are liable, inflammation only excepted, are always so obscure in their origin, that they are seldom or never perceptible, even to the patient herself, till they have made considerable progress" (307–8). This may go some way in explaining why vernacular medical manuals often eschewed discussing ovarian disease altogether. John Ball's (1704? – 1779) *The Female Physician: Or, Every Woman Her Own Doctress* (1770), for example, aimed towards women as well as young practitioners, gave no mention to the ovaries at all (iv).

Despite this most practitioners were cognisant that ovarian disease did often occur and some elected to address the matter in more detail. The young surgeon and anatomist Charles Bell (1774–1842), writing at the end of the century when he was assisting his brother John (1763–1820) in the teaching of anatomy in Edinburgh, appeared, like Manning, relatively unconcerned with promulgating novel knowledge about the ovary. However Bell, no doubt influenced by his brother, who insisted upon the relevance of anatomical teaching to the everyday practice of surgery (Gordon-Taylor and Walls 1958, 9), believed there was one condition practitioners were likely to encounter in their work and to which they needed to be alert: "Of all the parts of the female pelvis," he wrote "the ovaries are most frequently diseased; though, in reference to practice, the knowledge of them is unimportant, if we except that of dropsy, so frequently occurring" (Bell 1798, 89). "Dropsy" was the term used to describe most kinds of swelling of water, serum, or air found throughout the body. Dropsical tumours were considered common, the bread-and-butter of medical practitioners, and what the historian Charles Rosenberg has described as a "familiar yet frightening clinical phenomenon" (1992, 3). Yet dropsy also harboured distinctly extraordinary qualities. Its chief effect, the gradual augmentation of one or sometimes multiple body parts, meant that in advanced cases its unchecked growth caused a vast swelling of the sufferer's body. Extreme cases saw what amounted to a parasitical destruction of their insides as organs became entirely transformed into dropsical swellings. Some people appeared to be more predisposed to the disease than others, none more so than women whose wateriness seemed to make them more prone (Monro 1756, 14). But dropsy could seemingly attack any part of the body and indeed anybody. Gender was just one possible factor in a condition that was far reaching in society: age, class, and lifestyle were all at some time or another pinpointed in its causation.

Humoral imbalances, however, were generally understood as the root of all forms of dropsy and as such the disease was usually approached holistically. William Withering's *An Account of the Foxglove and Some of Its Medical Uses* (1785), the most notable work to be produced on dropsy in the eighteenth century, relied heavily upon this framework, as most accounts of dropsy did. In it Withering (1741–99) publicized his successful experimentation with the diuretic effect of *Digitalis* which, he argued, effectively cured many forms of the disease. But his work also demonstrated that some forms of dropsy, notably that of the ovary, did not respond to its effects. Structural peculiarities were held responsible; dissections of dropsical ovaries showed that the disease almost always presented in an encysted form, where the ovary transformed into a multitude of small fluid-filled sacs. This made it almost impossible to treat the disease by the usual means of medical compounds to re-integrate the fluid into the bodily circulation; "the ovarium dropsy defies the power of medicine," Withering starkly concluded (1785, 203). This led to a common perception among practitioners that "there is no species of Dropsy worse than that of the ovaries in women" (Mead 1751, 142).

The difficulties in treating the disease meant that dropsical ovaries often grew to a huge size, permitting the condition to be conceived of, and described as, monstrous. The ovary, it seemed, had a peculiar disposition towards distension caused by its lymphatic and spongy composition that made it "calculated for allowing the stagnation of fluids" (Hamilton 1792, 127). Unlike dropsy of the womb, which was thought to reach its maximum volume at around six or seven months before beginning to diminish, there was no timescale for dropsy of the ovary. In most cases it simply continued to slowly grow until it killed the patient (Lumsdaine 1792–3, 67). This prospect gave the disease an unnerving quality. The abnormal size of anything, not least the human body, was not just something around which ideas of monstrosity could be constructed; it was a fundamental way in which the monstrous was defined. In a meeting of the Royal Society in the summer of 1784, John Hunter (1728–93) communicated a report from Philip Meadows Martineau (1752–1829), a young surgeon from Norwich, recounting Martineau's interactions with a local pauper woman named Sarah Kippus who had recently died. For the last twenty-five years of her life Kippus had laboured under a dropsical swelling of the abdomen from which, over that time, an extraordinary 6631 pints of watery fluid had been withdrawn by paracentesis, (or "tapping" as it was more commonly known), whereby a trocar was inserted into the abdomen to draw off the fluid. When Martineau first met her just three years before her death he was horrified by what he saw; Kippus's belly had grown so huge that her face was now almost wholly obscured and her appearance was "truly deplorable, not to say shocking" (Martineau and Hunter 1784a, 1). Upon her death, the woman's dissected body proved to be almost as unwieldy as it had been in life, with Martineau forced to draw off some seventy-eight pints of fluid before he could reach the abdominal cavity. Only then was he able to locate the source of the swelling to the left ovary, which had converted into two large sacs engulfing almost the entire abdomen. This extraordinary case was a prime example of how a dropsical swelling could develop in the ovary and grow to such a size that it then destroyed the organ it emerged from. Because of this, practitioners often struggled to find the right language to describe such cases, at times using "ovary" interchangeably with "tumour" to communicate the curious transformation taking place (Yonge and Sloane 1706, 2390).

The changes that diseased ovaries underwent were a productive example of the type of morbid anatomy Matthew Baillie wished to integrate more fully into British medicine. Baillie was vocal about the need for anatomists to identify those diseases where "alterations in the structure take place" (1793, i). The chance to do so was not lost on Martineau, who accompanied the Kippus case with an ontologically complex hypothesis about the interrelationship between pathological swellings and the bodies in which they occurred. The case, Martineau believed, was an intriguing example of "the provision which is made in every animal for the preservation of life" (Martineau and Hunter 1784a, 6). This preservation instinct, he argued, meant that the body's structure adapted to accommodate disease. He noted that around the dropsical ovary found in Kippus's body, the peritoneum had prodigiously thickened and even ossified in some places, forming a protective layer. This went some way towards explaining how her belly had continued to grow exponentially. Martineau marvelled at this process, describing it as "not less wonderfull than beautifull" (Martineau and Hunter 1784a, 7). Interestingly, though, these particular observations were omitted from the version of his account published in the *Philosophical Transactions*, suggesting that either John Hunter or perhaps more likely, the powers that be at the Royal Society, were less taken by his theory (Martineau and Hunter 1784b, 471–6).

The chronic nature of ovarian dropsy problematized the boundaries between physiology and pathology. But so too did the frequency with which the condition occurred. This made it difficult to establish what exactly should be considered a normal ovary: "the change of condition, which these disorders produce in the *ovaria,* has often deceived anatomists; and made them mistake the true structure of these parts," the French physician Jean Astruc (1684–1766) noted (1767, 14). Indeed, it seemed there was a decided changeability to the structure of the ovary – even in its healthy state – which made it vulnerable to disease. Thomas Denman (1733–1815), England's leading man-midwife in the last decades of the eighteenth century, speculated that the organ's vesicular structure might explain the prevalence of dropsy, with the cyclical formation of small liquid-filled capsules within the organ possibly giving it an innate disposition to the disorder (Denman 1794, 125). Charles Bell also drew attention to the alterations the ovary underwent, particularly as women aged, when their ovaries were subject to a number of changes, becoming increasingly solid, enlarging with fluid or shrinking. However Bell, like others, seemed to come into difficulties when defining the pathological ovary; "Their changes can scarcely be considered as disease," he opined, before going on to describe them as just that (1798, 89). Whatever the case, the frequency with which ovaries altered in structure suggested that the preternatural was in some sense natural to the organ.

"I Find Myself As Full As At The Nine Months": Mistaking Dropsical Ovaries for Pregnancy.

As Lisa W. Smith has highlighted, for eighteenth-century practitioners signs of pregnancy, particularly in the first few months, were ambiguous (Smith 2010, 72); confusion as to whether a woman was pregnant or suffering from disease occurred frequently. Because of its appearance, ovarian dropsy was the condition most likely to be confused with pregnancy. This brought with it a number of problems. Practically, it meant that the grim possibility of a surgeon erroneously performing paracentesis on a pregnant woman always loomed; socially, it led younger, unmarried women to a place of considerable vulnerability in which the spectre of illegitimacy was raised by their swollen bellies. The Plymouth surgeon James Yonge (1647–1721) recounted such a case, a thirty-year-old woman from Deal, in a letter to Sir Hans Sloane (1660–1753) in 1706. Sloane reported to the Royal Society:

> Ad 1696: A Virgin of thirty fell into a periodical fever and afterward a total suppression of her *Menstrua*; which soon followed with a pain and tumour on the right side of her belly, which grew and increased ... till it became bigger and harder than that of a woman in her last month. When it had grown a full year, it began to soften, and then the censorious people who suspected her thought her in a dropsie. (Yonge and Sloane 1706, 2389)

Judgment then was dependent on a number of actors and not only the medical practitioners, although they remained authoritative in deciding whether pregnancy had occurred or not. Others also observed and interpreted the swollen bellies before them. In the Deal case, only as the woman's belly continued to grow beyond the usual nine months did dropsy become accepted by the local community as a more likely scenario than an illegitimate pregnancy. There were the women's own beliefs too: often cases of ovarian dropsy continued to grow unchecked by medical attention because the woman involved not only assumed pregnancy from the visible changes occurring to her body but also because she *sensed* the quickening of her unborn child (Morgagni 1769, 535). In situations like this where pregnancy was just one possible cause of bodily change, a woman's sensibilities could often be valued as a part of the interpretive process (McClive 2002, 227).

This tangling of disease, pregnancy, and promiscuity was exemplified in a case brought to the attention of French practitioners by physician Désiré-Auguste Chifoliau (c. 1757–1810) in 1781. During the mid-decades of the eighteenth century, France led the way in surgery and obstetrics, and the thriving correspondence cultures of organizations like l'Académie Royale de Chirurgie (est. 1731) and la Société Royale de Médecine (est. 1778) – the archives of which have no real equivalent in Britain – reveal in detail dozens of cases of ovarian disease that were discussed among French practitioners. Chifoliau's case involved a young woman of twenty-two who, according to the physician, "loved a young man desperately" and who had been devastated when he died. Upon learning of his demise the woman had fallen into a "black melancholy," an allusion to the classical idea of lovesickness as a humoral affliction, associated particularly with an excess of black bile (Dawson 2008, 20). Soon after, a noticeable augmentation of her abdomen had begun to show itself "in a way that gave rise to suspicions of pregnancy" before she eventually died (Chifoliau 1781, 1). The patient's situation, young and affianced, was precarious in light of her swollen belly and Chifoliau's pronouncement of dropsy of the ovary after examining her body was crucial in extinguishing suspicions of pregnancy among her family. Strikingly, the way Chifoliau presented the case intimated a connection between the patient's heartache and her ovary's imitation of pregnancy, in which a monstrous growth had formed instead of the true conception that might have occurred upon her intended marriage. This fitted with contemporary ideas that the emotions were connected to the parts of generation, in particular the continued belief that uterine disorders were the cause of hysteria (Churchill 2012, 201). However, the ovary was also beginning to be incorporated into this schema. Jean Astruc singled out the peculiar effect of the "passions of love" on the ovary, which could be exacerbated if coupled with "fear, shame and surprize," and which led Astruc to conclude that such ovarian afflictions were more common in young unmarried women and widows (1762, 233). This drew upon the popular notion that the women most subject to hysteria were those whose sexual passions were in some way disappointed or unfulfilled (Ball 1770, 15). But significantly Astruc repositioned the disorder to the ovary and by doing so made the ovary rather than the womb the troubled seat of unfulfilled sexual potential.

While these blurred boundaries between ovarian dropsy and pregnancy could render individual cases less than clear, practitioners at times utilized the links between the two to convey understandings of the former. Most obviously this was done by deploying the stages of pregnancy as a means of illustrating the way dropsy looked; those with advanced cases of the disease were often described as having an abdomen the size of that in the eighth or ninth month of pregnancy. This partly reflected the ambiguities between the two conditions that practitioners initially met with, and where pregnancy was often the more likely scenario. But in lieu of a better description, the analogy remained useful even when ovarian dropsy had been more definitively identified. The two conditions were further intertwined by prevailing beliefs that pregnancy could play a role in turning ovaries dropsical; difficult labours especially, were often attributed as a cause (Denman 1794, 125; Smellie 1764, 154). When pregnancy and dropsy did occur at close intervals, the result could be an unpredictable body. A rare patient account, probably sent to William Hunter in the mid- to late decades of the century, recorded the plight of an unnamed but well-educated young woman who described both the physical and emotional toll of labouring under dropsy, probably ovarian, as well as multiple pregnancies. From soon after her marriage both had occurred frequently and often concurrently. By the time she wrote the account of her illness, the woman suspected herself to be both on her third pregnancy as well as highly dropsical, her body almost overcome by the twin growths – one fetal, one its monstrous mirror – within her. She found herself "as full as at the nine months, tho not six months gone, which makes me almost helpless" ("A Dropseycall Case" nd). Her words suggested the disturbing possibility of a boundless, ever expanding pregnancy, a body beyond the control of both medicine and nature. Like the fat bodies described in Sarah Toulalan's chapter in this collection, the dropsical body was disruptive to normality. Significantly this was also a female body, still culturally imbued with the power to make monsters through maternal impression (Wilson 2002, 5; Daston and Park 2001, 330). If uncontrollable dropsies defied bodily order, they did so all the more when they sprang from the ovary. The discovery of the ovary's egg-producing function gave the ovary meaning as just that: the organ that *produced* the seed of life, in contrast to the womb, the role of which was to act as the *vessel* in which the embryo grew, expanding as it expanded. Growth of any sort in the ovary could only ever be a distorted copy of what was expected to occur in the womb.

Imitation or Imperfect Generation? Ovaries Containing Hair, Teeth, and Bone

There was one form of ovarian disease which proved to be particularly puzzling and where the experiences of medical practitioners clashed directly with contemporary questions on the nature of generation. These were enlarged ovaries which upon dissection of a woman's body were found to contain a variety of tissues supposedly foreign to the organ, such as hair, teeth, and bone. This disease – at times described as a form of dropsy, at others as an entirely different condition – was relatively uncommon. Nonetheless the bizarre nature of these tumours meant that specimens were frequently to be found in anatomical collections (Denman 1794, 133), while textual and visual descriptions of them abounded in the medical literature. When in 1771 the surgeon Benjamin Gooch (1708–76) discovered such an entity upon dissection of a pregnant patient who had died from the disease, his description of the jumble of tissues he was confronted with relied on a rich mixture of language that evoked animal, human, and non-organic qualities. The tunica of the ovary was likened to a "thick leather bag" within which was "a lump the bigness of a turkey's egg, in substance like hog's lard." At the bottom of the ovary were found "two distinct irregular bones," with a number of teeth fixed to them. Most bizarrely of all, mixed in with this was a large quantity of hair which "twisted and curled in a wonderful manner, some of which exceeded a foot in length, and had evidently bulbous roots" (Gooch 1773, 113–15). Gooch provided an illustrated plate of the ovary, believing that the image could "give more adequate ideas of it than cou'd be verbally conveyed" (1773, xxi) (figure 15.1).

Such ovaries were usually detected only upon dissection, as most did not give rise to symptoms that differed greatly from those of the more familiar type of ovarian dropsy. This distanced the condition from concerns of curing towards questions of where in the scale of generation – if at all – these tumours belonged. Like the fleshy tumours known as "moles" that formed in the womb – described in *The Whole of Aristotle's Compleat Master-piece* as "an inarticulate piece of flesh without any form; and therefore differs from monsters, which are both formata and articulata" – the dropsical ovary was monstrous but not a monster (83). Unlike moles, however, which were more usually assumed to be the product of sexual intercourse, the question of whether these matter-filled ovaries were a form of embryonic development was a source of contention. The seventeenth-century anatomist Edward Tyson (1651–1708) believed them to be the remains of an embryo which had been unable to form properly. For Tyson this meant the entities lay somewhere between the animal and vegetable kingdoms, too garbled to be considered truly human and better understood as something closer to a vegetative life, created in lieu of a true fetus (Birch and Tyson 1683, 284). Not dissimilar was a theory espoused by Astruc during the middle of the eighteenth century that further aligned pathological change to generation. Astruc believed the entities to be putrefying embryos which had erroneously embedded themselves and then died in the ovary. Contrary to Tyson then, Astruc's theory allowed for the spark of animal life to have once existed before death occurred, after which there took place a reversal of the natural generation process, where the embryo degenerated into a tumour (Astruc 1767, 60–2).

Both views took as their starting point that the disease was in some way related to conception, an idea that was pervasive throughout the eighteenth century. Yet neither was persuasive enough to prevent competing theories emerging. James Yonge was one early voice to express dissatisfaction with such explanations; the case involving the thirty-year-old woman from Deal, described above, was one where the ovary had been found to contain teeth, hair, and bone. Here the "very nice and strict scrutiny of jealous eyes" among the local community, which had judged the woman a virgin, proved useful to his premise that the formation of these human parts did not rely on sexual intercourse; thus natural philosophers could turn neither to preformationist nor epigenetic theories of generation for answers (Yonge and Sloane 1706, 2391). Even ovist preformation, which

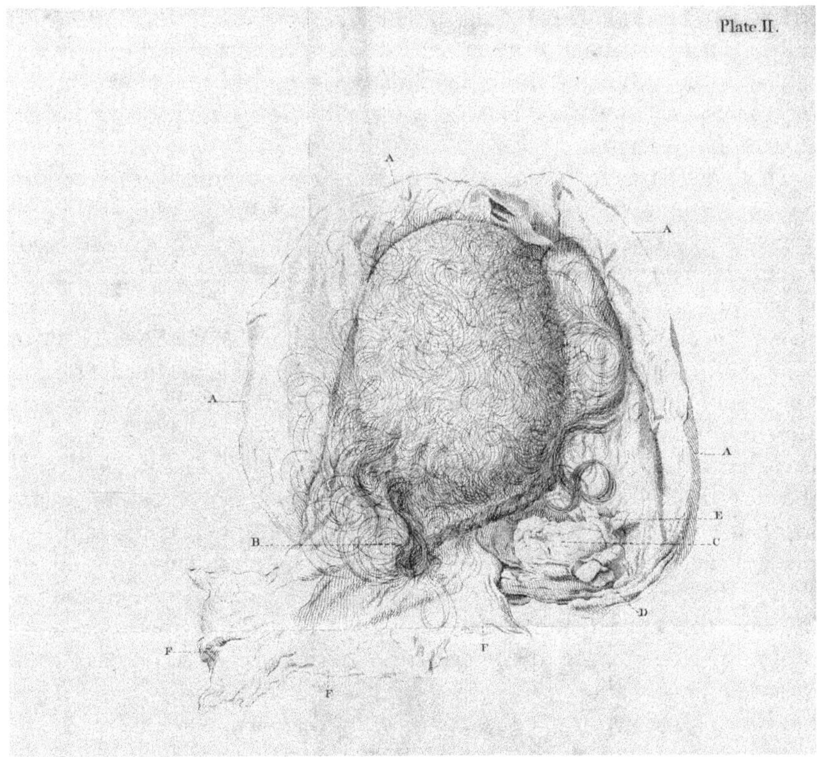

Figure 15.1 Illustration of a dropsical ovary "of which were contained many extraordinary appearances." From a case in B. Gooch's *Medical and Chirurgical Observations as an Appendix to a Former Publication* (London and Norwich: G. Robinson and R. Beatniffe, 1773), table III. The dissected ovary was found to contain bone, vast quantities of hair as well as a number of teeth (labelled in the image D and E). Courtesy of Wellcome Library, London.

allowed for the structure of a fetus to already be formed in an egg before sexual connection, could not explain these tumours, for while often containing perfect parts, as a whole they formed a disordered and chaotic mess which contradicted the pre-ordained perfection supposed by preformation. Furthermore the theory might be able to account for the structure of these masses without the male influence, but it could not account for their expansion without semen, which ovists believed provided the spark that activated fetal growth. Other theories came and went too. One surgeon conjectured that the tooth he had discovered in the ovary of his deceased patient could not possibly have been formed within the organ and instead speculated that it had been swallowed while the tumour was growing, piercing the ovary and amalgamating with the diseased mass (Cheston 1766, 47).

That these strange masses defied prevailing philosophies of generation did not go unnoticed by medical men, some of whom crowed at the powerlessness of established theories to explain what was truly a *medical* conundrum. Yonge chastised those who simply classified such growths as monstrous *Lusus Naturae* rather than explaining them, warning that such an approach was increasingly antiquated (Yonge and Sloane 1706, 2391). In 1787 the Irish physician James Cleghorn (c. 1764–c. 1826) issued a similar judgment in a paper communicated to the Royal Irish Academy. Cleghorn, who had become intrigued by these monstrous ovaries, openly scorned the French natural philosopher Comte de Buffon (1707–88) for his rejection of the idea that a fetus could exist in the ovary or even that teeth, bones, and hair had ever been found in the ovary. For Cleghorn this was characteristic of the general disregard theorists had for facts: "Monsieur le Comte de Buffon, finding it difficult to account for the formation of a foetus in the ovarium, like a true theorist, seems to reject the fact altogether ... thinking it of more consequence to establish his own theory than to propagate the knowledge of truth" (1787, 74–5). Even the eminent Buffon, Cleghorn implied, was fazed by the material reality of morbid anatomy.

In 1789 there appeared in the *Philosophical Transactions of the Royal Society* a paper by Matthew Baillie which provided the most sophisticated and most public challenge yet to the idea that these tumours were formed from conception. The body of a girl aged around twelve or thirteen had been brought to Baillie for dissection. Upon opening the girl's right ovary he had been startled to find a mass of hair and bones. Having always accepted the dominant view that conception was the cause of this condition, Baillie nonetheless asserted that the girl's age, intact hymen, and underdeveloped womb suggested otherwise (Baillie 1789, 6–7). His rather fortunate position as the nephew of John and William Hunter not only gave his account good standing but also the opportunity to connect it with one of John Hunter's cases where a tumour filled with similar matter had been extracted from underneath an eyebrow (Baillie 1789, 8). Baillie thus provided what seemed to be clear evidence that tissue growth could occur without sexual activity.

This assertion was not in itself controversial – after all Baillie was not the first to venture such a theory. But the young anatomist built on the idea to cautiously stretch the concept of generation beyond the connection of male and female, suggesting that ovaries had "some power within themselves of taking on a process which is imitative of generation, without any previous connection with a male" (1789, 4). Baillie resisted describing the resulting masses as genuine forms of generation, instead depicting them as the product of a process highly emulous of generation, an action in the ovary sympathetic to the true reproduction that occurred in the womb. Nonetheless by doing so he appeared to raise the puzzling prospect of self-generation within the female body. This displeased some contemporaries, who recoiled from ascribing the ovaries such power. Andrew Duncan's influential *Medical Commentaries* welcomed the publication of Baillie's findings, declaring the author "ingenious" and conceding that "there is no reason for supposing the generation of hair and teeth, in the fatty substance found in the ovarium ... was the effect of any connection with the male." But the journal would not endorse Baillie's analogy to generation, stating that "perhaps a conjecture, more simple than any supposed action of the ovarium itself, imitative of generation, maybe suggested with respect to their production" ("An Account" 1791, 280). The *Critical Review* was more unequivocal in its disdain for Baillie's argument. It had previously taken issue with what it saw as Baillie's use of anatomical curiosities to attempt "to say something new and ingenious" (*Philosophical Transactions* 67, 1789, 61) and it now took offence at his utilization of a monstrous ovary to speculate upon the nature of generation. While Baillie's words "may appear to be philosophical ... they are in reality, words without meaning," it warned (*Philosophical Transactions* 68, 1789, 418). This was quite the opposite of Yonge and Cleghorn's ruminations that empirical observations had been overlooked in investigations into monstrous ovaries. On the contrary, Baillie, who had substantially altered his view of the ovary based on the case, was being accused by the *Critical Review* of making a lackadaisical attempt at philosophizing which relied merely on observation of the abnormal. Thus the journal questioned not only the usefulness of this particular case in explaining generation, but of morbid anatomy as an epistemological system when applied to the philosophically loaded organs of generation.

A Pathologized Organ: The Ovary beyond the Eighteenth Century

In 1827 Karl Ernst von Baer (1792–1876) experimentally identified the mammalian ovum. Increasingly, it was also accepted that eggs existed in the ovary before conception, and gradually medical men began to perceive the ovary as having more importance than the womb in governing femininity. This was reinforced at the tail end of the century by new understandings of the organ's internal secretions, which appeared to exercise power over the female sexual characteristics (Sengoopta 2000). Squeezed between the re-conceptualizations of the organ's physiology in the seventeenth and nineteenth centuries, the eighteenth century may appear a somewhat less dramatic period in the history of the ovary. Yet it was during this time that the diseased ovary at least, was ascribed with characteristics that still resonate strongly today. Chaotic, deceptive, and at times astonishing, it generated monstrosity in the female reproductive system and defied both bodily order and medical control. In particular, the ability of the organ to stretch to an enormous capacity and develop matter seemingly unnatural to it suggested striking powers of both growth and transformation which left medical men struggling to define what a normal ovary was. This perception of the ovaries in Enlightenment medicine speaks to broader motifs of deformity that have been examined by historians, not least the close alignment of monstrosity to femininity (Nussbaum 2000, 49–50). In general, though, diseased ovaries were not "monstrous" in the way the term is often understood in the context of eighteenth-century medicine. They were not quite in the realm of monstrous births, for example, nor did they particularly expose cultural attitudes towards the disabled. However, precisely because they tested the boundaries of pathology and of otherness, they were conceived of as worthwhile objects of inquiry.

The early to mid-decades of the nineteenth century saw radical and controversial developments in the treatment of ovarian disease, with the growing use of abdominal surgery to remove large tumours. The comparatively rapid progression of ovarian surgery at this time, compared to other types of abdominal surgery, has often been framed in relation to the rise of a "science of woman" during the nineteenth century, when understandings of women as defined by their reproductive and sexual organs began to more obviously manifest in medical and surgical practices (Moscucci 1993). But it can be attributed as much – if not more – to the practical difficulties long encountered by medical practitioners in treating ovarian disease.

Indeed, the treatment of ovarian tumours has remained distinctive in being problematic. Outcomes for ovarian cancer have tended to be poor in comparison to many other cancers because most malignant ovarian tumours are only diagnosed once the disease is advanced (Jasen 2009, 491; National Institute for Health and Care Excellence 2011, vii). Only very recently have survival rates begun noticeably to improve, probably due to increased recognition of what have long been considered the vague symptoms of early ovarian cancer (Kmietowicz 2012, e7861). Frequency and visibility also remain familiar characteristics. Ovarian cysts are today recognized as a common condition in women, and indeed the term "cyst" is sometimes used to describe the follicle in which the ovum is contained while it is developing (Grimes et al. 2011, 2). That a normal aspect of ovarian function is described in this way – in language interchangeable with that of disease – compels us to reflect upon the pathologization of the female reproductive system that continues today. Furthermore, the capacity of some ovarian tumours to grow to an enormous size if left untreated, as well as their occasional tendency to grow teeth, hair, and bone (a condition known today as a dermoid cyst or teratoma), continues to engender curiosity and disgust even if their causes are better understood: we have only to look at the lurid reports of giant ovarian tumours that crop up in the news from time to time to recognize their continued shock value (Springer 2007). Even the confusion between ovarian disease and pregnancy remains problematic. As recently as 2007 the magazine *Marie Claire* published an article entitled "They Told Me I Was Pregnant, But It Was Ovarian Cancer," which featured a number of young women who were initially told they were pregnant before later discovering that their abdominal growth was in fact the result of a cancerous ovarian tumour (Landau 2007). Ambiguities between the two conditions remain even with the powerful diagnostic technology of today.

Historians of medicine have tended to focus more on monsters than the monstrous and the differences between the two are rarely nuanced. Whereas the former relies on an understanding that life exists, or once existed, the monstrous can potentially be embodied in almost anything, extant or non-extant. In the eighteenth century dropsical ovaries were significant in troubling this boundary because their relation to life and to generation was unclear. Dropsy of the ovary, far from being a run-of-the mill disease category of easy understanding, stretched the medical imagination, forcing anatomists, philosophers, and practitioners to consider the changes it was possible for the ovary to undergo. By doing so they fundamentally shaped conceptions of what the ovary's role in the female body should be and – perhaps more significantly – what it should not be.

REFERENCES

Aitken, J. 1784. *Principles of Midwifery, or Puerperal Medicine*. Edinburgh: Edinburgh Lying-In Hospital.

"An Account of a Particular Change of Structure in the Human Ovarium by Matthew Baillie." 1791. *Medical Commentaries* 5:271–81.

"The Anatomy of the Human Gravid Uterus Exhibited in Figures by William Hunter." 1774. *The Critical Review, Or, Annals of Literature*. 38:408–12.

Astruc, J. 1762. *A Treatise on the Diseases of Women*. Vol. 2. London: J. Nourse.

Astruc, J. 1767. *A Treatise on the Diseases of Women*. Vol. 3. London: J. Nourse.

Baillie, M. 1793. *The Morbid Anatomy of Some of the Most Important Parts of the Human Body*. London: J. Johnson.

Baillie, M., and Hunter, J. 1789. *An Account of a Particular Change of Structure in the Human Ovarium from the Philosophical Transactions*. London.

Ball, J. 1770. *The Female Physician: or, Every Woman Her Own Doctress*. London: L. Davis.

Bell, C. 1798. *A System of Dissections, Explaining the Anatomy of the Human Body, the Manner of Displaying the Parts, and Their Varieties in Disease*. Edinburgh: Mundell and Son.

Berkowitz, C. 2013. "Systems of Display: The Making of Anatomical Knowledge in Enlightenment Britain." *British Journal for the History of Science* 46 (03): 359–87. http://dx.doi.org/10.1017/S0007087412000787.

Birch, S., and E. Tyson. 1683. "An Extract of Two Letters from Mr. Sampson Birch, an Alderman and Apothecary at Stafford, concerning an Extraordinary Birth in Staffordshire, with Reflections Thereon by Edw. Tyson M.D. Fellow of the Coll. Of Physitians, and of the R. Society." *Philosophical Transactions of the Royal Society* 13: 281–4. http://dx.doi.org/10.1098/rstl.1683.0039.

Burton, J. 1751. *An Essay Towards a Complete New System of Midwifry, Theoretical and Practical*. London: James Hodges.

Cheston, R.B. 1766. *Pathological Inquiries and Observations in Surgery, from the Dissections of Morbid Bodies. With an Appendix Containing Twelve Cases on Different Subjects*. Gloucester: R. Raikes.

Chifoliau, J.-G. 1781. Observation: dilation monstrueuse d'un ovaire compliqué d'anasargue. Mémoires, observations et correspondance médicale adressés à la SRM. SRM 190, d.1 n. 4. Paris: Académie Nationale de Médicine.

Churchill, W.D. 2012. *Female Patients in Early Modern Britain: Gender, Diagnosis, and Treatment*. Farnham: Ashgate.

Cleghorn, J. 1787. "The History of an Ovarium, Wherein Were Found Teeth, Hair and Bones. By James Cleghorn M.B. Communicated by Robert Perceval M.D." *Transactions of the Royal Irish Academy* 1:73–89.

Cunningham, A. 2010. *The Anatomist Anatomis'd: An Experimental Discipline in Enlightenment Europe*. Farnham: Ashgate.

Daston, L., and K. Park. 2001. *Wonders and the Order of Nature, 1150–1750*. New York: Zone Books.

Dawson, L. 2008. *Lovesickness and Gender in Early Modern English Literature*. Oxford: Oxford University Press. http://dx.doi.org/10.1093/acprof:oso/9780199266128.001.0001.

De Graaf, R. (1672) 1972. *Regnier de Graaf on the Human Reproductive Organs: An Annotated Translation of "Tractatus de Virorum Organis Generationi Inservientibus" (1668) and "De Mulierum Organis Generationi Inservientibus Tractatus Novus" (1672)*. Translated by H.D. Jocelyn and B.P. Setchell. Oxford: Blackwell Scientific Productions.

Denman, T. 1794. *An Introduction to the Practice of Midwifery*. Vol. 1. London: J. Johnson.

A Dropseycall Case: An Account of Her Condition, Including Treatment Prescribed by William Hunter. (nd) Papers of William Hunter. MS Hunter H8. University of Glasgow Special Collections, Glasgow.

Gooch, B. 1773. *Medical and Chirurgical Observations, as an Appendix to a Former Publication*. London and Norwich: G. Robinson and R. Beatniffe.

Gordon-Taylor, G., and E.W. Walls. 1958. *Sir Charles Bell: His Life and Times*. Edinburgh and London: E & S Livingstone Ltd.

Grimes, D.A., L.B. Jones, L.M. Lopez, and K.P. Schulz. 2011. "Oral Contraceptives for Functional Ovarian Cysts." *Cochrane Database of Systematic Reviews* 9:CD006134. http://onlinelibrary.wiley.com/doi/10.1002/14651858.CD006134.pub4/abstract. Accessed 4 December 2014.

Hamilton, A. 1792. *A Treatise on the Management of Female Complaints, and of Children in Early Infancy*. Edinburgh and London: Peter Hill and John Murray.

Hunter, W. 1774. *Anatomia Uteri Humani Gravidi Tabulis Illustrata. The Anatomy of the Human Gravid Uterus*. Birmingham: John Baskerville.

Jasen, P. 2009. "From the 'Silent Killer' to the 'Whispering Disease': Ovarian Cancer and the Uses of Metaphor." *Medical History* 53 (4): 489–512. http://dx.doi.org/10.1017/S0025727300000521.

Jordanova, L.J. 1985. "Gender, Generation and Science: William Hunter's Obstetrical Atlas." In *William Hunter and the Eighteenth-Century Medical World*, edited by W.F. Bynum and R. Porter, 385–412. Cambridge: Cambridge University Press.

Kmietowicz, Z. 2012. "Death Rate from Ovarian Cancer in England Has Fallen by a Fifth since 2001." *British Medical Journal* 345: e7861. http://dx.doi.org/10.1136/bmj.e7861.

Landau, M.D. 2007. They Told Me I was Pregnant, But It Was Ovarian Cancer. *Marie Claire*, 11 June. Accessed 4 December 2014. http://www.marieclaire.com/health-fitness/news/ovarian-cancer.

Lumsdaine, J. 1792–3. Notes on Lectures on Midwifery, given by Alexander Hamilton. Lumsdaine Papers. Vol. 1. MS 45919. British Library, London.

Manning, H. 1771. *A Treatise on Female Diseases*. London: R. Baldwin.
Martineau, P.M. and J. Hunter. 1784a. An Extraordinary Case of a Dropsy of the Ovarium, with Some Remarks. By Mr. Philip Meadows Martineau, Surgeon to the Norfolk and Norwich Hospital; Communicated by John Hunter, Esq. F.R.S. Journal Book Original. JBO/31. Royal Society, London.
Martineau, P.M., and J. Hunter. 1784b. "An Extraordinary Case of a Dropsy of the Ovarium, with Some Remarks. By Mr. Philip Meadows Martineau, Surgeon to the Norfolk and Norwich Hospital; Communicated by John Hunter, Esq. F.R.S." *Philosophical Transactions of the Royal Society* 74: 471–6. http://dx.doi.org/10.1098/rstl.1784.0040.
McClive, C. 2002. "The Hidden Truths of the Belly: The Uncertainties of Pregnancy in Early Modern Europe." *Social History of Medicine* 15 (2): 209–27. http://dx.doi.org/10.1093/shm/15.2.209.
Mead, R. 1751. *Medical Precepts and Cautions*. London: J. Brindley.
Monro, D. 1756. *An Essay on the Dropsy and Its Different Species*. London: D. Wilson & T. Durham.
Morgagni, G. 1769. *The Seats and Causes of Diseases Investigated by Anatomy*. Vol. 3. Translated by B. Alexander. London: A. Millar and T. Cadell, and Johnson and Payne.
Moscucci, O. 1993. *The Science of Woman: Gynaecology and Gender in England, 1800–1929*. Cambridge: Cambridge University Press.
National Institute for Health and Clinical Excellence. 2011. *Ovarian Cancer: The Recognition and Initial Management of Ovarian Cancer*. London: National Institute for Health and Clinical Excellence. https://www.nice.org.uk/guidance/cg122.
Nussbaum, F. 2000. "Dumb Virgins, Blind Ladies, and Eunuchs: Fictions of Defect." In *Defects: Engendering the Modern Body*, edited by H. Deutsch and F. Nussbaum, 31–53. Ann Arbor: University of Michigan Press.
Philosophical Transactions of the Royal Society of London 78 for the year 1788 Part II. 1789. *The Critical Review, Or, Annals of Literature* 67:56–64.
Philosophical Transactions of the Royal Society of London 79 for the year 1789 Part I.1789. *The Critical Review, Or, Annals of Literature* 68:413–20.
Pinto-Correia, C. 1997. *The Ovary of Eve: Egg and Sperm and Preformation*. Chicago: University of Chicago Press. http://dx.doi.org/10.7208/chicago/9780226669502.001.0001.
Rosenberg, C. 1992. "Preface to S.P. Peitzman: From Bright's Disease to End-Stage Renal Disease." In *Framing Disease: Studies in Cultural History*, edited by C. Rosenberg and J. Golden, 3–19. New Brunswick, NJ: Rutgers University Press.

Sengoopta, C. 2000. "The Modern Ovary: Constructions, Meanings, Uses." *History of Science* 38:425–88.

Smellie, W. 1764. *A Collection of Cases and Observations in Midwifery. By William Smellie, M.D. To Illustrate His Former Treatise, or First Volume, on That Subject*. Vol. 2. London: D. Wilson.

Smith, L.W. 2010. "Imagining Women's Fertility before Technology." *Journal of Medical Humanities* 31 (1): 69–79. http://dx.doi.org/10.1007/s10912-009-9097-1.

Springer, J. 2007. "Woman's 93-Pound Tumor Mystery." *Today*, 5 March. Accessed 12 December 2012. http://www.today.com/id/17464957/ns/today-today_health/t/womans--pound-tumor-mystery/#.VH-RCBB-QTB.

Wagner, D. 2011. "Visualisations of the Womb through Tropes, Dissection and Illustration (circa 1660–1774)." In *Book Illustration in the Long Eighteenth Century: Reconfiguring the Visual Periphery of the Text*, edited by Christina Ionescu, 541–72. Newcastle: Cambridge Scholars Publishing.

The Whole of Aristotle's Compleat Master-piece, in Three Parts: Displaying the Secrets of Nature in the Generation of Man. 1780. London.

Wilson, P.K. 2002. "Eighteenth-Century 'Monsters' and Nineteenth-Century 'Freaks': Reading the Maternally Marked Child." *Literature and Medicine* 21 (1): 1–25. http://dx.doi.org/10.1353/lm.2002.0014.

Withering, W. 1785. *An Account of the Foxglove and Some of Its Medical Uses: with Practical Remarks on Dropsy, and Other Diseases*. Birmingham: M. Swinney.

Yonge, J., and H. Sloane. 1706. "An Account of Balls of Hair Taken from the Uterus and Ovaria of Several Women; By Mr. James Yonge, F.R.S. Communicated to Dr. Hans Sloane, R.S. Secr." *Philosophical Transactions of the Royal Society* 25 (305–12): 2387–92. http://dx.doi.org/10.1098/rstl.1706.0040.

16 Intestinal Chaos: Tapeworms, Dead Flesh, and Reproduction during the Eighteenth Century

LIANNE McTAVISH

I photographed Jacques Fabien Gautier d'Agoty's anatomical painting while visiting the storage areas of the Musée des beaux-arts in Dijon. The curator explained that ten similar panels had entered the collections of the Académie des sciences, arts et belles-lettres de Dijon – of which the artist was a member – in 1774, offering compelling versions of the printed illustrations in his *Anatomie des parties de la génération de l'homme et de la femme* of 1773. The mezzotints produced by Gautier d'Agoty for anatomical atlases have received scholarly attention, and are typically discussed in terms of either the artist's collaborations with such anatomists as Joseph-Guichard Duverny and Antoine Mertrud, the aesthetic effects of the large colourful plates, or the contributions made by the images to advancements in knowledge about the human body (Lowengard 2006; Anderson, Barnes, and Shackleton 2011). The representations created for the publication dedicated to generation and pregnancy, including a printed version of the image of the uterus shown below, are further addressed within scholarly accounts of the history of childbirth, which is why the curator showed the painted panels to me. After writing a book on the visual culture of childbirth in seventeenth-century France, I was eager to learn more about eighteenth-century material (McTavish 2005). I eventually published work focusing on how a long-standing emphasis on the fleshly and mysterious womb was displaced by a medical concern with the potentially constraining bones of the pelvic region during the eighteenth century, when pregnancy was increasingly measured and mechanized, and generally described in obstetrical treatises as a set of normal and abnormal outcomes instead of a series of unique cases that defied standardization (McTavish 2010). Yet as I stood gazing at renditions of pregnant women and dissected fetuses in Dijon, my attention was drawn towards the meaty hollow entrails shown resting on top of and strangely inseparable from the uterus. What role, if any, did they play in early modern theories of reproduction?

This chapter was inspired by my attempts to answer that question, which quickly moved beyond straightforward considerations of maternal nutrition towards broader and frankly more challenging approaches to the generative body during the eighteenth century. To my surprise and slight disgust, following the trail of intestines in early modern sources ultimately led me to two different but not entirely unrelated subjects: intestinal worms and the preservation of corpses. Like other scholars of the early modern body, I had to overcome my initial reluctance in order to explore and begin to grasp this material. When historian Barbara Duden, for example, examined the eighteenth-century notebook of German physician Johann Storch, she struggled to understand his strange accounts of beneficially open sores and agreeable head lice (Duden 1991). Along similar lines, I had to set aside my assumption that tapeworms were always bothersome parasites that had invaded human bodies. Before and throughout the eighteenth century, such worms were mysteriously difficult to discern and classify. Attracting attention from philosophers, medical practitioners, and naturalists alike, intestinal worms were dissected, drawn, collected, and displayed in various formats. Multiple theories were proposed about the sources of their generation and growth, shedding further light on early modern understandings of fertility.

Anatomists developed various methods to preserve dead bodies and body parts during the eighteenth century, sometimes through drying flesh. These efforts were characterized as a battle to save bodies from such forces of decay as the worms that would otherwise devour them, starting with the vulnerable guts that were most liable to putrify first. Scholars who study the history of the body, researching the socially and culturally specific understandings of both flesh and the experience of it, have long regarded the corpse with particular interest. The printed and written representations of anatomical dissection are repeatedly addressed in the literature, alongside a more recent upsurge of attention to corpse medicine, which features the early modern reuse and consumption of dead body parts in medical practices, especially *mumia*, the medicinal corpse matter sometimes associated with dried Egyptian mummies (Sawday 1995; Park 2006; Sugg 2011; Noble 2011). In the second section of this chapter, I address the status of human flesh as food – a topic already broached in my descriptions of hungry tapeworms – but I also consider the practices related to the preparation of bodies and body parts for visual display. I

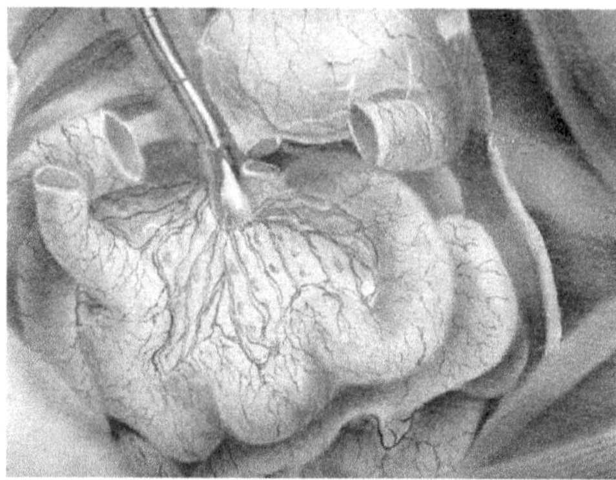

Figure 16.1 Anatomical painting showing female reproductive organs, detail. Fabien Gautier d'Agoty, 1774. oil/canvas, 60 x 200 cm. Dijon: Musée des beaux-arts.

highlight the anatomical specimens produced by Honoré Fragonard, a French man who was born in Grasse in 1732, and licensed as a surgeon in 1759. Fragonard gained renown for his preparations of both animal and human corpses, displayed at the national veterinarian school, located just outside of Paris, where he was its director and a professor of anatomy. Around twenty examples of Fragonard's handiwork, made between 1766 and 1771, remain on view at the Musée de l'École nationale vétérinaire d'Alfort, better known by its popular name, Le Musée Fragonard. One of the oldest collections in France, it suffered much neglect after the Revolution, but has been rediscovered, leading to a refurbishment of the museum and a few publications devoted to Fragonard's anatomical career (Simon 2002; Degueurce 2011). I contribute to this ongoing work by exploring the artistic and technical elements of his process to argue that by making the dead seem alive, Fragonard's dried figures provided him with a kind of procreative power and, perhaps more important, a demonstrable ability to control all-pervading worms.

Intestinal Fertility

In the 1780s the German physician Marcus Elieser Bloch entered a heated debate by arguing that tapeworms were generated within human bodies, not introduced via air, food, or water. Drawing on the dissections and microscopic investigations he had undertaken, Bloch insisted that humans were born filled with worm semen, which if provided with the ideal growing conditions would develop into creatures liable to cause insomnia and constipation (Bloch 1788, ix). Like other early modern authors, this physician portrayed the presence of tapeworms within the digestive tract as at once an intrinsic component of human existence and the potential cause of unwelcome illness in need of medical remedy. Bloch also categorized the worms he discovered – calling one "intestinal chaos" – and provided admirable images of them in his treatise. The sixth plate in his book, for instance, features carefully labelled views of different kinds of *taenia solium*, or solitary tapeworms (124–5). It exemplifies the physician's research methods by comparing those found in different species, including humans and dogs, while featuring microscopic views of their heads and tails to highlight the themes of digestion and excretion that recur throughout the text.

Bloch also took great care to defend his position with regard to a subject that continued to puzzle various philosophers and medical thinkers. How had such worms come to be present in their apparent hosts: from external sources, by internal causes, by means of a divine plan, or in a manner consistent with the mechanical order of things? Bloch drew on his extensive experimentation with the intestinal parasites found in humans and fish, among other examples – he would become a renowned ichthyologist – claiming that he had not only examined the worms with microscopes, looking assiduously for their eggs, but had also boiled and chilled particular specimens, testing their reaction to temperature and noting the conditions causing their demise (38–40). The German physician concluded that such worms were designed to live in intestines and could not be found outside of them, refuting earlier authors who had claimed that fully formed worms entered host bodies, including William Buchan, who suggested that children were infected with worms from the milk of their wet nurses (49). Bloch then listed twelve carefully delineated proofs against the external introduction of intestinal worms, asserting that tapeworms were found in young children and even miscarried fetuses, and that because such worms could easily withstand the digestive liquids and muscular actions of the stomach, they were naturally suited to live there, dying quickly once removed from the body of the selected host. Bloch finally concluded that because certain types of intestinal worms were innate to specific animals and could not be found elsewhere, they could hardly have been randomly introduced from exterior sources (82–95). The physician thereby insisted on a particular kind of spontaneous generation, not that which historian John Farley has characterized as "abiogenesis," the belief in the creation of living things from non-organic matter, which had been entirely dismissed

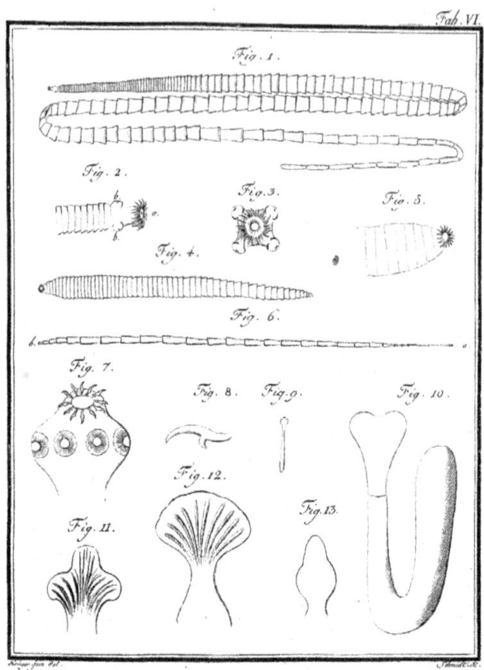

Figure 16.2 Tapeworms. M.E. Bloch, *Traité de la génération des vers des intestins et des vermifuges* (Strasbourg: J.G. Treuttel, 1788), plate VI, engraving. Courtesy of Wellcome Library, London.

by the eighteenth century, but that produced by "heterogenesis," or the belief that organic matter was capable of generating living things, a position finding support well into the nineteenth century (Farley 1972, 96).

One of the authorities that Bloch both drew from and attempted to refute was the French physician Nicolas Andry de Boisregard, who published an important treatise called *De la génération des vers dans le corps de l'homme* in 1701. On the topic of the generation of worms, Andry was an externalist, arguing that intestinal worms were formed inside the human body from seed that had entered through the acts of eating, drinking, or breathing (Andry 1701, 9). According to Andry, all animals stemmed from semen and eggs and could not spontaneously spring to life from rotting matter as suggested in ancient theories of *abiogenesis*. Yet the world was literally teeming with visible as well as invisible insects – still a broad category that at the time included flies, worms, and some amphibians – as had been revealed by the microscope, and their seed could easily enter human bodies (1). Andry confirmed that worm eggs and semen could also be introduced by means of the blood or breast milk of parents, making it possible for a fetus to foster worms, which would grow as quickly as the fetus itself (27–8). The enclosure of these worms in eggs that were then heated appropriately would ensure their generation.

The engravings that Andry commissioned for his treatise are distinctive from those included in Bloch's later publication. Whereas the engraver of Bloch's plates stressed the removal of the worms from their intestinal environment, presenting them in a rigid diagrammatic format meant to promote comparative scrutiny on the part of viewers, Andry's artist used subtle cross-hatching to model in three dimensions a lengthy tapeworm that is largely intact – one of its sections, labelled G has been opened for view – and hung as if to dry in a natural setting complete with trees and plants to insist on its presence outside of the intestinal tract. The image below invokes not only the convention in anatomical treatises of showing flayed human bodies standing within landscapes, notably in the 1543 publication by Andreas Vesaluis, but also frames the worm as an integral part of its environment, not unlike the work of German entomologist Maria Sibylla Merian, who portrayed butterflies in varying stages of development alongside their food sources in early watercolours as well as in her *Metamorphosis Insectorum Surinamensium*, published in 1705. Comparing the illustrations in the books by Bloch and Andry does more than reveal changing artistic styles or representational conventions; it indicates how each author worked with collaborators to make visual arguments that would bolster his theoretical claims. Andry's image positions the viewer in nature, standing alongside the physician who is present in the explanatory written text that fills the right side of the plate, to observe a remarkable tapeworm. In contrast, the engraving made for Bloch places the viewer above rows of dissected specimens, looking down on them in a manner that mimics microscopic observation and invites the comparison of shapes and forms, referring to the author's experimental methods while suggesting that artistic intervention has been kept to a minimum.

My engagement with these and other treatises revealed that the study of tapeworms was an important part of the fabrication of reproductive knowledge throughout the eighteenth century, contributing to discussions of the respective roles of semen and ova and lending weight to the various positions taken on theories of, among others, spontaneous generation. The rich, contradictory, and often fantastical early modern discussions of

On ne sçauroit, par le secours de la dissection, appercevoir aucun organe dans les
vers plats. On est venu à bout d'en découvrir
dans celuy cy, par le moyen d'une eau qui l'a
déchargé d'une humeur dont il estoit plein, et
à rendu visible les conduits qu'on y voit mar-
quez. ils sont dessinez avec une grande
exactitude. C'est un ver de la 2.e espece. voyez
pag. 73 du Liv. de la gener. des vers.
A. Vaisseaux disposez en forme
de peignes.
B. Intervalle entre les dens de ces peignes, vis à vis chaque Mammelon.
C. Rosettes formées par le contour
des vaisseaux. Les portions qui
composent ce ver ont, comme dans
tous les autres vers de la même
Espece, un costé qui recoit la portion
qui le suit et un autre où il est em-
boetté luy même dans la portion
qui le precede, Ces rosettes ne se
trouvent que du costé qui est en
boetté, Ce qu'il est important de
remarquer pour connoitre la
structure de ce ver.
D. Inegalité coudée.
E. la mesme inegalité veüe par
dessous.
F. Mammelons naturellement
ouvers.
G. Portion plus evasée que les
autres, et où l'on ne remarque point
de vaisseaux.
H. fente dans le milieu
de cette portion evasée.
Ce sont peut être là des
minuties, mais c'est sou-
vent dans les plus peti-
tes choses que la nature
paroit d'avantage.

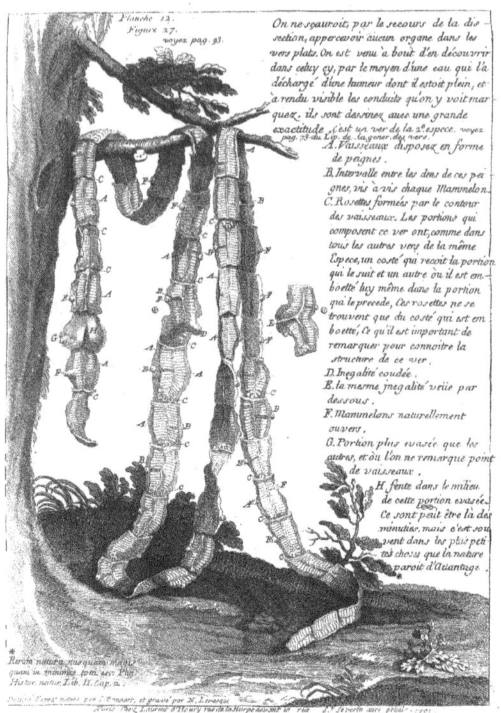

Figure 16.3 Tapeworms. N. de B. Andry, *De la génération des vers des intestins et des vermifuges (Strasbourg: J.G. Treuttel, 1701), plate XII,* engraving. Courtesy of Wellcome Library, London.

reproduction in terms of preformation, *emboîtement*, ovism, or spermism have long attracted the interest of scholars, as indicated by the work of Bowler and Pranghofer in this volume (Fissell 2004; Keller 2007; Porter and Hall 1995; Roger 1997). A substantial academic literature recognizes the role played by "worms" – widely construed during the eighteenth century to include so-called animalcules and microorganisms – in these ongoing debates, highlighting the microscopic observations of seemingly omnipresent "worms" made by Anton van Leeuwenhoeck (Palm 1989; Ruestow 1983). A recent study by Justin E.H. Smith, for instance, contends that the philosophical thought of Gottfried Wilhelm Leibniz was fundamentally influenced by the research of both van Leeuwenhoeck and English naturalist Robert Hooke. Smith argues that the microscopic revelations of these men encouraged, among other things, Leibniz's doctrine of "worlds-within-worlds," which holds that matter lacks any ultimate or indivisible parts (Smith 2011, 144). To a lesser degree, the eighteenth-century research that specifically addresses tapeworms has also been assessed in modern scholarship, notably in the analysis of Andry's apparent devotion to both spermism and *emboîtement* by Clara Pinto-Correia (Pinto-Correia 1997, 32, 75–6). Yet historian of biology John Farley has arguably undertaken the most thorough account of tapeworms in his historical account of spontaneous generation, asserting that the rise and fall of beliefs in *heterogenesis* accorded with the waxing and waning of ovism before concluding that "in the fifty years following 1780, the more expert one was on parasitic worms, the more likely one was to embrace the doctrine of spontaneous generation" (Farley 1972, 106). Farley contends that a considerable amount of scholarly attention was paid to tapeworms during the eighteenth century precisely because intestinal parasites provided a conundrum that both thwarted and invited research. Unlike the experiments conducted during the seventeenth century by Francesco Redi – he disproved the theory of *abiogenesis* by showing that maggots did not develop in meat kept protected from flies – living tapeworms could not be isolated from their host, nor could their selected hosts be deprived of food or water (97). Tapeworms were thus very "good to think with" during this period.

I enrich these discussions of eighteenth-century tapeworms by glancing away from the apparently central question of how they reproduced, to consider the locations in which they flourished, especially human intestines. Precisely what role did human entrails play in the generation of omnipresent worms? Andry claimed that the eggs and semen deposited everywhere by insects of all kinds would sometimes meet under the right circumstances, allowing generation to occur – another version of the panspermism discussed by Bowler in this volume (9–15). The warm human body would seem to provide a convenient nesting area for such nascent creatures, but in reality only certain kinds of worms would be harboured within particular bodies, depending on the temperament and conditions of that flesh. One issue was poor digestion (15). Andry argued that worms fed on what he called "superfluities," or food that was not fully consumed, a problem for those who overindulged in milk or such sweets as honey and melons, not to mention spongy mushrooms, which were liable to rot and provide the "corrupt" sustenance preferred by worms (24, 164). His theory explained why a fetus could also be replete with worms, because it was often not able to digest the abundant food received within its mother's belly from multiple sources, including its umbilical cord, mouth, and pores, creating ideal growing conditions for worm eggs (27–8). Although Bloch disagreed with Andry's claims that free-floating worm eggs entered human bodies from external sources, he confirmed that eating habits played a major role in the ability of tapeworms to thrive within the intestines. An individual who drank hot liquids and primarily ate moist food with little fibre, Bloch argued, would enfeeble the bile in a way that diminished the force of the stomach and the intestines, thus facilitating the augmentation of *glaires* or viscous fluids that could sustain worms (105). The German physician identified young boys as generally more subject to worms than their elders, for they were not yet able to digest their food fully, thereby providing ready meals for the kinds of worm that would have literally died of starvation within the entrails of more active male adults (13).

Despite writing at opposite ends of the eighteenth century, both Andry and Bloch linked human intestines with various qualities; they could be strong and effective, working with just the right amount of sour and dry fibrous substances, or they could be weakened and passive, overfilled with superfluous sweetness. The authors drew from a long-standing interpretation of Galenic humoral theory that viewed the lack or excess of a particular bodily fluid (blood, black bile, yellow bile, or phlegm) as a primary cause of illness. Since the stomach played a role in the incorporation of food and the separation as well as eventual removal of excrement, its digestive function was central to the maintenance of health in the form of balanced humours. Yet as literary scholar Michael Schoenfeldt has pointed out, during the early modern period the entire human body was in many ways approached as a giant stomach that incorporated foreign substances and discharged excess by means of feces, urine, sweat, hair, nails, and mucous (Schoenfeldt 1997, 245). Tapeworms thus thrived on the body's general failure, which could be understood in physical as well as moral terms. Schoenfeldt's contention that the stomach "was a primal site for the exercise of ethical discrimination and moral virtue" in early modern culture is invoked when both Andry and Bloch advocate a moderate diet based on self-control rather than self-indulgence (257). Andry argued that it was best to avoid worms by eating properly and avoid excessive sexual activity, thinking, or studying, which could all interfere with the digestive process (179); if already present then worms could be alleviated by bleedings, and by imbibing drinks made of lemon, garlic, and white wine (246). Bloch further suggested that those filled with tapeworms should drink a mixture of dried orange peel, *quassia* (likely *quassia amara* or "bitter wood," a shrub from Surinam, among other places, which was used as an insecticide), and thickened beef bile, mixed with cinnamon water (105). This concoction would help to undermine the moist and excessive humours that worms enjoyed by delivering drying, bitter, and digestive ingredients, the latter most evident in the introduction of bile from another animal. Among Bloch's suggestions for killing or driving out intestinal worms, he advised drinking cold water first thing in the morning, an act that would chill the stomach and intestinal canal to render them less hospitable to worms (114).

Both Andry and Bloch subtly gendered their discussions of tapeworms. In Andry's account, the over-abundant female body endangered the fetus, recalling Buchan's fear that wet nurses could provide infants with polluted milk (28). In addition to instances in which women acted as sources of contamination, both Andry and Bloch suggested that the bodies infested with worms were feminized, either weakly unable to resist the temptation of overindulgence, or laden with moist, excess humours, characteristics more closely associated with female bodies than with those of healthy men. During the eighteenth century, female menstruation remained linked with women's special need to purge the excess humours that their often cold and sluggish bodies were unable to consume (McClive 2000). Along these lines, young boys were more like women than men when they did not "burn up" all of their food, experiencing ill effects by being furthermore incapable of purging this superfluity through regular blood loss. The boys' bodies were thus compromised by providing food for bodily inhabitants, a further feminization which had them playing the maternal role of nourishing a dependent creature. Such associations of tapeworm infestation with pregnancy were made more directly when Andry reported, for example, that he had been called to assist a lady of quality who was experiencing the food loathings and cravings typical of a pregnant woman, as well as a swollen belly and cessation of menstruation. Although different physicians and even midwives had unanimously deemed the woman pregnant, her distress continued until death and an autopsy finally revealed that she was filled, not with a child, but with "un grand amas d'eaux & un verplat, qui occupoit toute la langueur des boyaux" [a large amount of water and a flat worm that occupied the entire length of her intestines] (118). In this case, all of the signs of pregnancy were present, including the physical sensation of interior movement, which according to Duden was the surest evidence of pregnancy during the eighteenth century, indicating that the fetus had quickened and was potentially ensouled (Duden 1993). When male clients reported feeling similar movements within their bodies to such physicians as Andry and Bloch, they reinforced the correlation between the presence of tapeworms and the embodied sensations of pregnancy.

Male pregnancy was not impossible during the early modern period. In *Le progrès de la médecine*, a journal published in 1697, French physician Claude Brunet described a case in which a Cistercian monk conceived a child in his right testicle after engaging in "lively caressing of the lower parts" with a nun. The physician went on to report another remarkable case, in which a Flemish man had mocked his wife while she was in the throes of labour and then found himself with a swollen right buttock, which grew for nine months and eventually produced a son (Brunet 1697, 62–5). Brunet argued that both situations supported the theories of the animalculists; male seed was clearly replete with "tiny animals" able to become embryos independently of women, especially in such passionate circumstances. The author wondered why men did not become pregnant more often, but finally concluded that they were inconvenienced by birth, suffering greater pain than women. Women's organs were simply more disposed to childbirth, despite men's capacity for it.

Such scholars as Kirk Read, Raymond Stephanson, and Sherry Velasco have studied how early modern men adopted a form of "masculinized maternity," enhancing their academic prowess by associating themselves with both breastfeeding and the gestation of ideas (Read 2002; Stephanson 1998; Velasco 2006). These negotiations of the gendered maternal role could verge on appropriation, as when early modern male writers portrayed themselves giving birth to prose and poetry or even breastfeeding their students. Other men strove to embody the physical symptoms of pregnancy, including those early modern French surgeons who described the bodily exhaustion they experienced while working as men-midwives within the lying-in chamber (McTavish 2005, 156–9). Still others insisted on a visible assertion of paternity: some Spanish husbands of newly delivered women took to their beds, demanding rest and service, in a ritual known as the *couvade* (Dawson 1929). Intestinal worms offered another instance for men to approach, consider, and literally sense pregnancy, "giving birth" to creatures that were both formed within and could be detached from them. One famous example of this potential for male-centred procreation is found in the *Journal de la santé*, a diary in which the royal physicians of the French King Louis XIV recorded daily the monarch's physical condition. In 1696 the king produced a half-foot long living worm, classified as "un ascaride lombirciode," and then, with the assistance of purgative medicine, produced equally large tapeworms in 1697, 1703, 1704, 1705, 1707, and 1709 (Degeuret 1924). Although the king's intestinal afflictions were blamed on his poor digestion – exacerbated by his melancholy humour and unfortunate fondness for melon – the descriptions of his production of impressive tapeworms recall scenes of birth.

Male authors of tapeworm treatises portrayed themselves in the guise of midwives who "delivered" their clients of worms, doing so with success if called to assist in time (Andry 1701, 87). This allusion to male midwifery continued when such men as Andry and Bloch offered advice about nutrition, attended to the fertile bellies of their clients, and eventually provided purges meant to assist in the expulsion of worms, some inspired by the famous emetic made from a certain male fern and delivered with success by a wise Swiss woman named Madame Morat (Andry 1701, 246; Bloch 1788, 115). Like male midwives who preserved in visual and material form the embryos, fetuses, and monstrous births that they encountered in the lying-in chamber, so too did tapeworm doctors reproduce images of "their" worms as described above, and claim them for the enrichment of personal collections. Andry admitted to preserving worm specimens from families who would have foolishly thrown them into the fire, while Bloch boasted of the hundreds of intestinal worms that he had stored in jars and carefully placed in his own cabinet (préface, 73). These displays were arguably another form of male (pro)creativity which articulated the owner's identity in relation to worms, but also showed how he had vanquished and claimed the right to manipulate the still mysterious and apparently ubiquitous creatures.

Teeming with Worms

Microscopic interventions by van Leeuwenhoeck, Hooke, and others suggested that small creatures, insects, animalcules, or entities otherwise known as "worms" populated every part of the world (Hooke 1665). For some early modern writers, the suggestion that human bodies were riddled with worms, both inside and out, was disturbing. Consider the discussion of pernicious worms by William Ramesey, court physician to King Charles II, in his *Helminthologia, or, Some physical considerations of the matter, origination, and several species of wormes* of 1668. According to him, worms could clearly take up residence beyond the body's entrails and stomach in their search for food: "For, if the matter of *worms* be thick, gross, viscid, and putrid humours, joyned with heat and moisture, and so quickned and rendred apt to receive a vital property; and if they be ingendred of every humour, (as you have heard) what part of the body of man can be free[?]" (Ramesey 1668, 5). Ramesey viewed unhindered worms as a kind of punishment from God, potentially the result of witchcraft, and certainly the cause of numerous illnesses.

Later writers reinforced this image of a human body filled with worms but did so in a more matter-of-fact and even positive manner. In 1699 the microscopist Nicolaas Hartsoeker asserted that "[Worms] have been found in all parts of the body," while in 1738 Friedrich Lesser argued that "man ... is a world in which a multitude of insects live" (Smith 2011, 147). Some thinkers went so far as to understand human bodies as fundamentally composed of worms. According to Smith, Leibniz himself took up a related position when faced with substantial evidence that "worms really are the elements of bodies," though unlike the more literal Lesser he understood corporeal substances as infinitely nested organic bodies that were "worm-like" (146). In any case, this corporeality was not necessarily linked with disease, just as worms did not always cause sickness when they inhabited the entrails of humans for Andry, who assumed that in sanguine people such worms "just float like those saved in vinegar and do not cause any pain" (101). Bloch went further by insisting that because worms were naturally designed to live in animal bodies, they were a necessary part of a harmonious world, in which every living creature served as food for another (82). Intestinal worms would be disturbing primarily to those whose over-indulgence and weakness had rendered them incapable of balancing their humours and managing a cooperative coexistence with the omnipresent worms that fed on and within them.

It is striking that many of the sources discussed in this chapter feature images of the human body as a food source. Lesser phrased this idea vividly by claiming that "our whole body is nothing more, so to speak, than a butcher-shop, providing meat to an infinity of insects" (Smith 2011, 147). Although microscopic revelations of microorganisms undoubtedly promoted this view of a material human body that continually interacted with parasites, the notion that human flesh was fit for consumption was really nothing new. Early modern Europeans had long consumed as medicine the flesh and excretions of the human corpse by collecting, transforming, and reusing matter from both mummified and newly dead bodies. Seemingly all manner of bodily products could be redeployed for healing purposes: urine, feces, blood, fat, and bone, as well as *mumia*. Literary scholar Richard Sugg describes how human remains were stolen, purchased, distributed, and sold throughout Europe, with the apparent cannibalism of these bodies justified by distinguishing it from the reputedly more aggressive forms of consuming human flesh practised by the natives of South America (Sugg 2011, 113–34).

The idea that omnipresent worms fed on the excess, corrupt, putrid, or otherwise decaying material within the human abdomen was furthermore in keeping with the empirically observable degradation of human bodies shortly after their death. Recycling the body's excretions or even using entire corpses meant intervening to consume that body before parasites could do the same; it required that the body be preserved from its ultimate destruction by worms, often through the application of drying agents. In fact, many of the methods employed to save the dead body and its parts were based on the same principles that physicians advised for keeping in check the worms inside the living body. Bloch advised diminishing the body's viscous fluids as the best first step before taking further action against worms (109), while Andry advocated that his clients avoid sweet foods, used either onion juice or a bit of old urine to chase worms from their ears, and administered to them various drying mixtures to assist in the removal of excess humours before they corrupted, including such ingredients as lemon, garlic, and *verjus* (the juice of unripened grapes) (220, 229). At the same time, both men conserved tapeworms they had "delivered" from clients by placing them in jars of vinegar or drying them in the oven (Andry 1701, 73; Bloch 1788, 42). Excess moisture was linked with the decay of both living and dead bodies as medical practitioners strove to contain the effects of the voracious worms that competed for control of those bodies.

Thinking about the preservation of living and dead bodies in tandem can shed new light on the dried anatomical preparations that flourished during the eighteenth century. Along with the medical uses of dead body parts, increasing importance of anatomical dissection, and veneration of saintly body parts as relics, during the early modern period surgeons and physicians collected just about anything produced within or by the human body – tumours, fetuses, tape worms, syphilitic ulcers – drying them out or preserving them in jars filled with spirits, for display in more or less private collections. As described by Pranghofer, the Dutch physician Frederik Ruysch is best known for his fetal skeleton sculptures, but he was also a master of drying blood vessels and treating them with varnish, displaying dead bodies to provide viewers with medical as well as moral lessons (Knoeff 2008, 4). Other medical men became famous for their own anatomical methods, including Claude-Nicolas Le Cat, Giuseppe Flajani, and Regnier de Graaf, a Dutch physician and anatomist also discussed by D.N. Wagner in this volume, who in his *Treatise Concerning the Generative Organs of Men* (1668) dared anyone doubting his claim that the *vasa deferentia* had considerable communication with the seminal vessels to come to his home where: "We shall demonstrate this not in the organs of brutes but in those of various human males which we always keep inflated and dried out in our museum" (de Graaf 1668, 34, cited by Stephanson 2004, 80). Along similar lines, the *écorchés*, or flayed figures created by Honoré Fragonard displayed his anatomical knowledge in the form of dried flesh. What's more, he explicitly contextualized them within ongoing efforts to manipulate the relationship between human flesh and worms. In a letter written in 1792 to the Assemblée Nationale, Fragonard insisted that his specimens were unrivalled in Europe because they were "inattaquables par les vers destructeurs" [unassailable by destructive worms] (Degueurce 2008, 40).

The most striking surviving *écorché* by Fragonard, called *The Horseman*, shows a fully articulated man mounted on top of a horse. In anatomical terms, the preserved bodies are primarily designed to show the myology or musculature of the two figures, and offer a suitable subject for a veterinary school, portraying the hierarchical relationship between man and beast. Yet the display is often discussed in aesthetic terms by contemporary scholars who recognize its theatrical elements, especially the horse which is posed in full gallop. Descriptions by eighteenth-century visitors indicate that the staging of these figures in the collections at the school was even more elaborate than the current version, with additional props – the rider, for instance, had held a whip in his right hand. The figural group was furthermore surrounded by a ring of tiny skeletal horses ridden by fetal skeletons also holding whips (Degueurce 2011, 132). This selection of figures carries layers of meaning, referencing, among other things, Roman emperors, Italian *condottiere*, and French noblemen. The broader scene calls to my mind a more recent work, namely *The Portrait of Chancellor Séguier*, painted in 1660 by Charles Le Brun, then Director of the Royal Academy of Painting and Sculpture in Paris. As a creative anatomist, Fragonard both invoked and altered this well-known academic composition, drawing attention to his artful invention of staged bodies.

Fragonard invited critics and admirers alike simply to look at and judge his displays, which were open to the public. He never recorded his painstaking methods, despite boasting about the ability of his specimens to withstand worms. The materials and techniques he used have nevertheless been reconstructed by Christophe Degueurce, curator of the Fragonard Museum, who has undertaken scientific analyses of the chemicals and pigments used in the specimens (2008). According to him, Fragonard followed many of the embalming techniques increasingly elaborated in instructive treatises such as that of Jean-Joseph Sue, a well-known French anatomist,

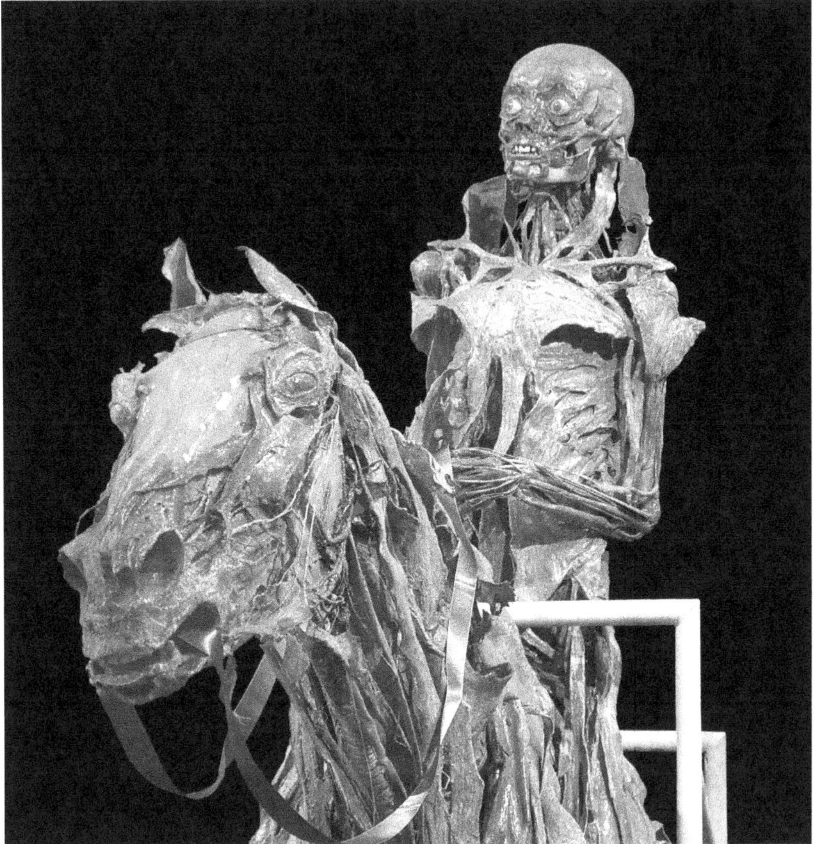

Figure 16.4 Honoré Fragonard, *The Horseman*, 1766–71, *écorché*, Paris: Musée de l'École nationale vétérinaire d'Alfort.

called *L'abrégé de l'anatomie du corps de l'homme*, first published in 1748. In accord with Sue's advice, Fragonard selected the freshest possible corpses of young flexible people with little body fat – the mounted horse rider, for instance, was a twelve-year-old boy – who had died of causes other than a debilitating disease or disfiguring execution. This preference was also in keeping with the desire for obtaining a mummy from a youth who had died violently, based on the belief that a sudden death would preserve the body's healing properties (Noble 2011, 3). The selected body was then washed, shaved, and warmed by immersion in a tank of hot water for several hours, so that it could be opened, its blood removed and replaced with preservative substances. As indicated by Wagner in this volume, injecting dead bodies was not a new method – anatomist Jacopo Berengario da Carpi had used water to reveal communications between vessels, Jan Swammerdam introduced wax, and Ruysch substituted a secret recipe that was finer than wax but solidified at room temperature – but Fragonard mixed mutton tallow and pine resin with the essence of turpentine and essential oils. Unlike Sue, who injected the vascular systems of his specimens with a coloured mixture of wax, animal fat, and plant resins, Fragonard did not add pigments to his recipe. Instead, he placed the more fully dissected body in a liquid bath filled with water and alum, and then dehydrated it in an immersion of alcohol and other corrosive substances, anywhere from eight to fifteen days. Afterwards the anatomist positioned the body into the desired pose inside a wooden framework, waiting until the alcohol evaporated. Only after all the supports, including threads, pads of horsehair, pins, pieces of card, or small sticks, were removed, and the *écorché* was completely dried, did Fragonard paint it, using vermillion for the arteries, ash or Prussian blue for the veins, and carmine for the muscles. The entire body was then coated with a white varnish that included Venice turpentine, adding a glossy finish that was visually appealing.

I have described this labourious process as elaborated by Degueurce (2008) at some length in part because it reveals how the anatomist transformed bodies into something resembling sculpture. In that sense, Fragonard's work bears comparison with that of Jean-Honoré Fragonard, the anatomist's cousin of the same age, who was born in the same town, yet rose to greater fame during the eighteenth century as a prolific painter and print maker in demand at the Bourbon court for such decorative works as *The Swing* (1767). Though scholars have recently taken pains to differentiate between the two similarly named Fragonards, I contend that there are interesting connections between them that surpass aesthetic effects and include those of process (Le Guay 1989). Like his painter cousin, the anatomist Fragonard prepared and mixed pigments, considered the various postures of the human body as well as its overall composition and expressiveness for an audience, and finally sealed the finished product with a varnish whose recipe was probably provided by the painter Fragonard because it was also applied to the surfaces of his canvases. Both Fragonards additionally relied on an intimate knowledge of the nude human body, which they strove to display in a "lifelike" manner by conveying its movement. As indicated by the galloping horse, the anatomist typically selected excited postures, including the famous dancing fetuses – one is described as performing a jig – which troubles some contemporary viewers, though such works were apparently regarded with a kind of sentimental admiration during the eighteenth century (Simon 2002, 72). On one hand this focus on expressive movement can be explained as a continuing flourish of technique, drawing attention to the anatomists' masterful intervention, but it is also in keeping with anatomical tradition. The Italian physician Berengario da Carpi showed dissected corpses as if they were alive during the sixteenth century, encouraging viewers to feel more comfortable about looking at dead bodies by revealing those bodies in the act of inviting the viewer's gaze (Sawday 1995, 84–5). For Fragonard, the body in motion also displayed the mechanics of movement, something of less interest to earlier anatomists.

More important for our discussion, the anatomist Fragonard maintained an image of the lively human body by protecting it from parasites, a crucial element of his preservative methods, but also one that required ongoing attention. Sue warned that in order to ensure that anatomical pieces would not be eaten by worms or mites during the summer months, it was necessary to return to them on a regular basis, treating the dried body parts with spirits or "l'huile de therebentine," a protective tree resin. This attention was especially important at the beginning of May, when insect eggs began to hatch and "one should be most afraid that anatomical pieces would be eaten away by worms" (Sue 1765, 259). The ability to maintain dead flesh against the continual onslaught of worms over a long period of time was indeed a point of pride for Fragonard, whose letter to the Assemblée Nationale explicitly stated that his anatomical preparations had survived unscathed for thirty years. This longevity was also praised in 1802, when Karl Rudolphi, a Swedish naturalist who wrote on the subject of parasitic worms, visited Fragonard's cabinet and marvelled at the excellence of its contents' condition (Degueurce 2011, 29). All the same, worms were not always the enemies of anatomists, for these creatures could be deployed to remove the flesh from skeletons by consuming it, a preservative method potentially more effective than the alternative option of boiling the bones (Sue 1750, 162–3). Just as worms could exist in relative harmony within the bodies of hosts healthy enough to contain them, so too could worms be helpful agents in the preservation of corpses if properly managed by vigilant anatomists.

Dried anatomical specimens provided evidence of their maker's intimate tactile and visual knowledge of the human body, but also revealed an ability to intervene and prevent that body from decaying via consumption by worms, even after death. Continual efforts were required in order to maintain the (relative) integrity of those bodies, and anatomists interacted physically with their collections in order to do so, while also handling them for other reasons, as suggested by de Graaf's offer to demonstrate anatomical truths with the dried reproductive parts in his museum. In this way, such medical men moved more fully into the realm of collectors, an identity that rests on the displacement of objects from one context into another. As French theorist Jean Baudrillard and other museum critics have argued, collectors typically relish the masterful experience of controlling and manipulating objects, undercutting their original meanings and values to reshape new ones (Baudrillard 1994). In this respect Fragonard was an effective collector of dead bodies, for he remade and re-enlivened those bodies, re-generating them into artistic forms that signified differently than had the originals, consequently evoking responses of admiration and sympathy rather than disgust from early modern visitors to his cabinet. On one hand, these visitors could hardly be shocked by the prospect of altering and consuming dead flesh, for it was common practice at the time. On the other hand, they may well have taken sheer delight in the way in which Fragonard's technically proficient *écorchés* cheated death by displaying lively movement, but perhaps even more so, by preserving human flesh in the face of its threatened consumption by voracious worms.

Conclusions

My encounter with representations of intestines at the Musée des beaux-arts in Dijon ultimately led me to broaden my research on reproduction to include such unexpected topics as tapeworms and dead flesh. These subjects nevertheless returned me to the heated debates about the principles of generation that arguably reached their height during the eighteenth century. Research suggested that worms were everywhere, living in and on human bodies in a way that challenged the very definition of those bodies. Attending to what we would now consider parasites – which are perhaps better labelled "co-habitants" – revealed the human body as a site for the gestation and subsequent formation of worms. To a certain degree, this understanding of the human body as a fertile site for the production and nutritional sustenance of others was considered natural, with worms becoming bothersome only when their host was replete with corrupt, moist humours. Anti-verminous medical treatments were meant to dry and expel those humours, for the most part hoping to manage and control the worms rather than completely rid the body of them. My exploration of the ambivalent relationship between humans and worms foregrounded the striking materiality of early modern flesh, providing another way to perceive the goals of and responses to eighteenth-century dried anatomical specimens, including those pro-created by the fertile hands and mind of Honoré Fragonard. At the time, his work was recognized for its technical virtuosity, artistry, and lively appeal to viewers. It was also praised, however, for its ability to withstand the inevitable onslaught of worms, a crucial point that may well be lost to the modern audiences now simultaneously puzzled and fascinated by his *écorchés* at the Musée Fragonard.

REFERENCES

Anderson, J., E. Barnes, and E. Shackleton. 2011. *The Art of Medicine: Over 2,000 Years of Images and Imagination*. Chicago: Chicago University Press.

Andry, N de B. 1701. *De la génération des vers dans le corps de l'homme*. Amsterdam: Thomas Lebrail.

Baudrillard, J. 1994. "The System of Collecting." In *The Cultures of Collecting*, edited by J. Elsner and R. Cardinal, 7–24. Cambridge, MA: Harvard University Press.

Bloch, M.E. 1788. *Traité de la génération des vers des intestins et des vermifuges*. Strasbourg: J.G. Treuttel.

Brunet, C. 1697. "D'une grossesse d'home [*sic*]." *Le progrès de la médecine* (Paris), 62–5. Paris.

Dawson, W.R. 1929. *The Custom of Couvade*. Manchester: Manchester University Press.

Degueret, E.H.R. 1924. *Histoire Médicale du Grand Roi*. Paris: Librairie Marcel Vigne.

Degueurce, C., S. Vo Dhui, J. Bleton, P. Hugon, L. Cadet, and A. Tchapla. 2008. "Un mystère: la technique de conservation mise en oeuvre par Honoré Fragonard." *Bulletin de la Société française d'Histoire de la Médecine et des SciencesVétérinaires* (Kiev) 8:40–57.

Degueurce, C. 2011. *Fragonard Museum: The Écorchés*. New York: Blast Books.

Duden, B. 1991. *The Woman beneath the Skin: A Doctor's Patients in Eighteenth-Century Germany*. Cambridge, MA: Harvard University Press.

Duden, B. 1993. *Disembodying Women: Perspectives on Pregnancy and the Unborn*. Translated by L. Hoinacki. Cambridge, MA: Harvard University Press.

Farley, J. 1972. "The Spontaneous Generation Controversy (1700–1860): The Origin of Parasitic Worms." *Journal of the History of Biology* 5 (1): 95–125. http://dx.doi.org/10.1007/BF02113487.

Fissell, M. 2004. *Vernacular Bodies: The Politics of Reproduction in Early Modern England*. Oxford: Oxford University Press.
Hooke, R. 1665. *Micrographia*. London: Martyn and Allestry.
Keller, E. 2007. *Generating Bodies and Gendered Selves: The Rhetoric of Reproduction in Early Modern England*. Seattle: University of Washington Press.
Knoeff, R. 2008. "Animals Inside: Anatomy, Interiority and Virtue in the Early Modern Dutch Republic." *Medizinhistorisches Journal* 43:1–19.
Le Guay, P. 1989. *Les deux Fragonard*. Paris: Un film de CFC Production.
Lowengard, S. 2006. Industry and Ideas: Jacques-Fabien Gautier or Gautier d'Agoty. In *The Creation of Color in Eighteenth-Century Europe*, 586–612. New York: Columbia University Press.
McClive, C. 2000. "Bleeding Flowers and Waning Moons: A History of Menstruation in France, c.1495–1761." PhD Diss. University of Warwick.
McTavish, L. 2005. *Childbirth and the Display of Authority in Early Modern France*. Aldershot: Ashgate.
McTavish, L. 2010. "Practices of Looking and the Medical Humanities: Imagining the Unborn in France, 1550–1800." *Journal of Medical Humanities* 31 (1): 11–26. http://dx.doi.org/10.1007/s10912-009-9099-z.
Noble, L. 2011. *Medicinal Cannibalism in Early Modern English Literature and Culture*. New York: Palgrave Macmillan. http://dx.doi.org/10.1057/9780230118614.
Palm, L.C. 1989. "Leeuwenhoek and Other Dutch Correspondents of the Royal Society." *Notes and Records of the Royal Society of London* 43 (2): 191–207. http://dx.doi.org/10.1098/rsnr.1989.0014.
Park, K. 2006. *Secrets of Women: Gender, Generation, and the Origins of Human Dissection*. New York: Zone.
Pinto-Correia, C. 1997. *The Ovary of Eve: Egg and Sperm and Preformation*. Chicago: University of Chicago Press. http://dx.doi.org/10.7208/chicago/9780226669502.001.0001.
Porter, R., and L. Hall. 1995. *The Facts of Life: The Creation of Sexual Knowledge in Britain, 1650–1950*. New Haven, CT: Yale University Press.
Ramesey, W. 1668. *Helminthologia*. London: John Streater.
Read, K. 2002. "Mother's Milk from Father's Breast: Maternity without Women in Male French Renaissance Lyric." In *High Anxiety: Masculinity in Crisis in Early Modern France*, edited by K.P. Long, 71–92. Kirksville, MO: Truman State University Press.
Roger, J. 1997. *The Life Sciences in Eighteenth-Century French Thought*. Translated by R. Ellrich. Stanford: Stanford University Press.

Ruestow, E.G. 1983. "Images and Ideas: Leeuwenhoek's Perception of the Spermatozoa." *Journal of the History of Biology* 16 (2): 185–224. http://dx.doi .org/10.1007/BF00124698.
Sawday, J. 1995. *The Body Emblazoned: Dissection and the Human Body in Renaissance Culture*. London: Routledge.
Schoenfeldt, M. 1997. "Fables of the Belly in Early Modern England." In *The Body in Parts: Fantasies of Corporeality in Early Modern Europe*, edited by D. Hillman and C. Mazzio, 240–61. New York: Routledge.
Simon, J. 2002. "The Theater of Anatomy: The Anatomical Preparations of Honoré Fragonard." *Eighteenth-Century Studies* 36 (1): 63–79. http://dx.doi .org/10.1353/ecs.2002.0066.
Smith, J.E.H. 2011. *Divine Machines: Leibniz and the Sciences of Life*. Princeton: Princeton University Press.
Stephanson, R. 1998. "The Symbolic Structure of Eighteenth-Century Male Creativity: Pregnant Men, Brain-Wombs, and Female Muses." *Studies in Eighteenth-Century Culture* 27 (1): 103–30. http://dx.doi.org/10.1353/ sec.2010.0084.
Stephanson, R. 2004. *The Yard of Wit: Male Creativity and Sexuality, 1650–1750*. Philadelphia: University of Pennsylvania Press.
Sue, J.J. 1748. *L'abrégé de l'anatomie du corps de l'homme*. Paris: Pierre-Guillaime Simon.
Sue, J.J. 1750. *Anthropotomie, our l'art d'injecter, de dissequer, d'embaumer et de conserver les parties du corps humain*. Paris: Cavellier.
Sue, J.J. 1765. *Anthropotomie, our l'art d'injecter, de dissequer, d'embaumer et de conserver les parties du corps humain*. 2nd ed. Paris: Cavellier.
Sugg, R. 2011. *Mummies, Cannibals, and Vampires: The History of Corpse Medicine from the Renaissance to the Victorians*. New York: Routledge.
Velasco, S. 2006. *Male Delivery: Reproduction, Effeminacy and Pregnant Men in Early Modern Spain*. Nashville, TN: Vanderbilt University Press.

17 A Bit Exposed: Displays of Male Genitals

DARREN N. WAGNER

The Georgians had a remarkable penchant and talent for anatomy. At first glance, their overt interest in morbid displays of bodies and body parts seems at odds with the polite modesty characteristic of that era's culture of sensibility.[1] Yet, as the historian of life sciences Anita Guerrini argues, anatomy and sensibility were mutually informed and dependent (2006, 12). That relationship was particularly evident in regards to those body parts that grated modesty and piqued curiosity the most: genitals. Both eighteenth-century anatomy and sensibility were committed to a physiological understanding of generation and sexuality premised upon fluids. Scholars have continued to stress the importance of humoral perceptions of bodily fluids, especially blood, in eighteenth-century generative medicine (Laqueur 1990; Haggerty 1999, 84; Smith 2010; Evans 2012; and see Toulalan in this volume). But animal spirits formed the physiological line between sexuality and sensibility. They were believed to be an ethereal fluid that was "distilled in the brain, and thence communicated by the nerves to the whole body" (Willis 1980, 54), providing sense and initiating movement. Sensibility, sexuality, and generation hinged upon these extremely fine and protean spirits as they connected the reproductive organs to the rest of the body and mind. In sensibility, animal spirits explained physical reactions like blushes, tears, or swoons and mental responses like distractions, shocks, or moods that individuals with delicate or refined minds and constitutions experienced.[2] In generation, they contributed to seed, provided sensation, conveyed desire, caused arousal, participated in conception and gestation, and figured prominently in venereal disorders. This sexual/sensible physiology was especially evidenced by male genitals. The anatomical techniques of injecting and inflating male sexual organs using syringes profoundly influenced both medical and literary ideas and representations of bodies and sexuality. In medicine syringes became a central model for how male organs of generation worked – particularly penises – whereas in literature syringes became a phallic metaphor used to critically engage medicine and sexuality. Various kinds of eighteenth-century authors used this association of syringes and penises to examine how sexuality and generation involved the body and mind within the context of sensibility's physiology. As this chapter concludes, perspectives about penises working like syringes controlled by the motions of animal spirits highlighted questions about male sexual volition.

Of the several studies of eighteenth-century anatomical museums, none have exclusively focused on male genitalia.[3] Recent scholarship on anatomies of female reproductive organs, such as Ludmilla Jordanova's *Sexual Visions*, has shown how social elements like gender politics critically influenced medical understandings and approaches. Yet, in anatomical displays and texts, male organs of generation regularly featured alongside and in complement to female organs. Texts on midwifery, generation, and venereal disease generally attended to both female and male bodies. Only in a few specialized obstetrical texts and settings more typical of the latter part of the century were female reproductive organs exclusively presented. This chapter reorients this current historiographical focus to include displays of male reproductive organs, which is essential for a full and just perception of sexuality, generation, and gender in eighteenth-century anatomical culture.

Anatomical activities and ideas concerning male genitalia had a significant relationship with non-medical representations in literature. In particular, the literary adoption of a metaphoric syringe-penis in language and imagery shows the wider dissemination of that anatomical practice in society and non-medical cultures. To use cultural historian Dror Wahrman's term, tracking this idea's dissemination from anatomy to literature indicates its "resonance" (2008, 592). In some cases – particularly of the legal sort – medical practitioners and experts directly introduced the idea that penises act like syringes into non-medical discourse. But, most influentially, literary authors adopted phallic syringe metaphors in both obscene and polite genres. This circulation in print reveals the important role syringes and anatomical preparation played in engendering perceptions of male organs of generation as autonomic: mechanical parts filled and vitalized by animal spirits.

Penises and Testicles for Show and Sale

"It is not always that a penis can be thus completely and beautifully injected," lamented the German anatomist-physician Lorenz Heister. "It frequently happens, that the matter of the injection, thrown in at the vein of the back of the penis, makes its way out by the urinary passage" (1752, 476). This instructive advice accompanied an engraved plate showing a human penis "injected with crude quicksilver" (474) (figure 17.1). Injection, as with other emerging anatomical techniques like inflation and different mountings, was a highly valued and sought-after skill. By the late seventeenth century anatomical preparation was a fine craft that expressed aesthetics, supplied markets, entertained spectators, edified pupils, and investigated the form and function of human bodies. Although Heister allowed that "even miscarriages of this kind are not without their use: we discover by this the communication that there is between the urinary passage and the veins of the penis," his chagrin at a botched preparation is evident (476). Injections and inflations offered more than insight into the physiology, pathology, and anatomy of generation. Heister related a deep appreciation for the beauty of these preparations. His fellow anatomists, both in Leiden and further abroad, similarly appreciated such preparations for their craftsmanship and beauty. As McTavish details in the preceding chapter, anatomical displays could assume various meanings depending on how they were created, shown, and viewed. Preparing male genital organs, such as injecting testicles or erecting a flaccid and morbid penis by injection or inflation, particularly showed anatomical skill and discovered physiological features.

Instrument modifications, embalming methods, dissection practices, anatomical jargon, and display styles rapidly developed after the 1650s, and particularly in relation to the organs of generation. These organs represented an area of new and exciting research, wherein anatomists established their names and legacies. Yet, anatomists not only *made* their names by researching genitals, they *gave* their names. From the late seventeenth to the late eighteenth century, a significant cohort of anatomists achieved such an honour: Highmore's body, Graafian follicles, Poupart's ligament, Cowper's glands, Littre's glands, Bartholin's glands, tunica Ruyschiana, Fallopian tubes, and the Wolffian duct. Ruysch gained more international and royal recognition for his special, secret preservation fluid. Renown was also seized by those who excelled at injections. Accolades were given to anatomists like Adriaan van den Spiegel, Francis Glisson, Giovard Bidloo, and William Cowper for corrosion casting (injecting vasculature or a potential space with a hardening fluid then dissolving the remaining soft tissue, leaving only the form of the injection). Numerous others achieved notability by injections and inflations from the mid-seventeenth century till the close of the eighteenth century, when endeavour and innovation in those anatomical techniques dwindled (Cole 1921, 287, 335).

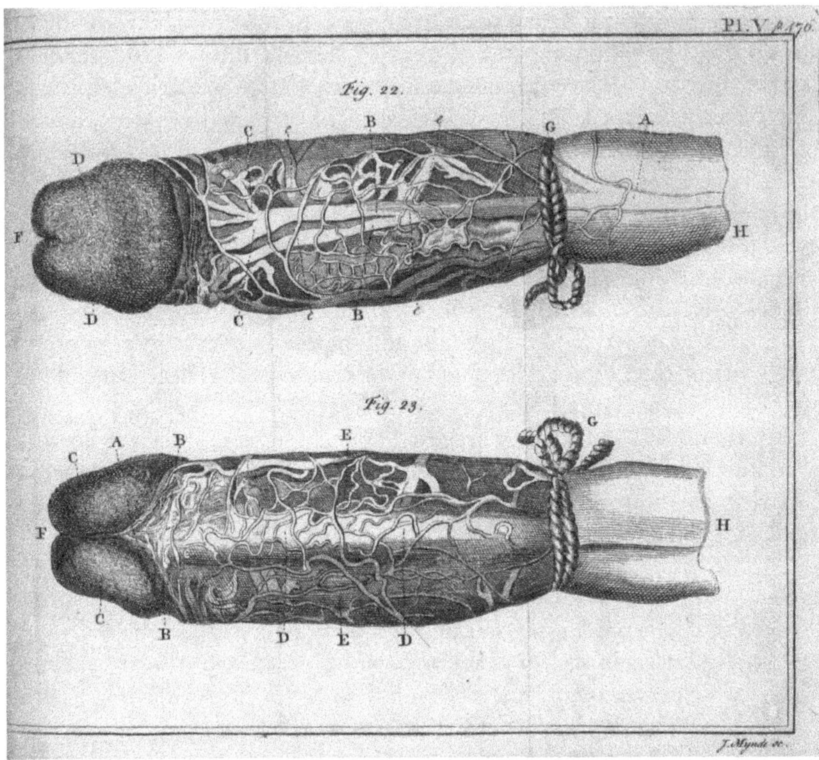

Figure 17.1 The human penis with its veins, and the cavernous substance, injected with crude quicksilver. L. Heister, *A Compendium of Anatomy* (London: W. Innys et al., 1752), 476, plate V. Courtesy of the Thomas Fisher Rare Book Library, University of Toronto.

But during their heyday, injections and inflations were vigorously used in experiments on genitalia. Anatomists inflated various structures and cavities, tweaking and measuring the process of drying and preserving. They also tried injecting numerous substances besides mercury: tin, lead, bismuth (and other metals), talc, plaster of Paris, alcohols (including brandy and wine), various waxes, oil of lavender, starch, turpentine (and other resins), urine, and animal extracts, including fat, suet, tallow, and spermaceti. Liquids were coloured with cinnabar, verdigris, vermillion, red oxide of lead, carmine, and indigo. Syringes underwent several modifications by anatomists, medical practitioners, and – because of their interest in mechanical principles of pump and suction – natural philosophers. Such modifications included new sizes and materials, filling without removing the nozzle, fine-point and curved nozzles, flexible outflow pipes made of leather, increased watertightness, and plungers with greater smoothness and delicacy (figure 17.2). The growing use of syringes in anatomy corresponded to their growing use in medicine, especially in reproductive and sexual therapies. Medical application led to further modifications, like the sex-specific "*Yard* Syringe" and "*Womb* Syringe," as the English surgeon John Marten described (1708, 46). For inflation, pipes, bellows, and syringes conveyed air into organs, and different varnishes preserved those tissues once dried, as McTavish describes. Although some anatomists guarded their experiments, methods, and improvements as secrets, others freely shared their discoveries to aid understandings of generation and further their personal reputations.

Another, more reputable, surgeon Thomas Gibson published his own and other anatomists' procedures and discoveries, which included careful instructions about inflating penises that Reinier de Graaf had originally published (Stephanson 2004, 73–8).

> Let the Yard be prepared thus: First gently squeeze the blood out of it, which it always has in greater or lesser plenty, and then put a little Tube into the spongy substance, namely in at that end which is next to the *Os pubis*; and let the Cavity of the *Penis* be half fill'd with water by the help of a Syringe, and shake the *Penis* with the water in it: pour out that bloody water, and fill it again with clear, and so three or four times till the water is no longer stain'd with blood. Then betwixt two linen clothes squeeze out what water is in the Nervous bodies, and at length blow up the *Penis* so long till it have its natural bigness; in which posture if you will keep it, you must tye it hard. When the *Penis* is thus distended and dried, you may examine it as you please. (1682, 126)

Aside from an eye for scientific examination, aesthetic taste significantly directed such preparations of penises, as suggested by Gibson's advice to enlarge the specimen to "its natural bigness." Such aesthetic sense corresponded to an ideal pursued by anatomists and natural philosophers: to "approach the *pura Naturalia*, in our Description and Expression" (*A Philosophical Essay on Fecundation* 1742, 13). Instruction in method and a particular aesthetic for these preparations were further disseminated through engraved illustrations. For instance, figure 17.3 from James Drake's 1707 treatise *Anthropologia Nova* visually demonstrates how to inflate a penis, showing where to insert the blow pipe and where to place ligatures to capture the air. Preparing, displaying, and representing any

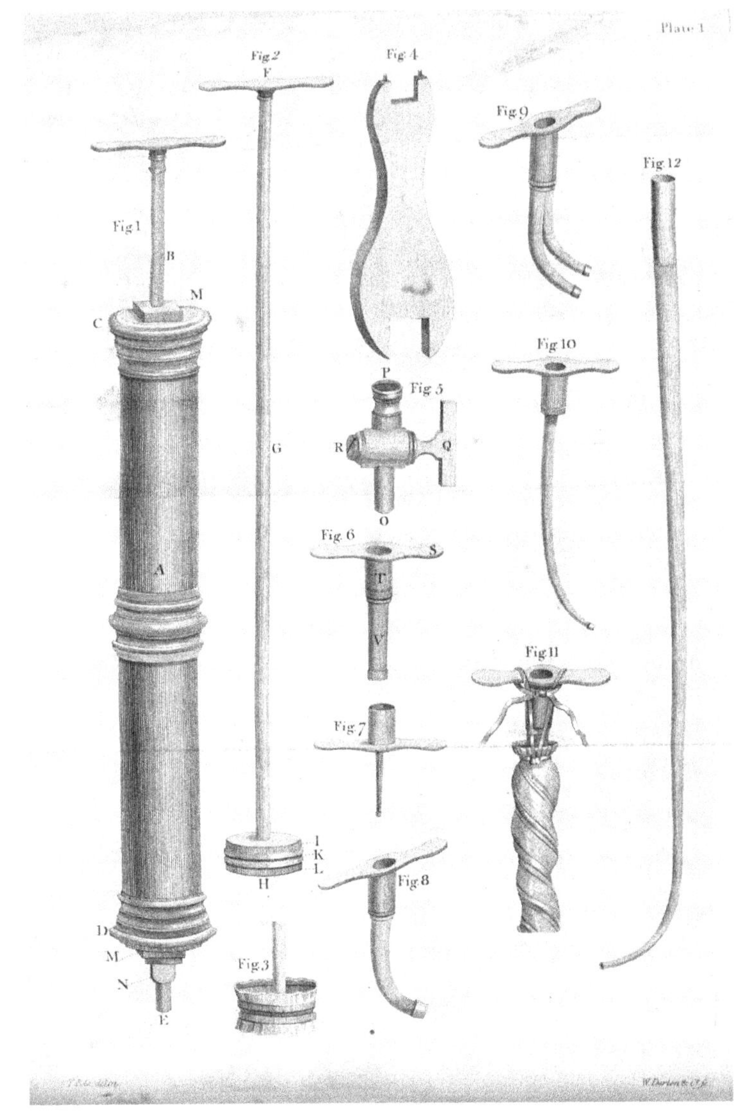

Figure 17.2 Illustrations of a brass injection syringe manufactured by W. Darton and Co. Pole, *The Anatomical* Instructor; *Or, an Illustration of the Modern and Most Approved Methods of Preparing and Preserving the Different Parts of the Human Body, and of Quadrupeds* (London: Couchman and Fry, 1790), plate I. Courtesy of the Royal College of Surgeons of England.

body part was (and is) a highly selective process. In late seventeenth- and early eighteenth-century illustrations, models, or preparations of genitals particular features were intentionally emphasized by the anatomist or engraver. Such was the case in the choice of bright dyes in the wax penis shown in figure 17.4. This injected preparation gives a sense of engorgement while highlighting the distinction between the *corpus spongiosum* and *corpus cavernosa* through the contrast of vermillion and brown dyes. Anatomists intentionally made these dissected male organs to be eye-catching and gaudy in hopes of eliciting observation and comment.

For instance, both a demonstrator's pride and intents on the public's curiosity are evident in the 1741 advertisement for "A Likeness of the Human Penis Prepared with a Waxen Injection Displaying Some New Anatomical Discoveries"[4] (figure 17.5). This exhibit was part of a small but very visible eighteenth-century museum market for anatomical preparations that often featured cadaveric penises, uteruses, testicles, breasts, and other such reproductive organs (Lieske 2001, 69). Two such exhibits in London were Rackstrow's Museum in Fleet Street and the more temporary exposition of Monsieur Desnoues's preparations, both of which dedicated several displays to human genitalia. Several different advertisements published in the 1730s described Desnoues's wax works, the collection first being shown in Somerset House, then offered at auction at the Great Room, and later exhibited at the corner of Durham-Yard, all in the Strand (*A Catalogue of Several Curious Figures of Human Anatomy in Wax* 1736; Cock 1736; Thomson 1739). The auction held in May of 1736, conducted by the aptly named Mr Christopher Cock, was advertised by one such catalogue, which doubly served as a ticket for viewing the collection, priced at one shilling. This advertisement, like the others, used surprising technical anatomical language. Lot 31, for example, showed "the Figure of a Man" that included "the spermatick Vessels to the Testicles, the differing Vessels from the *Epididymis* to the *Vesiculae Seminales* into the *Urethra*" (Cock 1736, 12–13). Such technical jargon conferred a learned tone to the exhibit – entirely empirical, gentlemanly, and separate from low concerns. Promoting civility further, both 1736 catalogues specify that gentlemen were to view the exhibit on alternating days of the week from the ladies. While the exhibit seems to have an equally represented and intermixed display of both sexes' reproductive organs, viewing these objects was done one gender at a time. Such attempts to show genitalia in a respectable and modest manner betray awareness that the exhibit contained erotic material. Successful exhibitors tactfully used sexual curiosity to draw crowds to see natural curiosities.

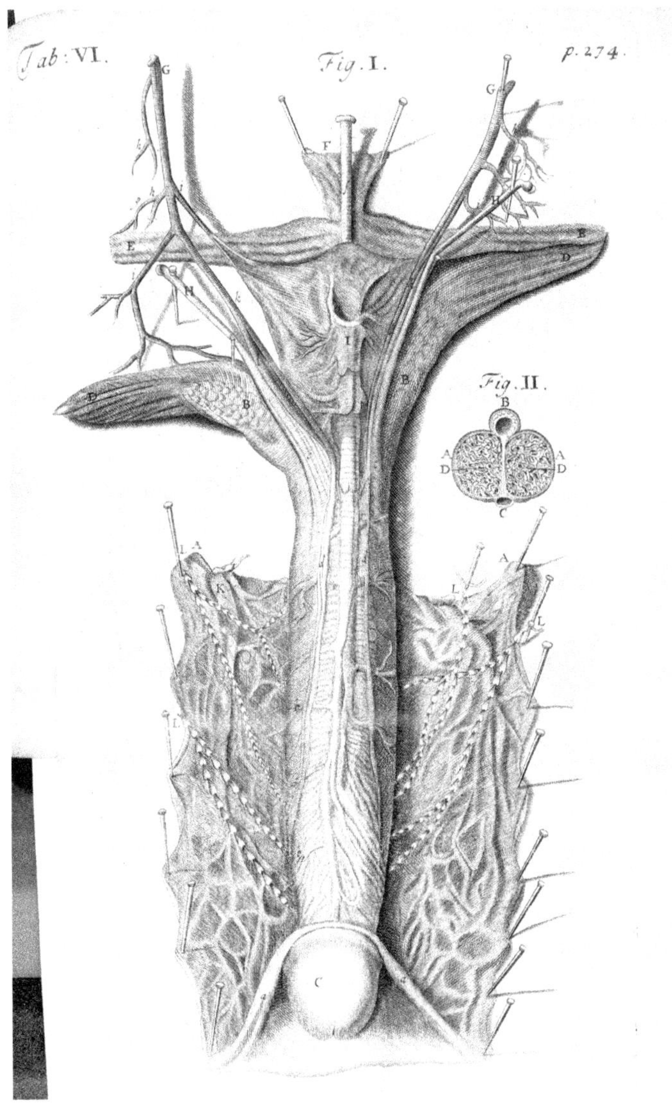

Figure 17.3 Engraving of the "Fore-part of the Human *Penis* prepared with *Mercury*" (fig. I) and the "two *Corpora Cavernosa Penis*, and that of the *Urethra*, after a Transverse Section, when Inflated and dry'd" (fig. II). J. Drake, Anthropologia Nova: *Or, a New System of Anatomy*. 2nd ed. Vol. 1 (London: W. Innys, 1707), 273–5. Courtesy of Wellcome Library, London.

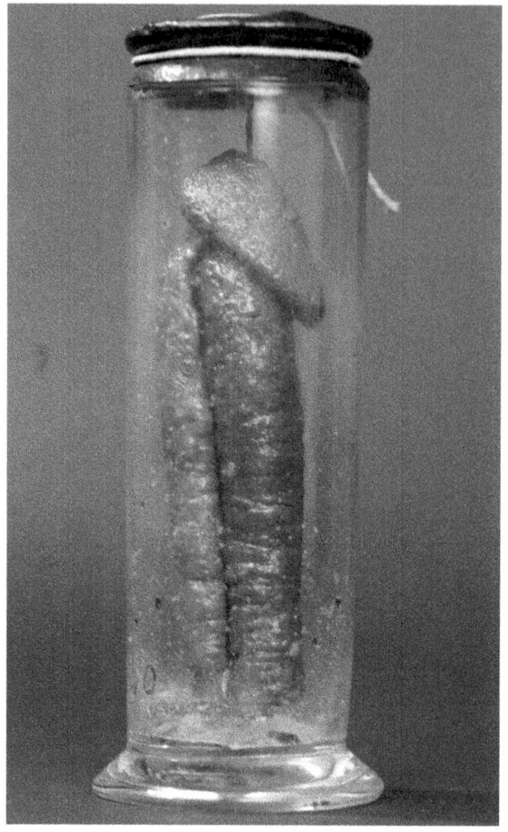

Figure 17.4 A wax-injected human penis dyed in two tones, vermillion and brown, and prepared by John Hunter. Courtesy of the Museum of the History of Science, University of Oxford.

However, erotica was not the central intent or trade of these and other exhibits of anatomized genitalia. Rackstrow's Museum, for instance, consistently featured reproductive organs, which, according to a 1784 advertisement catalogue, amounted to a third of its total anatomical displays. Nonetheless, Rackstrow's attention to human genitalia was not unusual for anatomical collections of that time, and, as Matthew Craske adroitly argues, previous "derisive assessments" of that exhibit as being pornographic are not accurate (2011, 75). Representations of genitalia also appeared in anatomical treatises, on *écorché* statues, on wax models, and in

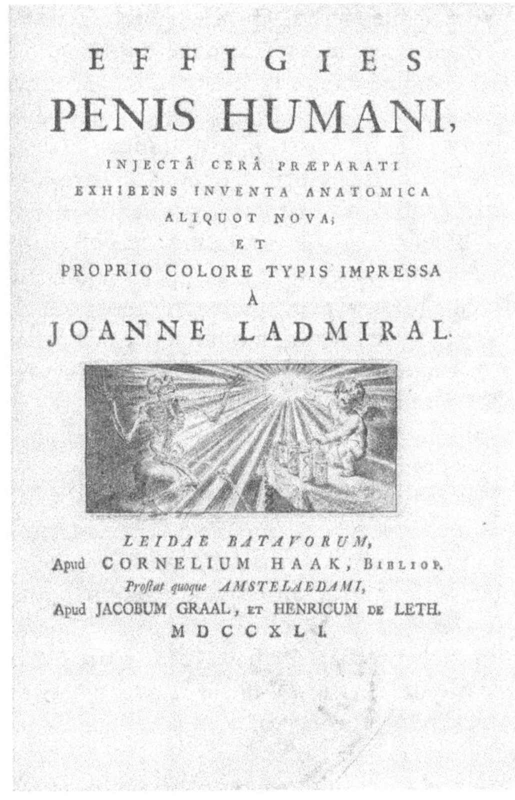
EFFIGIES
PENIS HUMANI,
INJECTÂ CERÂ PRÆPARATI
EXHIBENS INVENTA ANATOMICA
ALIQUOT NOVA;
ET
PROPRIO COLORE TYPIS IMPRESSA
À
JOANNE LADMIRAL.

LEIDAE BATAVORUM,
Apud CORNELIUM HAAK, BIBLIOP.
Proſtat quoque AMSTELAEDAMI,
Apud JACOBUM GRAAL, ET HENRICUM DE LETH.
MDCCXLI.

Figure 17.5 A 1741 advertisement by Joanne Ladmiral for Bernard Siegfried Albinus's exhibition of a wax-injected human penis. This sheet accompanied a striking coloured mezzotint by Ladmiral of dissected human testicles. Courtesy of the Wellcome Library, London.

glass jars in and around London for viewing by all manner of audiences. In eighteenth-century anatomical culture, boundaries between medical and erotic, licit and illicit, edifying and sensational, were muddled and rarely mutually exclusive – reminiscent of that period's colourful spectrum of medical practices and diverse medical marketplaces.[5] As Craske observes, there is a tendency "to produce a politically tidy account of gender dynamics in eighteenth-century anatomical spectacle" (2011, 79), which accounts overlook the nuances and complexities of that anatomical culture. Rackstrow's specimens, like those shown by esteemed anatomists, raised eyebrows and shocked the modest. But these displays of genitalia gained general legitimacy and acceptance through their edifying role: Rackstrow's hosted medical courses and, in the 1770s and 1780s, a midwifery clinic.

The blend of sexual curiosity, experimental design, anatomical craft, and higher learning added value to preparations of male genitalia when sold to collectors. The 28th of April, 1769, was advertised as the first of a two-day auction of a surgeon's anatomical preparations and paraphernalia held "At *Essex-House* in *Essex-Street*, in the *Strand*" (Paterson 1769, 1). Surveying the catalogue of mounted body parts and anatomical instruments, one is struck with how many preparations of both female and male genitalia were on sale. A simple dry mounted injected penis went for two shillings, and a wet mount of an injected glans penis was taken at four (2, 7). A larger dry mount that included part of the pelvis, penis, urethra, prostate gland, seminiferous vesicles, and bladder, all shown in "their natural State of Connexion," fetched ten shillings and six pence (3). For surgical instruction, there was a "compleat Preparation of the Parts concerned in Lithotomy," which cost a considerable one pound, nine shillings (3). For the anatomist in the crowd, perhaps the most interesting object was a testicle of a horse with "Part of the Epididymis fill'd with Quicksilver, and a Portion of the Vesicula Seminalis from the same inflated" (2). A similar injected testicle preparation had recently been at the centre of a highly publicized dispute between William Hunter and Alexander Monro *secundus*, and an anatomical collector may have happily parted with the two shillings being asked.

Both prominent mid-eighteenth-century anatomists, Hunter and Monro came to loggerheads over certain discoveries, and most importantly about who first successfully injected an epididymis and seminiferous tubules with mercury, thereby demonstrating the nature of the lymphatics. As Charles Ambrose recently chronicled, this print-based dispute quickly grew into a family feud, involving Alexander's brother Donald Monro, their father Alexander Monro *primus*,[6] and William's brother John Hunter. Monro *secundus* claimed that "On the 9th of *January* 1753, in attempting to make such a preparation, I was so lucky as to impel the quicksilver still farther into the seminal ducts than Dr. HALLER had done; making it fill, for a considerable length, a very great number of the serpentine ducts of the *testis*" (1758, 6). Monro gave further proof by insisting, "This preparation was publicly demonstrated, the very next day, to the Gentlemen attending the College of Anatomy at *Edinburgh*" and that "above a year and a half thereafter, I printed an account of this preparation, with figures" (6) (figure 17.6). William's priority claim also followed a demonstration of an epididymis filled with mercury, one which he had filled, and one which John had filled. This mercury preparation revealed the delicate continuity of the epididymis with the seminiferous tubule, described as follows:

> About the beginning of November 1752, in presence of Mr. Galhie and some others, I injected the *vas deferens* in the human body with mercury, and by that means filled the whole epididymis, and the tubes that come out from the body of the testis to form it; and observed, in this operation, that the mercury continued to run, and the body of the testis to become gradually more turgid and heavy for some time, after the external parts were completely filled. (Hunter 1758, 437)

These competing claims about testicle injections, along with other discovery disputes, provided for a seven-year-long paper war that included plagiarism accusations, defamatory remarks, and personal defences. Hunter gained the last word by publishing several witness accounts testifying to the public demonstration of his mercury injected epididymis.

For over a century anatomists endeavoured to entirely inject a testicle's epididymis and seminiferous tubule. As Francis Cole described, De Graaf was "the first to figure an injecting syringe of the modern pattern, and is credited with having injected mercury into the spermatic vessels" (1921, 297), which he showed in *De Virorum Organis Generationi Inservientibus* in 1668 (figure 17.7). William Cowper detailed this preparation in his 1698 anatomy text *Anatomy of Humane Bodies*, which included an engraved plate illustrating testicular anatomy (figure 17.8). Figure 1 on the lower right was described as showing "the Blood-Vessels of the Testicle call'd *Vasa Praeparantia*, as they Appear before any Injection or Inflation is made into them" (102). Cowper presented these non-inflated, non-injected vessels as truer representations of what was seen on the dissecting table, rather than what was in a living person. By the early eighteenth century, Herman Boerhaave reported injecting a boar's testicles, which animal subject was chosen because his gonads were "very large in Proportion to his Body" (1746, 54). Boerhaave's colleague Ruysch also injected seminiferous tubules (50). Although these injections met with some success, Boerhaave confessed that "even to the present Day we have been able to inject only a few arterial Branches spread upon the membranous Partitions of the Testicle" (65). Cole recounted how for Ruysch, two exceptions to his theory of "vascular autocracy were admitted – the ovary and testis, the fabric of which Ruysch was never able to prepare by injection" (1921, 306). Many other anatomists also attempted to inject testicles to reveal their structure

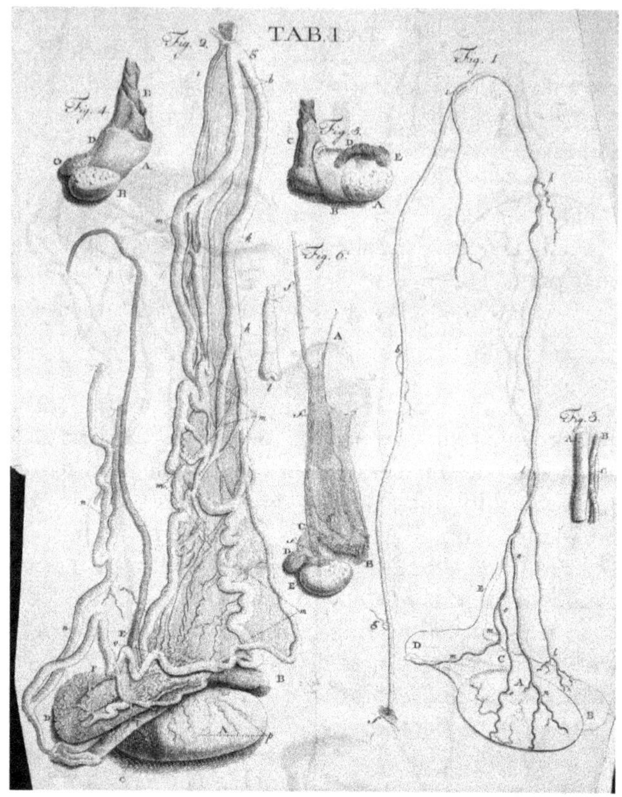

Figure 17.6 Testicular preparations made by Alexander Monro *secundus*, from his *Dissertatio Medica Inauguralis, De Testibus et de Semine in Variis Animalibus* (Edinburgh: G. Hamilton and J. Balfour, 1755); fig. 2 in the engraving particularly shows the mercury-injected ducts of a testis. Courtesy of the Thomas Fisher Rare Library, University of Toronto.

and form; the history of failed attempts made such a preparation a tempting and crowning achievement for both Hunter and Monro.

Hunter was particularly pleased with that preparation he injected in November of 1752, and kept it for several years. A similar injection graced John Hunter's anatomical collection, which, in the current-day Hunterian Museum in Lincoln's Inn Fields in London, stands out as the most ornately presented item (figure 17.9). That preparation of a boar's epididymis at once represents anatomical craftsmanship, experimental innovation,

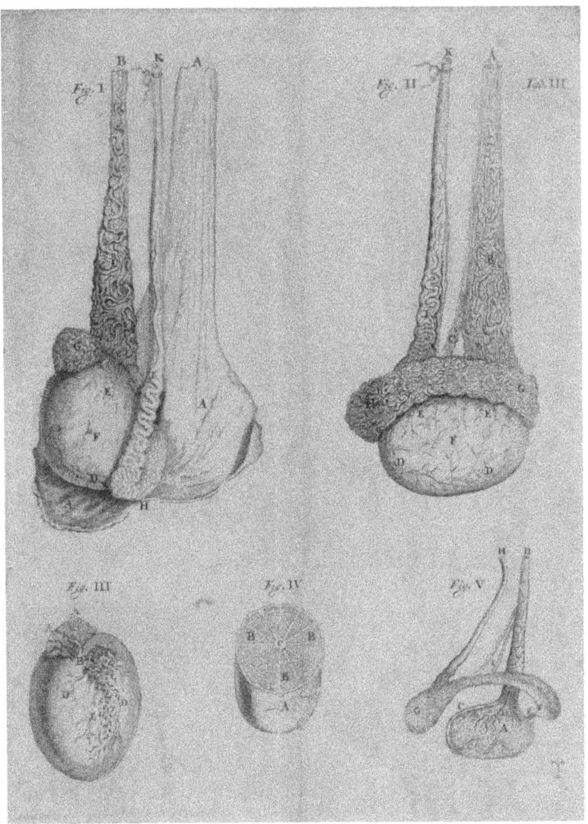

Figure 17.7 Engravings of testicles from R. de Graaf, *De Virorum Organis Generationi Inservientibus, De Clÿsteribus et de Usu Siphonis in Anatomia* (Leiden and Rotterdam, 1668), table III. Courtesy of the Hunterian Museum at the Royal College of Surgeons of England.

and a personal vindication. It is said that John Hunter displayed this piece not in his museum collection but in his dining hall. With its ornate gilt frame and intricate setting, this object seems more like a delicate piece of jewellery; its appearance shows the value imbued in such anatomical preparations of genital material. Such is this anatomical preparation that only the initiated could surmise what body part moulded its shape. Yet, its display and setting represented to the knowing viewer and owner the culmination of that long-sought-after anatomical accomplishment.

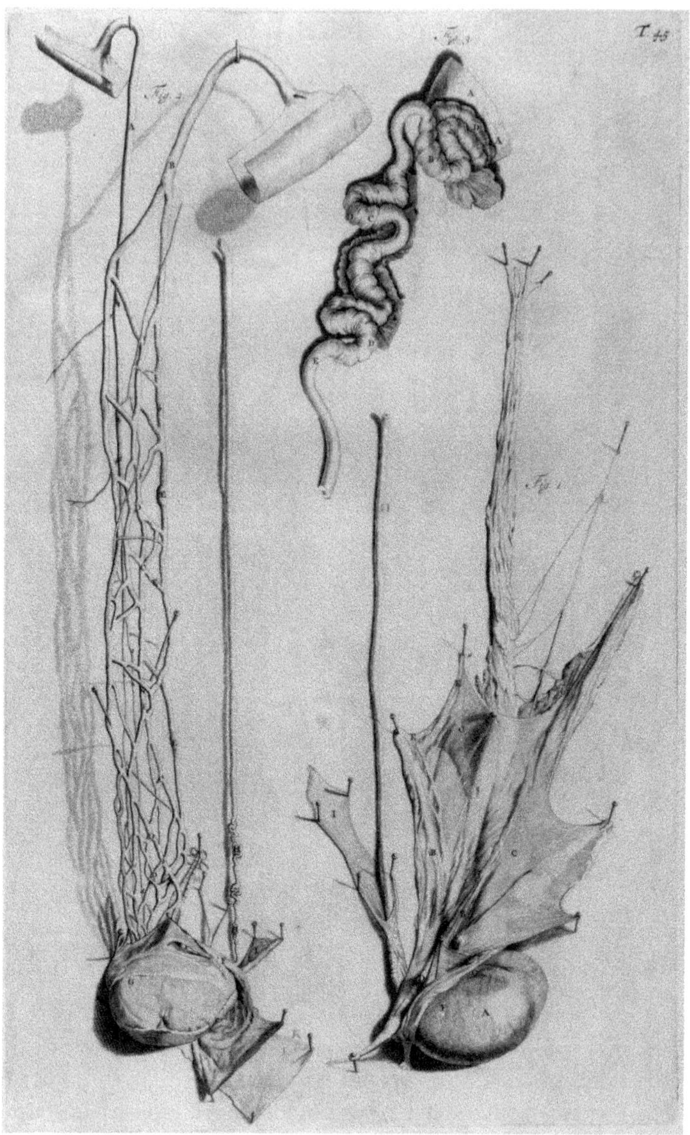

Figure 17.8 Engraving of testicular tissue dissected and manipulated with pins and magnification but specifically not inflated or injected. W. Cowper, *The Anatomy of Humane Bodies with Figures* (Oxford: S. Smith and B. Walford, 1698), table 45. Courtesy of the Thomas Fisher Rare Book Library, University of Toronto.

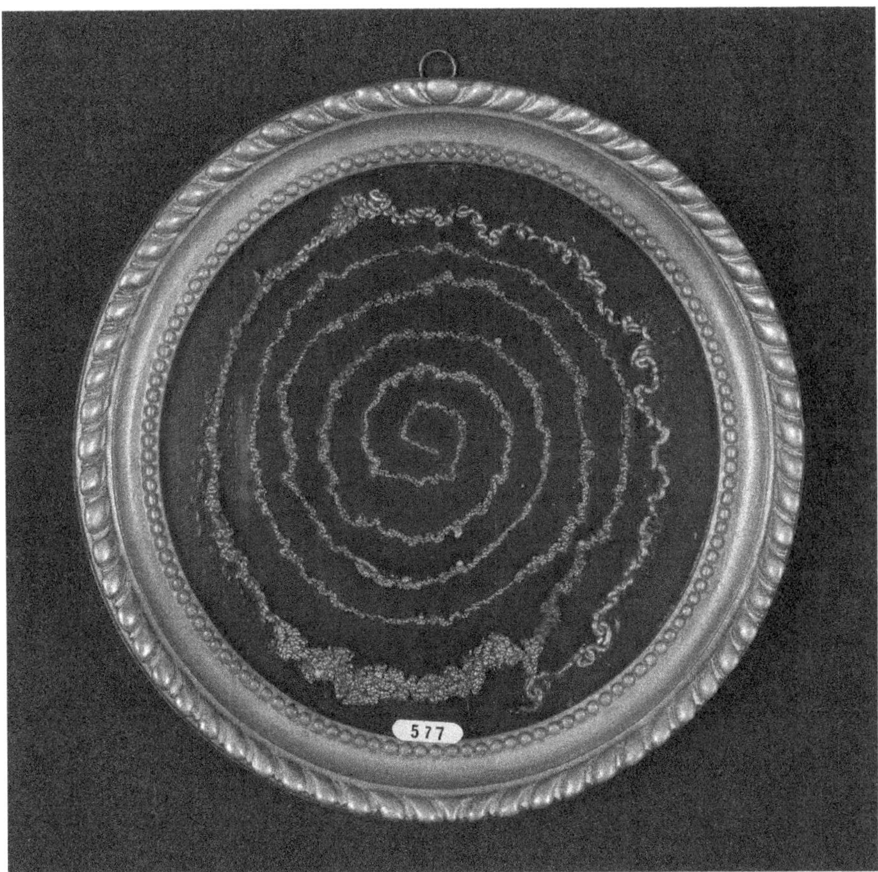

Figure 17.9 Mercury-injected boar epididymis in the original gold-painted wood frame from John Hunter's collection. Courtesy of the Hunterian Museum at the Royal College of Surgeons of England.

Spirits, Blood, and Erections

Peaking mid-century, dissecting and preparing genitalia progressively informed anatomical, physiological, and pathological understandings of generation. Anatomists, and subsequently a wider public, viewed inflations and injections as demonstrating how genitalia worked. These highly reproducible techniques showed the form of genital organs, circulation of blood and spirits, the maternal/fetal divide in the placenta, the intricate connections within genito-urinary tracts, and the nature of the lymphatic system. But, a particular point of fascination was the physiology of erection and ejaculation. These physiological displays were particularly convincing and influential because, as the art and science historian Julie Hansen suggests, "Representation, and demonstration – the witnessing of a phenomenon with replicable results – is essential to its acceptance into the larger cultural body of knowledge" (1996, 671). Anatomists had more ready success at injecting and inflating penises for demonstrating the form and function of erection. Boerhaave noted that Jan Swammerdam first showed "that the true Cause erecting the Penis was, the arterial Blood filling the three cavernous Bodies" (1746, 85). Likewise, the surgeon, physician, and anatomist Sir Edmund King investigated not only "the connexion between the vas deferens, seminal vesicles, and urethra by injections," but also how "the penis can be erected after death by injecting the internal iliac artery" (Cole 1921, 300). Those anatomical techniques displayed the physiology of the male penis, especially how the circulation of fluids filled that organ and connected it to the body and mind.

Anatomists conceptualized two male sexual processes in terms of these preparation techniques: penile engorgement was akin to the process of inflation or injection, and ejaculation paralleled a syringe's squirt. These understandings not only reinforced the role of animal spirits in sexual arousal, but neatly accommodated those ethereal spirits with an increasing attention to mechanics and circulation. These mechanistic interpretations, as Emily Booth suggests, led anatomists to be "guided by a concern to discover the physical evidence of a hydraulic system for the conveyance of spirits" (2005, 106). Thomas Bartholin, the eminent Danish natural philosopher and anatomist, depicted nerves as "conduit pipes" and the brain as a pump, which dilated to draw "vital Spirit with arterial blood out of the Carotick Arteries, and Air by the Nostrils" and contracted to force "Animal spirits into the Nerves" (1668, 322, 135). Boerhaave described how prostatic fluid could "lubricate the Urethra almost like an Oil" (1746, 77). Applying these mechanical terms to penises conjured up images of a syringe. The seventeenth-century Dutch anatomist Isbrand van Diemerbroeck gave an early account of this blood and spirits physiology of erection, and its analogy to a syringe.

> When the Animal Spirits, with the hot Arterious Blood, flow more plentifully into it out of the Nerves and Arteries, then the Yard grows hot and extends it self: but when the Spirits cease to flow into it, then the more copious

> Blood and Spirits already within it, are suckt up by the little Branches of the small Veins, and then the Yard falls again. Now that the Yard is extended by the influx of Blood and Spirits, is easily demonstrated in Bodies newly dead: for if you immit Water through a Syringe thrust into the Orifices of the Veins, and then force that Water forward toward the nervous Bodies, we shall find the Yard to be extended in the same manner, as we find it stiffen'd in those that are alive by the Influx of Blood and Animal Spirits. (1694, 151)

Van Diemerbroeck, like his contemporaries, perceived preparing an erect morbid penis using a syringe and water as being "in the same manner" as an erection in vivo.

Other body parts, however, were also analogized to syringes. For example, the physician John Cook suggested that "the Heart is a wonderful Machine like unto Syringes, serving to propel the Blood over the whole Body, and so is the fountain of all our Heat and Motion" (1730, 36). Yet, associations between syringes and penises were more pervasive. One reason was that inflation/injection became the model for the physiology of erection. Gibson described how the "Nervous bodies" of the penis "puff up like Bellows when the Yard is erected" (1682, 133). A mixture of blood and animal spirits rushed into the spongy tissue, distending the organ just like inflating it with air or injecting it with fluid. Yet anatomical demonstrations of erections had a major limitation in that they did not replicate the crucial stimulating power of animal spirits.

Understandings of male organs of generation based on mechanics and fluids located the mind's will or volition in the animal spirits. The English physician, theologian, historian, anatomist, and notable Epicurean Walter Charleton expounded how "the Animal Spirits, whose subtility makes them to approach neerer to the nature of the Soul, and whose sudden influx through the Nerves, into the body of the Muscle, causeth a swelling or distention, and so a contraction thereof, and consequently a change of Figure in the member" (1659, 186). The soul, as the "Regulating Faculty," impressed itself upon the fine and sensible animal spirits, which moved through the nerves, physically impressing the soul's commands onto the muscles of the body (190). Like Charleton's description of "swelling and distention," the Oxford professor, physician, and anatomist Thomas Willis described how venereal sensation in the genitalia made "Spirits flock thither," causing engorgement, perpetuating pleasure, and conveying desire back to the mind (1684, 158). Injections and inflations, according to anatomists, replicated that surge of animal spirits and blood during arousal, which affirmed notions of a mutual nervous influence between the groin and the brain.

However, sometimes the animal spirits circulating through genitalia became excited without the mind; arousal could be spontaneous and involuntary. Often described as the most sensible part of the body, sex organs represented a vulnerability to external influences that could incite lascivious feelings and lustful ideas, which threatened to overcome cool reason. This understanding of animal spirits and the organs of generation – of mechanics and fluids – embodied concerns about free will, sexual behaviour, public decorum, and mankind's sinful nature.

These physiological, philosophical, and moral concerns were not limited to discussions among the medically educated; rather, these ideas were openly presented to the lay public, particularly through anatomical displays. To return to Rackstrow's Museum, their catalogue descriptions of the anatomical works on show included detailed commentary on sexual physiology. Entry number 16 specifies "that a larger quantity of blood is thrown into the Penis by the Arteries, than the veins are capable of returning in a given time; in consequence of this, the Penis begins to swell" (Rackstrow's Museum 1784, 10–11). Entry 18, which was a wax representation of a woman's parts of generation, offers more strangely in-depth comments about the physiological and philosophical ideas connected with viewing these preparations. It details how the clitoris "probably conveys similar impressions, or affections, to a Woman, with those conveyed by the Penis to a Man" (12). Such commentary directly compared the sexual anatomy, physiology, and experiences of the two genders while drawing attention to how genitalia affected thought, volition, and behaviour. Although anatomists presented their preparations and descriptions of penises as true reflections of physical realities or "after nature," in actuality, such representations pointedly responded to prevailing social anxieties and cultural preoccupations about male sexuality. Several medical authors cited concerns about male reason succumbing to irrational sexual desires, which led to loose living and social disorder. These concerns were inextricably bound with representations of male sexual reproduction in the animal spirit physiology, depictions of sensibility, and anatomical demonstrations. As Catherine Wilson suggests, new technologies and procedures do not drive "discovery by themselves," but rather these "new technologies and procedures come to be valued and exploited only in the context of certain hopes and expectations" (1995, 71). That animal spirits coursed through nerves, crucially connecting the mind and genitals, became imprinted on the experiments, preparations, and observations involving injections and inflations. Yet, the association of syringes and male genitalia gained much wider influence as the terms and ideas of anatomical injections and inflations were appropriated by literary authors for metaphoric descriptions of the sexual and sensible body.

Male Sexuality, Sensibility, and Syringes

> The Doctor her half Sainted,
> For Cures controuling Fate;
> That has warm Engines planted,
> At many a Postern gate:
> If *Peggy* once were ill,
> And wanted his Skill,
> He'd soon bring her to Death's door;
> By Love made blind,
> Slip from behind,
> And make his Injection before. (D'Urfey 1719, 130)

This verse from the ballad "Pretty Pegg of Wandsor," set to a tune in B minor, mocks the widespread therapeutic use of glister syringes as perverse. The poem contains several typical bawdy metaphors: penises as engines, vaginas as postern gates, and orgasms as dying. Coitus and semen were prescribed in both earnest and jest as a cure, most frequently for greensickness, as many eighteenth-century ballads depict. But in this ballad excerpt the most prominent trope is the Doctor's injection. Such lewd figurative meanings for "syringe" corresponded to both a mounting suspicion towards the morals of medical practitioners, such as quacks and man-midwives, and a growing association between that instrument and penises, as presented in medical and anatomical discussions.

According to Gordon Williams's *Dictionary of Sexual Language and Imagery in Shakespearean and Stuart Literature*, the use of glister syringe as a metaphor for penis dates back as early as 1536 (1994, 601–3); by the seventeenth century, this metaphor was common stock. For instance, a couple of other early eighteenth-century satires use Syringe as a comic name for surgeon figures.[7] These caricatures reflected how, as the surgeon Thomas Bayford observed, it was "a time when the use of injections is so much in vogue," particularly for treating venereal complaints (1773, 9). The linguistic register associated with syringes, including terms and ideas of injecting and squirting, was used in imagery and descriptions of male sexual organs, fluids, and actions. This kind of language signified a broader literary adoption of physiological ideas about nervous and sexual fluids moving between the brain and, the otherwise, mechanical male genitals.

Even early in the century, the sexual sense of syringes and injections had become firmly established in non-medical discussions. *The Works of the Earls of Rochester, Roscommon, Dorset, &c.* that Edmund Curll published early in the century was bound with a collection of bawdy works called *The Cabinet of Love*, which included "The Delights of Venus." That poem employs a standard erotic narrative, in which an experienced woman gives a virgin maid detailed sexual advice. The piece concludes with the maid praising her tutor:

> She taught me first the Raptures which proceed
> From the Injection of Man's gen'rous – . (1714, 24)

Seed was invested with animal spirits that, as suggested by this couplet and contemporaneous medical writings, endowed pleasure upon contact with the sensitive genital organs. A new emphasis about the function of male members as seminal injectors, in both non-medical and medical writings, possibly corroborate Tim Hitchcock's suggestion of a significant increase in "forms of phallo-centric, penetrative sex" in eighteenth-century England (Hitchcock 1996, 85).

Prose writings also explored these syringe metaphors and ideas about animal spirits and seed. In a scene from *The History of the Amours of the Marshal de Boufflers*, the incorrigible rake and eponymous protagonist is upbraided by his laundress, Judith, "O what a pretty sort of Clyster you were about to apply to me!" (D.P.E., 1726, 212). Through a figurative use of clyster, Judith accuses de Boufflers of attempting anal sex with her. When pressed about this transgressive attempt, de Boufflers offers to try "the proper place where such Applications ought to be made." The trope continues as a verb with de Boufflers commenting "Let us try whether I can Syringe you right there or not" – he does. In this episode, the syringe metaphor as a euphemism enables the discussion of an offensive kind of sexual conduct, which would otherwise have incurred some censure. But, the same metaphor was also used as a direct and technical expression of transgressive sexual acts, particularly in criminal cases. In May of 1722, the fifteen-year-old James Booty was tried in court for the rape of five-year-old Ann Milton (*Select Trials* 1742, 198–201). During the proceedings, a witness surgeon Mr Holloway was asked "Do you think she [Ann Milton] could have been infected in that Manner, if there had not been an *Emissio Seminis*?" (199). Holloway reasoned that such a "Disease may be communicated by the Emission of an infectious Matter, without a seminal Injection" (191). Many other court testimonies of medical specialists invoked a similar usage of "injection."[8] The trial of George Duffus for sodomy concluded that "The Spermatick Injection not being proved, the Court directed the Jury to bring in their Verdict *Special*" (*Select Trials* 1742, 107). During the eighteenth century, "Spermatick Injection" equated to the legal categorization of "Emissio Seminis," which was a determination of whether an ejaculation occurred and a requisite proof for many rape and sodomy cases. On several occasions medical practitioners witnessing in trials of sexual crimes directly introduced their understanding and language linking syringes with male organs of generation.

Other literary descriptions of male genitalia in terms of hydraulic mechanisms explored more deeply the implications for sensible bodies and minds. John Cleland's notorious erotic novel, *Memoirs of a Woman of Pleasure*, or *Fanny Hill*, shows the penis-syringe trope to be firmly entrenched in the mid-century's erotic register. For instance, one episode wherein Fanny copulates with her lover describes, "I touched that sweetly critical point, when scarce prevented by the spermatic injection from my partner spurting liquid fire up to my vitals, I dissolved, and breaking out into a deep drawn sigh, sent my whole sensitive soul down to that passage where escape was denied it, by its being so deliciously plugged and choked up" (Cleland 2001, 161). More than merely resorting to medical jargon for variation's sake, Cleland's erotic imagery and depictions of sexual bodies were profoundly physiological. For example, Cleland described how Fanny and her fellow prostitute Louisa arouse an unwitting lad's erection: "by all the irritations we had used to put the principles of pleasure effectually into motion, and to wind up the springs of its organ to their supreme pitch; and it stood accordingly stiff and straining, ready to burst with the blood and spirits that swelled it" (199–200). This portrayal, like many others in *Fanny Hill*, recalls a physiology of erection based on mechanics, blood, and spirits that medical figures like Swammerdam, Boerhaave, and Bartholin had previously described. This borrowing from the physiological register also appears in Cleland's depictions of ejaculation. A later episode involves Fanny's "whole spirits of life and sensation, rushing impetuously to the cock-pit ... and clustering to a point there" as her gallant "spouted" into her "a potent overflow of the balsamic injection" (189). Again, spirits and injections are employed, but the ejaculate is described as balsamic. Elsewhere Fanny relates a man's "oily balsamic injection mixing deliciously with the sluices in flow from me" (120). Boerhaave had likewise defined semen as a "thick balsamick Humour" (1746, 70), which referred not only to the fluid's consistency but to its soothing quality. One explanation for *Fanny Hill*'s debt to medical and anatomical discussions is that Cleland had an active interest in those disciplines. But his interest was part of a greater movement, wherein literary authors generally referred to physiological ideas to explore sexual and sensible bodies.

This erotic syringe trope made another notorious appearance in a novel that Cleland deemed as bawdy that "gives no sensations" – Laurence Sterne's *The Life and Opinions of Tristram Shandy, Gentleman* (Cash 1992, 92). Sterne levelled many satirical pokes at medicine, anatomy, physiology, mechanical philosophy, and especially in reference to (man-) midwifery. Early in the novel while Tristram is still being birthed, the obstetrical theme widens to include a short argument about baptismal squirts.[9] Squirts were used for cases "in which a mother cannot deliver her child, and in which the child is held in its mother's womb in such a way that it cannot make any part of its body appear, which ... would be a case, according to the Rituals, to baptize it" (Sterne 1978b, 103).[10] This religious interference in obstetrical matters, especially while wielding an injecting tool, corresponds to the "parallel between the conduct of male accoucheurs and that of the Catholic clergy," which the controversial historian A.D. Harvey has rightly observed (2001, 56). Sterne continued ridiculing these squirt baptisms by asking "whether, after the ceremony of marriage, and before that of consummation, the baptizing all the HOMUNCULI at once, slap-dash, by *injection*, would not be a shorter and safer cut still" (1978a, 69–70). This procedure, he suggested, would be done "*par le moyen d'une* petite canulle, and, *sans faire aucun tort a le pere*" (1978a, 70).[11] As in much of *Tristram Shandy*, theories of generation, male sexuality, and the physiology of sensibility are the backdrop to this segment about squirts. With a wink and a nod, Sterne introduced syringes and allowed their many meanings – medical, mechanical, sexual, and sensible – to dawn on the knowing reader.

Legacies of Spirits and Syringes

Syringes became more than just figurative phalluses: they were adapted to be both sexual and reproductive devices. Those seeking to enhance their private pleasures could benefit from squirting dildos. In the lewd book *A New Atalantis for the Year One Thousand Seven Hundred and Fifty-Eight*, such a device was acquired and used by the lascivious young maid Tonzenie, who took her sexual cues from reading "Ovid's Art of Love, Rochester's works, and the Memoirs of a Woman of Pleasure" (1758, 52). While Tonzenie pleasured herself, her French maid, who was "well skilled in such practices, would in the moment of rapture, dart a warm injection; nay, sometimes artfully gird it to her loins, and act the man with her young mistress" (1758, 52–3).[12] Physiological descriptions, figurative associations, and these dildos that mimicked male ejaculations foreshadowed the first documented human artificial insemination, which John Hunter designed using a syringe. A man who had a hypospadias and could not impregnate his wife was advised by Hunter to "be prepared with a syringe fitted for the purpose, previously warmed; and that, immediately after the emission had taken place, it should be taken up by the syringe, and injected into the vagina, while the female organs were still under the influence of the coitus" (Home 1799, 8). This move to insemination by manual injection was not a giant leap; preceding decades of anatomical practices, literary imagery, and erotic devices portended this mechanical replacement of a penis in experiment.

Around the same time as Hunter's experiment, William Smellie (the encyclopaedist, not the man-midwife) asserted that male and female genitals without nerves and spirits "convey nothing more than the idea of an automaton, or self-moving machine" (1790, 78–9). For most of the eighteenth century, animal spirits embodied the non-mechanical, non-material, and active elements essential to human generation and sexual physiology. That fluid occupied a central role in the function of male organs of generation, a role which was reinforced by the hydraulic qualities emphasized through penis-syringe analogies. But Smellie also deemed animal spirits a "subject covered with darkness, and which all the efforts of human powers will probably never bring to light" (1790, 81). Efforts to illuminate these animal spirits were rapidly diminishing even before Smellie's words made print. Electricity assumed the role of animal spirits in nerve experiments, reproductive physiologies, sexual therapies, and experimental demonstrations. At the close of the century, the dominant physiological understandings of male organs of generation – a simple combination of mechanical parts and spiritous fluid – fell from favour, although the register of animal spirits would linger in erotic and sensibility literature.

NOTES

1 See Ferrari for a discussion of the relationship between eighteenth-century sensibility and anatomy (1987, 50–106).

2 See Haigh (1976), McMaster (1988), Mullan (1988), Stephanson (1988), Barker-Benfield (1992), Van Sant (1993), and Rousseau (2007).

3 See Knoeff for an analysis of male testes and penises prepared by Ruysch (2012, 43–58).
4 Translation by Andrew Klein.
5 For the early modern medical marketplace in England, see Jenner and Wallis (2007, 1–23).
6 For the anatomical career and techniques of Alexander Monro *primus*, see Lawrence (1988).
7 See *Democritus, the Laughing Philosopher's Trip into England* (London, 1723); *The Adventures of a Kidnapped Orphan* (London, 1747).
8 A 1727 case brought against Thomas Padget of Fulham for the rape of five-year-old Catherine Burchet found the accused guilty because a shared infection suggested "an Injection had been made on the Orifice" (Trial of Thomas Padget 1727).
9 In the seventeenth century, squirts and syringes were interchangeable terms. However, squirts increasingly referred specifically to the religious tool.
10 Quoting a translation of "Memoire" from *The Life and Opinions of Tristram Shandy, Gentleman*, ed. J.A. Work (New York: Odyssey Press, 1940).
11 Translated as "by means of a little injection-pipe, and, without doing any harm to the father" (Sterne 1978b, 106).
12 Also referred to by Harvey (2001, 44).

REFERENCES

Ambrose, C. 2007. "The Priority Dispute over the Function of the Lymphatic System and Glisson's Ghost (the 18th-Century Hunter-Monro Feud)." *Cellular Immunology* 245 (1): 7–15. http://dx.doi.org/10.1016/j.cellimm.2007.02.015.

Barker-Benfield, G.J. 1992. *The Culture of Sensibility: Sex and Society in Eighteenth-Century Britain*. Chicago: University of Chicago Press.

Bartholin, T. 1668. *Bartholinus Anatomy.* London: N. Culpeper and A. Cole.

Bayford, T. 1773. *The Effects of Injections into the Urethra, and the Use and Abuse of Those Remedies....* London: J. Whiston.

Boerhaave, H. 1746. *Dr. Boerhaave's Academical Lectures on the Theory of Physic*. Vol. 5. London: Innys.

Booth, E. 2005. *"A Subtle and Mysterious Machine": The Medical World of Walter Charleton (1619–1707)*. Dordrecht: Springer. http://dx.doi.org/10.1007/1-4020-3378-8.

Cash, A. 1992. *Laurence Sterne: The Later Years*. London: Routledge.

A Catalogue of Several Curious Figures of Human Anatomy in Wax. 1736. London.

Charleton, W. 1659. *Natural History of Nutrition, Life, and Voluntary Motion ....* London: H. Herringman.
Cleland, J. (1748–9) 2001. *Fanny Hill; or Memoirs of a Woman of Pleasure.* Edited by P. Wagner. London: Penguin.
Cock, C. 1736. *A Catalogue of Several Curious Figures of Human Anatomy in Wax.* London.
Cole, F.J. 1921. "The History of Anatomical Injections." In *Studies in the History and Method of Science*, vol. 2, edited by C.J. Singer, 285–343. Oxford: Clarendon Press.
Cook, J. 1730. *An Anatomical and Mechanical Essay on the Whole Animal Oeconomy.* London: W. Meadows.
Cowper, W. 1698. *The Anatomy of Humane Bodies with Figures.* Oxford: S. Smith and B. Walford.
Craske, M. 2011. "'Unwholesome' and 'Pornographic': A Reassessment of the Place of Rackstrow's Museum in the Story of Eighteenth-Century Anatomical Collection and Exhibition." *Journal of the History of Collections* 23 (1): 75–99. http://dx.doi.org/10.1093/jhc/fhq018.
De Graaf, R. 1668. *De Virorum Organis Generationi Inservientibus, de Clÿsteribus et de Usu Siphonis in Anatomia.* Leiden and Rotterdam: Hack.
"The Delights of Venus." 1714. In *The Works of the Earls of Rochester, Roscommon, Dorset.* 4th ed., 11–24. London: E. Curll.
D.P.E. 1726. *The History of the Amours of the Marshal de Boufflers.* 2nd ed. London: E. Mory.
Drake, J. 1707. *Anthropologia Nova: Or, a New System of Anatomy.* 2nd ed. Vol. 1. London: W. Innys.
D'Urfey, T. 1719. "Pretty Pegg of Wandsor." In *Songs Compleat, Pleasant and Divertive; Set to Musick.* Vol. 2, edited by H. Playford, 128–31. London: printed by W. Person for J. Tonson.
Evans, J. 2012. "'Gentle Purges corrected with hot Spices, whether they work or not, do vehemently provoke Venery': Menstrual Provocation and Procreation in Early Modern England." *Social History of Medicine* 25 (1): 2–19. http://dx.doi.org/10.1093/shm/hkr021.
Ferrari, G. 1987. "Public Anatomy Lessons and the Carnival: The Anatomy Theatre of Bologna." *Past & Present* 117 (1): 50–106. http://dx.doi.org/10.1093/past/117.1.50.
Gibson, T. 1682. *The Anatomy of Human Bodies Epitomiz'd.* London: M. Flesher.
Guerrini, A. 2006. "Alexander Monro Primus and the Moral Theatre of Anatomy." *Eighteenth Century* (Lubbock, TX.) 47 (1): 1–18. http://dx.doi.org/10.1353/ecy.2007.0018.

Haggerty, G. 1999. *Men in Love: Masculinity and Sexuality in the Eighteenth Century*. New York: Columbia University Press.
Haigh, E. 1976. "Vitalism, the Soul, and Sensibility: The Physiology of Théophile Bordeu." *Journal of the History of Medicine and Allied Sciences* 31 (1): 30–41. http://dx.doi.org/10.1093/jhmas/XXXI.1.30.
Hansen, J.V. 1996. "Resurrecting Death: Anatomical Art in the Cabinet of Dr. Frederik Ruysch." *Art Bulletin* 78 (4): 663–79. http://dx.doi.org/10.2307/3046214.
Harvey, A.D. 2001. *Sex in Georgian England: Attitudes and Prejudices from the 1720s to the 1820s*. London: Phoenix Press.
Heister, L. 1752. *A Compendium of Anatomy*. London: W. Innys et al.
Hitchcock, T. 1996. "Redefining Sex in Eighteenth-Century England." *History Workshop Journal* 41 (spring): 72–90. http://dx.doi.org/10.1093/hwj/1996.41.72.
Home, E. 1799. *An Account of the Dissection of an Hermaphrodite Dog*. London.
Hunter, W. 1758. "Facts Relating to the Dispute between Dr. Hunter and Dr. Monro." In *The Critical Review: or, Annals of Literature. By A Society of Gentlemen*, vol. 4, edited by T. Smollett, 437–9. London: R. Baldwin.
Jenner, M.S.R., and P. Wallis. 2007. "The Medical Marketplace." In *Medicine and the Market in England and Its Colonies, c. 1450–c. 1850*, edited by M.S.R. Jenner and P. Wallis, 1–23. Basingstoke: Palgrave Macmillan. http://dx.doi.org/10.1057/9780230591462.
Jordanova, L. 1993. *Sexual Visions: Images of Gender in Science and Medicine between the Eighteenth and Twentieth Centuries*. Madison: University of Wisconsin Press.
Knoeff, R. 2012. "Sex in Public: On the Spectacle of Female Anatomy in Amsterdam around 1700." *L'Homme: Europäische Zeitschrift für feministische Geschichtswissenschaft* 23 (1): 43–58.
Laqueur, T. 1990. *Making Sex: Body and Gender from the Greeks to Freud*. Cambridge, MA: Harvard University Press.
Lawrence, C. 1988. "Alexander Monro *Primus* and the Edinburgh Manner of Anatomy." *Bulletin of the History of Medicine* 62 (2): 193–214.
Liekse, P. 2011. "'Made in Imitation of Real Women and Children': Obstetrical Machines in Eighteenth-Century Britain." In *The Female Body in Medicine and Literature*, edited by A. Mangham and G. Depledge, 69–88. Liverpool: University of Liverpool Press.
Marten, J. 1708. *A Treatise of all the Degrees and Symptoms of the Venereal Disease, in both Sexes.* 6th ed. London: S. Crouch et al.
McMaster, J. 1988. *Reading the Body in the Eighteenth-Century Novel*. Basingstoke: Palgrave Macmillan.

Monro, A. 1755. *Dissertatio Medica Inauguralis, de Testibus et de Semine in Variis Animalibus.* Edinburgh: G. Hamilton and J. Balfour.

Monro, A. 1758. *Observations, Anatomical and Physiological, wherein Dr. Hunter's Claim to some Discoveries is Examined.* Edinburgh: Hamilton, Balfour, and Neill.

Mullan, J. 1988. *Sentiment and Sociability: The Language of Feeling in the Eighteenth Century.* Oxford: Oxford University Press.

A New Atalantis, for the Year One Thousand Seven Hundred and Fifty-Eight. 1758. 2nd ed. London: M. Thrush.

Paterson, S. 1769. *A Catalogue of Anatomical Preparations and some Anatomical Apparatus, the Property of a Surgeon (Who has declined Lecturing).* London.

A Philosophical Essay on Fecundation: Or, an Impartial Inquiry into the First Rudiments, Progression and Perfection, of Animal Generation .... 1742. London: J. Roberts.

Pole, T. 1790. *The Anatomical Instructor; Or, an Illustration of the Modern and Most Approved Methods of Preparing and Preserving the Different Parts of the Human Body, and of Quadrupeds.* London: Couchman and Fry.

Rackstrow's Museum. 1784. *A Descriptive Catalogue (Giving a Full Explanation) of Rackstrow's Museum.* London.

Rousseau, G.S. 2007. "Temperament and the Long Shadow of Nerves in the Eighteenth Century." In *Brain, Mind and Medicine: Essays in Eighteenth-Century Neuroscience*, edited by H. Whitaker, C.U.M. Smith, and S. Finger, 353–69. New York: Springer. http://dx.doi.org/10.1007/978-0-387-70967-3_26.

Select Trials at the Sessions-House in the Old Bailey, for Murder, Robberies, Rapes, Sodomy.... 1742. Vol. 1. London: Printed by J. Applebee for J. Hodges.

Smellie, W. 1790. *The Philosophy of Natural History.* Vol. 1. Dublin: W. Porter. http://dx.doi.org/10.1037/14228-000.

Smith, L. 2011. "The Body Embarrassed? Rethinking the Leaky Male Body in Eighteenth-Century England and France." *Gender & History* 23 (1): 26–46. http://dx.doi.org/10.1111/j.1468-0424.2010.01622.x.

Stephanson, R. 1988. "Richardson's 'Nerves': The Physiology of Sensibility in *Clarissa*." *Journal of the History of Ideas* 49 (2): 267–85. http://dx.doi.org/10.2307/2709500.

Stephanson, R. 2004. *The Yard of Wit: Male Creativity and Sexuality, 1650–1750.* Philadelphia: University of Pennsylvania Press.

Sterne, L. (1759–67) 1978a. *The Life and Opinions of Tristram Shandy, Gentleman. The Florida Edition of the Works of Laurence Sterne.* Vol. 1. Edited by M. New and J. New. Gainesville: University Press of Florida.

Sterne, L. (1759–67) 1978b. *The Life and Opinions of Tristram Shandy, Gentleman. The Florida Edition of the Works of Laurence Sterne.* Vol. 3. Edited by M. New and J. New. Gainesville: University Press of Florida.

Thomson, G. 1739. *Syllabus. Pointing Out Every Part of the Human System … the Anatomical Wax-Figures, of the Late Monsieur Denoue.* London: J. Hughs.

Trial of Thomas Padget for Rape, 22 February 1727. *Old Bailey Online*. Reference Number: t17270222-72.

Van Diemerbroeck, I. 1694. *The Anatomy of Human Bodies*. Translated by W. Salmon. London: W. Whitwood.

Van Sant, A.J. 1993. *Eighteenth-Century Sensibility and the Novel: The Senses in Social Context*. Cambridge: Cambridge University Press.

Wahrman, D. 2008. "Change and the Corporeal in Seventeenth- and Eighteenth-Century Gender History: Or, Can Cultural History Be Rigorous?" *Gender & History* 20 (3): 584–602. http://dx.doi.org/10.1111/j.1468-0424.2008.00538.x.

Williams, G. 1994. *A Dictionary of Sexual Language and Imagery in Shakespearean and Stuart Literature*. London: Athlone Press.

Willis, T. 1684. *Dr. Willis's Practice of Physick.* London: T. Dring; C. Harper; and J. Leigh.

Willis, T. 1980. *Thomas Willis's Oxford Lectures, compiled by R. Lower and J. Locke*. Edited by K. Dewhurst. Oxford: Sandford.

Wilson, C. 1995. *The Invisible World: Early Modern Philosophy and the Invention of the Microscope*. Princeton: Princeton University Press.

PART FOUR

Attitudes, Tropes, Satire

18 The *Aristotle* Texts, Sex, and the American Woman

MARCIA D. NICHOLS

America in the late eighteenth century witnessed a proliferation of print discourse on reproduction. American printers both reissued influential British texts on the subject and published new works from American pens. It seems likely that a scarcity of medical professionals combined with a dispersed population made home health guides particularly relevant for American readers. Moreover, the increasing intrusion of male professionals into women's reproductive health, coupled with the isolation of frontier living, began to break down traditional female networks. This situation perhaps made midwifery and child rearing guides especially appealing. Thus, Mason Weems, the book agent of Philadelphia printer Matthew Carrey, offered many medical titles to his rural clients, including British midwifery guides by Alexander Hamilton and Thomas Denman, as well as American midwifery guides by Samuel Bard and William Dewees (Letters of Weems/Carrey). Despite the prevalence of these new scientific works, one name remained a popular cheap-print alternative in the catalogues of itinerant booksellers – *Aristotle's Masterpiece*. However, there were actually two distinct versions of this hoary tome available in America (*Aristotle's Complete Masterpiece* [herein Version C] and *Aristotle's Masterpiece Completed* [herein Version B]), and each of these was grounded in opposing ideals or types of women. At this time two different concepts of female sexual nature were in play – the new concept that understood women as naturally chaste and modest, and the traditional older one that understood women as naturally lascivious (Godbeer 2002; Lyons 2006; Foster 2006; Zagarri 2007; Bloch 2003; Block 2006; Klepp 2009; and see Peakman and Watkins in this volume). *Aristotle's Complete Masterpiece* (Version C), with its scurrilous doggerel and jesting tone, would seem to be more in tune with the traditional concept of female sexual nature, the one that saw most women as "no better than she should be." However, beginning in the 1780s, American printers began reissuing *Aristotle's Masterpiece Completed* (Version B). With its more sober tone and emphasis on female modesty, it would seem to be meant to appeal to the emerging belief in female sexual continence. I will briefly sketch these two "types" of women before examining how the differences between each version of the *Aristotle* texts fit into these separate discourses on feminine sexuality and bodily sex.

Sex and the American Woman

In the eighteenth century, ideas about femininity were in flux. According to many thinkers of the Scottish Enlightenment, the "natural" modesty, chastity, and passivity of women made them the vessels of morality, progress, and civilization. Stadial histories of human progress envisioned women's sexual reluctance as channelling men's passions into technological and scientific achievements; hence, women's status as matrimonial property became the telltale sign of the state of a civilization's progress. Through a woman's influence alone could men morph from beasts to gentlemen. As Roy Porter explains, "The privatization of women as exclusive personal belongings thus accorded them a role, however passive, in social progress; for as wives they could inspire the ripening of male sentiments and passions, even if they hardly developed into higher beings themselves. The sex was thus instrumental in bringing about the ends of progress" (2003, 260). A woman's ability to civilize derived from her role as not only a wife, but also as a moral mother, which reflected the belief that mothers should dedicate themselves to nurturing and educating their children. "Natural" moral maternity was reconceptualized as the primary role for women, motherhood, childrearing (Schiebinger 1993; Leavitt 1986; Bloch 1978), and maternal breastfeeding (see Boon's chapter in this volume). Whether written by women or by medical men, home health manuals were important vehicles in promulgating these ideas. For instance, in *Advice to Mothers* (1809), William Buchan describes a mother as "her who faithfully discharges the duties of a parent – whose chief concern is the well-being of her infant – and who feels all her cares amply repaid by its growth and activity" (Buchan 1809/1972, 3). This woman had no cares outside of her offspring.

During the same period, employment opportunities for women were truncating in response to changing economies, as local systems began moving from largely self-sustaining domestic economies into part of the emerging capitalistic consumer economy. In many areas, production moved from home to workplace, effectively reducing some women's ability to earn.

Nevertheless, fashion also played a decisive role in the changes in women's work. As a consumerist economy developed, women were increasingly styled as the consumer. The leisure of its female members became a way for a family to put on fashionable airs. Increasingly, daughters were not sent out to learn trades, even that of housewifery. At the same time, reformers called for better female education, primarily for this new leisured middle class of women (Hill 1989; Crane 1994; Karlsen and Crumpacker 1984).

Decreasing employment opportunities also affected the practice of women's health care. Whereas earlier traditional medical care had been a central part of housewifery and specialized care had fallen to midwifery, in this new era the idea that women had insight into their own health and bodies was being superseded by male authority grounded in "heroic" medicine. Even in rural communities on the American frontier, like the Kennebec Maine region of midwife Martha Ballard, the generations of formally trained man-midwives had made inroads into the birthing room and into women's health care in general (Ulrich 1990). Midwives were increasingly portrayed as inept – dangerous even – unless under the tutelage and direction of male physicians. Pioneering accoucheurs declared women's health – soon to be dubbed "gynaecology" and "obstetrics" – their conquered province, saved from the barbarity of meddlesome women.

Nevertheless, new ideals of domesticity did not go uncriticized. Many women in Britain and the newborn United States made protests such as Mary Wollstonecraft's in her *Vindication of the Rights of Women* (1792), claiming that marital slavery was being inaccurately described as benevolent social progress. American women actively read and debated the ideas of Wollstonecraft. In post-Revolutionary America, as Rosemarie Zagarri explains, "the concept of women's rights took on a life of its own. A widespread public debate ensued over what it meant for women to have rights and whether women shared the same rights, including political rights as men" (Zagarri 2007, 42). In various print media, men and women discussed and debated women's intellectual, spiritual, and political equality with men. Wollstonecraft's plea for better education found an especially receptive audience in the new nation. Annis B. Stockton wrote that women's "faults" were caused by "*education*, not our *sex*."

> … the source which makes the female mind
> Too oft appear but puerile and blind;
> How many would surmount stern custom's laws,
> And prove the want of *genius* not the cause;
> But that the odium of a *bookish fair*,

> Or *female pedant*, or "*they quit their sphere*,"
> Damps all their views, and they must drag the chain,
> And sigh for sweet instruction's page in vain. (Stockton 1995, 89–90)

Women could be intellectually equal to men if given the chance; however, the rare woman who attempted to improve her mind faced scorn and mockery from men themselves, thus resulting in the reductive teleology that kept women intellectually inferior to men. Stockton's poem asks the male reader to help women out of this bind by ceasing to damn those who sought self-improvement. Many other American writers, including Charles Brockden Brown and Judith Sargent Murray, agreed with Stockton's assessment (Branson 2001). Indeed, as moral motherhood became the dominant feminine ideal, women's education took on a political urgency – the uneducated mother would not be able to provide her sons with the proper guidance and upbringing that would ensure they would grow into responsible citizens.

The change in women's economic and social roles necessitated a similar change in how female sexual nature was understood. Traditionally, women had been seen as sexually voracious, in need of male dominance to keep their appetites in check. Although this idea did not disappear, as the concept of biological sex difference emerged, "natural chastity" became located in the female body. Wollstonecraft declared, "As a sex, women are more chaste than men; and as modesty is the effect of chastity, they may deserve to have this virtue ascribed to them in rather an appropriated sense" (Wollstonecraft 1792/1992, 235). Wollstonecraft and others blamed faulty education for women's sexual frailty. Girls needed to be educated as intellectual beings, rather than encouraged to be coquettish spectacles, if their chastity was to be ensured. Wollstonecraft was not alone in her concern to make girls less seducible. Much of the cultural anxiety about non-marital sexual activity can be traced to the actions of actual women. In Revolutionary America, women were engaging in extramarital intercourse in apparently record numbers. At this period in Philadelphia illegitimacy rates were on the rise (Lyons 2006, 73), and in New England "between 30 and 40 percent of brides" were pregnant (Godbeer 2002, 228). Yet, at the same time birth rates were steadily declining among white women in the North, suggesting a growing use of family planning methods (Klepp 2009), and perhaps indicating that premarital or extramarital sex was even more widespread than the number of births suggest. As Clare Lyons expresses it, for perhaps the first time, "Pursuing sexual pleasure for its own sake could be envisioned" (2006, 73). Women of the lower orders visibly engaged in extralegal marital practices such as private marriage, self-divorce, and remarriage. Across the social spectrum practices like bundling – individuals of the opposite sex sleeping together while at least partially dressed, and characterized by one scholar as "nocturnal courting" – seems to have been commonplace. Discursively, bawdy humour in cheap and ephemeral print helped normalize such behaviour (Lyons 2006; Godbeer 2002). However, more polite discourse tended to condemn female sexual laxity. For instance, medical writers identified unregulated sexual practices as a source of health problems, while seduction novels lingered over the regret-filled deaths of their wayward heroines. In either case, cheap-print readers would seem to have had the choice of an *Aristotle* text that subscribed to whichever version of female sexual nature they preferred.

The Many Faces of Aristotle

The group of texts identified as *Aristotle's Masterpiece*, a motley collection of folk remedies and sex advice, was hands-down the best-selling English advice book in the eighteenth century. It had "gone through at least forty-three editions by 1800, and quite probably scores more now unrecorded or lost" (Porter 1994, 136). Although scholars sometimes treat the various versions as a largely monolithic text, lumping the several distinct titles and editions together (Fissell 2003a; Fissell 2003b), in the eighteenth century there were at least three distinct versions of *Aristotle's Masterpiece* (not to mention *Aristotle's Complete Midwife*, *Aristotle's Problems*, and *Aristotle's Last Legacy*). These versions are different in tone and implied an audience. Although this chapter is only concerned with the two later versions (*Aristotle's Complete Masterpiece* [1795] and *Aristotle's Masterpiece Completed* [1788]), a brief description of all three versions is in order.

The original *Aristotle's Masterpiece* (Version A) was originally published in 1684 and seems to have largely fallen out of print by the 1720s. This text purported to address a female audience to inform them about sexual intercourse, conception, and childbirth. Despite the later reputation of the *Aristotle* books as bawdy (Bullough 1973; Beall 1963; Wagner 1988; Porter 1985), this text takes a pious, even Puritan tone, quoting *Paradise Lost*: "God out of the abundance of his Goodness, sent forth his Holy Spirit, who Dove-like, with mighty out-spread Wings, sat brooding on the Vast Abyss, and made it Pregnant" (*Aristotle's Masterpiece* 1694/1986, i). Moreover, the text advocates companionate marriage as early as the 1680s. As scholars have long pointed out, the text is largely a collection of traditional humoral medical wisdom; however, there does seem to be an awareness of scientific innovations – namely, embryology and William Harvey's declaration that all life came from ova.

A second revised and altered version, *Aristotle's Masterpiece Completed* (Version B) appears to have been first published in 1697. It fell out of print in the 1720s but had a revival in the late eighteenth century. Also addressed to a female audience, Part 1 focused on marriage, intercourse, and birth while Part 2 focused on female complaints, from menstrual problems to postpartum care. Part 1 of Version B was substantially derived from the original. Mary Fissell identifies John Sadler's *The Sick Woman's Private Looking Glass* (1636) as the primary source for Part 2, "A Private Looking Glass" (2003a, 63). As an ordered consideration of female complaints from menstrual problems to postpartum care, Version B was the most reader-friendly and possibly useful of the three versions.

These two versions were eclipsed by the substantially different third version, *Aristotle's Complete Masterpiece* (Version C). Its tone attempted to be witty, even urbane. Although it still seemed to expect its heterogeneous audience of men and women to be primarily interested in marital and procreative sex, it had lost all of the piety of the previous versions. Indeed, this is the version that contained the infamous doggerel verses, giving it a levity not found in the other two. Moreover, it went beyond a simple marital and sexual health guide. The first half focused on sexual health and pregnancy, but the second consisted of a treatise on physiognomy and a collection of fanciful medicinal recipes (such as "man's skull prepar'd" for epilepsy). Moreover, while the changes are subtle, it registers an increased awareness of and comfort with the current embryological theories of ova and what would come to be called sperm. In what follows, I will look in more detail at the differences between the two *Aristotle* texts available to American readers, versions C and B.

Version C

By far the most well-known and successful version of the *Aristotle* books was the third published, *Aristotle's Complete Masterpiece* (Version C). According to the *English Short Title Catalogue* (ESTC), it was first printed in 1702, and was then reprinted nearly every year either in Britain or America well into the early nineteenth century. This version was most likely the *Aristotle* book the young people were reading, over which a scandal erupted in Jonathan Edward's Northampton, Massachusetts parish in 1744. Some young men were reading at least two books "about women's having children[n]," and, armed with illicit knowledge, they teased young women in the parish about knowing their "secrets" (Johnson 1932, 44). Pointing out that young women were present at many of the readings, Ava Chamberlain observes that "reading became flirting, even incipient foreplay" among the young people of Edwards's congregation. This shared reading had gone on for at least five years before Edwards got wind of it and put a stop to it (Chamberlain 2002). For Edwards, this heterosocial exploration of sexual knowledge was clearly dangerous. Let us examine the contents to discover what these playful young people might have learned.

The treatise itself begins with a description of male and female genitalia, replete with Latin and medical (or quasi-Latin and quasi-medical) terminology. The anatomical information provided is all traditional stuff, much the same as that found in Nicholas Culpeper's *Directory for Midwives* (1651) or Jane Sharp's *The Midwives' Book* (1671/1999). Despite its grounding in a surpassed medical paradigm, however, Version C still engages with Enlightenment debates on embryology and perceptions of biological sex. The language partially embraces Harvey's revolutionary declaration that life comes from ova but, at the same time, does not entirely relinquish the older terminology of female seed. Thus, Version C seems to be a transitional text in the historical switch from a one-sex to a two-sex model (Laqueur 1990). The ovicular language is part of a two-sex discourse that saw male and female bodies as radically different, whereas the language of female seed used a Galenic model of the body, which Thomas Laqueur identifies as one-sex. Version C fluctuates between these two positions, suggesting that for eighteenth-century cheap-print readers, male and female bodies were both homologous and radically different – and women could be lascivious or chaste depending upon the discursive situation.

The embryological debates about sperm and eggs had important implications for the understanding of female sexual nature. The idea that women were egg-producers derives from the publication of *De Generatione* (1651), in which William Harvey revolutionized embryology and the science of sexual difference by rejecting both the Galenic theory that life came from a mixture of male and female seed and the Hippocratic and Aristotelian theories that male seed acted upon female matter (menstrual blood) to create life, to declare instead "that all animals whatsoever, even the viviparous, and man himself not excepted, are produced from ova" (Harvey 1989, 170). Although Harvey did not discover the egg in the ovary, he maintained that male seed, through "contagion," was the prime efficient that sparked ova into epigenetic development. The ovum was independent of the uterus, which was merely a vessel to contain and protect the ovum after fertilization. As part of his evidence against Galen's theory of female seed, Harvey argued that

> the females of all lower animals, and all women, do not experience any such emission of fluid, and that conception is nowise impossible in cases where it does not take place, for I have known several, who without anything of the kind were sufficiently prolific, and even some who after experiencing such an emission and having had great enjoyment, nevertheless appeared to have lost somewhat of their wonted fecundity; and then an infinite number of instances might be quoted of women, who, although they have great satisfaction in intercourse, still emit nothing, and yet conceive. (Harvey 1650/1989, 298–9)

By pointing out that orgasm, and female ejaculation during orgasm in particular, seemed to have no influence whatsoever on conception, Harvey set in motion the line of thinking that, by the nineteenth century, had separated orgasm from pleasure and pleasure from conception, at least in women. As Patricia Crawford describes, "It was much easier to argue in the eighteenth century that good women did not enjoy sex" (1994, 87).

The contradictory explanations of biological sex are perhaps best highlighted by one of the unique features of Version C – the bits of scurrilous doggerel that wittily summarize each section. The content of the poems often cut against the information in the text itself. For example, the poem summarizing the section on female anatomy contradicted the two-sex model just laid out:

> Thus the Womens secrets I have survey'd,
> And let them see how curiously they're made:
> And that, tho' they of different Sexes be,
> Yet in the whole they are the same as we:
> For those that have the strictest Searchers been,
> Find Women are but Men turn'd Out side in:
> And Men, if they but cast their Eyes about,
> May find they're Women, with their Inside out. (Version C 1749/1986, 23)

This poem presented a one-sex view of the body, equating male and female bodies. However, the chapter itself presented male and female as incommensurable through the separate production of sperm and eggs respectively (although the clitoris was still described as a female penis). This seeming contradiction is not evidence so much of sloppy editing as it is of the human ability to accept and hold contrary notions. The female body could be incredibly different from the male *and* incredibly the same. Perhaps more unsettling for the male reader, the final couplet reduced his sense of masculine privilege by describing his genitals as inverted female genitals. He might simply be a woman in disguise and not a man at all!

Nevertheless, the doggerel affirmed masculine superiority. The tone of the poem was that of condescension, an expert teaching the ignorant. Women were directed not to examine themselves, but to look into this male-authored text to learn about themselves, obviating female self-knowledge. In medical discourse at large, men declared that women did not possess bodily secrets that only they could discern. No longer could women rely on their own sensations to determine if they were pregnant or if the child had quickened. Such knowledge had to be verified by male experts. In contrast, the poem on male genitalia lauded male sexuality:

> And thus Man's noble parts describ'd we see,
> For such the parts of Generation be;
> And they that carefully surveys, will find,
> Each part is fitted for the Use design'd.
> The purest blood, we find, if well we heed,
> Is in the Testicles turn'd into Seed,
> Which by most proper Channels is transmitted,
> Into the Place by Nature for it fittest:
> With highest Sense of Pleasure to excite
> In amorous Combatants the more Delight
> For Nature does in this great Work design
> Profit and Pleasure, in one Act to join. (Version C 1749/1986, 14–15)

The focus shifted from anatomical description to a celebration of male sexual conquest, a shift in concert with the entrenching belief in men's sexual prerogative (Foster 2006; Block 2006). The poem seems designed to encourage male readers to seek the "Profit and Pleasure" promised in the poem by having sex with and impregnating a woman. For male readers, self-knowledge needed experiential verification. In contrast, for female readers, because their truth was hidden from sight, it came from reading *Aristotle's Complete Masterpiece* (Version C) – or perhaps from having it flirtatiously read to them.

Moreover, the attitude towards coitus in Version C was somewhat liberatory. While marital sex was still praised as a gift from God, the text also seems to wink and smile at extra- or premarital sex. In Version C women's sexual continence was always suspect: "a Virgin her Desires can't smother,

/ But restless is, till she be made a Mother" (Version C 1749/1986, 29). In fact, because women's sexual urges were so powerful, the text explained how to detect virginity, even if the hymen was missing – a concern perhaps not unwarranted given the commonality of bundling and rising bastardy rates. Version C, in keeping with libertine stories, argued that although some brides were wrongly accused of impropriety, it was more likely for women to trick unwitting husbands with false virginity. These women,

> not having an Opportunity to enter into a married State ... have anticipated the Pleasures of Matrimony, and lost their Virginity before hand, and yet, perhaps, have afterwards pretended to bring their Virginity to a Marriage Bed by which means many an honest Man has been deceived, and meretricious Women escap'd with Impunity ... (Version C 1749/1986, 30)

It was more likely for a husband to be deceived than an innocent woman to be wrongly accused. In the latter scenario only the bride suffered unjustly whereas, in the former, the injustice was double: the woman escaped *and* an "honest Man...deceived" (Version C 1749/1986, 30). The text even described how one "courtesan" used comfrey roots to fake virginity (Version C 1749/1986, 33), providing specific details on astringents not included even in pornographic texts like *The School of Venus* (1680) or *Fanny Hill* (1749). This titillating tidbit spoke to both men and women – it told men how to detect fake virginity, yet it told women how to fake it.

Despite such condemnation of non-virgin brides, a carpe diem attitude competed with the moral outrage. For example, although "Virginity ... is the Boast and Pride of the fair Sex," the text seemed to approve of women's desire to "put it off" as soon as they could be "honestly rid of it" because if "they keep it too long, it grows useless, or at least loses much of its Value" (Version C 1749/1986, 30–1). An old virgin was a stale virgin, and not nearly as desirable to men as pubescent girls. However, Version C did not condone debauching virgins, but rather pressuring them to early marriage instead. Moreover, erotic desire in both sexes was described as a positive. At odds with the prevailing attitudes of the day, Version C even condoned masturbation (whose only drawback was that it destroyed the hymen), and was willing to wink at sexual indiscretions that did not lead to pregnancy or other flagrant consequences.

In fact, Version C was willing to wink at women who committed adultery. Although a man had no excuse to neglect or cheat on his wife, because "her Husband may make use of her" even if she were barren, surprisingly, the reverse was not true. An impotent man "ought not to marry; nor if he does he must be contented if he finds his Wife seeking that Satisfaction which he is incapable of giving. 'Tis true, for a Woman to supply her Husband's Defects is contrary both to Honour and Virtue; but where a Woman doth break the bounds on such occasion, the Fault will lie in a great Measure at the Husband's Door" (Version C 1749/1986, 52–3). Because spouses owed each other due benevolence, an adulterous wife of an impotent man was more forgivable than an adulterous husband of a barren woman. However, this caveat is missing from several editions that I have examined, suggesting that many editors disagreed with this claim enough to excise it. Moreover, adulterers were warned that after straying from the marital bed, they "will find at last they leave a Sting behind"; in other words, monogamy was best because it protected against venereal disease (Version C 1749/1986, 21).

By and large, Version C portrayed marital sex positively. The underlying assumption was that spouses engaged in procreative intercourse, and because Version C blended the various theories on conception, both parties needed to be equally aroused and willing to maximize conception. Version C gave advice on aphrodisiacs and how to set up a romantic evening. However, it went further by offering actual advice on foreplay, providing poetic examples of lagnolalia – dirty talk – in order to increase both partners' arousal. A few lines should suffice to give an ample idea of the rest: "My Rudder, with thy bold Hand, like a try'd, / And skilful Pilot, thou shalt steer; and guide / My Bark in Love's dark Channel" (Version C 1986, 37–8). Poems such as this one give insight into the kind of flirting those Northampton young men and women were engaging in, and why Edwards was so shocked by their behaviour. Interestingly, this poem was retained in even the most expurgated copies of Version C printed over the long eighteenth century. Perhaps because it metaphorically described marital copulation, it was not considered inappropriate reading for either gender. Nevertheless, one suspects that the shared reading of passages like this would have been alarming to the Reverend Edwards.

Also in keeping with the medical trends of the day, Version C was more open to the presence of men in the birthing chamber. The chapters on labour offered the standard public service announcement reminding midwives that to cause the death of infants or mothers either through lack of skill or deliberately, would "assuredly be call'd to Account for it before a higher Tribunal" (Version C 1749/1986, 61). The midwifery chapters provided detailed instructions on how to deliver the child, both in normal labour and in complicated ones. The text assumed that a male "Operator" might be delivering the woman during a difficult labour. Although Version C was written right on the cusp of the forceps revolution, continental men-midwives like Hendrik van Deventer and François Mauriceau had a following among medical men and the extended Chamberlain family had been quietly using the forceps for decades. Men-midwives, or accoucheurs as they were often called, were on the rise. As the century progressed, man-midwives had become acceptable, normal, and even fashionable. Their activities gradually slipped the birthing process out of the hands of women (Wilson 1995; Cody 2005; Leavitt 1986).

This change is perhaps best illustrated in an American edition of Version C, with the legend "Solely for the Use of Midwives" printed on the bottom of the title page, published by Isaiah Thomas of Worcester, MA, in 1795 (Version C 1795). He simplified the sections on difficult and unnatural labour to remove the distinctions between the different types, and completely excised the instructions on how to deliver in emergency situations like convulsions or hemorrhages, how to deliver footling, and how to deliver a dead child. Presumably all of these situations were to be strictly handled by male practitioners, who would not need such a homely advice manual as the *Complete Masterpiece* (Version C). Thomas, who also reprinted many cutting-edge obstetrical works by renowned men-midwives like Thomas Denman, Alexander Hamilton, and William Smellie, likely felt he was doing the next generation a favour by keeping such dangerous knowledge out of the hands of hubristic midwives who might be tempted to go it alone.

Version C was the first of the *Aristotle* texts to include two sections not connected with reproductive health, a section on physiognomy, and a collection of medical recipes. Part 3, "Displaying the Secrets of Nature relating to Physiognomy," would seem to serve little purpose in a midwifery guide. It offered standard astrological guidance on interpreting a person's character through their physical attributes and demeanour and, in the most complete versions, included woodcuts of an astrological map of the face, a palmistry diagram, and the zodiac man. Like the earlier sections of the book, it also included couplets and bits of doggerel to sum up and conclude each section. As one might expect, this section of Version C was often abridged by editors. Some editions lack the woodcuts; some excise the poetry; others are missing entire sections of the complete physiognomy. When cramped for space, editors seemed to turn their scalpels to this incongruous part.

"The Family Physician," purported to be translated from Hippocrates in the introduction, made up the fourth and final part of the *Complete Masterpiece* (Version C). It was a list, in no particular order, of recipes for various ailments as disparate as epilepsy, worms in children, or nosebleeds. Some of the cures were standard and practical, like using an ointment of "hog's lard" to ease hemorrhoidal pain; others smacked of the occult. This section also was often abridged, with the number of recipes ranging from over seventy to a mere ten or so, depending entirely, it seems, on how many pages a printer needed to complete a signature.

The final two, apparently anomalous, sections reflected the intended heterogeneous audience of Version C. Male readers might expect more than merely a witty, sexy treatise on childbearing. The physiognomy guide could aid him in his day to day business and dealings, informing him whom to trust and whom to avoid with a quick glance at pate or palms. For the same reason, it would appeal to female readers as they looked for employers or navigated the marriage market. Version C's attempts at witty urbanity and its permissive tone towards a variety of sexual behaviours seem to be in tune with the growing sense of sexual liberty in eighteenth-century America. At this time, fornication and bastardy were decriminalized, or at least not prosecuted as frequently, and an increasing number of brides stepped to the altar already mothers-to-be. Nevertheless, new ideals of female sexual continence and moral motherhood were growing in popularity. A revival of the more modest *Aristotle's Masterpiece Completed* (Version B) occurred to cater to this new ideal.

Version B

Why would printers dust off and reprint an outmoded, old-fashioned, out of print women's health guide, first in Edinburgh, the belly of elite medical training, and then in New York, home of many Scottish-trained physicians and the second American medical school? Chronologically, *Aristotle's Masterpiece Completed* (Version B) was the second version to appear, with the earliest known publication in 1697. Like the original *Aristotle's Masterpiece*, Version B seems to have been overshadowed by the meteoric success of *Aristotle's Complete Masterpiece* (Version C), disappearing from the *English Short Title Catalogue* after 1717. However, unlike the original *Masterpiece*, the *Masterpiece Completed* (Version B) enjoyed a revival, first in Scotland then in North America in the 1780s and1790s.

So why did printers begin reissuing *Aristotle's Masterpiece Completed* (Version B)? On the one hand, this question might be answered in commonsensical commercial terms. Male-authored health guides for families and/or women were abundant, popular, and, no doubt, lucrative. Reprinting an older book, with a recognizable and trusted name, was a cheap way for a printer to enter the market. Even for American reprinters, the small size of Version B gave it less overhead than reprinting another sure-seller like Buchan's massive *Domestic Medicine*. Moreover, a "new" version of *Aristotle's Masterpiece*, such as the copies of Version B reprinted and sold by the Flying Stationers Company (a group of peddlers), would be nearly guaranteed to spark some interest among cheap-print consumers who perhaps could not afford the $2.50 for *Domestic Medicine*. Nevertheless, I do not think this consideration alone is enough to account for the multiple editions produced at the close of the eighteenth century. Rather, I think it was the need for an *Aristotle* text with a more demure tone that came closer to the new feminine ideals emerging in the latter half of the eighteenth century than that found in Version C.

Aristotle's Masterpiece Completed (Version B) offered women an idea of their bodies and "natures" that was no longer found in the more polite medical guides of the day. Though companionate marriage had become the ideal in most writings, Version B offered a positive image of goodwifery, a role that a growing emphasis on middle-class leisure was endangering. Nevertheless, the image of the "goodwife" might be rehabilitated in the emerging image of the domestic angel. The woman reading Version B would find herself described as mistress of the kitchen and therefore mistress of the boudoir, able to arouse or subdue her husband's ardour through careful culinary planning. Though the first part of Version B was nearly identical to the original, there were subtle changes, such as fewer expensive and exotic ingredients. The recipes on the whole tended to be more homey and practical, perhaps reflecting the cheap-print status of the text. However, the recipes for treating the various ailments of pregnancy included expensive ingredients like nutmeg, musk, mace, cloves, and, of course, laudanum, although by the end of the eighteenth century, all of these items were more common than when the source text was written. Unlike polite medical guides, which offered almost no advice on fertility, Version B offered many recipes and culinary suggestions that promised not only to affect libido, but also to increase or decrease fertility.

Part 2 of Version B was unique to the *Aristotle* books. It was a systematic description of the female reproductive system and the various ailments women could suffer in it, as well as the more typical explanation of pregnancy and labour. It was "A Private Looking Glass for the Female Sex" and had none of the scurrilous mockery found in Version C. Giving detailed information on menstruation, pregnancy, and female diseases, this section was perhaps the most useful for those women isolated on the frontier. Although it listed signs of conception, it also gave them a malleable test to distinguish pregnancy from retention of the courses to prevent women from "becom[ing] murderers of the fruits of their own bodies" (Version B 1788, 88). Women were advised to drink honey and water before bed, which would cause them pain in their stomachs if they had conceived. If no pain ensued, they were told how to treat this ailment with bloodletting and home-made medicines. One of the physics included mugwort (Version B 1788, 63–3), long used as a labour-inducer and emmenagogue (Riddle 1997, 32). This chapter put women in control of their fertility by enabling them, on the one hand, to determine if they were pregnant – knowledge that physicians denied them – and, on the other, to decide whether or not to remain pregnant – a choice physicians no longer allowed them to make. Birth rates in the early American republic steadily declined for most demographic groups, at least in part because moral motherhood required an intensive investment in the rearing of a small number of children (Klepp 2009). In order to meet this new domestic ideal, women had to take charge of their fertility. It is quite possible that some women did turn to some version of *Aristotle* for this type of information.

Version B also provided information about a variety of female diseases not usually addressed in polite health manuals. Most polite health manuals confined themselves to menstrual disorders, *fluor albus*, and illnesses experienced during pregnancy and possibly childbed. They were silent on diseases included in Version B, such as "The Suffocation of the Mother," a type of hysteria caused by "retained" or "corrupted seed" (i.e., sexual frustration); prolapsus of the vagina or uterus; and diseases we would likely diagnose as cancer ("schirrosity of the womb" and "dropsy of the womb") (Version B 1788, 71–9). Most of the suggested medicines actually compare favourably with the regimens recommended for these diseases in male textbooks, although Version B lacked the reliance on heavy metals like mercury or lead that medical men would have liberally employed. These diseases were the province of medical men, not midwives nor women's home remedies. Version B's inclusion of these diseases offered an alternative to women who did not choose to consult with a medical man, or whose geographic isolation made it impossible to consult with one. Women in isolated frontier areas could turn to this cheap text for the advice that would have been unavailable in a more expensive, "scientific" work.

In keeping with this self-reliant ethos, the instructions for what to do when labour commenced were directed to the labouring woman herself, reinforcing that this was a book meant for women readers, and one that respected their autonomy and gave them at least some control over their bodies. When a woman found herself in labour, she should "send for a skilful midwife, and that rather too soon than too late; and against which time, let her prepare a pallet, bed or couch, near the fire, that the midwife and her assistants may pass round, and help as occasion requires, having a change of linen ready, and a small stool to rest her feet against, she having more force when they are bowed, than when they are otherwise" (Version B 1788, 87–8). This was not a woman under the care of a man-midwife, instructed to lie on her left side to preserve both their modesty. This was a *labouring* woman, heroically struggling with the birth, supported half-upright by midwife and attendants. Natural, breech, and multiple births were all described as being handled by the midwife. Only in "Case of Extremity" such as hemorrhage or convulsions does the text presume a male "Operator." In the pages of Version B, birth remained firmly in the hands of women. Of course, it is likely that rural and/or poor women, who were unlikely to have available the services of a man-midwife, were the primary purchasers of Version B. This text would have reflected their reality more so than a polite guide written by a male physician. Nevertheless, the frontier conditions broke down traditional female networks. Traditionally, mothers, grandmothers, older sisters, and other female relatives or friends would have instructed a newly expectant mother on how to prepare for childbed. But as families scattered across the vast edges of the growing nation, family members and female friends became too distant to offer such advice and support (Hoffert 1989). Thus a literate woman might turn to advice books for help, and Version B would have been perhaps the least expensive option available.

On a final note, American versions of Version B included abridged versions of the "Physiognomy" and "Family Physician" of the *Complete Masterpiece* (Version C). Perhaps printers needed to fill up the last few pages, or perhaps they were hoping to cash in on the popularity and widespread appeal of the latter version. We will never know for certain. Nevertheless, their inclusion seems even more out of place in the *Masterpiece Completed*, giving a curious ending to what is otherwise a fairly straightforward and serious medical advice book. *Aristotle's Masterpiece Completed* was not cutting-edge or fashionable, but the possibility of agency and autonomy it offered seemingly found consumers in the Early Republic, as it stayed in print during the first two decades of the nineteenth century.

Backlash and the Need for a New *Aristotle*

For Americans in the late eighteenth century, in high and low print, the fundamental truth about female sexual nature was debated. Two versions of female sexual nature were at discursive odds. The first, more traditional view understood women as naturally lascivious and found discursive expression in bawdy humour and songs. It also gained credence from the seeming sexual laxity of the times, as evidenced by the decreasing legal regulations of extramarital sexual practices and the openness with which private marriage, self-divorce, and remarriage were practised. At the same time, a new concept of female sexual nature was being articulated. This version promoted the idea that women were naturally chaste and modest and located these attributes in the bodily sexual difference between male and female. It envisioned women as the civilizing force whose influence as mothers would guide and shape the Republic through the proper upbringing of their sons.

Cheap-print American women readers could chose an *Aristotle* text that fit with their belief about female sexual nature. The two versions of *Aristotle's Masterpiece* discussed here were each embedded in differing concepts of feminine nature. Version C embraced a permissive sexual ethos, whereas Version B, though chronologically older, was invested in a belief in female chastity in better harmony with the emerging ideals of domesticity and moral motherhood of the time. Indeed, it seems likely that Version B came back into print to provide a cheap alternative for women invested in these ideals. Both texts remained popular in the last decades of the eighteenth century and into the nineteenth. As the revolutionary fervour waned, however, the sexual permissiveness in Version C increasingly fell out of favour, as did the text itself. Its levity and the transitional wavering between a one- and two-sex model would have increasingly seemed outmoded and uncouth. But the fortunes of Version B were also on the decline. Scientific discourse had gained more authority and its views on the female body, women's health, and proper medical treatment (not to mention proper practitioners) were at growing odds with the information found in Version B. Version B invested women with an authority to diagnose and treat themselves that medical practitioners sought to deny them. Moreover, the culture at large was beginning to frown upon any stepping beyond what was articulated as women's proper sphere. As Zagarri has demonstrated, the early nineteenth century witnessed a backlash against women's active participation in the public sphere. Not only did domesticity and moral motherhood increasingly become the only option for women, but also proper domesticity and maternity was conceptualized as requiring male guidance to keep it in check. Thus, it is not surprising, then, that by the 1820s, both Versions C and B were superseded by a new version of *Aristotle's Masterpiece* (Version D), one completely rewritten to fit its medical advice and sexual ethos into the emerging Victorian ideal of women as pure, domestic angels.

Research for this chapter was generously made possible by a Mellon Fellowship from the Library Company of Pennsylvania and a Mellon Fellowship in Early American Literature and Material Texts Dissertation Fellowship from the McNeil Center for Early American Studies. My research consisted of the careful reading and comparison of versions of the *Aristotle* texts held at the Historical Medical Library at the College of Physicians of Philadelphia, the Library Company of Philadelphia, and the Royal College of Surgeons of England. Copies looked at include nine versions of *Aristotle's Masterpiece Completed* (Version B), thirteen versions of *Aristotle's Complete Masterpiece* (Version C), and seventeen versions of *The Works of Aristotle*, which contained either Version C or a nineteenth-century edition of *Aristotle's Masterpiece* (Version D) not addressed in this chapter. I also examined those versions available on *Eighteenth Century Collections Online* (ECCO), *Early English Books Online* (EEBO), and *Early American Imprints*. The dates of these texts range from 1684 to 1900, and places of publication include London and various American cities, including Worcester, Philadelphia, New York, and others.

REFERENCES

Aristotle's Complete Masterpiece. Version C (1749) 1986. Edited by Randolph Trumbach. New York: Garland.

Aristotle's Complete Masterpiece. Version C 1795. Worcester, MA: Isaiah Thomas.

Aristotle's Masterpiece. Version A (1694) 1986. Edited by Randolph Trumbach. New York: Garland.

Aristotle's Masterpiece Completed. Version B 1788. New York: Flying Stationers Company.

Beall, O.T., Jr. 1963. "*Aristotle's Master Piece* in America: A Landmark in the Folklore of Medicine." *William and Mary Quarterly* 20 (2): 207–22. http://dx.doi.org/10.2307/1919297.

Bloch, R.H. 1978. "American Feminine Ideals in Transition: The Rise of the Moral Mother, 1785–1815." *Feminist Studies* 42:101–26.

Bloch, R.H. 2003. "Changing Conceptions of Sexuality and Romance in Eighteenth-Century America." *William and Mary Quarterly* 60 (1): 13–40. http://dx.doi.org/10.2307/3491494.

Block, S. 2006. *Rape & Sexual Power in Early America*. Chapel Hill: North Carolina University Press.

Branson, S. 2001. *Those Fiery Frenchified Dames: Women and Political Culture in Early National Philadelphia*. Philadelphia: University of Pennsylvania Press.

Buchan, W. (1809) 1972. "Advice to Mothers." In *The Physician and Child-Rearing: Two Guides, 1809–1894*, edited by Charles E. Rosenberg, 1–125. Boston: Joseph Bumstead.

Buchan, W. (1785) 2014. Domestic Medicine. 2nd ed. On AmericanRevoltion.org. The JDN Group. http://www.americanrevolution.org/medicine.html

Bullough, V. 1973. "An Early American Sex Manual, or, Aristotle Who?" *Early American Literature* 7 (3): 236–46.

Chamberlain, A. 2002. "Bad Books and Bad Boys: The Transformation of Gender in Eighteenth-Century Northampton, Massachusetts." *New England Quarterly* 75 (2): 179–203. http://dx.doi.org/10.2307/1559763.

Cleland, J. 2001. *Fanny Hill, or Memoirs of a Woman of Pleasure (1749)*. Edited by Gary Gautier. New York: Modern Library.

Cody, L.F. 2005. *Birthing the Nation: Sex, Science, and the Conception of Eighteenth-Century Britons*. Oxford: Oxford University Press.

Crane, E.F. 1994. Introduction to *The Diary of Elizabeth Drinker by Elizabeth Drinker. ix–xxv*. Boston: Northeastern University Press.

Crawford, P. 1994. "Sexual Knowledge in England, 1500–1750." In *Sexual Knowledge, Sexual Science: The History of Attitudes to Sexuality*, edited by Roy Porter and Mikulás Teich, 82–106. Cambridge: Cambridge University Press.

Culpeper, N. 1651. *Directory for Midwives or a Guide to Women in Their Conception, Bearing, and Suckling Their Children*. London: Peter Cole.

Fissell, M. 2003a. "The Aristotle Texts in Vernacular Medical Culture." In *Right Living: An Anglo-American Tradition of Self-Help Medicine and Hygiene*, edited by Charles E. Rosenberg, 59–87. Baltimore: Johns Hopkins University Press.

Fissell, M. 2003b. "Hairy Women and Naked Truths: Gender and the Politics of Knowledge in 'Aristotle's Masterpiece.'" *William and Mary Quarterly* 60 (1): 43–74. http://dx.doi.org/10.2307/3491495.

Foster, T.A. 2006. *Sex and the Eighteenth-Century Man: Massachusetts and the History of Sexuality in America*. Boston: Beacon.

Godbeer, R. 2002. *Sexual Revolution in Early America*. Baltimore: Johns Hopkins University Press.

Harvey, W. 1989. *On Generation*. In *The Works of William Harvey*, translated by Robert Willis, 151–518. Philadelphia: University of Pennsylvania Press.

Hill, B. 1989. *Women, Work and Sexual Politics in Eighteenth Century England*. Montreal: McGill-Queen's University Press.

Hoffert, S.D. 1989. *Private Matters: American Attitudes toward Childbearing and Infant Nurture in the Urban North, 1800–1860*. Urbana: University of Illinois Press.

Johnson, T.H. 1932. "Jonathan Edwards and the 'Young Folks' Bible.'" *New England Quarterly* 5 (1): 37–54. http://dx.doi.org/10.2307/359489.
Karlsen, C.F., and L. Crumpacker. 1984. Introduction to *The Journal of Esther Edwards Burr* 1754–1757. 3–42. New Haven, CT: Yale University Press.
Klepp, S.E. 2009. *Revolutionary Conceptions: Women, Fertility, and Family Limitation in American 1760–1820*. Chapel Hill: North Carolina University Press. http://dx.doi.org/10.5149/9780807838716_Klepp.
Laqueur, T. 1990. *Making Sex: Body and Gender from the Greeks to Freud*. Cambridge, MA: Harvard University Press.
Leavitt, J.W. 1986. *Brought to Bed: Childbearing in America 1750–1950*. New York: Oxford University Press.
Letters of Weems/Carrey. 1803–10. The Library Company of Philadelphia. Philadelphia, PA.
Lyons, C.A. 2006. *Sex Among the Rabble: An Intimate History of Gender & Power in the Age of Revolution, Philadelphia, 1730–1830*. Chapel Hill, NC: University of North Carolina Press.
Porter, R. 1985. "'The Secrets of Generation Display'd': *Aristotle's Master-Piece* in Eighteenth-Century England." In *Tis Nature's Fault*, edited by Robert Purks Maccubbin, 1–21. Cambridge: Cambridge University Press.
Porter, R. 1994. "The Literature of Sex Advice before 1800." In *Sexual Knowledge/ Sexual Science: The History of Attitudes to Sexuality*, edited by Roy Porter and Mikulás Teich, 134–57. Cambridge: Cambridge, University Press.
Porter, R. 2003. *Flesh in the Age of Reason: The Modern Foundations of Body and Soul*. New York: Norton.
Riddle, R. 1997. *Eve's Herbs: A History of Contraception and Abortion in the West*. Cambridge, MA: Harvard University Press.
Schiebinger, L. 1993. *Nature's Body: Gender in the Making of Modern Science*. New Brunswick, NJ: Rutgers University Press.
"The School of Venus." (1680) 2004. In *When Flesh Becomes Word*, edited by Bradford K. Mudge, 1–57. Oxford: Oxford University Press.
Sharp, J. (1671) 1999. *The Midwives Book*. Edited by Elaine Hobby. Oxford: Oxford University Press.
Stockton, A.B. 1995. "To the Visitant *from a Circle of Ladies, on Reading His Paper* No. 3 *in the* Pennsylvania Chronicle." In *Only for the Eye of a Friend*, edited by Carla Mulford, 89–90. Richmond: University of Virginia Press.
Ulrich, L.T. 1990. *A Midwife's Tale: The Life of Martha Ballard, Based on Her Diary, 1785–1812*. New York: Vintage.
Wagner, P. 1988. *Eros Revived: Erotica of the Enlightenment in England and America*. London: Paladin.

Wilson, A. 1995. *The Making of Man-Midwifery: Childbirth in England, 1660–1770*. Cambridge, MA: Harvard University Press.
Wollstonecraft, M. (1792) 1992. *A Vindication of the Rights of Women*. Edited by Miriam Brody. New York: Penguin.
Zagarri, R. 2007. *Revolutionary Backlash: Women and Politics in the Early American Republic*. Philadelphia: University of Pennsylvania Press.

19 Eve's Choices: Procreation, Reproduction, and the Politics of Generation in *Paradise Lost*[1]

CORRINNE HAROL AND JESSICA MacQUEEN

In John Milton's Protestant epic *Paradise Lost* (Milton (1667) 2008), it is always assumed that eventually Adam and Eve will have children, but God's famous utterance, "be fruitful and multiply" (King James Bible, Genesis 1:28), is not represented in *Paradise Lost* as a command to be obeyed but rather as a natural eventuality: God offers a "blessing" that humans will "be fruitful, multiply" (Milton (1667) 2008, VII.530–1). The question of obedience in the poem is usually discussed in terms of the prelapsarian mandate to abstain from eating the fruit of the tree of knowledge. This mandate to obedience is a negative injunction, involving the one thing that may not be done. Adam and Eve do perform activities in the garden, including agricultural labour, but they do not conceptualize these activities as acts of obedience insofar as they are not mandated by God.[2] As far as Adam knows, when we first see them in Book IV, God asks "no other service" of the first humans than that they abstain from eating the fruit of the tree of knowledge (IV.420). The first humans do not produce offspring in the prelapsarian garden, and their only act of obedience is not to eat the fruit. We will argue that although Eden is largely a scene of fertile abundance, human life in the garden revolves around an ethos of abstinence: Adam and Eve's control over their desire to eat the fruit and their management of fertility both vegetable and human. The "inabstinence" of Eve in eating the forbidden fruit causes their fall from grace (XI.476), and as a result humans move from the fertile garden, which must be managed by Eve's labour and her abstinence, to a fallen world in which Eve's "seed" and her consent to bear progeny are central to the historico-spiritual frame of reference that structures meaning in that world (X.180). In short, we read *Paradise Lost* as a complicated engagement with female reproductive agency.

The poem famously claims to "justify the ways of God to men" (I.26); we read this not so much as promising to justify the original creation or the punishment for Eve's disobedience but rather to justify the physical and theological laws of the fallen world of early modern England. This world relies on humans choosing to labour and to reproduce. In contrast with the negative injunctions of the prelapsarian world, the injunction to obedience in the fallen world has primarily active elements: Adam and Eve, as a sign of their obedience, must perform specific tasks, and they must, congruent with a theory of obedience, suffer while doing them. The specific things the curse demands of them are precisely the things that were natural but not matters of theological concern before the fall: Adam must choose to labour upon the earth and Eve must choose to bear children in "sorrow" (X.193). This chapter, then, reads the poem as a justification for those human activities – male labour and, especially, female reproduction – that lacked a mandate and a justification in prelapsarian Eden.[3] Via the poem's pre- and postlapsarian structure, the Puritan revolutionary and anti-monarchist Milton reconfigures the theological question of obedience for an emerging secular Protestant modernity. He does this by positing that these two different worlds function with different physical and theological laws, which, as we will argue, hinge upon two very different theories of generation. These two versions of generation, which we call procreation and reproduction, are based in scientific and theological controversies surrounding preformation and epigenetics that were prominent in Milton's early modern England. By drawing on these controversies, the poem articulates a view of human reproductive agency that supports Milton's anti-monarchical political leanings and his Protestant vision of human political agency.

As a Puritan writer, Milton's depiction of human generation, and specifically Eve's role in it, participates in the Protestant Reformation's reconfiguration of maternity and femininity. The Virgin Mary, the ideal Catholic woman, offered a model of procreation that was sacred, in that women could view their childbirth experiences as connecting them to Christ – both in terms of a woman having given birth to Christ and in terms of female labour pains as microcosmic of Christ's suffering. The Reformation was marked by a concerted effort to de-emphasize and desacralize Mary and often returned to Eve as the exemplar of mundane femininity. Eve's disobedience and inabstinence provided misogynist writers renewed occasion for blaming women for the fall and for representing childbirth as the painful punishment for sin. As Mary Fissell has argued, once female generation lost its miraculous character "making babies became a physical process like any other" (2004, 72), and women, in terms of both their sexuality and their fertility, were increasingly associated in negative terms with Eve. Thus, by the time Milton was writing *Paradise Lost*, the shame of female sexuality and female suffering in childbirth had long been conceptualized as effects of the fall, punishment for humanity's, and especially women's, disobedience.[4] Milton's epic reconfigures this discourse in order to imagine human generation as a part of the historical process that will redeem original sin.

Paradise Lost was written on the cusp of the new Enlightenment ideas about human generation that are discussed in this book, and Milton's reconceptualization of the theological status of human sexuality and generation was made possible by these scientific debates. These scientific debates over generation allowed Milton to theorize generation in a way that accords it importance within the terms of an emerging secular (i.e., Protestant and disenchanted) culture.[5] In other words, *Paradise Lost* deploys controversies about how children are conceived and born in order to re-imagine why, theologically and culturally, they should be conceived and born. There were a number of models of generation available to Milton in seventeenth-century England, and those scientific theories almost inevitably correlated with a writer's theological and political beliefs. The central debate was between preformationist and epigenetic theories of generation (Keller 2007; Laqueur 1992; Pinto-Correia 1998; Roe 2003). This debate was complicated, with many nuances, but the essential difference was that preformationists believed that God had created (preformed) all life forms at the beginning of creation. Epigeneticists, by contrast, believed that new forms of life were created de novo from undifferentiated matter (Pinto-Correia 1998, 2). The different versions of birth put forth in *Paradise Lost* do not follow one single scientific model of generation: Eve's birth from Adam's side, Satan's claim that he is self-begotten, Sin springing from her father's head, the teeming multitude of animals that crawl out of Earth's womb fully formed are all variations in representations of birth that suggest Milton was engaging in the debates surrounding generation. So we are not arguing that the poem offers a consistent or original scientific view. Rather, we explore how it deploys certain aspects of the scientific debate in order to justify Milton's politico-theological theories about human choice and obedience.

Because we are mapping scientific ideas about generation onto the pre- and postlapsarian structure of *Paradise Lost*, we mark this shift with a nominal one: we associate prelapsarian Eden with procreation and postlapsarian human life with reproduction. These terms are controversial and not fully specific to the argument we make; nonetheless, they do help us to outline the general contours of the shift we see. By procreation, we mean generation as preformationist, inevitable, spatial, and part of divine creation. By reproduction, we mean generation as epigenetic and entailing choice, generation that is historical, secular, and central to human political culture. We use the term generation neutrally, to refer to the creation or production of progeny outside of these scientific and ideological inflections.[6] We argue that Milton describes a prelapsarian world where generation is steeped in the metaphysical monism of preformationism and a postlapsarian world marked by a vitalist epigenetic model of human generation.[7] We associate procreation with divine right monarchy in which masculine creation is both mystified and supremely important, while we see reproduction as demystifying and thereby de-emphasizing divine creation in favour of human political agency, including female agency. In *Paradise Lost*, prelapsarian generation is asexual, non-biological, mysterious, and part of God's original creation, while postlapsarian generation is treated as scientifically and politically logical and requiring human agency (both sexual and political), while also being part of God's plan. In using this language, we are also signalling a shift to a postlapsarian world organized around a capitalist division of labour and reproduction. Our focus on the ways that the poem's pre- and postlapsarian structure re-imagines human labour and generation tracks the transformation in Adam from a reluctant labourer who is the inevitable patriarch of a monistic universe to a labourer who chooses to suffer in order to "sustain" himself and to "earn rest" (X.1056; XI.375). More importantly, we trace Eve's transition from a labourer who manages fertility via abstinence and gardening to a woman who embraces the historico-spiritual importance of her reproduction.

Paradise Lost, as many scholars have noticed, clearly emphasizes that the prelapsarian garden is both extraordinarily fertile and a site of human labour.[8] God's original act of creation in the performative utterance "let the earth bring forth" immediately results in the earth "straight / Opening her fertile womb teemed at a birth / Innumerous living creatures, perfect forms, / Limbed and full grown" (VII.451, 453–6). This original instance of generation is scientifically preformationist and parthenogenic: God is the creator, and there are no developmental or biological processes involved. In the garden "nature multiplies / Her fertile growth" (V.318–19), and reptiles, fish, and fowl all participate in this magical multiplication. Adam and Eve are often described as having a symbiotic relationship with this fertile garden through their eating and their labour: "after no more toil / Of their sweet gardening labour than sufficed / To recommend cool zephyr, and made ease / More easy, wholesome thirst and appetite / More grateful, to their supper fruits they fell" (IV.327–31). Sometimes, a more instrumental logic governs life in the garden. Adam and Eve, for instance, must perform certain tasks in the garden for their own comfort. They must clean up "unsightly" "blossoms" if they "mean to tread with ease" (IV.630–2), and they must maintain the garden paths "as wide / As [they] need walk" (IX.245–6).[9] In these cases, human labour in the garden arises in response to human needs, but the garden's needs retain pre-eminence, as is evidenced by the fact that Adam and Eve must "Ask riddance" of the blossoms before amending the garden for their own comfort (IV.632). The prelapsarian garden offers another logic of labour, one that is even more external to human need: humans pick fruit not only for their nutritional and sensual needs but also because humans are needed to "Help to disburden nature of her birth" (IX.624). Humans are a kind of midwife to the earth; their humble labour of disburdening via eating and gardening serves the earth's material comfort. Such "disburdening," however, only makes the earth more "fruitful" (V.319–20), creating a need for more labour.

Eve is expected to bear progeny that will manage this growing workload, but despite the fact that she is hailed the "mother of mankind" she is generally depicted not as a mother but as a labourer (V.388). Although Adam and Eve often work together in paradise, Eve is the more dedicated and ingenious labourer, and her labour is specifically contrasted with her procreative function. She is the one we see propping up flowers, storing up fruit to increase its flavour, and preparing food to serve the archangel Raphael (IX.427–33; V.321–30). This scene of domestic meal preparation is particularly telling of the sexual division of labour between the first pair, where Adam reclines in the shade of his "cool bower" while Eve hurries about the garden selecting the choicest fruits to present to their heavenly visitor (V.300).[10] While Adam and Raphael are deep in conversation, Eve retreats to her garden to tend her flowers. This is Eve's garden, described as her "nursery" (VIII.46), almost as if a substitute for children, and it would have been her responsibility to name and rank the flowers here. Eve's reign over this garden is made explicit when Satan stalks her and sees "the hand of Eve" in the landscape (IX.438); her "handiwork" (Knott 2005, 79), the physical impression of her gardening labour is rendered visible in the plants she cultivates. Moreover, Eve's primacy as the garden's central labourer is underscored in her desire for efficiency, as evidenced by her suggestion that she and Adam divide their labours. Adam responds to this suggestion by asserting that God did not intend their work to be toil and by insisting on the importance of pleasure and amorous distraction in conjunction with labour. Eve is concerned that working together detracts from the pair's productivity, and so, "[Their] day's work brought to little ... the hour of supper comes unearned" (IX.224–5). This scene of negotiation leads Teresa Michals to argue that Eve's labour maintains order in the garden but disrupts the marital hierarchy, "leading to the disorder of a domestic Adam and an entrepreneurial Eve" (1995, 511). We will argue that Eve's suggestion that their work be divided in order to increase the efficiency of their manual labour functions as a means to forestall procreation and reveals Eve's alienation from the ecological harmonization of labour, obedience, and fertility in the garden.

Human procreation is assumed to follow the same logic of natural multiplication that God has envisioned for all living things, as David Glimp has argued (2003, 145–80); in Book VII Raphael explains to the first pair that God has also "blessed" them by saying "Be fruitful, multiply, and fill the earth" (VII.530–1). However, the multiplication of humans has a special status in the garden because it has not yet occurred and because its purpose is imagined as a way to manage or "Subdue" the multiplication of the rest of nature (VII.532).[11] Because Adam and Eve do not yet have children while all other creations seem already to be multiplying, "uncropped" fruit falls to the ground in Eden faster than the pair can manage it (IV.731).[12] The "scant" work of the first humans will suffice, Adam and Eve acknowledge, only "till younger hands ere long / Assist us" (IV.626; IX.246–7). The earth's fertility necessitates a larger labour force, one that depends upon what we now call reproductive labour but which *Paradise Lost* represents as an inevitable part of God's plan. Eve is referred to as "mother" (V.388), but otherwise, the references to children in the prelapsarian garden are surprisingly devoid of interest in the process of their creation. When children are mentioned, it is frequently in terms of the synecdoche "hands": "till more hands" and "till men / Grow up to their provision, and more hands..." are examples of how future generations are referenced in the garden (IX.207, 623). Human progeny, and especially Eve's role as mother of these offspring, is repeatedly explained as a natural and inevitable response to the fertility of the rest of the earth. Raphael, for example, addresses Eve: "Hail mother of mankind, whose fruitful womb / Shall fill the world more numerous with thy sons / Than with these various fruits the trees of God / Have heaped this table" (V.388–91). Although here progeny are referred to in human terms as "sons" (V.389), they are nonetheless seen in relation to fruits, as part of the ecology of the garden. The agent of procreation is Eve's womb, acting (synecdochically) seemingly of its own initiative. The "magical numbers" of multiplying human procreation are evidence of "divine vision" because human procreation will balance earth's fertility and serve its need for disburdening (Pinto-Correia 1998, 274–301). Marxist feminists such as Silvia Federici (2004) would see such generation for the sake of labour as typical of capitalist discourse, in that human generation is mystified, assumed to be natural, a force of creation, and not a form of labour itself: in short, procreation not reproduction. In Milton's garden, human procreation is linked to a kind of manual labour (the hands to pick fruit), but both human labour and human procreation are imagined as inevitable and natural, a part of the ecology of God's creation, not a matter of choice and not connected to human spiritual destiny.

This logic of human procreation in the garden follows preformationist science in several ways. The language of multiplication suggests that generation does not produce something de novo but rather follows God's plan. The fact that it is specifically hands that are multiplied also follows preformationist logic: hands are a synecdoche – taking the part for the whole implies the kind of microcosmic participation in the macrocosm upon which the metaphysics of preformationism rests. In the debate between preformationist and epigenetic models of generation, the formation of particular body parts was always at issue: preformationists believed that each part always existed in its final form, while epigenetic theorists proposed a developmental model. That the offspring of Adam and Eve are depicted as hands who will support the handiwork of Eve – that is, that they are imagined as body parts who exactly replicate the function of their parents' body parts – implies a preformationist logic, one steeped in the similarity of physiology and functionality among all humans and one that sustains the ecology of God's original creation. These hands are also spatially rather than temporally connected: the offspring of Adam and Eve are imagined not as future generations but rather as the means by which the earth will "fill" with humans (V.389), just as the garden has already filled with animals and plants.

This has made critics wonder why no such human multiplication takes place in the garden, and several theories have been floated.[13] Most critics follow the logic that the poem enacts and supports a positive form of marital sexuality in the garden. But if Adam and Eve are having sex, it is not clear why human generation has not happened. Milton was a leading proponent of conjugal intimacy as having spiritual and psychological benefits outside of generation, so it is possible that they are having sex but not (yet) fertile and that this would have been seen as quite natural by Milton.[14] It is also possible that Adam and Eve are practising some form of abstinence; after all, as John Rogers has argued, before *Paradise Lost* Milton experimented, in his life and in his writings, with the attractions of various forms of abstinence (1998, 93–7). The incestuous and tortuous depiction of Sin's procreative experiences in Book II would support the possibility that *Paradise Lost* is against procreative sexuality. It is also possible that Adam and Eve are practising some form of contraception, which would seem to be heretical in terms of the logic of the poem, where married sexuality is supposed to be fruitful, inevitable, and beneficial to the earth. But seventeenth-century England maintained an extensive system of contraception (Federici 2004, 92; McLaren 1984, 62–3, 87, and 182; Mies 1999, 54), and its cultural signifiers are present in the poem's representation of Eve. Eve's gardening and food preparation expertise could be read as an indication of her capacity for using herbs for contraception (Knoppers 2011, 140–64), linking her activities to those of early modern witches (Van den Berg 1986). Moreover, when Satan whispers in Eve's ear he is described as a toad, an animal frequently envisioned as the witch's consort (Federici 2004, 194). Finally, disobedience itself was associated with contraception in seventeenth-century England (McLaren 1984, 59).

But we do not need extra-textual information about early modern contraception and misogyny to imagine that Eve is responsible for the couple's lack of progeny. Eve, we argue, reveals the lack of justification for human generation before the fall, for she is both highly attuned to the physical laws of the garden and yet decidedly non-procreative herself, both in terms of her own birth and in terms of her gardening. God forms Eve in response to Adam's specifically human desire for companionship, and her birth does not follow a parthenogenic or a preformationist model of procreation, because shaping a rib into a human form is decidedly not preformationist. Along this line, Susan McDonald (2000) has argued that Eve's birth is described in the language of Caeserean section. Eve's birth is thus the first instance of reproduction in the garden, and it prefigures her lack of progeny in the garden as well as the disobedient act that will exile her and the reproductive choice that will redeem her. In terms of her relation to the garden's procreativity, Eve employs strategies – outside of mere manual labour or its reproduction – for addressing problematic fertility in the garden. Eve manages the garden not with any effort to generate offspring but rather with ingenious techniques of cultivation that function as a sort of assisted reproductive therapy. At first, Adam assists her in this project of cultivation. The pair encourage appropriate sexuality by "[leading] the vine / To wed her elm" and in directing the vine with her "adopted clusters, to adorn / [the elm's] barren leaves" (V.215–19). The cultivation of fruit is thus a corrective procedure to "check / Fruitless embraces" (V.214–15), and so the deviant sexuality of wandering vines is rerouted through the pair's cultivation methods. They manage the garden's procreative excess by restricting inappropriate sexuality and by encouraging married procreation in the garden, thereby resolving both the promiscuity and the infertility that evidently exist in Milton's version of paradise. Their gardening labour upholds a reproductive ideal of fertile monogamy; it corrects barrenness and enforces fertility; it also prevents the garden's fecundity from growing wild. In so doing, the agricultural labour of the first pair transforms wild procreative multiplication into managed reproductive fertility. In short, the agricultural labour of Adam and Eve is explicitly and repeatedly linked to the management of fertility: the first humans live in a garden described as a magical place of procreative, fertile abundance, and yet their labour is associated with reproductive techniques.

Eve approaches her own generative capacities with similar strategies of management. As we have argued earlier, Eve understands the need to have children as a function of the need for more manual labourers to tend the earth, and she understands that generation can be cultivated or prevented. Thus, when she suggests to Adam that they divide their labour, she can be seen as making a choice to be non-procreative via practising abstinence for contraception in two senses. First of all, and as Adam laments, their separation for the purposes of work inhibits their "sweet intercourse," the "looks and smiles" of "love" that are central to his sense of their relationship (IX.238–40). Adam refers explicitly to the mental and discursive pleasures of love, but his sensual language here (and Milton's larger defence of "Social communication") suggest that marital sexuality is at stake in Eve's desire to divide their labour (VIII.429). By separating from Adam, Eve avoids the sexual intercourse that might lead to pregnancy and progeny. And second, when Eve suggests that they separate in order to increase the efficiency of their labour, this is a way of undermining the necessity to generate or multiply "hands" to help manage the garden (IX.207). Eve's choice to divide her labour from Adam's is itself a form of reproductive choice, as Diane McColley (1972) has argued.[15] If hands are needed mainly to garden, then increasing the productivity of their work will forestall the need for additional hands. "[T]ill more hands" materialize (IX.207), Eve reasons, she will maximize the efficiency of her work in the garden by dividing her labour from Adam's. Eve's choice to separate in order to work more thus means both that they do not have time for the amorous interludes that Adam desires and that it would be possible for their physical labour to become efficient enough to offset the earth's need for more hands. Tellingly, Adam refers to Eve's impulse here as a form of "good works" – the poem's sole reference to the controversial theological idea that human activity can have an effect on spiritual destiny (IX.234).[16] Eve's choices and her actions – her agricultural labour, her desire to be more efficient at it, and her concomitant avoidance of procreation – are, in Adam's critical invocation of good works, not sacred but rather secular practices, goodly perhaps, but things indifferent to God, who has made the garden for their pleasure and who asks for only one sign of obedience. In the prelapsarian garden, procreation is assumed to be inevitable and obedience is measured by inaction and abstinence – by not eating the forbidden fruit. Eve's efforts to bring good works into the garden suggest that her choices, even before she eats the fruit, conflict with God's preformationist logic of procreation, because they are choices that aspire to affect both spirituality and the garden itself.

Preformationist science correlates with a philosophy of divine right monarchy, in terms of both human generation and knowledge. Preformationism suggests that God, as father, determined all offspring and established all knowledge, including what humans could know. Preformationism as epistemology and philosophy has the advantage, as Shirley Roe has argued, of not needing a teleological explanation: because everything is already formed by God, cause is more important than outcome or purpose (2003, 149–56). Epigenetic theory challenged the biological connection between a father and his offspring, and thus it was part of the challenge to patriarchy as divine right. Epigenetics theorizes a developmental process that is not predetermined and that recognizes the female's role in generation. Jennifer Mensch (2013) argues that what is at stake in the debate over epigenesis is not only reproductive agency but knowledge itself; Kant's Enlightenment theory of knowledge as developmental, according to Mensch, is based in the developmental logic of epigenesis. Preformationist and epigenetic theories of generation thus map onto different models of politics, knowledge, and justification.

These political and epistemological differences play out in *Paradise Lost*'s famous temptation scene. In response to the serpent's claim that eating the fruit transformed him for the better, Eve's only explanation for her refusal to eat the fruit is that she cannot eat because God as patriarch has commanded her not to. Eve links the patriarchal mandate to a preformationist logic of birth when she says that the prohibition against eating the fruit is the "Sole daughter of [God's] voice" (IX.653). Thus she justifies her obedience via a preformationist emphasis on generation as cause. Satan counters this logic of cause with promises of effect, saying that eating the plant has transformed his sense of reason. Satan claims that he can now "discern / Things [not only] in their causes," but he can even "trace the ways / Of highest agents" (IX.681–3). He points to the garden, where Eve's handiwork is clear, and claims that "this fair earth," which is "Warmed by the sun, producing every kind," is productive of its own accord, and thus he argues, in an epigenetic logic, that not "all from [the Gods] proceeds" (IX.719–21). Satan's "persuasive" words seem to be "impregned / With reason ... and with truth" (IX.737–8); the use of a metaphor of generation, "impregned," to describe knowledge and rhetoric and moreover a metaphor that implies agency and development makes Satan's logic even more clearly epigenetic. According to Satan, the epigeneticist, things can be transformed; ways (or paths) can be traced; and nature is not predetermined by God. Eve, born outside of preformationist logic, attentive to the fertility of nature, and already capable of reproductive management, can articulate the proscriptive preformationist mandate to obey, but she also readily understands Satan's epigenetic logic. Thus, Eve's eating of the fruit is part of a continuum whereby she was born and develops in ways that are contrary to God's logic of preformation, which assumes both procreation and knowledge to be preformed. Thus in this pivotal scene of temptation, Eve's alienation from preformationism makes possible her disobedient act of inabstinently eating from the tree of knowledge. Satan and Eve are not the poem's only converts to epigenesis. Milton is also using an epigenetic logic in his great Protestant epic, as his whole project aims to "justify the ways of God to men" (I.26), which is itself a postlapsarian goal because it moves from first causes to the ways of the future. One of the main things, we have been arguing, that is justified in *Paradise Lost* is the need to generate humans. Postlapsarian human generation as epigenetic is justified by the poem theologically: it is the means by which Christ will redeem humanity and thus whereby humans will be justified with God.

We have traced here the strong connection between Eve's agricultural labour and the fertility of the garden, and thus of her own imagined future fertility, by way of setting up a larger argument about Milton's justification for the physical and theological laws that govern the fallen world, a world that depends upon Adam's labour and Eve's "seed" (X.180). Before the fall, Eve is prohibited from eating the fruit, but otherwise her actions have no theological implications. She makes choices about labour and generation, but these choices are things indifferent to her salvation as well as things that belie her agency over the natural or political world: God's garden simply continues to grow wild at a rate well beyond her capacity to labour. We argue that Eve's abstinence as an agricultural labourer in the prelapsarian garden is connected to the specificity of her disobedience – her inabstinent act of desiring knowledge – and to the specific injunctions of the curse that structures the fallen world the poem will justify: that Adam must labour to sustain himself and that Eve must choose to bear children both in submission to Adam's "will" and "In sorrow" (X.195). Interestingly, these two different forms of labour are explicitly hierarchized by the poem's justification of postlapsarian human culture: Eve's reproductive labour is especially important for the historical and spiritual destiny of humans while Adam's agricultural labour does not figure centrally in the panorama of human history that Michael lays out for him at the poem's end. In Book XI, Michael tells Adam that God's plan (before the fall) had been that Eden would have been the "capital seat" from which "had spread / All generations, and had hither come / From all the ends of the earth, to celebrate / And reverence thee their great progenitor" (XI.343–6). Thus the plan for human generation before the fall assumed a world organized spatially, with Adam as the monarchical centre and the source of its generative capacity. But after the fall Adam is "brought down / To dwell on even ground now with thy sons" (XI.347–8), and the orientation of generation becomes temporal instead of spatial, a patrilinear model concerned with future generations instead of a patriarchy centralized around geographical spread.

We are, thus, tracing a shift not just from procreation to reproduction, but also from a world operating under the logic of natural spatial multiplication from a monarchical centre to one organized by the logic of contingent linear history – that is, from one in which political structure is given to one in which human action can effect historical and political change. The anti-monarchist Milton, writing shortly after the restoration of the Stuart monarchy in 1660, does not make a case against monarchy inherently, but rather he represents the historicity of political structures and links that historicity to different logics of generation. Milton is clearly not engaged in nostalgia when he aligns monarchy with prelapsarian forms of human procreation. Rather, this association – of both divinely ordained monarchy and divinely ordained human multiplication as prelapsarian – allows him to imagine a postlapsarian culture in which sorrow and punishment are not the only outcomes of the fall. This postlapsarian culture is more epigenetic than preformationist, both in terms of generation and politics, because it offers the possibility that something will be created de novo. The scientific epigenetic argument allowed Milton to link his theory of postlapsarian obedience to a non-monarchical political structure: humans make something new, biologically and politically, when they act in accordance with God's will. This creation of the new, then, stands somewhere between a fully creationist theory and Thomas Hobbes's entirely artificial view of political organization, in which political organization arises ex nihilo from a state of nature via human agency.[17] In *Paradise Lost,* the choice to reproduce is linked to the choice of political structures, and both are seen as part of the new reality of a postlapsarian world, in which neither political structures nor human generation is divinely ordained but in which humans making the choice to act in accordance with God's will might produce something historically new but not completely original – de novo but not ex nihilo.

The postlapsarian envisioning of human offspring thus differs sharply from the prelapsarian assumption that humans will procreate. If prelapsarian Eden lacks a compelling logic to support the procreation that is assumed to be inevitable, then part of what happens after the fall is the reverse: postlapsarian reproduction is not assumed to be part of the original plan of God's creation, and in fact it operates under a disincentive, "sorrow" (X.195), but it is part of the spiritual and historical destiny of humankind: a descendant of Eve (her seed) "shall bruise / The serpent's head" (X.1031–2). By contrast with the way that prelapsarian offspring are imagined as "hands" (IV.629), "seed" suggests epigenesis (X.1031), described by Thomas Laqueur as a "rationalistic and somewhat more vitalist" model "in which matter was not merely inert substance to be worked on by God's laws" (1992, 175). While there were many theories of seed in the debates over generation (Laqueur 1992, 25–62), and while seed does not necessarily preclude a preformationist logic, we argue that within the context of *Paradise Lost*, "seed" introduces a new scientific, historical, and theological logic for generation (X.1031). In the prelapsarian garden, there is no need for planting seeds. God as "sovereign planter" has already planted the garden and blessed its multiplication (IV.691). Eve manages the garden's fertility, but she does not plant anything new. Her obedience is measured by what she does not do, and her offspring are imagined as preformed in order to share her labour of cultivation. After the fall, instead of being seen as "hands" or "innumerable" beings (IV.629; VII.156; and VIII.297), the offspring of humans are referred to for the first time as "children" and "things living" (X.194; XI.160). These terms suggest a developmental logic – children will mature into adults – and thus a generational logic – they are not temporally coexistent with their parents. As living beings, the offspring of Adam and Eve are imagined to have dignity and agency not afforded to the prelapsarian hands. While hands are mere multiplication of the same in service of the unending task of gardening in order to sustain the garden's ecology, "things living" suggests both that Eve's seed will develop into something different from Eve herself and that these living beings will affect the ecology and the history of the world (XI.160). This suggests a view of human agency neither totally free nor totally determined. As William Shullenberger describes it, Eve comes to accept her role in human generation "as eschatological privilege" (1992, 170). Milton was not an ovist – that is, he did not exclude male seed from generative capacity. In fact, in the history that Michael lays out for Adam, male seed, especially Abraham's seed, frequently plays a crucial role in the future. It is therefore even more striking that Eve's seed (even if not Eve herself) is granted such historical and syntactic agency – Eve's seed will "bruise the head of Satan" (XII.430). The significance of this action could not be more emphatic: aside from God's original creation of the world, the birth of Christ – via the seed of Eve – is the most significant world-historical event in a Christian world view.[18]

Thus we argue that Eve's development unfolds in terms of a reproductive agency that takes her from an abstinent gardener alienated from God's plan to the willingly fertile "mother of mankind" (V.388). Eve's disobedience in eating the fruit of the tree of knowledge is the hinge between the prelapsarian abstinent gardener and the postlapsarian justified mother. Eve's development is intellectual as well as biological: before the fall she is abstinent both sexually and intellectually, while her intellectual analysis of whether to reproduce is key to the postlapsarian world. When the first pair begin to understand the implications of the curse, their main concern is over the suffering of future generations: Adam asks "what can I increase / Or multiply, but curses on my head?" (X.731–2). Now that death is possible and thus that the future is made possible, the pair are invested in thinking about future generations and both the suffering and salvation that rest on their decision to reproduce. Eve, whose understanding of fertility has been established, knows that generation is a matter of choice; the choice to reproduce is presented as the right choice, and the inevitable choice, but it is importantly an active choice, and one that offers compensation rather than punishment: her "Pains" in "child-bearing" will be "soon recompensed with joy" (X.1051–2). Eve suggests that the possibility exists to not have children. She considers both abstinence as contraception and suicide, which the introduction of death after the fall makes possible, as potential alternatives.[19] Eve's analysis of their potential responses to the curse reveals the fact that, unlike with the first covenant, made before she was born, her consent to reproduce must be freely willed; moreover, the reason for reproduction is clear, and her actions will affect history. So, Milton reconfigures Eve from a sinner and a sufferer to a political subject of God and an agential historical figure, one who responds with active obedience to the postlapsarian logic for producing offspring.

This is why it is crucial that in the postlapsarian world of *Paradise Lost*, the emphasis is on Eve's seed, while Adam is viewed as a labourer, not a "progenitor" (XI.346). While Rogers argues that seventeenth-century vitalism "necessitated feminism"(1998, 15), Eve Keller is much less sanguine about a feminist epigenesis, seeing in the development of epigenetic theories over the course of the long eighteenth century a decreasing possibility for female agency (2007, 101–24). The small temporal window in which female agency matters in terms of the history of epigenesis is, for Keller, merely a transition, which quickly gives way to the egg's "autonomy" (2007, 117), inevitably represented as male. Milton, however, lingers over this moment of female agency, by locating both the first political act of consent and the salvation of humanity in the first pair's decision to reproduce. The question of epigenetic agency and temporality is viewed by Keller as ontogenetic – focused on the developmental process of the individual and thus invested in liberating the developing male egg, not the mother (2007, 101–24). We are arguing that *Paradise Lost* links this ontogenetic process to a phylogenetic one. *Paradise Lost* was written in the historical moment when patriarchy was giving way to modern forms of political agency and when epigenetic theory was beginning its fitful ascent, and it situates Eve's decision to have children, early in the Old Testament, as constitutive of the promise of a New Testament. As such, the poem is situated in that phylogenetic moment – and indeed it is about that phylogenetic moment – when female agency over reproduction has a world-historical importance. Eve's choice to reproduce is rationalized and recompensed by God's promise, it is unrepresented in the poem, and it is usually overlooked by critics more interested in Eve's subjection or in Adam's intellectual and vocational supremacy. Nonetheless, in *Paradise Lost*, the quintessential question of female choice – reproductive choice – is precisely the difference between pre- and postlapsarian life, and it is "justif[ied]" rather than commanded (I.26). The transformation of Eve's procreative abstinence into reproductive consent is thus central to Milton's vision of secular modernity.

NOTES

1 This essay was supported by a grant from the Social Sciences and Humanities Research Council. The authors would like to thank Sarah Ellenzweig,

Raymond Stephanson, the anonymous readers at UTP, and the audience at the 2012 *Canadian Society for Eighteenth-Century Studies* conference for helpful comments on earlier drafts.

2 Diane Dreher (1991) sees their gardening as vocation instead of obedience. John Knott asserts that Adam and Eve's gardening is "acting on God's mandate" and their efforts to subdue nature "can be seen as a means of enacting obedience to God" (2005, 78, 81).

3 With a few exceptions, particularly David Glimp (2003) critics have not focused on reproduction in the poem. Michael Lieb (1970) takes this discounting of reproduction the furthest, by reading all the references to it as metaphors for something more important. Historians of sexuality and obstetrics Louis Schwartz (2009) and Susan McDonald (2000) have looked at the historical relevance of Milton's depiction of birth but have not produced interpretations of the poem.

4 Eve Keller shows how ideas about generation shifted, from thinking about women as Eve to thinking about them as Christ. She shows how when "women suffer in pain for a purpose," they may be seen as acting "not in the stain of Eve but in imitation of Christ" (2007, 79). See also Colin Atkinson and William Stoneman (1990) and Charlotte Otten (1993).

5 Keith Thomas (1971) and Charles Taylor (2007) see the disenchantment of the world as central to secularization. Talal Asad (2003) argues that secularization is protestantization and that the very notion of agency invoked by this paper (and by the epigenetic scientists) is Protestant.

6 Keller points to the unsuitability of employing "reproduction" in late sixteenth- and early seventeenth-century English contexts; the word "became current" she notes, "only after the physiological processes from conception through birth came to be understood within the context of mechanism" (2007, 191 n. 1). Allison Muri (2010) disputes this history. We do not presume to be offering any evidence in this debate.

7 On Milton's monism and vitalism, see John Rogers (1998). Keller distinguishes vitalist and mechanical theories of epigenesis (2007, 143–6). We are associating *Paradise Lost* with the vitalist strain.

8 Teresa Michals sees Eve's gardening labour as a challenge to Adam's sovereignty and the reproductive mandate as solving this problem (1995, 510–11). On the importance of work in the garden, see also Dreher (1991), Kevis Goodman (1997), Laura Knoppers (1991), Knott (2005), Barbara Lewalski (1969), Anthony Low (1983), and Joanna Picciotto (2010).

9 See Knott for further analysis of Adam and Eve's gardening labour. Knott describes Eve as a "master gardener" (2005, 74), and he argues that her labour is both mandated and completely inadequate to the wildness of the garden.

10 This dinner party scene has been discussed at length by Ann Torday Gulden,

who argues that this scene is a defining instance of the division of labour in the poem and that Eve's domestic labour is elevated rather than demeaned by Milton (2003, 137, 141).

11 Glimp argues that the procreation in Eden, including the potential procreation of humans, is all part of "God's wealth"; "On the one hand," he argues, "future offspring are one among many elements of divine wealth, a part of Eden's abundance; on the other hand, Eve's children are implicated in the management of Eden's abundance, understood not as wealth but as potential waste" (2003, 145–80). This is true enough, but it is also the case, we argue, that human offspring are imagined as the moderators of unchecked growth.

12 Horace Jeffrey Hodges (2011) links the language of uncropped versus cropped to virginity versus death and sexual corruption, and he argues that Satan and Eve, who embody the qualities of cropped fruit, are necessary to God's plan.

13 James Grantham Turner discusses the theological explanations for the lack of reproduction in the garden (1987, 98–106). Kent Lehnhof (2000) argues that because Adam and Eve are unfallen and therefore complete (like angels), our fallen idea of sex would not make sense for them. Karma de Gruy (2012) makes a similar argument about angelic desire and sex. John Savoie argues, in direct contrast with our point, "before the fall Adam and Eve have conventional sexual intercourse that would lead naturally to pregnancy, children, family, and a fully realized society" (2011, 161). Mandy Green (2005) makes a case for Eve's virgin status in the garden.

14 In *The Doctrine & Discipline of Divorce,* Milton argues that the primary reason for marriage is the "apt and cheerfull conversation of man with woman" and that "the purpose of generation" is "but a secondary end in dignity, though not in necessity" (1644, 2). On this topic, see also Lewalski (1974).

15 McColley (1972) argues that Eve's prelapsarian choices offer her dignity and prefigure her choice of reproduction as obedience.

16 See Joan Bennett (1983) for a discussion of good works, antinomianism, and political agency in *Paradise Lost.*

17 For a full elaboration of this difference between Milton and Hobbes, see Victoria Kahn (2004).

18 For a discussion of the various ways that "seed" was linked to an ambivalence about human agency, see Rogers (1998, 39–61). For a related analysis, see also Jonathan Golberg, who links "seed" to a Lucretian anti-procreative world view that prevails in the garden and in heaven (2009, 179–209).

19 Christopher Bond links Eve to Persephone via this "desire for sexual barrenness" after the curse (2009, np).

REFERENCES

Asad, T. 2003. *Formations of the Secular: Christianity, Islam, Modernity*. 1st ed. Stanford: Stanford University Press.
Atkinson, C.B., and W.P. Stoneman. 1990. "'These Griping Greefes and Pinching Pangs': Attitudes to Childbirth in Thomas Bentley's *The Monument of Matrones* (1582)." *Sixteenth Century Journal: Journal of Early Modern Studies* 21 (2): 193–203. http://dx.doi.org/10.2307/2541049.
Bennett, J.S. 1983. "'Go': Milton's Antinomianism and the Separation Scene in *Paradise Lost*, Book 9." *Publications of the Modern Language Association of America* 98 (3): 388–404. http://dx.doi.org/10.2307/462278.
Bond, C. 2009. "'Proserpin Gathering Flowers': A Miltonic Simile in Its Mythic Context." *Milton Studies* 50:106–24.
de Gruy, K. 2012. "Desiring Angels: The Angelic Body in *Paradise Lost*." *Criticism* 54 (1): 117–49. http://dx.doi.org/10.1353/crt.2012.0001.
Dreher, D.E. 1991. "Milton's Warning to Puritans in *Paradise Lost*: Another Look at the Separation Scene." *Christianity and Literature* 41 (1): 27–38.
Federici, S. 2004. *Caliban and the Witch: Women, the Body, and Primitive Accumulation*. Brooklyn, NY: Autonomedia.
Fissell, M.E. 2004. "The Politics of Reproduction in the English Reformation." *Representations* (Berkeley, CA) 87 (1): 43–81. http://dx.doi.org/10.1525/rep.2004.87.1.43.
Glimp, D. 2003. *Increase and Multiply : Governing Cultural Reproduction in Early Modern England*. Minneapolis: University of Minnesota Press.
Goldberg, J. 2009. *Milton's Angels. The Seeds of Things: Theorizing Sexuality and Materiality in Renaissance Representations*. New York: Fordham University Press. http://dx.doi.org/10.5422/fso/9780823230662.001.0001.
Goodman, K. 1997. "'Wasted Labor'? Milton's Eve, the Poet's Work, and the Challenge of Sympathy." *ELH* 64 (2): 415–46. http://dx.doi.org/10.1353/elh.1997.0013.
Green, M. 2005. "The Virgin in the Garden: Milton's Ovidian Eve." *Modern Language Review* 100 (4): 903–22.
Gulden, A.T. 2003. "Milton's Eve and Wisdom: The 'Dinner-Party' Scene in *Paradise Los*t." *Milton Quarterly* 32 (4): 137–43. http://dx.doi.org/10.1111/j.1094-348X.1998.tb00611.x.
Hodges, H.J. 2011. "Fruit Uncropt and Fruit Cropt: Unnoticed Wordplay in *Paradise Lost?*" *Milton Quarterly* 45 (4): 252–7. http://dx.doi.org/10.1111/j.1094-348X.2011.00299.x.
Kahn, V. 2004. *Wayward Contracts: The Crisis of Political Obligation in England, 1640–1674*. 1st ed. Princeton: Princeton University Press.

Keller, E. 2007. *Generating Bodies and Gendered Selves: The Rhetoric of Reproduction in Early Modern England*. Seattle: University of Washington Press.

Knoppers, L.L. 1991. "Rewriting the Protestant Ethic: Discipline and Love in *Paradise Lost*." *ELH* 58 (3): 545–60. http://dx.doi.org/10.2307/2873455.

Knoppers, L.L. 2011. *Politicizing Domesticity from Henrietta Maria to Milton's Eve*. Cambridge: Cambridge University Press.

Knott, J.R. 2005. "Milton's Wild Garden." *Studies in Philology* 102 (1): 66–82. http://dx.doi.org/10.1353/sip.2005.0002.

Laqueur, T. 1992. *Making Sex: Body and Gender from the Greeks to Freud*. Cambridge, MA: Harvard University Press.

Lehnhof, K.R. 2000. "'Nor Turnd I Ween': *Paradise Lost* and Pre-Lapsarian Sexuality." *Milton Quarterly* 34 (3): 67–83. http://dx.doi.org/10.1111/j.1094-348X.2000.tb00621.x.

Lewalski, B.K. 1969. "Innocence and Experience in Milton's Eden." In *New Essays on Paradise Lost*, edited by Thomas Kranidas, 86–117. Berkeley: University of California Press.

Lewalski, B.K. 1974. "Milton on Women – Yet Once More." *Milton Studies* 6:3–20.

Lieb, M. 1970. *The Dialectics of Creation: Patterns of Birth & Regeneration in Paradise Lost*. Amherst: University of Massachusetts Press.

Low, A. 1983. "Milton, *Paradise Regained*, and Georgic." *Publications of the Modern Language Association of America* 98 (2): 152–69. http://dx.doi.org/10.2307/462043.

McColley, D.K. 1972." Free Will and Obedience in the Separation Scene of *Paradise Lost*." *SEL: Studies in English Literature, 1500–1900* 12 (1): 103–20.

McDonald, S. 2000. "'Wide Was the Wound': Caesarean Section and the Birth of Eve." In *Living Texts: Interpreting Milton*, edited by Charles Durham and Kristin Pruitt, 80–98. London: Associated University Press.

McLaren, A. 1984. *Reproductive Rituals: The Perceptions of Fertility in England from the Sixteenth Century to the Nineteenth Century*. London and New York: Methuen.

Mensch, Jennifer. 2013. *Kant's Organicism: Epigenesis and the Development of Critical Philosophy*. Chicago: University of Chicago Press.

Michals, T. 1995. "'Sweet Gardening Labour': Merit and Hierarchy in *Paradise Lost*." *Exemplaria: A Journal of Theory in Medieval and Renaissance Studies* 7 (2): 499–514. http://dx.doi.org/10.1179/exm.1995.7.2.499.

Mies, M. 1999. *Patriarchy and Accumulation on a World Scale: Women in the International Division of Labour*. 2nd ed. London: Zed Books.

Milton, J. 1644. *The Doctrine & Discipline of Divorce: Restor'd to the Good of Both Sexes, from the Bondage of Canon Law*. London.

Milton, J. (1667) 2008. *Paradise Lost*. Edited by S. Orgel and J. Goldberg. Reissue. Oxford: Oxford University Press.

Muri, A. 2010. "Imagining Reproduction: The Politics of Reproduction, Technology and the Woman Machine." *Journal of Medical Humanities* 31 (1): 53–67. http://dx.doi.org/10.1007/s10912-009-9102-8.

Otten, C.F. 1993. "Women's Prayers in Childbirth in Sixteenth-Century England." *Women & Language* 16 (1): 18–21.

Picciotto, J. 2010. *Labors of Innocence in Early Modern England*. Cambridge, MA: Harvard University Press.

Pinto-Correia, C. 1998. *The Ovary of Eve: Egg and Sperm and Preformation*. 1st ed. Chicago: University of Chicago Press.

Roe, S.A. 2003. *Matter, Life, and Generation: Eighteenth-Century Embryology and the Haller-Wolff Debate*. Cambridge: Cambridge University Press.

Rogers, J.H. 1998. *The Matter of Revolution: Science, Poetry, and Politics in the Age of Milton*. Ithaca, NY: Cornell University Press.

Savoie, J. 2011. "'That Fallacious Fruit': Lapsarian Lovemaking in *Paradise Lost*." *Milton Quarterly* 45 (3): 161–71. http://dx.doi.org/10.1111/j.1094-348X.2011.00289.x.

Schwartz, L. 2009. *Milton and Maternal Mortality*. Cambridge: Cambridge University Press. http://dx.doi.org/10.1017/CBO9780511581175.

Shullenberger, W. 1992. "Sorting the Seeds: The Regeneration of Love in *Paradise Lost*." *Milton Studies* 28:163–84.

Taylor, C. 2007. *A Secular Age*. 1st ed. Cambridge, MA: The Belknap Press of Harvard University Press.

Thomas, K. 1971. *Religion and the Decline of Magic*. New York: Scribner.

Turner, J.G. 1987. *One Flesh: Paradisal Marriage and Sexual Relations in the Age of Milton*. Oxford University Press.

Van den Berg, S. 1986. "Eve, Sin, and Witchcraft in *Paradise Lost*." *Modern Language Quarterly* 47 (4): 347–65. http://dx.doi.org/10.1215/z00267929-47-4-347.

20 Making Babies: Eighteenth-Century Attitudes towards Conception, Reproduction, and Childbirth

JULIE PEAKMAN AND SARAH WATKINS

Moral, medical, scientific, and social ideas have long intertwined in attitudes to, and portrayals of, the human body, sex, and reproduction. This chapter examines the different ways in which generation was understood and portrayed in medical texts, sex advice manuals, midwifery texts, erotic pamphlets, and popular magazines, and show how these views often conflicted and shifted during the long eighteenth century. It also looks at how, in the face of emerging new medical claims, there was a simultaneous desire to hold onto old ways and ideas. In an attempt to understand these parallel, yet often opposing, stances, the medical orthodox line emanating from male physicians is compared to reproductive texts authored by women.

Meanwhile, as male medical men purported to offer the "official" line, popular pamphlets and articles in magazines emerged to challenge these ideas. Female-authored midwifery manuals occupied a middle ground between the two; these manuals tended to cling to the personhood of the pregnant woman, treating her holistically, giving her identity and authority, but also attempted to prove the female midwives' own midwifery skills within an increasingly crowded – and masculinized – medical marketplace. While new ideas were adopted within these texts, there was a reliance on the natural and traditional suitability of women and their bodies for the task of childbirth.

Although many changes are evident in the structure and style of the texts, as Roy Porter pointed out, there is "little in the advice literature of 1680 or 1720 that is not rooted in medieval and Renaissance texts" (Porter and Hall 1995, 35).[1] Much of the advice contained within the medical and self-help manuals can be traced back through to Hippocrates, Galen, Soranus, and *Trotula*. The midwifery manuals of the 1670s are firmly rooted in their predecessors of the previous century and a half, such as Raynalde's

Byrth of Mankynde (1545), Guillemeau's *Childbirth, Or, The Happy Delivery of Women* (1612), and Culpeper's *A Directory of Midwives* (1656).[2] While these old theories continued to circulate in the eighteenth century (Needham 1959; Porter 1996, 154–73; Porter 1997, 211–32), physicians and midwives were beginning to question the role of certain elements in the process of generation (Tuana 1983, 130–52). While both menstrual blood and semen were seen to have an essential role in reproduction, different physicians placed varying degrees of importance on each. More original midwifery works in England can be said to start with Edmund Chapman's *An Essay on the Improvement of Midwifery* of 1733 (Wilson 1995, 6). After this date, man-midwife authored texts were at the cutting edge of discovery and knowledge, forging a new understanding of the female reproductive body, which had wider social implications. Alongside these ran popular sexual advice medical manuals such as the anonymous *Aristotle's Master-Piece* and Nicolas Venette's *Conjugal Love Reveal'd* – both published many times – which offered advice to the layperson on sex and reproduction, and often retained a more conservative element. However, with technological advances, particularly that of the microscope, old ideas were being constantly challenged. Consequently, theories on the process of conception, reproduction, and gestation were becoming increasingly chaotic.

This change affected both the understanding and portrayal of the female body and was influenced by several specific but interlinked trends. First, the professionalization of medicine encouraged professional rivalries to develop, giving rise to methods and treatments, often opposing the ancient sources. Second, an increase in the number of medical men interested in midwifery was part of this trend, and they squeezed out women's traditional knowledge in new male-authored textbooks. Third, new methods of scientific investigation into the human body (and the scientific "proof" of female inferiority) brought new insights that seemed to root the woman more firmly in the home; she was now seen to be designed for domesticity and maternity, and her body was best understood and managed by the male authorities around her. Fourth, the interest in demographic growth and the evolving passive maternal ideal gave a new emphasis to activities for women which best suited them. A shift occurred over the century in the perception of women from sexually rapacious to passive bodies, devoid of sexual desire. Fifth, in direct contrast to this, the traditional view of female lasciviousness continued to reverberate through contemporary popular culture. Finally, an explosion in print culture meant that more people were publishing their opinions about reproduction and childbearing than ever before. Often these queries on childbirth were eroticized and the female body became a focus of sexual ideas. This erotica was often euphemistic, full of double-entendres and intended as jest, but the authors' satirization of the medical fraternity, with its new-fangled theories, might be rooted in traditional – even conservative – thinking.

Midwifery Texts

Although men wrote most of the midwifery manuals, female voices came through. Both used case histories in their texts to put increased emphasis on the skill of the practitioner, and to assert medical authority (Keller 2007, 179–82). However, there is a distinct difference between the practices and beliefs of male and female practitioners of midwifery. The texts represent different genres with different target audiences. Often, medical men wrote explicitly for their male students, while female midwives wrote for other women. Female midwifery writers were much more likely to direct their advice to the expectant mother herself (Fife 2004, 190, 192), as Margaret Stephen did, addressing her book *Domestic Midwife; Or, the Best Means of Preventing Danger in Child-Birth Considered* (1795) to "any woman who is, or may be a mother" (1795, 3; Fife 2004, 187). Women were increasingly excluded, as university education was deemed requisite and women too weak for such knowledge (Martensen 1994, 121–3; Fife 2004, 186). Those texts written in the earlier part of the period combine information about childbirth with instruction in anatomy, tips on conception, and childcare, as well as moral exhortation (Sharp 1671/1999). As the eighteenth century progressed, midwifery manuals became more strictly focused on the event of childbirth itself, leaving all the ancillary information such as genital anatomy, conception, and childcare, to popular books such as *Aristotle's Master-Piece*, and *Conjugal Love Reveal'd* (1720), both published in multiple editions. The texts discussed here illustrate this struggle over the suitability of the female body for childbearing, and who was best equipped to manage the process.

For both male and female writers reproduction was considered one of the prime duties of women, and it was assumed that a married woman would want children. The midwife Jane Sharp, writing in the 1670s, thought it "a kind of self-destroying not to be willing to leave some succession" (128). Over a century later Martha Mears, herself a midwife and a mother, wrote in her book *The Pupil of Nature* (1797): "We must hasten to convince the timid female, that the very state, at which she has been taught to tremble, brings her nearer to the perfection of her being" (4). To conceive a child, according to Sharp, both husband and wife should enjoy their sexual couplings; mutual orgasm was necessary for conception to occur. If there was a lack of love between husband and wife the "Seed never mixeth as it should" (79). This opinion was the norm in reproductive texts up until the later seventeenth century. Within thirty years of Sharp's manual being published, however, female orgasm had been rendered unnecessary for conception. The physician John Pechey wrote in his *The Complete Midwife Enlarged* (1698, 43) that women did not emit any seed, an opinion found in popular works such as later editions of *Aristotle's Master-Piece* (1690, 15). This negation of the necessity of women's pleasure allowed for the portrayal of a more passive image of womanhood, devoid of sexual feeling.

The passivity of women was reinforced by new anatomical investigations into the skeleton, which were picked up on by midwifery texts. In the 1730s these investigations had made differences between men and women visible in their very bones (Schiebinger 1986, 53). This new understanding of the physicality of women gave impetus to their domestication; they were now seen to be specifically designed for "the domestic engagements of superintending the oeconomy of a family," according to Hugh Smythson in his work *The Compleat Family Physician* (1781). Smythson concluded that "from the delicacy of their frame, and their domestic sedentary employments [women] are subject to many diseases for want of a proper portion of air and exercise" (421, 418). Women were placed in a double bind, suited only to a lifestyle that actually weakened them further.

It was the pelvic bones that particularly interested the midwifery practitioners. The pelvis "may be esteemed the foundation on which all the other parts are sustained" according to man-midwife Thomas Denman in *An Introduction to the Practice of Midwifery* (1788, 2). The eminent man-midwife William Smellie began his text *A Treatise on the Theory and Practice of Midwifery* (published between 1752 and 1764) with a description of the structure and form of the pelvis, telling his readers that the "pelvis in women is wider than in men" (1790).[3] Plates of the pelvis are included in his text, providing a new set of imagery for the education of his students. Thomas Cooper MD also included a series of plates in his work *A Compendium of Midwifery* (1766, between 8 and 9). Although female authors were less likely to inform readers with drawings, they too talked about the form of the pelvis, and its role in childbirth (Stephen 1795, 65; Nihell 1760b, 6–7). The midwife Sarah Stone referred to the pelvic bones throughout her manual *A Complete Practice of Midwifery* (1737), and specifically referred to a post-mortem of a pregnant woman she had attended, noting in particular the small space left in the pelvic cavity by the fetus (128–9). Margaret Stephen forthrightly acknowledged the usefulness of this information in her midwifery manual of 1795: "A clear knowledge of these bones, enables the midwife to practice her art with more judgement and safety, than she would otherwise do" (25). As, in her opinion, difficult births were most often caused by a disproportion between the child's head and the mother's pelvis, understanding the anatomy of the area was vital for midwifery practitioners (64). Both male and female practitioners drew on the authority gained from being familiar with this new research. While men presented themselves as natural authorities, the women midwives presented themselves as keeping up with the new research, and incorporating it into their practice.

With the entrance of male physicians into the arena of midwifery, discussions about the unsuitability of the female body for reproduction emerged which had not been evident in the earlier midwifery texts. In the male-authored texts, this sometimes took the form of discussion about problems caused by obstructions in the vagina. The female body came to be seen as something to be examined, accessed, and penetrated under the scrutiny of male midwives. This can be seen in William Smellie's detailed explanation of an examination of a young married woman: "I then directed her to lean forwards on the back of a chair, and seating myself behind, attempted to examine the uterus by the vagina, when I found the entrance obstructed." In these texts, the hymen became problematic and the excising of the hymen was considered permissible, if not essential, if full access to the female body was to take place. He continued,

> Through the persuasion of the mother, she consented to have the parts inspected; and being laid supine upon a couch, I separated the labia, when I perceived the hymen ... effectually obstructing the introduction of the penis. Having snipped this attachment asunder, I introduced my finger into the vagina. (1790, 173)

Intervention in disposing of the hymen was seen as necessary not just for inspection but also prior to the birth, as the physician, surgeon, farrier, and man-midwife Henry Bracken noted in *The Midwife's Companion* (1737). He described a case of a woman who retained her hymen, even after falling pregnant. This was approached as a problem in need of rectification, as he explains: "We snipped it in sunder with a Pair of Scissors, when she was in Labour" (16).

Even the hymen of young women and girls well below the age of menarche became a medical concern in the male-authored midwifery manuals. On a much younger patient, a girl aged five or six, who had already been unsuccessfully "twice opened by a surgeon" to rectify her imperforate hymen, Smellie snipped the hymen then "gradually dilated, first with my little finger, and then with the forefinger, until I could touch the os uteri," and stopped the flesh re-uniting by inserting a tent (1790, 174). In another of Smellie's cases, a teenage girl complained to her father of symptoms pursuant with menstruation but with no evacuation of blood. The father "immediately perceived it was occasioned by an imperforated hymen. This he forthwith opened with a lancet, which was instantly followed by a discharge of about three pints and a half of blood" (175). In these cases, the young women are utterly passive, their bodies are mere objects to be manipulated by the examiner – the overriding aim is to make the body penetrable. In these texts, the female body is seen to need male intervention if they are to be made fit for the purpose of childbearing. However, women writers diverge from male midwives in that there are no comparable discussions in the texts written by women, and they see little need for manipulation or intervention. The lone example is Jane Sharp who tells of a woman whose too-narrow passage was rectified by "a Chirugeon [who] made the Orifice wider, and she was by that means happily brought to bed of a Son" (203). No more detail is considered necessary.

Female midwives frequently objected to women being the objects of male scrutiny and experimentation. In her book, *A Treatise on the Art of Midwifery* (1760), midwife Elizabeth Nihell criticized the procedure in lying-in hospitals, where labouring women were placed with their "thighs raised and expanded ... feet drawn to posteriors, and kept steady in that position ... under the eyes of a male practitioner, with his helpers ... only for the experiments of a *forceps*" (237). A woman's body deserved some privacy according to the women writers, and it was generally thought indecent for men to want to be peering and poking at women who were not their wives. Nihell was very much opposed to the "utter impropriety of men addicting themselves to this occupation" (*A Treatise*, 1760a, 85). Margaret Stephen was clear that any touching "is to be made in as private a manner as possible: the patient should lie on the bed, on her left side, and she should be covered with the bed-cloaths" (30). While these women may well have been seeking to protect their own livelihood against the encroachment of man-midwives, they expressly believed that women's dignity was being affronted by constant male interference. Furthermore, female-authored midwifery texts stress that most women have normal births. Margaret Stephen reiterated this point throughout her manual; in her experience, "perhaps one woman in some hundreds may be found, who from disease, mal-conformation of the pelvis, or some lusus naturae in the foetus, requires the aid of an obstetric surgeon" (10). In the overwhelming majority of births, the labouring woman required little assistance, and that assistance could be more than adequately provided by a female midwife – the female body is seen as fit for both the purpose of giving birth and assisting at the event.

The nature of what constituted appropriate insertions was debated in the texts, and reflected the professional struggle between male and female midwives. Elizabeth Nihell took exception to Smellie's advocacy of inserting fingers into the anus to feel for the child's head through the rectal wall. She wrote: "But how such a thought could enter into a man's head I cannot conceive, as thrusting his fingers there, for any beneficial purpose" (*An Answer* 1760b, 19). She was also adamant that given time, the bodies of the mother and child would work together, as the child's head slowly moulded itself to fit through the mother's pelvis (*A Treatise*, 1760a, 275). However, criticisms were not necessarily split along gender lines; they could also reflect other professional rivalries. Sarah Stone complained of an ignorant midwife who "in opening the outer gate, (as she call'd it) was the way, said she, to help the inner," meaning that to help the cervix dilate the midwife had stretched the anus (1737, 24). When deemed necessary, though, a skilled midwife should intervene; Stone explained how, when presented with a difficult breech delivery, she "dilated the *Matrix*," "broke the Waters, and slipt my finger in the Bending of the Child's Thigh ... and so deliver'd her in less than three minutes" (98). Only where a mother or baby was in difficulty was intervention required.

How and when instruments, particularly forceps, were used for extracting the child during labour was a contentious issue. Horror stories started to emerge of the havoc wreaked by inept men extracting babies with undue force, damaging mother and baby in the process. Women were not necessarily asked whether they consented to their use either; it was sometimes assumed they were not capable of making an informed judgment. Smellie actually counselled his students to introduce their instruments into the birthing room by stealth:

> let him spread the sheet that hangs over the bed, upon his lap, and, under that cover, take out and dispose the blades on each side of the patient; by which means he will often be able to deliver with the forceps, without their being perceived by the woman herself or any other of the assistants. (1790, 84)

This would avoid alarming a woman, and allow the man-midwife to get on with his work unopposed. Female midwives did not find this covert behaviour acceptable. Margaret Stephen had herself trained with a former pupil of Smellie, but completely disagreed with this deceit. She wrote that the forceps "*never* must be used without acquainting" the woman (Stephen 1795, 18, 68). Stephen also cautioned against "the forwardness with which young men, in the practice of midwifery, use instruments in laborious cases," unable to differentiate a normal birth from a difficult or potentially dangerous one (54). She related a cautionary tale of an inexperienced doctor attempting a forceps birth on a long but normal labour that resulted in the death of the child. His eagerness to introduce instruments was disastrous (54–62). Stephen believed that, although forceps could be of "the greatest utility," and "delivery with instruments has saved some lives … the instances in which they have done service, will never compensate for the mischief done by their unnecessary and mal-application" (67–8). Similarly, Nihell eschewed the use of instruments for extracting the child, preferring the hands as infinitely kinder (1760b, 4–5). Her claim that women were naturally more dexterous, with supple and safe hands (1760a, 68) was not new, but one that intensified with men's increased presence in the birthing chamber. The unnaturalness of man-midwifery and his use of instruments to deliver children, she believed, were "outrages to Nature," responsible for the murder of women and children (1760b, 25). Other practices appalled Nihell; she particularly disagreed with Smellie's idea of puncturing the pudenda if it became excessively stretched during labour. His theory was that such a method would apparently bring relief to the woman. Nihell responded: "The scheme of *puncturing* the *pudenda*, however, must be a pretty amusement for a *pudendist*, whatever is the greater suffering for it afterwards to the deluded woman, that will submit to it" (1760b, 16).

Male and female writers of midwifery texts also exhibited different attitudes to pain. Margaret Stephen acknowledged the "anguish of childbirth." In her estimation, manually stretching the vagina, inserting the hand and putting the fingers into the cervix were all painful procedures, and only those who had gone through childbirth could "say, what it would be to have this practised upon themselves" (37). Sarah Stone, while allowing that some intervention was necessary, wrote that it should be carefully done with regard to the woman's pain and suffering. She acknowledged that childbirth was painful and stressed that despite what certain man-midwives might write: "'tis to be observed, when the hand is in the body, and in motion, it creates great pain to the Woman" (42). Women writers empathized with their patients claiming direct experience, while using an assuring tone to their readers. Men could be far less sympathetic to the suffering of women in childbirth. Physician Stephen Freeman in his book,

The Ladies' Friend (1788), dismissed the pain felt when the midwife's hand is put up into the womb: "Poh! That is a groundless fear; you cannot hurt the woman by passing your hand into the womb" (319).

Older midwifery manuals detail the perennial problems of knowing true from false conception, and knowing when true labour was taking place. According to Sharp, the woman patient herself could not be relied on to know; only a skilled practitioner could tell (159–60). As more man-midwives took up practice, the question of who had the better knowledge was cast differently. Female midwives needed to show that women had more knowledge by virtue of their sex. Sarah Stone included examples. In one case, she was called to attend a woman who thought her labour had begun, but Stone was sure that actually the woman only needed to move her bowels. By giving the woman a medicinal remedy, the pains were stopped. In another case, the pains were actually the early symptoms of smallpox; in yet another, the woman was advised that she had colic, but unfortunately she didn't heed Stone's advice and called a second midwife in, who forced the labour resulting in the delivery of a dead child (Stone 1737, 97, 87–91). While these examples served to establish Stone's skill and experience, she included examples where midwife and patient work together. One experienced mother was able to relate how her latest labour differed, allowing Stone to assess the problem and ultimately facilitate a successful delivery (140). Margaret Stephen allowed the woman some agency during the labour; she found "no occasion to confine the patient to any particular posture, until the time comes in which she must be assisted; she may sit, lie, or walk, as inclination leads" (35). Self-interest on the part of the practitioners encouraged the extolling of their own capabilities, but the women authors used their gender to advantage by addressing the women readers as allies, not merely patients. The women in their texts are more active, contributing to the process of reproduction, not just passively awaiting a male practitioner's intervention. Man-midwives tended to focus on themselves as practitioners, treating a pregnant body; the personhood of the patient is largely absent, and the woman is rarely addressed directly.

Erotic Satires

Scientific theories on conception, pregnancy, and childbirth emanated from the Royal Society, an institution which had been founded "for Improving Natural Knowledge." Its findings were published in the pamphlet *Philosophical Transactions*, the first in 1665, and it would continue to run throughout the eighteenth century. As early as 1677 (not published until

1679),[4] in a letter to the Royal Society, Antoni van Leeuwenhoek had described his findings of "spermatic worms" (spermatozoa) and "animalcule" viewed under his improved microscope; he noticed the multitudes of animalcules in rainwater as "seeds" being carried up when rainwater evaporates in the heat of the sun to be returned to earth as rain. Christiaan Huygens confirmed his findings of sperm, along with Nicholaas Hartsoeker (inventor of the screw barrel simple microscope) who in 1694 reported his belief that tiny humans existed in sperm.

Around the same time as developments were occurring in medical understandings of conception, reproduction, and childbirth, a specific form of satire surfaced which questioned these new hypotheses. These satires came in the form of suggestive erotica published as articles in magazines and in pamphlets for a public who was increasingly dubious about the claims of physicians and scientists. The satires acted as a platform for debate and were used as a tool to question the more outlandish theories emerging in science and philosophy, while simultaneously using ideas about pregnancy and childbirth as a place where secrets of the female sex might be gleaned.[5]

All three satires examined here were probably written by "Sir" John Hill (1714–75).[6] Hill was a prolific, unscrupulous man who managed to combine a serious study of medicine and botany with writing satirical erotica. He studied botany, and was employed by both Lord Petre and the Duke of Richmond in the arrangement of their gardens and collection of dried plants. He also ran a column as "The Inspector" in the *London Daily Advertiser and Literary Gazette*, which Isaac D'Israeli decried as a highly scandalous chronicle (Rousseau 1960; Rousseau 1982; Rousseau and Haycock 1999, 377–406).[7] He knew various members of the Royal Society, including Martin Folkes, Sir Hans Sloane, Henry Baker, William Watson, and James Parsons. Although Folkes and Baker had acted as his patrons introducing Hill to the Royal Society, Hill failed to obtain the requisite number of votes to allow him entry. As a result of his rejection by the society, while he was editor of *British Magazine* (1746–50) he wrote scurrilous pieces condemning the Royal Society while attacking his former patrons, Folkes and Baker, in a publication entitled *A View of the World of the Royal Society* (1751). He also ridiculed the Society's *Philosophical Transactions*, a journal to which he had contributed only a couple of years previously. Despite his knack of upsetting eminent colleagues, Hill was recognized for his serious works including a translation of Theophrastus's *History of Stones* (1746), his *General Natural History* (1748–52), a catalogue of animals, vegetables, and minerals, *The Vegetable System* (1759), and *Exotic Botany* (1759). He corresponded with the Earl of Bute, and with Linnaeus to whom he dedicated *The Sleep of Plants and Cause of Motion in the Sensitive Plant Explain'd* (1757). He was also the first to connect cancer to tobacco in a little-known pamphlet *Caution against the Immoderate Use of Snuff* (1759).

All three erotic satires were published in 1750 and depicted fantastical ideas on reproduction and female sexual behaviour in parodies on female self-fertilization, while simultaneously deriding the contemporary scientific world. The first tract, *Lucina Sine Concubitu,* went under the pseudonym "Abraham Johnson" and was "a letter humbly address'd to the Royal Society"; the second was *A Letter To Dr. Abraham Johnson on his new schemes for the propagation of the human species* by "Richard Roe"; the anonymous third was entitled *A Dissertation on Royal Societies. Occasioned by the late pamphlets of Dr. Abraham Johnson and Dr Richard Roe.* The pseudonyms thus tie them all together. They examine four main concerns which were circulating among scientists in contemporary debate: first, the diminished role of women in reproduction; second, the need for female orgasm as a necessary prerequisite for conception; third, the problem of unwanted offspring; and fourth, the entry of both science and the male physician into the female domain of childbirth (Donnison 1977; Porter 1997; Wilson 1985).

Lucina Sine Concubitu was published both as an independent chapbook (selling for one shilling) and as an article in *British Magazine*, March 1750. Further editions followed and translations were made into French and German, a testimony to their popularity at home and abroad. The narrator is portrayed as a physician practised in "Man-Midwifry," a breed of men regarded by the wealthier clients as more knowledgeable than female midwives. In a parody of the reproductive process, he claims that women have no need for men and aims to prove "by most Incontestable Evidence, drawn from Reason and Practice, that a Woman may conceive and be brought to Bed without any Commerce with Man." He attests to a discovery "entirely new, and which I am sure will equal anything that has been offered to the World since Philosophy has been a Science" ("Johnson" [Hill] 1750, 1).

The need for male involvement in conception is questioned in the same fashion that contemporary scientists were questioning the contribution of the female in the reproductive process. While the role of the female was being diminished by scientists, the narrator turns their theories on their head, dispensing with the male role altogether. The narrator ponders alternative methods of fertilization, this time following writers of ancient erotica; he quotes Virgil's suggestion that offspring can be born without coition:

The Mares to Cliffs of rugged Rocks repair,
And with wide Nostrils snuff the western Air:
When (wondrous to relate) the Parent Wind,
Without the Stallion, propagates the Kind. (13)

Aristotle had originally deemed mares sexually wanton; they were said to chase stallions in order to satisfy their sexual urges. If not impregnated by a stallion, the mares would be fertilized by the wind (Schiebinger 1996, 163–77). Taking up this idea, the author suggests that if mares become pregnant without coition, through sniffing the air, then maybe the same could be done by women. He proposes that it is women who are the most fertile and likely carriers of fertility, not men, and to test his theory, he builds "a wonderful cylindrical, catoptrical, rotundo-concavoconvex Machine" which acts as "a kind of Trap to intercept the floating Animalcula in that prolific Quarter of the Heavens" ("Johnson" [Hill] 1750, 15–16). He concludes that the wind carries the Animalcula which women then inhale. Impregnation occurs resulting in the possibility that "a Woman may be with Child in a single State, consistently with the purest Virtue" (37).

Humorous jibes are directed at women on account of their sexual natures; the narrator suggests an altered state of affairs regarding female sexual licence. He proposes that, once parthenogenesis is understood, women will be able to sexually indulge themselves without fear of tarnishing their good names, and "it will be easy for a young Lady to lose her Maidenhead without losing her Character" (38).

Two contemporary issues – that of conception without the aid of a man; and that of pneumatic conception, or the notion of animalcula or "seeds" being propagated by air – are played out. The piece satirizes William Harvey who had already made an impact during the previous century with his book *De Generatione* (1651), in which he established the basic process for formation of life and had defined the production of eggs as common to all animals. Yet Harvey had also suggested that impregnation could be attained through magnetization, by conception of an idea or "contagion," asserting that "many animals, especially insects, arise and are propagated from elements and seeds so small as to be invisible (like atoms flying in the air), scattered and dispersed here and there by the winds; yet these animals are supposed to have arisen spontaneously, or from decomposition because their ova are nowhere to be found" (Gasking 1967, 19). The doctor in *Lucina Sine Concubitu* similarly queries a more recent assertion: "I began to question, why might not the Foetus be as compleatly hatched in the seminal Vessels of the Woman, as when it passes through the

Organs of both Sexes ... whether Animalcula did really float about in the Air, and slide down the Throat as he [Mr. Woolaston] described?" ("Johnson" [Hill] 1750, 11). Here, he is referring to William Wollaston (1660–1724) whose *Religion of Nature Delineated* (1722) was a popular book selling 10,000 copies "in a few years" and went through at least six editions by 1738. Wollaston had suggested the idea of pneumatic conception:

> If then the semina, out of which animals are produced, are as (as I doubt not) animalcula already formed; which, being dispersed about, especially in some opportune places, are taken in with aliment, or perhaps the very air; being separated in the body of the males by strainers proper to every kind, and then lodged in their seminal vessels, do there receive some kind of addition and influence; and being thence transferred into the wombs of the females, are there nourished more plentifully, and grow, till they become too big to be any longer confined. (Wollaston 1722, 65)

In an attempt to explain the female predicament, the narrator confesses that after reading the book,

> I was instantly thrown into a *Reverie*, and began to reflect with myself, that if such little Embryos, or *Animalcula* are so dispersed about, and taken in at the Mouth with Air or Aliment ... why might not the Foetus be as compleatly hatched in the seminal Vessels of the Woman, as when it passes through the Organs of both Sexes? ("Johnson" [Hill] 1750, 10–11)

A second erotic satire, *A Letter To Dr. Abraham Johnson, On the Subject of his new Scheme for the Propagation of the Human Species* (1750) parodied the scientist René-Antoine Ferchault Réaumur who had undertaken studies on eggs and embryonic chickens. A member for the Academy of Science in Paris, Réaumur, had written to the London Royal Society explaining his experiments. The results were published in *The Art of Hatching and Bringing Up Domestic Fowls by Means of Artificial Heat* (1750), according to the pamphlet, "an abstract of Réaumur's work communicated to the Royal Society January last by Mr. Trembley [possibly Abraham Trembley, a Swiss naturalists] translated from the French." Here, methods in Egypt of using "ovens which are very different sizes were described, but in general capable of containing from forty to forty-score thousand eggs" (Réaumur 1750, 4). Dung generated heat and so it was thought to be an easy way to propagate chickens. The pamphlet explains,

> Dung is indeed capable of acquiring a much greater degree of heat, than that which is necessary for the hatching of Eggs: and Mr. De Reaumur has put his eggs into an earthen pot, and lodges them in a layer of dung where they have almost stewed and parboiled. (12)

The experimenter in *A Letter to Dr. Abraham Johnson* similarly lays out his own experiment,

> I have plann'd out a spacious Area with Walks for the Ladies to take the Air upon, and with Ranges of my *artificial Uteri* disposed on every Side, into which they may at Pleasure drop their Load ... into hot Beds of Dung ... and other Receptacles of proportion'd Size, for the more corpulent of my Customers; in each of these I have placed a Basket of soft Cotton, and in each I have suspended a Thermometer, to certify me to the utmost Exactness of the Degree of Heat. ("Roe" [Hill] 1750, 18–20)

A world is proposed in which women could conceive without recourse to sex, and leave the incubation of their offspring elsewhere. Natural abortifacients were well-known in early modern England and used as a means of controlling fertility (McLaren 1984), and the doctor in the narration proffers a means of avoiding pregnancy altogether using contraception in the form of eaglestone; if tied to her leg, "or worn on any Part below the Seat of Impregnation" it would immediately bring on a miscarriage and "bring forth the little Embryo, of whatever Age, or under whatever Circumstances, it may be fix'd there" ("Roe" [Hill] 1750, 25–6).[8]

Overtly, the satire pokes fun at the more conventional view on women's modesty and ambitions of chasteness. The implication is that but for the moral regulations controlling women's sexual behaviour and the risk of pregnancy, women would revert to their natural state, embracing sexual practices. However, there is an underlying tension which suggests that this alternative world is being shown as a warning to men. Free from their burden of pregnancy and childbirth, women would be able to indulge their naturally libidinous yearnings undetected.

In March 1750, a third satire, *A Dissertation on Royal Societies. Occasion'd by the late pamphlets of Dr. Abraham Johnson, and Dr. Richard Roe*,[9] was published which described the Royal Society in a derogatory fashion as a "motley Mixture of all Kinds of men from the Fop to the Philosopher, from the Lord to the Mechanic," overseen by a President full of "imaginary Importance" ([John Hill] 1750, 17). The author further vilifies the

Royal Society declaring, "It was with strange Discontent that I found myself unable to discover ... the least Glimpse of those Talents which their Works speak them possessed of" (45). To ensure there could be little doubt as to the identity of the true author of the pamphlet, an advertisement had been placed in the front stating, "The recorder is admonished not to suppose these Letters the Product of either of those random Genius's Abraham Johnson or Richard Roe" (3).

If anyone was left in doubt as to the reason for these pamphlets, Hill made sure that his intentions were well known. In February 1750, the *British Magazine* (viz. Hill as editor), published "A Letter from Dr. Abraham Johnson To the Author of the British Magazine" declaring, "You are sensible, that the very last thing I was call'd upon to do, was to prove that a natural child might be born without the help of the father" (Hill, *British Magazine*, 1750, 216). Hill was amazed at the consternation the tract caused since he had no other ambition than "to tickle myself to make myself laugh," but it was obvious to readers that ridicule of the Royal Society and its experiments were at the heart of the matter. The following month, the *British Magazine* under the same title heading "A Dissertation on Royal Societies. Occasion'd by the late pamphlets of Dr. Abraham Johnson, and Dr. Richard Roe" again retold the story of *Lucina Sine Concubitu*, and asked disingenuously who was the author of these tracts; could it be "one author with two names?" Hill further connected himself with the papers by printing the article in the *British Magazine*, entitled "A *strange* Instance *given by Mr.* REAUMUR, *in his* Treatise *of the hatching of* Eggs" (*British Magazine* 1750, 216).

Conclusion

The portrayal of the female reproductive body in medical texts and scientific journals shifted during the eighteenth century. Some changes can be linked with developments within the medical profession which impacted on midwifery by increasing the role of men-midwives and consequently making the discourses about the female body more masculine. The language employed in midwifery manuals becomes more detached from the woman patient as a sentient being and more concerned with establishing the medical authority of the practitioner. The female-authored texts follow the same trend, but retain a greater awareness of the whole person. Changes are also linked with the new conception of women as sexually passive and maternal. As the female body was understood not to produce seed, the necessity of female orgasm was disposed of. The passive, seedless woman is portrayed in the texts, both literally and more obliquely as a passive body awaiting the intervention of men, without which her body is unfamiliar and unfit. The female body is increasingly represented as little more than its reproductive parts, whose regulation and penetration is now under masculine supervision.

Among these conflicting and chaotic discussions in the medical world, erotic satires acted as a leveller, parodying new theories on conception, pregnancy, and childbirth, and humorously re-establishing women's rights to the enjoyment of sex. The expectation of the writer would be that the readers would identify with his own prejudices – that scientists were above themselves in presenting new-fangled ideas, which sounded far-fetched and pretentious. The popularity of the texts, evident in their sales and translations, show that popular culture sometimes lagged behind the new theories of conception and childbirth being developed by the medical world, but reflected them in a ribald fashion as a form of mockery.

NOTES

1 See also Elaine Hobby's introduction in Sharp, 1671/1999, xvi, and Wilson 1995, 6.
2 See also *The Trotula*, 2002; *Soranus' Gynecology*, 1956; Lloyd 1983.
3 The 1790 edition contains the three volumes originally published between 1752 and 1764.
4 This had not been translated earlier because of regard for propriety and fear of the mention of sexual parts in vulgar words. Latin expressions were even used in the translations (Gasking 1967, 52).
5 I first explored these satires and themes in my book Peakman, *Mighty Lewd Books* 2003, 78–91; also see Rousseau 2010, 53–71.
6 According to George Rousseau, Hill took to calling himself "Sir" after 1774 when he received the order of Vasa from the king of Sweden (Rousseau 1960).
7 For more biographical information, also see George Rousseau 2012.
8 Eaglestones were hollow stones composed of several crusts, having a loose stone within, which were supposed at one time to be found in eagle's nests, to which medicinal values were attributed. Dent, ed. *Brewer's Dictionary of Phrase and Fable*, 15, 419.
9 This is also probably Hill, according to the BL Catalogue.

REFERENCES

Aristotle's Master-Piece. 1690. London: J. How.
Bracken, H. 1737. *The Midwife's Companion*. London: J. Clarke and J. Shuckburgh.
Chapman, E. 1733. *An Essay on the Improvement of Midwifery*. London: Printerd by A. Blackwell for A. Butterworth and J. Walthor.
Cooper, T. 1766. *A Compendium of Midwifery*. London.
Culpeper, N. 1656. *A Directory for Midwives*. London: Peter Cole.
Denman, T. 1788. *An Introduction to the Practice of Midwifery*. Vol. 1. London: J. Johnson.
Dent, Susie, ed. 2012. *Brewer's Dictionary of Phrase and Fable*. 19th ed. London: Hodder Education.
Donnison, J. 1977. *Midwives and Medical Men: A History of Inter-Professional Rivalries and Women's Rights*. London: Heinemann.
Fife, E. 2004. "Gender and Professionalism in Eighteenth-Century Midwifery." *Women's Writing* 11 (2): 185–200. http://dx.doi.org/10.1080/09699080400200304.
Freeman, S. 1788. *Ladies' Friend*. London.
Gasking, E. 1967. *Investigations into Generation, 1651–1828*. London: Hutchinson.
Guillemeau, J. 1612. *Childbirth: Or, The Happy Delivery of Women*. London: A. Hatfield.
[Hill, John]. 1750. *A Dissertation On Royal Societies In Three Letters from a nobleman on his Travels, to a Person of Distinction in Sclavonia, Containing An Account of an Assembly of a Royal Academy of Sciences at Paris. A Description Of A Meeting Of A Royal Society In London And A Coffee-House Conversation. With Explanatory Notes.* London: John Doughty.
[Hill, John]. 1750. "A Letter from Dr. Abraham Johnson To the Author of the British Magazine." London: *British Magazine*.
[Hill, John]. 1752. *Letters From The Inspector to a Lady*. London: M. Cooper.]
Johnson, Abraham [John Hill]. 1750. *Lucina Sine Concubitu*. London: M. Cooper.
Keller, E. 2007. *Generating Bodies and Gendered Selves: The Rhetoric of Reproduction in Early Modern England*. Seattle: University of Washington Press.
Lloyd, G.E.R., ed. 1983. *Hippocratic Writings*. London: Penguin.
Martensen, R. 1994. "The Transformation of Eve: Women's Bodies, Medicine and Culture in Early Modern England." In *Sexual Knowledge, Sexual Science: The History of Attitudes to Sexuality*, edited by Roy Porter and Mikulas Teich, 121–3. Cambridge: Cambridge University Press.

McLaren, A. 1984. *Reproductive Rituals: The Perception of Fertility in England from the Sixteenth Century to the Nineteenth Century*. London: Methuen.
Mears, M. 1797. *The Pupil of Nature; or Candid Advice to the Fair Sex*. London.
Needham, J. 1959. *History of Embryology*. Cambridge: Cambridge University Press.
Nihell, E. 1760a. *A Treatise on the Art of Midwifery*. London: A. Morley.
Nihell, E. 1760b. *An Answer to the Author of the Critical Review*. London: A. Morley.
Peakman, J. 2003. *Mighty Lewd Books: The Development of Pornography in Eighteenth-Century England*. Basingstoke: Palgrave.
Pechey, J. 1698. *The Complete Midwife Enlarged*. London: H. Rhodes, J. Philips, J. Taylor, and K. Bentley.
Porter, R., ed. 1996. *Cambridge Illustrated History of Medicine*. Cambridge: Cambridge University Press.
Porter, R., ed. 1997. *The Greatest Benefit to Mankind: A Medical History of Humanity from Antiquity to the Present*. London: HarperCollins.
Porter, R., and L. Hall. 1995. *The Facts of Life: The Creation of Sexual Knowledge in Britain, 1650–1950*. New Haven and London: Yale University Press.
Raynalde, T. 1545. *Byrth of Mankynde*. London.
Réaumur, R.-A. 1750. *The Art of Hatching and Bringing up Domestic Fowls by Means of Artificial Heat*. Dublin: George Faulkner.
Roe, Richard [John Hill]. 1750. *A Letter To Dr. Abraham Johnson, On The Subject Of His New Scheme For The Propagation Of The Human Species.* London: M. Cooper.
Rousseau, G. 2010. "Sexual Knowledge: Panspermist Jokes, Reproduction Technologies and Virgin Births." In *A Cultural History of the Human Body in the Enlightenment*, edited by Carole Reeves, 53–71. Oxford: Berg.
Rousseau, G. 2012. *The Notorious John Hill: The Man Destroyed by Ambition in the Era of Celebrity.* Bethlehem, PA: Lehigh University Press.
Rousseau, G.S. 1960. "The Much Maligned Doctor." *Journal of the American Medical Association* 8:103–8.
Rousseau, G.S., ed. 1982. *The Letters and Papers of Sir John Hill 1714–75*. New York: AMS Press.
Rousseau, G.S., and D. Haycock. 1999. "Voices Calling for Reform: The Royal Society in the Mid-Eighteenth Century – Martin Folkes, John Hill, and William Stukeley." *History of Science* 37 (118): 377–406.
Schiebinger, L. 1986. "Skeletons in the Closet: The First Illustrations of the Female Skeleton in Eighteenth Century Anatomy." *Representations* (Berkeley, Calif.) 14 (1):42–82. http://dx.doi.org/10.1525/rep.1986.14.1.99p01227.

Schiebinger, L. 1996. "Gender and Natural History." In *Culture of Natural History*, edited by N. Jardine, J.A. Secord, and E.C. Spary, 163–77. Cambridge: Cambridge University Press.

Sharp, J. (1671) 1999. *The Midwives Book, Or The Whole Art of Midwifery Discovered (1671).* Edited by Elaine Hobby. New York: Oxford University Press.

Smellie, W. 1790. *A Treatise on the Theory and Practice of Midwifery.* 3 vols. London: Alexander Cleugh and M. Watson.

Smythson, H. 1781. *The Compleat Family Physician.* London: Harrison.

Soranus' Gynecology. 1956. Translated by Oswei Temkin. Baltimore: Johns Hopkins University Press.

Stephen, M. 1795. *Domestic Midwife; Or, the Best Means of Preventing Danger in Child-Birth Considered.* London: S.W. Fores.

Stone, S. 1737. *A Complete Practice of Midwifery.* London: T. Cooper.

The Trotula. 2002. Translated by Monica H. Green Philadelphia: University of Pennsylvania Press.

Tuana, N. 1983. *The Less Noble Sex: Scientific, Religious and Philosophical Conceptions of Woman's Nature.* Bloomington: Indiana University Press.

Venette, N. c. 1720. *Conjugal Love Reveal'd.* 7th ed. London.

Wilson, A. 1985. "Participant or Patient? Seventeenth-Century Childbirth from the Mother's Point of View." In *Lay Patients and Practitioners: Lay Perceptions of Medicine in Pre-Industrial Society*, edited by Roy Porter, 129–44. Cambridge: Cambridge University Press.

Wilson, A. 1995. *The Making of Man-Midwifery: Childbirth in England 1660–1770.* London: University College London Press.

Wollaston, W. 1722. *Religion of Nature Delineated.* London.

21 Making the Rounds in the Old and New *Foundling Hospitals for Wit*: (Mis)Conceptions about Conceiving

DONALD W. NICHOL

Before Byron set the bar high for sexual revelation, Sir Charles Hanbury Williams (1708–59) was infamous for infecting his wife with syphilis, introducing the future Catherine the Great to her Polish lover, and penning sexually explicit satire. Regarded by Horace Walpole as the finest poet after Alexander Pope, Hanbury Williams was the creative force behind *The Foundling Hospital for Wit* (1743–9), a literary miscellany which spawned a sequel, *The New Foundling Hospital for Wit* (1768–73). The latter miscellany paid tribute to its founding editor and was published by John Wilkes's friend, the radical bookseller John Almon.[1] These two six-volume collections of poetry, prose, and parody took the pulse of foundlingism. This chapter makes the rounds of these satirical wards which reflected the rise in unwanted pregnancies in Britain during the long eighteenth century, both within and without the bonds of matrimony which, in turn, led to an alarming rise in abandoned newborns.

Britain's first real Foundling Hospital came about through the prolonged campaigning of Captain Thomas Coram (c. 1668–1751). Appalled by the all-too-common sight of helpless infants left to face the elements on the streets of London, Coram campaigned for seventeen years until George II signed the Royal Charter which gave the go-ahead to build a "Hospital for the Maintenance and Education of Exposed and Deserted Young Children" in 1739 which opened two years later.[2] With so much good will associated with the institution, it was only a matter of time before somebody satirized it. If deserted infants now had a place to go, then abandoned verses likewise deserved some form of literary shelter. The Foundling Hospital was a de facto admission of an underlying dysfunctionality in English society: more and more women were being impregnated by men who, for one reason (war; death) or another (reckless ne'er-do-wellism; already married), were not around to support their babies. Six years after the first *Foundling Hospital for Wit* started giving new life to literary strays, Mrs Deborah Wilkins was still offering to remove the newborn Tom Jones from Squire Allworthy's bed to the "Church-Warden's Door," giving him a fifty-fifty chance of surviving the night, "only a little rainy and windy," in the opening to Fielding's novel. The "Hussy its Mother," she thought, ought to be "committed to *Bridewel*, and whipt" (41). Fortunately, the good squire decided to adopt the baby and only banish the "esteemed" mother from the county.

The Literary *Foundling Hospital*

The first *Foundling Hospital for Wit* opened with a parody of the royal charter which gave the real Foundling Hospital, then in operation for two years, its mandate:

THE
ROYAL CHARTER
OF
Apollo and the *Muses*,
FOR
Establishing an HOSPITAL for the
Reception and Preservation of such
Brats of WIT and HUMOUR whose
Parents chuse to drop them.

By mimicking George II's royal proclamation, *The Foundling Hospital for Wit* displayed the insouciant sort of defiance Pope did, about the same time, in prefacing the 1743 *Dunciad* with a fake coat of arms over a mock royal proclamation which ordered Lewis Theobald "utterly to vanish, and evaporate," leaving "the said Throne of Poesy" vacant for the laureate, Colley Cibber (Pope, 5:252).[3] With a similar lack of concern about repercussions from the Lord Chamberlain, *The Foundling Hospital for Wit* announced this new home for unwanted literary creations with royal ventriloquism:

> WHEREAS our Trusty and Well-beloved Subject *Samuel Silence* Gentleman, in Behalf of great Numbers of *Mental Infants* daily exposed to Destruction, has by his Petition, humbly represented unto us, that many persons of WIT and HUMOUR of both sexes, being sensible of the frequent Murders committed on these beautiful Infants by the inhuman Custom of exposing them to

> perish and starve in the common News Papers, or to be bury'd and suffocated in Dunghills of Trash in the Monthly Magazines, have, by Instruments in Writing, declared their Intentions to contribute liberally towards the erecting and supporting an Hospital for the Reception and Preservation of such exposed and deserted Productions, as soon as We should be graciously pleased to grant our Letters Patent for that good purpose. (*FHW* 1: i–ii)

Samuel Silence was formally acknowledged "to be the sole Director, Proprietor, and Governour of this our *Hospital*" (ii). Abandoned poetical conceptions no longer needed to succumb to obscurity: with their new sturdier shelter, they now had a chance for a longer life than more ephemeral forms of the printed word could offer.

Fielding had good reason to be one of the first readers of the original *Foundling Hospital for Wit.* He was at Eton with the man assumed to be behind the mask of its editor and main contributor, Samuel Silence, i.e., Hanbury Williams, and they remained life-long friends.[4] The Battestins (who quote the first *Foundling* "brat" in full) suggest that Hanbury Williams witnessed the contretemps at Drury Lane between Fielding and the Irish actress Kitty Clive which inspired the very first poem in *The Foundling Hospital for Wit*: "*Verses occasioned by a Quarrel betwixt Mr.* F—ld—g *and Mrs.* Cl—ve, *on his intending her the Part of a Bawd, in his new Play called the* Wedding Day" (*FHW* 1:1; Battestin 361–2).

The second selection in this miscellany offers up "*A* SONG" (*FHW* 1:2) by Hanbury Williams (Adlard 122; Henke 279), composed in the ribald spirit of Tom D'Urfey whose licentious lyrics set the mood for many a copulation in the court of Charles II. D'Urfey's song, "When for Air I take my Mare," morphs from a horse-ride into a rhythmic copulation (which is attempted by Hanbury Williams's rider). D'Urfey's rider's mount "wriggles like a bride at night" with a motion that is "straight again, up and down, up and down, up and down, till she comes home with a trot, trot, trot, trot." Hanbury Williams's rider is too old to plant himself, let alone stay, in the filly's saddle:

> The Man so silly
> To think he's able,
> To back a Filly
> When old and feeble;
> Sighing,
> Toying,
> Grunting,

Mounting,
Scarce after all to his saddle can rise. (*FHW* 1:2)

The noun in the last line above is cited as an example of Hanbury Williams's use of "saddle" "as allusive of sexual riding" in which "lack of energy provides another dimension" "where an old man attempts 'to back a filly'" (Williams 3:1188). D'Urfey's rider resists being bucked: "When mane's seized, bum squeezed / I gallop, I gallop, I gallop, I gallop," but Hanbury Williams's old horseman cannot stay in the saddle: "Sudden she plunges, / Capers and lunges, / Off he is flung, and away Filly flies." Like the act of coition, D'Urfey's ride starts slowly and gallops to a climax, and "so ends the love of chase." As sung and grunted by The City Waites on their 1990 CD (track 18), *Thomas D'Urfey's Pills to Purge Melancholy*, "When for Air I take my Mare" rises to an ejaculatory leap followed by detumescence. Hanbury Williams's "SONG" ends like a sequel to D'Urfey's "pill" with words of advice to older men to take command.

Candid discussions about sexual intercourse took place long before Philip Larkin and Dr Ruth. Hanbury Williams carried on a voluminous and often peppery correspondence with Henry Fox, the future Lord Holland, another friend he met at Eton. On New Year's Day 1743, in a reply to Fox's "Perturbed letter" about his mistress, Hanbury Williams relayed a conversation overheard by his father-in-law between Lady Ethelreda Townshend (c. 1708–88) and Pope's friend, Robert Craggs Nugent (1709–88). Sitting between Lords Chesterfield and Cobham, Lady Townshend, who "speaks out and calls things by their Proper names," has the first word:

> Mr Nugent, I can't imagine How People ever came to imagine that you fuck well for my part to tell you the Truth I don't believe you fuck at all well. Now this was enough to dash a man before company, but as it happend my Father in law (who is very clever at repartee) had an answer ready that silenc'd her quite. Madam says he your Ladyship does me great injustice and besides that are very ungrateful for wherever I am I always declare that I believe your La[dysh]ip fucks more and better than any Woman in England. Now you know it was impossible for her to reply ... so her La[dysh]ip chang'd the discourse and ask'd my Father in Law whether he liked fucking in Condom. He told her not at all upon which said indeed If you would wet your Condom enough you would like it. For if a Condom is well Soak'd tis as good fucking with one as without one. (British Library: Add MSS 51390, ff. 102–3)

Such good advice on sexual hygiene came too late, if not ironically, for Hanbury Williams, who had undergone treatment for syphilis six months earlier. He infected his wife, Lady Frances, née Coningsby, youngest daughter of the first earl of Coningsby, without informing her. When her doctor diagnosed her condition, which, to her further mortification, became the talk of the town, she left the family home in Albemarle Street with their two daughters for good. The scandal did not adversely affect Hanbury Williams's political career: he served as MP for Monmouthshire (1734–47) and Leominster (1754–9), and was appointed to diplomatic missions between 1747 and 1757 in Dresden, Berlin, and St Petersburg where he acted as a go-between for his secretary (and future king of Poland) Stanislas Augustus Poniatowski and the soon-to-be Catherine the Great. His death at the age of fifty was hastened by his venereal disease.

He occasionally sent Fox drafts of poems and worked out ideas which found their way into verse. The topic of his letter to Fox, dated 9 July 1746, was "the D[uche]ss. of Manchester's Match" (BL: Add MSS 51391 f. 5v.) and hapless admirers who "fondled their dogs, Play'd with the monkey, and talked to the Parrot." This is a variation on the opening line of "Isabella: or, the Morning," one of Hanbury Williams's best poems: "THE monkey, lap-dog, parrot, and her Grace" (*NFHW* 1:2), a riff on Pope's "Men, Monkies, Lap-dogs, Parrots, perish all!" from *The Rape of the Lock* (Pope 2:193). Hanbury Williams winds up his letter with a post-script: "Pray tell Dicky that I hear that tho he had fortifyd thee [*sic*] Duchess very well, Husseys attack was a good one & that he fought well & gaind all his ground by Inches." Richard "Dicky" Bateman is one of the Duchess's admirers in "Isabella." Lady Isabella Montagu (d. 1786), daughter of John Montagu, 2nd Duke of Montagu, and Lady Mary Churchill, married William Montagu, 2nd Duke of Manchester, in 1723. When the duke died in 1739, his young dowager became one of the most desirable catches in the realm.

The fourth volume of *The Foundling Hospital for Wit* (1747) led with a clutch of poems about the duchess by Hanbury Williams, the first of which was enough to cause some consternation, so much so that the poet felt it wise to retire to rural Wales for a spell (and write a poem to that effect for the "Isabella" cycle). According to the *Oxford Dictionary of National Biography* entry by Mary Margaret Stewart:

> a poem he wrote but had never intended to publish, "An Ode to Fox, on the Marriage of the Duchess of Manchester," brought him trouble and deepened

his distress. The duchess of Manchester, widowed in 1739, married in 1743 Edward Hussey, an Irishman, but the marriage was kept secret until summer1746. The ode, while not uncomplimentary to the duchess, contained a stanza which was seen as a slur on the Irish. Williams – upset, partly because he had always supported the interests of Ireland – left London for Monmouthshire to avoid unpleasant confrontations with Hussey and his allies.

That is perhaps putting it mildly. The poem in question, "*An ODE to the Honourable* H— y F—x, *on the Marriage of the Du— —s of* M— —R *to* H—s—y, *Esq;*" begins:

CLIO, behold this charming Day,
The Zephyrs blow, the Sun looks gay,
  The Sky one perfect Blue;
Can you refuse at such a Time,
When *F—x* and I both beg for Rhyme,
  To sing us something new?

The Goddess smil'd, and thus begun:
I've got a pleasing Theme, my Son,
  I'll sing the conquer'd D— — —s;
I'll sing of that disdainful Fair,
Who, scap'd from *Scotch* and *English* Snare,
  Is fast in *Irish* Clutches. (*FHW* 4:1)

The fourth line of the third last stanza (below; italics mine) is undoubtedly insulting, but the damage may be somewhat mitigated in the last stanza by the fact that the most celebrated widow in the country chooses an Irish husband over an English one:

But careful Heaven design'd her Grace
For one of the *Milesian* Race,
  On stronger Parts depending;
Nature indeed denies them Sense,
But gives them Legs and Impudence,
  That beats all Understanding.

Which to accomplish, *H—ss—y* came,
Op'ning before the noble Dame
  His honourable Trenches;

Nor of Rebukes nor Frowns afraid,
He push'd his Way (he knew his Trade,)
And won the Place by Inches.

Look down, St. *Patrick*, with Success,
Like *H—ss—y's* all the *Irish* bless,
May they all do as he does;
And still preserve their Breed the same,
Cast in his Mould, made in his Frame,
To comfort *English* Widows.[5] (*FHW* 4:3)

In other words, size counts. Isabella, one of the few women in the eighteenth century who finds herself free to choose, opts for the best-hung mate. Such tropes as penis-as-battle-winning-weapon have been explored extensively in Raymond Stephanson's ground-breaking study of eighteenth-century phallocentricism, *The Yard of Wit*. Hanbury Williams merges English-versus-Irish with upper-versus-lower class in the debate over length, potency, and penetration power. Long before *Pride and Prejudice*, he presents us with an unacknowledged truth, the obverse of Jane Austen's much-coined phrase, that a young widow in possession of a good fortune must be in want of a stud.

A quarter of a century after the old series started, *The New Foundling Hospital for Wit* hit London with a splash. In 1768, names on the title-page like Charles Churchill, Thomas Potter, and John Wilkes would have enticed readers as they were linked to the mock-Satanic orgies at Medmenham Abbey (which came to be known as the Hell-Fire Club). It was the year of Wilkes's return from France, his determination to regain a seat in parliament, and the ensuing civil unrest. John Almon, the bookseller and probable editor, added frontispieces to each volume. The second volume (1768) opened with a writer witnessing Britannia being gang-raped. The frontispiece to the third volume (1769) satirized a blindfolded George III being led with the help of a nose-ring by his mother, the Princess Dowager, who sends a sexually provocative signal to her alleged lover, the Earl of Bute. While there seems to have been no basis for this rumour, such an image set the standard high for audacious scurrility in the wake of the Wilkes riots.[6]

Although he had been dead for nearly a decade, Hanbury Williams provided the segue between the old and new series: his "Isabella: or, the Morning" ushered in the first volume of *The New Foundling Hospital for Wit* in 1768. Williams mentions "Isabella" as the first of four new "*Town Scenes*" in a letter to Henry Fox on 6 June 1743. The next four poems in the new series all are foundlings in their own right. Thomas Potter's "Epigram on a Certain Lady's Coming into the Room at Bath, with a Diamond Crescent in her Hair" would certainly have been an unwanted "brat" in some quarters, particularly Gloucester Cathedral. Potter (1718–59) was the son of the Archbishop of Canterbury and said to be so rakish that even Wilkes was led astray by him.

CHaste Dian's crescent on her front display'd,
Behold! the wife proclaims herself a maid!
Come, fierce Taillard, or fiercer Julius come;
On this fair subject urge the contest home,
Pluck honour from this emblematic moon,
And solve the point which puzzles W— — —n:
This radiant emblem you may then transpose,
And give the horned crescent to the spouse. (*NFHW* 1:10)

One clue to this riddle is given in a corner of the frontispiece where the portrait of a clergyman rests over a legend reading, "N. to P.'s Works." William Warburton's "Notes to Pope's Works" were much ridiculed ever since the poet chose him to be his literary executor. The reference to Taillard is obscure although "Julius" seems to refer to Warburton's work on the emperor Julian published in 1751. Warburton was forty-seven when he married Gertrude Tucker, the eighteen-year-old niece of Ralph Allen, in 1746. The Warburtons had been married ten years when their first and only child, Ralph Allen Warburton, was born. The archbishop and his family had visited the Allens and Warburtons at Prior Park some nine months earlier. Rumours spread of an affair between Gertrude and the archbishop's prodigal son, Thomas Potter, who was twenty years younger than Warburton. Warburton was curiously silent about the birth of his son in his correspondence at the time. Warburton was elevated to the bishopric of Gloucester three years later. Potter, the alleged lover, father, and venomous epigrammatist, died in 1759. The epigram, laced with adulterous innuendo, relayed scandal that was a dozen years old.

The third entry, "Written under the Picture of Dr. Hayter, Bishop of Norwich," concerns the bishop's dismissal as governor of the Prince of Wales in 1752. Thomas Hayter (1702–62) was the natural son of Lancelot Blackburne, Archbishop of York (1658–1743), whom Pope had fingered as an adulterer in "Sober Advice from Horace." Even clergymen were imagined to be rutting in public places. Pope imagines Edmund Gibson, the Bishop of London (1669–1748), witnessing Thomas Sawbridge, Dean of Ferns and Leighlin (d. 1733), who had been accused, but not convicted, of committing rape:

> My Lord of *L*— —*n*, chancing to remark
> A *noted Dean* much busy'd in the Park,
> "Proceed (he cry'd) proceed, my Reverend Brother,
> "Tis *Fornicatio simplex*, and no other:
> "Better than lust for Boys, with *Pope* and *Turk*,
> "Or others Spouses, like my Lord of— —[York]." (Pope, 4:79, ll. 39–44)

The archbishop kept a mistress and fathered Hayter by another woman. His father evidently looked out for his illegitimate son: Hayter was consecrated Bishop of Norwich in 1749 and translated to London in 1761. According to Horace Walpole, the archbishop was formerly a buccaneer and "retained nothing of his first profession except his seraglio" (Pope 4:347). Fornication was preferable among clergy to sodomy, presumably because the act might result in the production of a child.

The fourth and fifth poems are linked: "A Simile" (*NFHW* 1:11–13) and "Doll Common" (1:13–16), which is subtitled "A Fragment. In Answer to the foregoing." "A Simile" follows the career of Corinna, an old-fashioned rustic girl:

> CORINNA, in the country bred,
> Harbour'd strange notions in her head,
> Notions in town quite out of fashion:
> Such as, that love's a dang'rous passion;
> That virtue is the maiden's jewel;
> And, to be safe, she must be cruel. (*NFHW* 1:11)

Such country girls sailing into society find it difficult to preserve chastity especially with a man in uniform:

> At length a troop of horse came down,
> And quarter'd in a neighb'ring town.
> The cornet, he was tall and, young,
> And had a most bewitching tongue.
> They saw and lik'd.

All's fair in love and war, and the tactics are much the same. The metaphors of seduction are cast in a distinctly military mould:

> The siege begun,
> Each hour he some advantage won.
> He ogled first; – she turn'd away; –
> But met his eyes the following day.
> Then her reluctant hand he seizes:
> That soon she gives him, when he pleases.
> Her ruby lips he next attacks: –
> She struggles; – in a while she smacks.
> Her snowy breasts he then invades:
> That yields too after some parades;
> And of that fortress once possest,
> He quickly masters all the rest.
> No longer now, a dupe to fame,
> She smothers or resists her flame,
> But loves without or fear or shame. (*NFHW* 1:11–12)

And so, the cornet penetrates the last bastion of Corinna's defence. The fifth poem, "Doll Common," is a Harlot's Progress with a twist. In this Hogarthian moral fable, Doll comes to town to sell her body for a living. Cælia, her friend from the country, tries to steer Doll along the path of virtue without success. Doll sells her wares in Hyde Park by day and the playhouses by night until time eventually catches up with her. While Doll's rates have been declining, Cælia's stock has risen through a good marriage and healthy offspring. Doll encounters Cælia with her children, Senegal and "twins of Indian mien," Louisbourg and Du Quesne, who represent the burgeoning empire. Her next child is to be named America, but the poem ends with Doll kicking Cælia in the womb, resulting in "black *abortion*" (*NFHW* 1:16).

Hanbury Williams borrowed a couple of characters from Swift – Strephon and Chloe – in "*A Lamentable* CASE. *Submitted to the* Bath *Physicians.*" The comic poem addresses the problem of sexual scheduling difficulties. Strephon comes home at night too drunk to perform; and, in the morning when he is sober, Chloe is still asleep.

> At Night, when *Strephon* comes to rest,
> *Chloe* receives him on her Breast,
> With fondly-folding Arms:
> Down, down he hangs his drooping Head,
> Fall fast asleep, and lies as dead,
> Neglecting all her Charms.

Reviving when the Morn returns,
With rising Flames young *Strephon* burns,
And fain, wou'd fain be doing:
But *Chloe* now, asleep or sick,
Has no great Relish for the Trick,
And sadly baulks his Wooing.

O cruel and disast'rous Case,
When in the critical Embrace
That only one is burning!
Dear Doctors, set this Matter right,
Give *Strephon* Spirits over Night,
Or *Chloe* in the Morning. (*FHW* 1:45–6)

The solution to a happy sex life in which both partners are satisfied lies in mutual compromise.

One of the most bizarre aberrations of reproduction was the case of Mary Toft (1703–63), who caused a sensation in 1726 by claiming she had given birth to fifteen rabbits (*ODNB*) and kept "producing" more until the method she used to hide rabbit fetuses in her vagina was discovered. Toft merits a mention in the second verse of a poem celebrating animals: "Ode To Lord Edgecombe's Pig" (*NFHW* 5:82–4). What makes this delightfully comical poem relevant here is the idea that staying well-connected with our barnyard friends can be beneficial to human reproduction:

Hail, pighog! by whose potent aid,
My L—d his health had, and employ!
My L—y too was brought to bed,
Heav'n bless it! of a chopping boy.
Event that Fame so sounded with her horn,
As scar'd the very infants yet unborn! (*NFHW* 5:84)

Living the life of a swineherd turns out to be good for his Lordship's potency. A plentiful supply of bacon, roasts, and pork pies is sufficient to get his juices flowing towards the creation of a strong male heir, "a chopping boy."

Robert Lloyd in his mock-Ovidian rhyming tale, *The New River Head*, which touches on the theme of unstoppable urination (not a reproductive problem per se, but wait), refers to Beroaldus (ll. 30–2) as an expert on female ailments. Philippus Beroaldus (1453–1505), who hailed from Bologna, Italy, published works by Cæsar and Florus, and wrote a *Chronicle* which quotes Hensler:

> No matter what illness a wench may suffer, she is called a leaky hussy (*fluss haiter Weibsbilder*) (*Rhoica*, weak), and the disease is called the woman's disease. Men who suffer from a copious flow of semen prematurely, suffer the same, says Benedetti, as the women with flux. And in common life, outside of the medical schools the ideas and names are naturally unintelligible. Beroaldus, who is no physician, also calls the disease the female disease, the men that were affected with it, the Gomorrhites of his time, he calls "leaky hussies." (Jelliffe 178)

After alluding to Lilliputian penis envy and Gulliver's method of extinguishing the palace fire, Lloyd connects Laurence Sterne's prurience in *Tristram Shandy* to Pope's *Rape of the Lock* and a racy rondeau he let slip in an unguarded epistolary moment:

> But to return – The tale is old;
> Indecent, truly none of mine –
> What *Beroaldus* gravely told;
> I read it in that sound divine.
> And for indecency, you know
> She had her fashionable turn,
> As prim observers clearly shew
> In t'other parson, doctor *Sterne*.
> Yet *Pope* denies it all defence,
> And calls it, bless us! Want of sense.
> But e'en the *decent Pope* can write
> * Of bottles, corks, and maiden sighs,
> Of charming beauties less in sight,
> Of the more secret precious hair,
> † "And something else of little size,
> You know where." (*NFHW* 6:147)

* Rape of the Lock
† Pope's Letters.

"That sound divine" might be Warburton as Lloyd seems to know that "t'other parson, doctor *Sterne*" had Pope's editor in mind as a model for Tristram's tutor. "Decent" Pope, Lloyd goes on to prove, had his indecent moments: the proto-Felliniesque imagery from the Cave of Spleen – "Men prove with child, as powerful fancy works, / And maids turn'd bottles, call aloud for corks" – and Belinda's "Hairs less in sight" pre-Freudian slip. Lloyd adapts the last lines from Pope's "Rondeau" – "And some Things, of little Size, / You know where" – which the poet included in a letter to Henry Cromwell on 24 June 1710. (Pope probably regretted committing this apparent reference to his tiny manhood to paper, but Cromwell's mistress, Elizabeth Thomas, guaranteed its survival by selling some of Cromwell's letters from Pope to Edmund Curll). Yet Pope's prefatory remarks exude considerable interest in sex: He was "in company with a Lady, who rally'd my Person so much, as to cause a total Subversion of my Countenance: some days after, to be reveng'd on her, I presented her with amongst other Company the following Rondeau on that occasion, which I desire you to show Sappho" (*Correspondence* 1:89–90). So Pope doesn't seem to have minded self-shrivelling humour.

Warburton comes under attack yet again in Wilkes's "*Notes on Mr.* Churchill's *Fragments of a Dedication to the B—of G—   —*" in 1769 (*NFHW* 3:89–105). One of the elephants in *The New Foundling Hospital for Wit* – a text lurking, but not in it – is *An Essay on Woman* which contributed to one of the most bizarre political scandals in British history (Sainsbury 152–62). Presumably vexed by the lack of sex in Alexander Pope's *Essay on Man*, Wilkes and Potter set out to correct the imbalance by penning the *Essay on Woman* (almost as if seen through the lens of *Sober Advice from Horace*). The title-page is said to have had a phallus on it; the hole where the phallus once was suggests that the (male) reader could inseminate the text (Cash 85; Hamilton 195). Wilkes incurred the wrath of both houses of parliament on the same day – 15 November 1763. He was on the hook for two charges: in the Commons he was accused of seditious libel for mocking George III's recent throne speech in *North Briton*, no. 45; in the Lords he was accused of blasphemous libel for attributing *An Essay on Woman*'s risqué commentary to William Warburton (Hamilton 193–246).

Warburton was evidently a favoured butt of the Medmenham monks. The authorship of the *Essay on Woman* remains uncertain, although evidence of execrable verse under Wilkes's name in *The New Foundling Hospital for Wit* suggests a collaborative effort. A dozen copies of the bawdy parody of the first epistle of Pope's *Essay on Man* were discovered during a search of Wilkes's home. Wilkes argued that these copies were for private circulation, presumably for the edification of his erstwhile Medmenham cronies. The exact authorship of *An Essay on Woman* remains a vexed question (we do not have enough proof that Potter composed it; and Wilkes's forte was not poetry). It could not be construed as a publication as it was never made available to members of the general public. The Secretary of State was in no mood for such semantic distinctions: the very existence of *An Essay on Woman*, whether seized legally or not, constituted an offence against a member of the House of Lords.

A copy of *An Essay on Woman* found its way into the hands of the Earl of Sandwich. Warburton was in attendance to witness one of the most unthinkable things that ever happened in the mother of all parliaments. The earl read parts of the obscene *Essay* aloud before the House of Lords:

> AWAKE, my Fanny, leave all meaner things,
> This morn shall prove what rapture swiving brings.
> Let us (since life can little more supply
> Than just a few good Fucks, and then we die)
> Expatiate free o'er that lov'd scene of Man;
> A mighty Maze! for mighty Pricks to scan ... (qtd in Hamilton, 213)

Hearing his name attached to footnotes on such subjects as female genitalia and how clergymen might increase their sperm counts could only have increased Warburton's outrage exponentially.

It must have seemed like divine providence to Warburton that Wilkes was shot in the groin the following day. Inspired by these extraordinary events, Churchill published *The Duellist* early in the New Year of 1764 which ends with jibes at Warburton as a cuckold. Churchill died while visiting Wilkes in France, bringing with him the proofs of his *Dedication to the Sermons* sarcastically addressed to Warburton. Wilkes prolonged Warburton's torment by publishing his "*Notes on Mr.* Churchill's *Fragment of a Dedication to the B— —of G— —*," in the 1769 volume *The New Foundling Hospital for Wit* (3:89–105). Here he names Warburton as well as his wife and makes a cruel joke about their son's paternity:

> The W— —*sett of features* might otherwise have convinc'd our children's children, that the most heavenly fire of the eye, and true dignity of aspect, may be tempered with grace and sweetness ... This loss is the more to be lamented, because the heir to his fortunes is unhappily not the heir to his

> graces. It is generally allowed that the boy does not in the least resemble him, but seems to be of quite another mould, or *Potter's earth*. (*NFHW* 3:93–4)

Ralph Allen Warburton would have been thirteen when *The New Foundling Hospital for Wit* told the world he was the product of an adulterous liaison between the Bishop of Gloucester's wife and the Archbishop of Canterbury's son. He died while still in his teens of consumption. There is no way of knowing whether he ever read the scandalous report about his paternity with that cruel play on "Potter's earth." Upon hearing of his son's death, Warburton went into a severe depression that lasted until his death in 1779. Following in the Duchess of Manchester's footsteps, Gertrude Warburton flouted social convention: she married her late husband's chaplain who was twenty years younger than she.

"Serio-Burlesque Canto"

The sort of national pride over penis length heralded in "*An ODE to the Honourable* H— —y F—x, *on the Marriage of the Du— —s of* M— —R *to* H—s—y, *Esq;*" pops up again in "Serio-Burlesque Canto on a certain Visc—ss at Brighth—" (*NFHW* 5:25–8). A hyphenate like Pope's "heroi-comical" *Rape of the Lock*, set in cantos), "Serio-Burlesque Canto" deals explicitly with a woman's attempt to get pregnant. Written in the spirit of Hanbury Williams (who died a dozen years earlier), it was composed especially for *The New Foundling Hospital for Wit* and has appeared nowhere else in print. Almon's successor, John Debrett, identified the initially anonymous author as the Right Honourable Temple Luttrell in the 1784 edition (*NFHW* 1:152) who is also credited with writing the "Ode to Lady Isabella Stanhope on her Birthday, written in 1768" (1:170). The viscountess, the former Lady Isabella Stanhope (1748–1819), was a daughter of General William Stanhope, 2nd Earl of Harrington, and Lady Caroline Fitzroy, a great-granddaughter of Charles II. In 1768 Lady Isabella married Charles William Molyneux, 8th Viscount Molyneux (1748–95), whose ancestors had come over with William the Conqueror. The bride and groom were both twenty. In the following year, Thomas Gainsborough's full-length portrait of Lady Isabella was unveiled at the inaugural exhibition of the Royal Academy to great acclaim. Between the date given on the poem – 18 July 1771 – and its first appearance in print in 1772, Isabella's husband was created 1st Earl of Sefton in the Irish peerage. Isabella's new title as countess is duly noted in the poem.

Brighthelmstone (soon to be abbreviated to Brighton) had recently become associated with the efficacies of sea-bathing thanks to Dr Richard Russell (1687–1759), author of *De Tabe Glandularie* (1750). This treatise, translated as *Glandular Diseases, or a Dissertation on the Use of Sea Water…* (1752), became popular enough to run to a sixth edition by 1769. The poem is prefaced with an "Argument," laying out Isabella's plight and Neptune's advice on how she might become pregnant in light of her husband's sperm's assumed lack of motility:

> Isabella at the approach of night descends to the seashore, and ent'ring the waves, offers up a petition to Neptune that she may conceive and bear a son – The God receives her courteously, praises her extreme beauty, and welcomes her to his domain; acquainting her that he had seen her consort, whose flimsey nerves and energick frame of body caused him to divine, that unless she found speedy relief at the Coterie, she must have recourse to his saline immersions: he rebukes her for not having sought him on the coasts of Ierne, whose brawny sons supply an energy of back so necessary to insure the efficacy of his waters – Then tenderly pressing the mount of love with each prong of his trident, there issue forth some balsamic drops; for the final power of which, he refers her to the approaching Installation of King Edward's Knights in the Castle of Windsor, where she is to perform a sacrifice to St. George. (*NFHW* 5:25)

A motto from Terence's *Eunuch*, "Color verus corpus solidum, et succi plenam!" (l. 231) – A natural complexion and a firm, juicy body – prepares us for the confrontation of female sensuality against male inadequacy. Viscount Molyneux would no doubt have been expected to demand satisfaction for the slur on his sexual potency by challenging the author to a duel had the poem not been anonymous. The seaside scene is reminiscent of Sandro Botticelli's painting *The Birth of Venus* (c. 1486): a fully formed beautiful nude, with long hazel tresses, one hand hiding her *mons veneris*, the other not quite hiding her breast:

> CALM was the sea – and silent was the night,
> And Dian's crescent shed a silver light,
> When Isabella threw her shift aside,
> And shew'd more charms than fifty hands could hide;
> One modest palm she o'er her centre held,
> While t'other the incroaching waves repell'd:
> Her hazel tresses from her shoulder flew,

To reach those happier locks in secret grew.
Her swelling breasts, mov'd by an inward tide,
The rudest efforts of the surge defy'd. –
Thrice had she plung'd her head, and wrung her hair,
When thus to Neptune she address'd a pray'r.

"Dian's crescent" hearkens back to Potter's epigram, but "fifty hands" lends a Rubenesqueness to her physique while those secret "happier locks" seem entwined with Belinda's "hairs less in sight" in Pope's *Rape of the Lock*. After wringing out the most alluring hair between Pope's Belinda and Rita Hayworth's Gilda, Isabella addresses Neptune, Roman god of the sea, associated with sexual potency and rain-giving fecundity:

Hail potent deity! whose briny flood
Has wrought such miracles on flesh and blood!
Who gave to Venus that creative seed,
From which all animals have life and breed!
So may its liquid joys refresh the w—b!
Nor be our globe one universal tomb!

The threat of human annihilation because of low sperm count made for a compelling carpe diem argument for a sexual free-for-all, but in this case Isabella desires impregnation.

Oh grant thy favours to a noble race!
I ask an offspring from my next embrace;
Not (like the waggoner in Æsop's tale,)
Invoke thy aid 'till human projects fail:
For I have Wilmot* and Lucretius† read:
Have con'd their lessons o'er at board and bed:
Nay, all the postures have I set in view,
That ever Aretin†† or C—d drew:
Have us'd the best endeavours I was able
On floor, – on carpet, – sofa, – chair, – and table,
In house, – in field, – in hay-loft, – and in stable.

The moral to Æsop's Fable LXXVII, "*The* Waggoner *and* Hercules," is not to bother the gods for assistance with jobs mere mortals can do by themselves, hence Isabella's listing of all the places she and her husband have tried to conceive (*Æsop* 57). John Wilmot, Earl of Rochester, is specified in a footnote while the 4th Book of Lucretius is particularly recommended along with Aretino's "De varies veneris Schematibus" (alternatively known as *I Modi* [*The Ways*], *The Sixteen Pleasures* or *De omnibus Veneris Schematibus*) – "concerning the different forms of love" – "with cuts." "Aretine's postures" (also mentioned in *NFHW* 1:124) was Italy's version of the *Kama Sutra*. Pietro Aretino's *Sonetti lussuriosi* was printed in 1524 accompanied by Giulio Romano's drawings engraved by Marcantonio Raimondi. Demand rose after the pope banned it; a second edition was prepared when all known copies of the first were burned (Foxon 1965 ch. 2). "C—d" may refer to John Cleland's *Memoirs of a Woman of Pleasure* which was issued in 1766 "with a set of elegant engravings." Clearly, Isabella has done her homework: they have tried everything short of in-vitro fertilization, including consultations at the College of Physicians:

> Yes, both my Lord and I have dealt in vain
> With half the faculty of Warwick-lane;
> Have tried empiric balsams – sov'rain props,
> I – Gibson's cordial; and he – Adden's drops.
> At length of ev'ry earthly hope bereft,
> From thy salubrious baths one chance is left.
> Full well I know at what a gen'rous rate,
> The subjects of thy empire propagate!
> Alas! I crave not their spermatick pow'r,
> That spawn by shoals – Impregnate ev'ry hour;
> To breed like shell-fish would be quite a *boar*:
> A brat in annual course – I seek no more:
> But, first an heir to fill my teeming b—y,
> Just such a chopping boy you gave to Sh—l—y. (*NFHW* 5:27)

The sea is one big soup of reproduction. Not wishing to become an octomom, Isabella prays for just enough "spermatick pow'r" from Neptune's bath to bear an heir and some spares. Samuel Gibson, druggist at the Angel and Crown in Lombard Steet, advertised his cure-all for man and beast, "true Cordial Horse Balls and Preparation of Antimony, adapted for the Use and Benefit of all, as well the Race as Cart Horse" in the *London Journal* (17 May 1729). Because of the high alcohol content, horses became addicted to Gibson's cordial; in "Serio-Burlesque Canto," it was intended to banish frigidity. Adden's drops were apparently the predecessors to today's male enhancements. The *Gazeteer and New Daily Advertiser* for 11 January 1770 published a letter from "E. Adden," to Dr

Smyth of Johnson's Court, Charing Cross, claiming he was cured of "a total imbecility of the parts of generation."[7]

Isabella's request causes a sensual tsunami. Neptune soon replies, likening Isabella to Amphitrite, wife of Poseidon, Neptune's Greek counterpart, and Venus.

> She spoke – the ocean to its centre shook,
> When Neptune cheer'd her with a gracious look!
> The arch of Iris on the waters shone,
> And girt around his loins a radiant zone.
>
> "Daughter (he said) – of beauty far above
> Our Amphitrit' – or ev'n the Queen of Love!
> O never have our temples held a shrine,
> So rich enchas'd! – of incense sweet as thine!"
>
> "Late as our Nereids waded on the beech,
> Thy smock-fac'd husband came within their reach;
> Nor need a virgin from his paths escape,
> In front no better furnish'd for a r—e,
> Than are those innocents – those puny imps
> Who paddle in yon shoals, and pick-up shrimps:
> Hence had I augur'd you must visit *me*
> Were you not enter'd of the Coterie." (*NFHW* 5:27–8)

Apart from being the publisher of *The New Foundling Hospital for Wit*, Almon was the official stationer and bookseller to the Coterie, the opposition club organized by Thomas Wildman, from 1764 (Thomas 107). The unprepossessing husband then makes an appearance.

> Ill have you done to chuse these southern banks,
> Where walks the sable prig, on spindle shanks,
> Burlesquing manhood (like a very ape
> Which grins to shew its teeth – and wears the shape;)
> Nor fish nor flesh, a creature dull and droney,
> Of doubtful sex, and call'd a *Maccaroni*.
> Where the fam'd Shannon pours his brazen urn,
> 'Ere morning's dawn we might have serv'd your turn,
> Mine is the vital heat, and humid source,
> The Images are stamp'd by spinal force. (*NFHW* 5:28)

English noblemen come off poorly as foppish macaroni, full of pretension, but lacking sex drive. If one of the Coterie members cannot give Isabella a son, she should lie down with a strong-backed Irish lover on the banks of the Shannon. When it comes to reproduction, DNA must be transmitted with "spinal force."

> With that – her hand he from the altar rais'd,
> And lo! its smoaking valves his trident graz'd:
> True Orient pearl, with lucid coral tipp'd,
> And in the purest flames of ether dipp'd;
> Nectareous spume kept oozing at the points,
> Shot thro' her veins, and thrill'd in all her joints:
> A gleam of extacy had reach'd her eyes,
> And sparks, like chrystal, bubbled from her th—s.
> "There (cries the God) is warmth and inclination:
> St. George will finish at the installation."
>
> Fair Isabella from the sea arose,
> And springing to the cliff, – put on her clothes. (*NFHW* 5:28)

The sea-god's trident brings Isabella to orgasm, her *mons veneris* overflowing with his "nectareous spume." Now that Neptune has planted the seed, the English husband (St George) can take over for what has been crudely referred to as sloppy seconds. Eighteenth-century attitudes towards impregnation had much in common with medieval beliefs: "Medical attitudes towards sex were far from puritanical, for sexual release was regarded as requisite for humoral balance, and female orgasm was widely believed essential for conception" (Porter 1997, 129). Something must have worked, for Isabella delivered a "chopping" heir,[8] William Philip, in the following year, their only child on record, but enough to continue the Molyneux line for two centuries. William Molyneux, 2nd Earl of Sefton (1772–1838), became known as Lord Dashalong for his rapid transitions between card-games and the race-track. Cronies with the Prince Regent, William managed to make it home often enough to sire four sons and six daughters, so the family line was at little risk of ending. His eldest son, the third earl, likewise had numerous progeny. With the death of Hugh Molyneux in 1972, the earldom became extinct. If a poem can be considered an aphrodisiac, then "Serio-Burlesque Canto" had "spermatick pow'r." "Serio-Burlesque Canto" predates James Graham's Celestial Bed, pitched to rich, infertile couples in 1779 (Porter, "James Graham"). Like her namesake in Hanbury Williams's poem, this Isabella was a relatively young widow, her husband having died in his forty-seventh year. She survived him by twenty-four years.

Both *The Foundling Hospital for Wit* and *The New Foundling Hospital for Wit* were reprinted in the eighteenth century, the latter by Almon's successor, John Debrett, of *Peerage* fame. Other collections pinched material from them, as seems to have been common. Jane Austen dipped into *The New Foundling Hospital for Wit* for the riddle Mr Woodhouse spins in *Emma*, originally asked by David Garrick, beginning "Kitty, a fair but frozen maid, / Kindled a flame I still deplore" (*NFHW* 4:104–5). Almon was an early fighter for freedom of the press, went to jail for printing the debates of the House of Commons, and has been treated in two monographs (Rogers, Stockdale) unlike Webb who has faded into obscurity. While so many writers like Swift, Pope, and Gay who left behind their literary rather than genetic codes, Almon and his wife Elizabeth Jackson (1737–81) had ten children. The figurative wards of the two *Foundling Hospitals for Wit* echo with bawling, beautiful, and forgotten verses like "Serio-Burlesque Canto" that celebrate fertility and deserve not to be forgotten by the adoptive parents of posterity.[9]

NOTES

1 The two *Foundlings* are cited as *FHW* and *NFHW*.

2 For more on the plight of foundling children and Coram's benevolent efforts, see Uglow, 325–39. The Foundling Museum, on the site of the original hospital which was demolished in 1926, opened in 2004 at 40 Brunswick Square by Coram's Fields, the park for children. The hospital provided support for 27,000 children between 1739 and 1954 (Wedd 3).

3 As *FHW*'s mock charter dates itself "on or before" 25 March 1743 (1: ii) and Pope's mock proclamation did not appear until the following October (Pope 5:248), it is possible that Hanbury Williams's parody inspired Pope's (whose influence on *FHW* may resonate from the poetic nursery of the 1728 *Dunciad* in lines like, "How Hints, like spawn, scarce quick in embryo lie,/How new-born Nonsense first is taught to cry" [Pope 5:67, *Dunciad* 1, ll. 57–8]).

4 As Foxon notes, "The canon of Sir Charles Hanbury Williams presents many difficulties," partly because a number of pieces included in the posthumous *Collection of Poems* in 1763 were not by him (*English Verse* 1:897). The same might be said of the editorship of *FHW*, which no biographers mention. Erstad notes: "Hanbury Williams was represented in contemporary

miscellanies such as Dodsley's *Collection of Poems: By Several Hands* (6 vols, 1748–58), *The New Ministry* (1742), *The Summer Miscellany, or, A Present for the Country* (1742), and *The Foundling Hospital for Wit*. It has been suggested that he acted as editor for the first volume of the last mentioned work under the pseudonym of Samuel Silence. In 'An Epistle to Fox' Hanbury Williams compares his poems to 'bastards, dropt about the town' (*Works*, II, 137)" (36).

5 Reprinted in Bell's *Classical Arrangement of Fugitive Poetry*, 18 vols. London: John Bell, 1796, 17:51.

6 Isobel Grundy, the foremost scholar on Lady Mary Wortley Montagu, whose daughter Mary became the wife of the Earl of Bute, does not believe an affair ever took place. According to Karl Wolfgang Schweizer's *ODNB* entry on Bute, the marriage "was by all accounts a happy union." They had eleven children.

7 I am grateful to Christine Jackson-Holzberg and Allison Muri for tracking down Adden.

8 In his 1755 *Dictionary*, Samuel Johnson defined "chopping" as "An epithet frequently applied to infants, by way of ludicrous commendation." Obviously, he was never a father. The only "Sh – ll – y" I could track down was Henrietta Shelley (1731–1809), who married George Onslow in 1753.

9 I am indebted to my graduate assistant, Rebeccah Hearn, for her vigilance in proofreading this at various stages.

REFERENCES

Adlard, J. 1975. *The Fruit of that Forbidden Tree: Restoration Poems, Songs, and Jests on the Subject of Sensual Love*. Manchester: Carcanet Press.

Æsop Naturaliz'd. 1756. 6th ed. London: John Ward.

Battestin, M., with R. Battestin. 1989. *Henry Fielding: A Life*. London and New York: Routledge.

Cash, A.H. 2000. *An Essay on Woman by John Wilkes and Thomas Potter: A Reconstruction of a Lost Book*. New York: AMS.

Cleland, J. (1749) 1766. *Memoirs of a Woman of Pleasure*. London: Ralph Griffiths.

The Correspondence of Alexander Pope. 1956. 5 vols. Edited by George Sherburn. Oxford: Clarendon Press.

Erstad, T.D.S. 1987. "The Works of Sir Charles Hanbury Williams." PhD thesis. Cambridge University.

Fielding, H. (1749) 2005. *The History of Tom Jones, a Foundling*. 4 vols. Edited by T. Keymer and A. Wakely. London: Penguin.

The Foundling Hospital for Wit. 1743–9. 6 vols. London: G. Lion (vol. 1, 1743), J. Lyon (vol. 2, 1743), W. Webb (vols 3–6, 1746–9).
Foxon, D. 1965. *Libertine Literature in England 1660–1745.* New York: University Books.
Foxon, D. 1975. *English Verse 1701–1750.* 2 vols. Cambridge: Cambridge University Press.
Jelliffe, S.E. 1916. "Notes on the History of Psychiatry. *The Alienist and Neurologist: A Journal of Scientific, Clinical and Forensic Neurology and Psychology.*" *Psychiatry and Neuriatry* 37:158–286.
Hamilton, A. 1972. *The Infamous Essay on Woman or John Wilkes Seated between Vice and Virtue.* London: André Deutsch.
Henke, J.T. 1979. *Courtesans and Cuckolds: A Glossary of Renaissance Dramatic Bawdy (exclusive of Shakespeare).* New York: Garland.
The New Foundling Hospital for Wit. (London: J. Almon, 1768–73). 2006. Facsimile edited by D.W. Nichol. 6 vols in 3. London: Pickering & Chatto.
Pope, A. 1939–69. *The Twickenham Edition of the Works of Alexander Pope.* Edited by John Butt. 11 vols in 12. London: Methuen.
Porter, R. 1997. *The Greatest Benefit to Mankind: A Medical History of Humanity from Antiquity to the Present.* London: HarperCollins.
Porter, R. 2004. "James Graham." In *ODNB.*
Rogers, D. 1986. *Bookseller as Rogue: John Almon and the Politics of Eighteenth-Century Publishing.* New York: Peter Lang.
Sainsbury, J. 2006. *John Wilkes: The Lives of a Libertine.* Aldershot: Ashgate.
Stephanson, R. 2004. *The Yard of Wit: Male Creativity and Sexuality, 1650–1750.* Philadelphia: University of Pennsylvania Press.
Stewart, M.M. 2004. "Sir Charles Hanbury Williams." *Oxford Dictionary of National Biography.*
Stockdale, E. 2005. *'Tis Treason, My Good Man! Four Revolutionary Presidents and a Piccadilly Bookshop.* New Castle, DE, and London: Oak Knoll Press and the British Library.
Thomas, P.D.G. 2002. *George III: King and Politicians 1760–1770.* Manchester: Manchester University Press. http://dx.doi.org/10.7228/manchester/9780719064289.001.0001.
Uglow, J. 1997. *Hogarth: A Life and a World.* London: Faber.
Wagner, G. 2004. *Thomas Coram, Gent. 1668–1751.* Woodbridge, Suffolk: Boydell Press.
Wedd, K. 2004. *The Foundling Museum.* London: The Foundling Museum.
Williams, G. 1994. *A Dictionary of Sexual Language and Imagery in Shakespearean and Stuart Literature.* 3 vols. London: Athlone Press.

22 Panspermist Jokes, Reproductive Technologies, and Virgin Births: Some Enlightenment *Luciniades*[1]

GEORGE ROUSSEAU

Freud, in one of his memorable pronouncements, decreed that jokes have a subconscious purpose that usually reveals the speaker's deep-layer intention, or ambivalence, about the joke's subject (Freud 1960).[2] Not all jokes, of course, deal with subjects; some extend to persons, including historical figures, and to events and abstract topics, and, nowadays, to "virtual" topics in cyberspace. The joke about historical epochs when I was a graduate student of literary history and theory in the United States in the 1960s was that earnest types became Victorianists, dripping sentimentalists Romanticists, and rollicky, fun-loving types (like me?) gravitated to the eighteenth century. It wasn't true, by a long shot; the Enlightenment had many faces to those who experienced or studied it. But the joke persisted and students then often selected their specialized fields according to these weird edicts, as if they were invincible myths.

More recently, psychoanalyst Jacques Lacan has located the genuine birth of human culture in the knowledge that heterosexual intercourse produces babies. Myths begin with this fundamental awareness, he claims, which is not exactly a "joke" but that functions as one (Lacan 1988). Lacan's "knowledge" invites further enquiry; if heterosexual intercourse leads to reproduction and necessarily involves the union of a sperm and egg, the ensuing joke is that culture itself can be undone without them, and this, presumably, is Lacan's point. But it is not at all clear what the "undoing of culture" means. Further analysis reveals that the issue is not pre-eminently biological: it is less a matter of one sperm and one egg – one customer to each – but rather that even when limited to *one* client per sperm and egg, the offspring is not created in, or reducible to, their exact image (Halberstam and Livingston 1995).[3] The "joke" is the maddening paradox that one and one do *not* equal one: the *one and only* created wholly in the likeness of its maker. Instead, *one and one* seems to equal many *others*, except for the similitude that a benevolent Nature, such as biology, ought to have decreed offspring in the likeness of its two makers.

Dr John Hill's (1714–75) panspermist jokes – the subject of this chapter – lie close to these linkages (Lemay and Rousseau 1978; Rousseau 2012). Hill's knowledge was that even the hierarchization of causes was incapable of separating out the body's role in reproduction from its (i.e., the body's) memorable part in politics, ideology, and technology. This is a complicated sequence, all the more so in that biographical Hill, about whom more momentarily, followed a generation of projectors – Defoe's, Swift's, the Scriblerians, projectors in the Royal Society – who proposed extravagant schemes for generation (Kerby-Miller 1950). In Dr Hill's version, technology was as important as the body: so the joke began and ended with the technological device – with his mad "wind-machines." His further joke, as we shall see, was the notion that Georgian procreative life could continue apart from biological reproduction. Viewed three centuries later it seems a plausible fantasy: the stuff of posthumanism (Gallagher and Laqueur 1987; Halberstam and Livingston 1995). Yet even empirically inclined mindsets today inquire how life can have continued without the heterosexual intercourse that produced babies. The slightest flicker reminds us that we have returned to Lacan's originating knowledge with this additional caveat: had Lacan lived on (he died in 1981) to turn posthumanist himself, he may have revised his "first classical principle" (bred in Freudian spirit about the birth of human culture in heterosexual reproduction) to *asexual* reproduction: i.e., reproduction by the *solitary* self. Odd as it appears, this asexual principle is a predominant view of recent posthumanists from Harroway and Halberstam (Halberstam and Livingston 1995; Badmington 2000; Weinstone 2004). They do not mean literal asexual reproduction: half jesters at heart, their posthumanist quip is that capitalism, culture, academia, and other professional institutions shape *reproduction* rather than babies (Halberstam and Livingston 1995: 17).[4] Ridley Scott's landmark posthumanist horror film *Alien* (1979) actually claims, capturing the spirit of Lacan's birth of cultures, that "the film works to take us outside of the logic of 'the human,' to imagine other (alien) systems of reproduction, other (alien) logics of identity," among which the asexual body is prime (Hurley 1995, 211). Among presentists of different persuasions asexual reproduction is a topic of interest.

The Reproductive Landscape

Hill's hoax about asexual reproduction was perpetrated at a moment in reproductive history when biology took a turn in dissociating female orgasm from generation. Thomas Laqueur has described this development in detail, even if his version of its historical profile has come under severe attack since he published it in 1987 (Laqueur 1987, 1–42; Laqueur 1990):

> Put briefly, the model of hierarchical difference, based on a set of homologies between male and female reproductive systems ... gave way to a model of complementary difference, which stressed the binary oppositions between the two physiologies. The hierarchical model that held sway from ancient times until the eighteenth century ... interpreted the female body as merely an inferior and inverted version of the male body, all of the woman's reproductive organs simply underdeveloped homologues of male organs ... Such a view assumed, moreover, that female orgasm, just like male orgasm, was necessary for generation and that orgasm derived from pleasurable stimulation. Laqueur traces ... [the new] reproductive biology stressing the opposition of male and female bodies, the woman's automatic reproductive cycle, and her lack of sexual feeling ... The new opposition of male and female turns into an opposition of desire and nondesire. Whereas it was thought normal for women to be ruled in all of their mental states by activities of their reproductive organs, it was also thought abnormal for them to have pleasurable sexual sensations. (Gallagher and Laqueur 1987, viii)[5]

Laqueur's theory poses all sorts of problems but nevertheless anticipates what is coming in mid-eighteenth-century human reproductive biology: the differentiation and diminution of each sex's contribution. That is, sperm and egg remain necessary but the female's role might be minimized to such a degree that orgasm is unnecessary for conception. Such reduction would not *equal* asexual conception (i.e., the notion that conception can occur without the congress of two sexes) but was construed as sufficiently proximate to overlap in the already confused popular imagination. Yet asexual conception struck most early Georgians as a contradiction in terms, or, at least, the stuff of myth and superstitious belief. Among the mid-century biologists in England, France, and the Netherlands it was an idea sorely to be ridiculed, as their debates of the 1740s demonstrate. If asexual conception had any basis in reality, which all biologists of credibility then doubted, its implication must be that women were somehow copulating under false pretences, thinking they were at least part, if not half, the cause of generation. But not even this constitutes the whole story. Before the one-sex / two-sex debates and later biological disputes in the 1740s about asexual conception, women putatively derived pleasure. But in any new biological model based on asexual generation, the effect of such forced copulation (forced because copulation will be unnecessary for generation) was reproduction *against* female wills. Only the male's volition will count because seed alone enables generation. In this model the consequential sequence is arousal, ejaculation, and attachment of sperm to egg, but not the role played by orgasm in conception.[6]

This context leads us to the essence of the yarn: Hill's tongue-in-cheek pretence and duplicity that asexual generation has scientific validity when he very well knows it has none. He deftly, and naughtily, removes female orgasm from the equation – the true precinct of contention – and substitutes for orgasm an absurd biology based on asexual reproductivity, intimating it is, in fact, the new biology of the up-to-the-minute theorists of generation. And he frames his prank in the form of a "*Letter Humbly Address'd to the Royal Society*" (*Lucina's* subtitle), as if he has made a startling new discovery worthy of debate – all this to mock à la Swift and Pope the pursuits of these learned gentlemen of science (Rousseau and Haycock 1999; Rousseau and Haycock 2000). Therefore, set the chronological dials to 1750 – when Hill publishes *Lucina Sine Concubitu* – and female orgasm no longer plays any part in generation. It has been wiped away. Yet how can Hill have imagined that anyone, let alone the Fellows of the Royal Society (FRS), would give a moment's thought to asexual generation? He could as the result of confusion and welter: when sufficient mystification enters into debates about a scientific model (think of our Big Bang controversies about the origin of the universe) even the most outlandish ideas can gain credence. Hill banks on just that, but erroneously in the end. He imagines his canard can be taken up because the theories of generation at mid-century have proliferated and become rampantly confused. Yet delve deeply into the history of mid-eighteenth-century biology and you discover that this is what our most competent historians of science have been documenting for a generation (Shorter 1985; Terrall 1996; Finucci and Brownlee 2001; Terrall 2011).

Or consider another analogy: Hill's panspermist hoax captured the reproductive landscape not dissimilarly from our posthumanist jokes about theory and jargon in a post-postmodern world run amok. Hill dares to purport that *cultural* birthing far exceeds the importance of biological reproduction in an overpopulated world, and that the institutions of cultural transformation are predominantly *asexual*. Non-posthumanists among us will wonder how this can be. The further posthumanist deceit within the analogy is that agents of transformation are not *quite* asexual – they are something else: Western capitalism, knowledge-based culture, the professions, the makers of knowledge – all "commingle" to "reproduce" culture.

Hill's spoof thus relied on different types of slippage. His title says all: *Lucina Sine Concubitu* – "Lucina conceives without a man": Lucina the old Italian goddess who brings children into the world and whose Roman cult fed into Juno's larger one elicited through polarized responses: anger and offence, versus uproarious laughter and hilarity. The satire's collective "furious" response came from Fellows of the Royal Society who were outraged at Hill's pot shots and dismissed *Lucina* as a depraved dunciadic lampoon (Rousseau 2012 65–82). A different response, which may be called the laughing reaction, interpreted Hill's satire as a stroke of wit about the reproductive body, and assumed his mischief to be that the essential nature of heterosexual intercourse was itself misunderstood. Traditional wisdom in this era held that the heterosexual body alone must be privileged for its role in human reproduction (Gallagher and Laqueur 1987). Yet now, in 1750, upstart-Hill comes along, exploiting the new ambiguity diminishing the female body and confusion about asexual reproductivity, and purports that neither the heterosexual nor sodomitical male body[7] was paramount, but an all-important *asexual* body. Two decades later, in the 1770s, John Hunter's artificial insemination will seem to be proof of Hill's visionary insight. But even without Hunter's imaginative technology of insemination Hill cleverly intuited what was coming, and saw what the FRS did not: that asexual reproduction *might* occur outside the female womb, as it does today. In 1750 these were very wickedly naughty ideas, and Hill thought nothing of espousing them as if visionary.

Sibly, Hunter, Sterne, and the Mechanics of Human Reproduction

Four years before the turn of the new century, when millenarian predictions ran high in 1796, one of the Enlightenment's most curious medical astrologers, Ebenezer Sibly, published a book as disturbing to his readers as Hill's had been in 1750. Their readerships differed – Hill wrote for metropolitan wits, gentlemen scientists, and other learned types, Sibly for diverse nonconformists and readers in far-flung parts of the realm – and even these two segments of readers had radically changed in a half century from 1750 to 1796, with Sibly's readers far more invested in magic, miracle, and superstition than Hill's had ever been. Even so, Sibly's *Medical Mirror* was weird, in form and content as well as for its explicit illustrations (Sibly

1796) (figure 22.1).[8] Polite readers judged Sibly's treatise on "the impregnation of the human female" – its subtitle – more pernicious than many French revolutionary tracts inciting readers to riot. Sibly's 198-page book discussed the reproductive organs, especially the anatomical penis and uterus, engraved them, and explained the "evolution of the human genitals" (1796, 35), following semen's pathway from its rise in the penis to its arrival, through coition, in the vagina; discussed the moment of conception when sperm and egg met for the first time; included illustrations of a cherubic nude male showing his genitals; and waxed lyrical on the anatomical female vagina. Sibly also traced the role of fantastical influences in biological reproduction: the moon, sun, and planets. He claimed the sun ("solar tincture") increased seminal discharge, while the moon enlarged the female's "fertility of menstrual discharge" (1796, 67), and explained, more generally, how important the genitals had been in human history (1796, 35ff). He pondered Hunter's "anatomy of the uterus in impregnation" (1796, 60ff), referring to Hunter's theories of reproduction, but not Hunter's 1776 experiments in artificial insemination, which Sibly appears not to have known.[9]

Reviewers reacted similarly to Hill's *Lucina* fifty years earlier; either dismissing it as unfit for polite discussion or neglecting it as the product of a diseased mind. Very few even deigned to survey its contents. Earlier in the century, Linnaeus had written about the "loves of plants" and Erasmus Darwin, the polymathic physician of Lichfield, had versified them in *Zoonomia* (1786). But these were inoffensive sallies into merry-May garden blooms, not explicit analyses of labia, wombs, and vaginas. If readers of Sibly in 1796 cried disapprobation, their attitude hardened Sibly in his view that esoteric astrological influences on fertility were justified and solidified his approach to parturition by explicit discussion of the organs of generation. Disapproval and neglect legitimized his book's title, "the medical mirror": he claimed merely to reflect through a prism, as it were, what he had seen inside the vaginal cavity. Sibly flaunted his "reproductive" erudition, and although the *Medical Mirror* contains no notes or index it enlists earlier authorities on these matters: Leeuwenhoek, Buffon, Maupertuis, Drake, Freind, Stahl, Cullen. Sibly presents himself as the contemporary "natural historian" of the organs of sexual reproduction, tracing the sexual "diseases Adam transmitted to posterity" (1796, 1).

My linkage of Hill and Sibly lies in their concealed jests, different though these were: slippage occurs in both books because their makers can touch a deep nerve in contemporary society without sacrificing their true intentions. Both authors can be by turns ironic and sarcastic, but neither ever surrenders belief in his theory. Nor was either aware of the

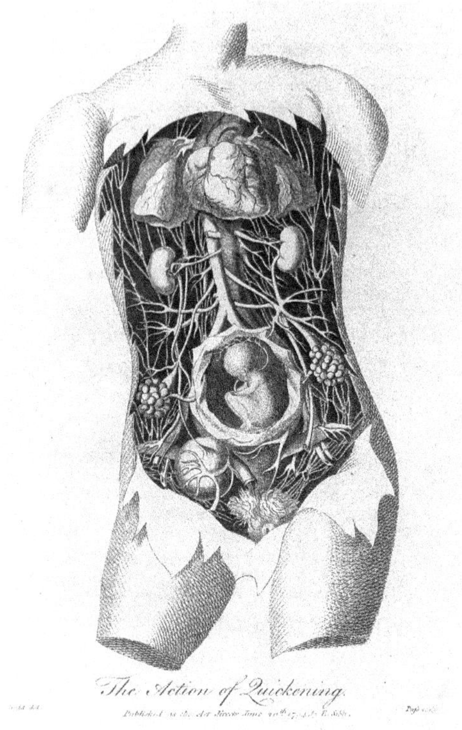

Figure 22.1 The action of quickening. Pregnancy at about the fourth month when the mother first feels the baby's movements (quickening). E. Sibly, *The Medical Mirror. Or Treatise on the Impregnation of the Human Female: Shewing the Origin of Diseases, and the Principles of Life and Death* (London, 1796), between page 116 and page 117. Courtesy of Wellcome Library, London.

moment in eighteenth-century reproductive technology when real science confronted jest and slippage. This was John Hunter's (1728–93) remarkable, even path-breaking, attempt at artificial insemination, and it was left to his brother-in-law, the controversial surgeon Sir Everard Home (1763–1832), to describe it for posterity. Home had remained closely associated with Hunter ever since he left Cambridge.[10] He had cultivated reproductive oddities, and would soon turn his attention to "hermaphroditical dogs," "sodomitical cats," and "deformed kangaroos" (1795; 1799).[11] His exposition of Hunter's attempts at artificial insemination dismayed members of the medical profession. Even Hunter was opposed to writing about Home's freaks within a milieu of advancing reticence about "private parts" and reproductive technologies. Home's biographers have adjudged his caution as justified, and despite being neither a Dr Hill nor a Dr Sibly Home's reputation remained untarnished at first (Foot 1794; Hunter and Home 1835; Dobson 1969). But Home went further: Hunter, according to him, apparently had been sought out by a husband whose wife was unable to conceive. Eager to help them, Hunter devised an infusion from the semen of a dog and injected her. *Mirabile dictu*, she conceived, and there Hunter rested his experiment in artificial insemination. Home waited ten years, until 1786, to write up his sensational story (Home 1786), which would have received different treatment under Hill's or Sibly's pen. Yet Home limited himself to Hunter's actual experiments, describing each event, explaining the physical interaction between (dog) sperm and female ovary in neutral terms, and delimiting his speculation about diseases arising from putrid male seed.[12]

Home's treatment continued to disturb British readers in 1786 who were preoccupied with other pressing matters, ranging from reports of revolution across the English Channel to fundamental instabilities at home. And even if they had not yet been introduced to Frankenstein (1818) – that other, awesome, contemporary marvel of reproductive technology – they had already been indoctrinated to other reproductive "indelicacies." Two decades earlier no less memorable a satirist than Laurence Sterne had opened his best-selling fiction, *Tristram Shandy*, on a similar theme: a description of the precise meeting of the sperm and egg at the moment of conception, having been conveyed through the genitals by the influential animal spirits. However ironic Sterne's treatment of the animal spirits' flowing through the penis and its attachment to the egg in the ovary, he made it plain from the first sentence of his cock-and-bull story that this subject was one of paramount importance: "I wish either my father or my mother, or indeed both of them, as they were in duty both equally bound to it, had minded what they were about when they begot me" (Sterne [1759–67] 1950, 1). No one knows whether Hunter read Sterne's ribald fiction taking a stand on these reproductive controversies, but it is ultimately beside the point: all three accounts – Sibly, Hunter, Sterne – corroborate that the mechanics of human reproduction, especially the moment of conception and physiology of genitals, were being widely discussed in the second half of the eighteenth century.[13]

Hill's earlier notion that human life could begin *asexually* – by a solitary person, or with the aid of machines and canine seminal injections, as in

Hunter's experiments – violated every providential principle, as well as it offended common sense. Yet miracle and progress permeated the air: anything was possible in that era collectively dreaming of perfection in many realms. Still, it was one thing to be put off by the prurient and pornographic – the idea that male and female private parts were now as available as the weather for public discourse – and another to uproot the fabric of Christian history with the fatuity that heterosexual intercourse was unnecessary for continuation of the species. Nevertheless, Hunter's experiments proved that the forlorn baker's wife could have children if she just foresook heterosexual intercourse. And by this demonstration he put on trial history's oldest act as if it were just another uncertain hypothesis.

Perhaps this is why Hunter knew better than to write up his experiments. An objective, if omniscient, observer of the whole scene might have recognized that technology was the villain far more than *phalli* and *pudenda*, biology's slippage then amounting to the notion that asexual conception was somehow more advanced, and progressive, than its heterosexual competitor. Furthermore, immaculate conception was by now centuries old, laden with layers of historical and theological significance. What was changed in the Georgian milieu, especially in Hill's mischievous lampoon intended as revenge, was the pathway of its reception.

Asexual Conception: A Doctrine of Winds and Embryos

The textual embodiment of Hill's hoax appeared in the form of a shilling book, as we have indicated. *Lucina* may now appear a somewhat obscure text, as the result of Hill's having disappeared from the radar by the turn of the nineteenth century, but *Lucina* was not obscure then. It was a prose satire of fifty pages, subtitled "A Letter Humbly address'd to the Royal Society," and signed "by Richard Roe," a nom de plume conjured for its alliterative ring.[14] "Roe" and his putative adversary "Abraham Johnson" are names Hill invented for the purpose of puffery. By 1753 Hill changed these aliases to female names as he entered a cross-gendered phase of his writing career.[15] He paid the London rogue printer Mary Cooper a fee to publish *Lucina* in January 1750, ingenious Cooper who had her own agenda contra authority; and even if she herself did not peruse Hill's lampoon, she basked in the promise of its bombshells that might make her famous. Under slightly more spiteful circumstances it may also have landed Hill in the pillory, so close had he come to treading too violently on a national institution, its president, and its fellows. Lesser deceits complemented greater ones in *Lucina's* appearance, and Hill-as-Roe cheekily inserted two jibes in his postscript (1750, 49–50). First, he announced that the FRS were diverted from replying to his "modest proposal" because London was threatened by three earthquakes on the eighth day of the first three months of 1750 (Rousseau 1968), and, second, he invited "All Ladies willing to breed [i.e., asexually] to favour me with their Companies [*sic*] before the 20th of *April* next" (1750, 50). He described himself as a "midwife" and country practitioner of "physic" who had "stumbled" upon his discovery when attending the "sick daughter of a Gentleman" whom he delivered of child without her "having had commerce with a man."

In the narrative the father confirmed his daughter's story. Startled, Hill claimed to have rummaged through natural philosophy and medical history for similar cases. In William Wollaston's (1659–1724) *Religion of Nature* (the edition of 1726), and specifically in the passages about traducianism (the entry of souls into bodies), Hill discovered the account of another young woman who bred by inhaling "seeds" (animalculae) that "served as a certain hot Bed for them to dilate and expand themselves" (Wollaston 1726). Hill paused at the notion of this type of asexual breeding, wondering whether seeds circulated through the air were "lodged in the Loins of Males" (1750, 9–10). He remembered how Lucretius explained these animalculae as dispersed during the atomic creation of the world, yet Wollaston omitted the Lucretian account. If in male loins, Hill wondered how they got into the wind? A fantasist might allow his imagination to run riot at the possibilities (onanism among them), but Hill looked for sources. He recalled passages in Virgil's *Georgics* where the west wind impregnated "certain Mares of his Acquaintance" (1750, 12).[16] Persuaded that these "floating Embryos" (1750, 13) permeated the air, he set about as a dedicated Newtonian projector to invent a machine capable of catching them: "a cylindrical, catoptrical, rotundo-concavo-convex Machine" (1750, 15).

Hill's narrator, still in the putative guise of an obscure, country, man-midwife, further recounts how he reached for his microscope to discover the "little Men and Women inside the animalcules."[17] He spent a further year repeating the experiments and concluded the likeliest explanation as "a Doctrine of Winds and Embryos" (1750, 17); wind, which in efficient Stoic fashion circulated all elements in the air over seven seas and continents, also scattered these "floating embryos." Still sceptical he located a sick chambermaid on whom to try his experiment: in Hunterian fashion yet without injecting her, Hill made her inhale millions of "floating embryos" collected in his machine (1750, 20). The chambermaid became pregnant, case proved, conception without a man, QED.

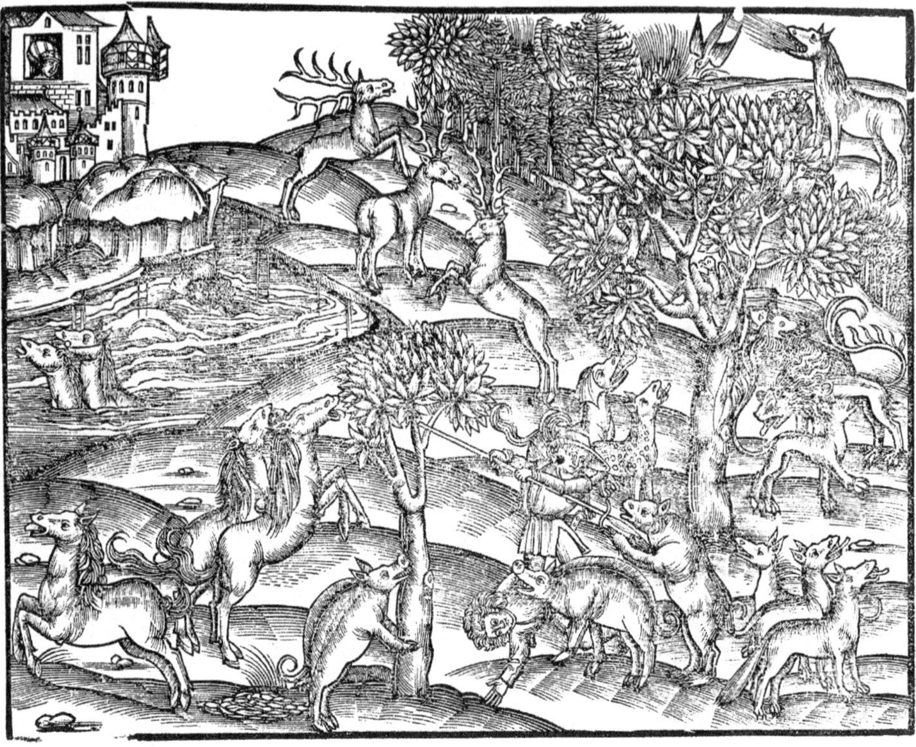

Figure 22.2 Rural scene from the Georgics. A mare (top right) impregnated by the west wind. Vergil, *Opera Vergiliana* (Paris 1515), cxix. Courtesy of Wellcome Library, London.

"Hill-Roe" ought to have ended his satire here but continues for another twenty pages (1750, 31–49), turning to his biographical hobby horses – Bishop Warburton, plagiarism, and venereal disease – without augmenting his case about the virtues of asexual, non-pleasurable, reproductive technology. He worried his readers would think he had "stolen the discovery" (the embryo-catching machines), so he ransacked ancient literature for immaculate conceptions apart from Mary's birth, in Galen, Hippocrates, and Ovid's *Fasti*, where Juno eats cabbage as the impregnated Flora sits hard by "ravaged by Zephyrus" (1750, 29) – the "fecund wind" that will impregnate her. This was the Ovidian passage Milton had in mind when versifying the same idea in *L'Allegro*: "The frolic Wind that breathes the Spring, /

Zephyr with Aurora playing," only to meet her once and "fill'd her with thee a Daughter fair,"/ So buxom, blithe, and debonair."

He also came upon another technological device: Antoine Réaumur's (1683–1757) chicken-breeding ovens reproducing avians without roosters (figure 22.3). Much was made of these ovens in Hill's generation, a technology as fraught as Hill's embryo-catching machines (Réaumur 1750a and 1750b).[18] About venereal disease Hill's man-midwife narrator waxes lyrical and pedantic by turns, first offering a potted history of it (1750, 41–5), paradoxically followed by descent into bathos in the name of sublimity, and claiming he elevated his style to describe the malady's terrific ravage on the human body. And he concludes these digressions with a dig at the ever-increasing tribe of cross-dressers, noting not all those clothed as women actually are women: "If all in female Shape (for I dare not call them all Women)..." (1750, 45). The last irrelevance has no place in his yarn about virgin birth, yet within three years biographical Hill will alter his all-male repertory of aliases to female, adopting "Susannah Juliana Seymour" as his favourite, another stunt in the art of self-puffery (Lemay and Rousseau 1978; Rousseau 2012).

Only when concluding, similar to the end of Swift's *Modest Proposal* (1729), does the narrator clinch his case about the benefits of immaculate conception by querying whether "single-distill'd Infants" will be as healthy as those "who pass thro' the seminal Vessels of both Sexes in the old way of Generation" (1750, 46). In real life the anatomically alert Hill was probably thinking of new ideas about the diminished role of orgasm in conception. He also sought to exploit theories of asexual generation: old-fashioned immaculate conception that sustained the logic of satiric *Lucina*. His conclusion is that asexually produced, and technologically induced, children will be vital: his new machine will procreate "Offspring robust and healthy" (1750, 46) as any generated in the old heterosexual way. Finally, he "will apply for a Patent" (1750, 47) to guarantee the trinity of "maidenly virtue," the abolition of matrimony, and the demise of sexually contagious diseases through his new "machine."

"Animalculists," "Ovists," "Preformationists," and Myths of Procreation

To call *Lucina's* 1751 reception cool is an understatement – it was icy. That powerful engine of sponsorship, the Royal Society, whose patronage biographical Hill needed if he were to advance, turned up the temperature of its fury. Dr James Parsons (1705–70), FRS and organizer of the famous

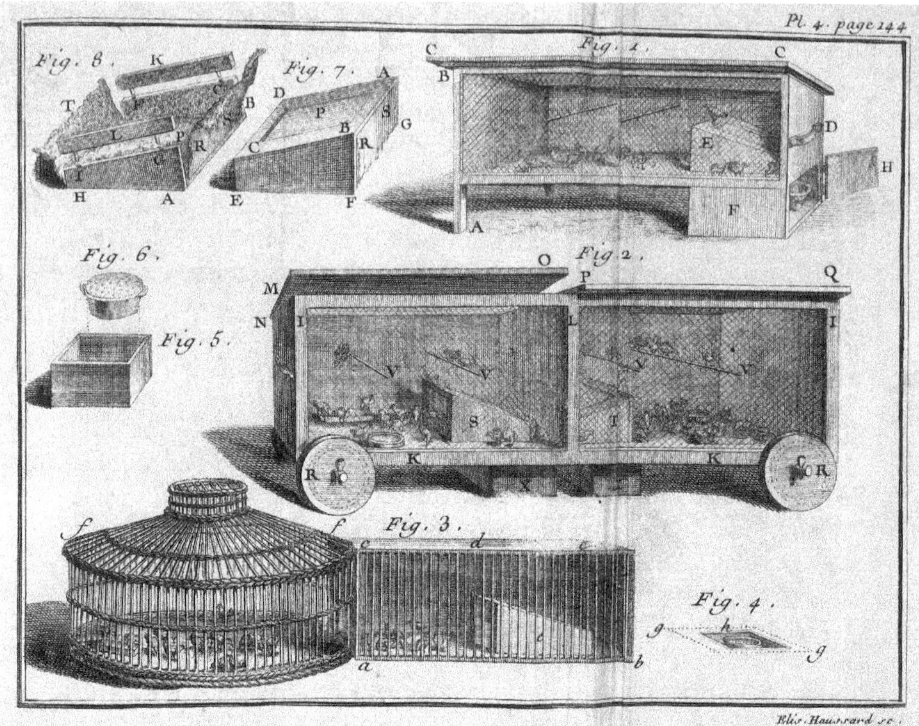

Figure 22.3 Chicken-breeding ovens. A. de Reaumur, *Pratique de l'art de faire éclorre et d'élever en toute Saison des Oiseaux Domestiques* (Paris, 1751), 144. Courtesy of Wellcome Library, London.

"Wednesday Circle," had himself been the author of a noted little treatise on "seeds" (Parsons 1745).[19] A decade older than Hill, he mentored him, now replacing cordiality with venom. *Lucina's* obsession with "seeds in the wind" could be interpreted as directed at Parsons. Parsons was imaginative, subtle, and never the run-of-the-mill FRS: by 1750 he had composed an insightful treatise on the anatomy of hermaphrodites (figure 22.4) interlinking anatomical and moral considerations (Parsons 1741; Parsons 1753) – no wonder Hill latched on to him. But now the gossip intensified, the rumours about overly ambitious, fact-falsifying, dust-licking Hill becoming rank. He was "written out" of their collective FRS memory and never again elected to their ranks. Within months a paper war began as FRS upon FRS attacked him, most often in letters dripping with calumny about this "maniac." *Lucina* was the checkerboard on which the dice of Hill's destiny was rolled. This was the biographical consequence, but another context than its reception demonstrates how closely attuned to the lineage of Hunter and Sibly, Hill's vision of Lucina – the mysteriously fertile maiden – was.

Its pivotal concept was male sperm and its configurations in the Enlightenment wars over reproduction. Without sperm Hill's "wind machines" are dysfunctional and Hunter's artificial insemination inexplicable. Male sperm, or spermatozoa, was widely being contested (Schurig 1780; Baker 1996): Ficino, Vesalius, and the Renaissance anatomists thought sperm resided in the blood, but Leeuwenhoek used his microscope in 1677 to detect these tiny particles which he christened "spermatozoa" and believed they contained life-giving properties necessary for generation, and that the womb, with its ovum, merely acted as a nutrient base, a temporary home. Other Dutch anatomists (especially Regnier de Graaf) concurred, as would Spallanzani almost a century later, all adhering to a view that "animalculae" inside the sperm were the "seeds of life" (i.e., they flowed in the sperm), hence the appellation "animalculists" for those who privileged sperm in procreation.[20] And it was not long before the female gonad was also explored as a rival site, as when Danish Niels Stensen conducted experiments and coined the word "ovary" to establish a rival camp of "ovists" or "ovulists" who attached equal importance to the female organ. Each group claimed to see a miniature organism present in the male or female genital organ. Ultimately the microscope – in 1750 still primitive and not yet widely compound – would tell the truth about these rival positions.

Another context, philosophic rather than microscopic, awaited consultation: the vexed topic of preformation versus differentiation. Aristotle had believed embryos developed by differentiation rather than having been *pre*formed. In this sense, he was neither animalculist nor ovist in the eighteenth-century sense, but "differentiationist." William Harvey, who discovered the circulation of the blood, followed Aristotle, but by approximately 1720 a rival camp of preformationists developed claiming that the "preformed organism" was already fully developed by the time the sperm met the egg. These preformationists could be either animalculists or ovists: they could think the fully preformed organism resided in the sperm or egg. The crucial element was opposition to Aristotelian differentiation or slow development of the embryo, rather than anatomical location based on gender. Two concurrent debates evolved: a) the importance of sperm versus egg and b) the existence or not of preformed

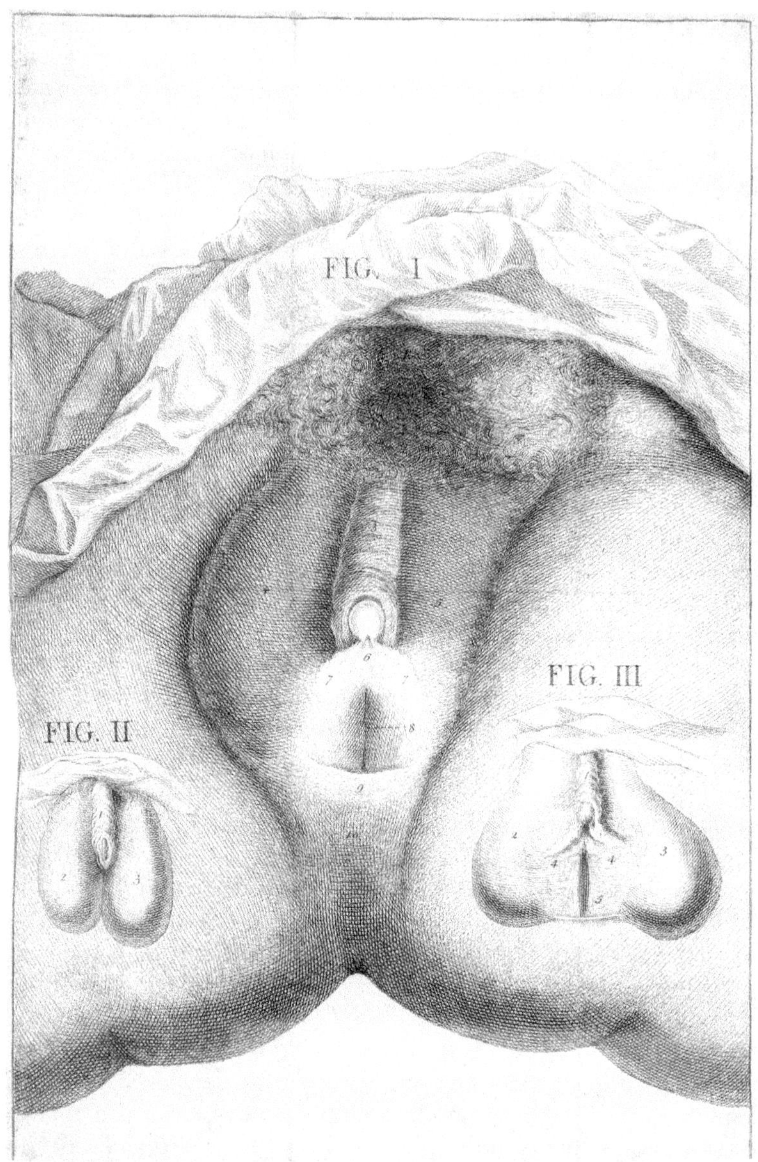

Figure 22.4 Hermaphrodite genitalia. J. Parsons, *A Mechanical and Critical Enquiry into the Nature of Hermaphrodites* (London, 1741), 156. Courtesy of Wellcome Library, London.

organisms. No wonder late historian of science Jacques Roger judged ours one of the most transformative moments in the whole history of generation, especially when viewed in the context of orgasm's role in heterosexual intercourse (Needham 1959; Roger 1997).[21] English microscopist and naturalist John Turberville Needham (1713–81) was one of Roger's foci, indeed well-known to Hill without whom *Lucina* may never have been written. Hill read Needham's treatise on generation (Needham 1749),[22] they informally collaborated, and – most crucial – Hill became partial to the animalculist-preformationist position (the antithesis of epigenesis) on which he based *Lucina*. As if this were insufficient, ambitious Hill tapped into another crest of the wave: the new, and often ridiculous, technologies of reproduction.

We have already commented on Leeuwenhoek's spermatozoa and the procreative theories of his Dutch colleagues in the 1670s, but we have not noticed that earlier attempts than Hunter's in the 1770s also dreamed of artificially inseminating eggs (Poynter 1968). As early as 1742 Italian anatomist Ludwig Jacobi pondered the possibility without injecting female mammals (Poynter 1968). A few decades later Spallanzani, professor of medicine in Pavia, injected toads with syringes, and again, in 1777–80, just when Hunter was inseminating the disappointed baker's wife, he syringed a spaniel bitch who gave birth to a litter of puppies (Poynter 1968).

Lucina was born in this milieu, naughty as it is to phrase it as such. If her biographical maker's anxiety included plagiarism and other forms of magpie-thievery, it was pilfering from the contemporary ferment of reproductive knowledge rather than from particular writers. The Jacobis, Spallanzanis, and Hunters were earnest in their endeavour to discover an artificial insemination capable of providing offspring to those incapable of having them. Even when their experiments are less literally interpreted – as flirtations with fantasy in the laboratory – there still is no jest, or slippage, in Hill's prankish sense.[23] Hill on the other hand perpetrated a colossal hoax on his brethren (FRS) who had failed to appreciate, he thought, his ability as a naturalist. In this slippage from serious laboratory attempts to half-baked "embryo-catching machines," Hill's "discovery" amounted to a nervous joke: the view that asexual conception heralded the future, for reasons including the denial of sexual pleasure altogether. The further irony is that Hill, despite having discovered nothing new in the laboratory of science and having allowed so much slippage to creep into these ideas, turned out to be as prophetic as these figures: asexual conception has rivalled artificial insemination, as contemporary commentators have commented in socio-ethical contexts.[24]

We have been silent about that other immaculate conception: the Virgin Mary's and the immaculate conception of her son, Jesus Christ. Mary's mother Anne (known as Saint Anne) was also alleged in scriptural tradition to have borne Mary virginally, as the iconographic tradition reveals (figure 22.5). But whereas Mary had two human parents (Anne and Joachim), the divine Christ had only one, the Virgin Mary, which raised all sorts of arcane questions in the early Middle Ages about their different forms of conception. These interrogated the necessity of two parents and two genders, as well as the bewildering biology of immaculate conception for the human Mary with just one parent. Yet the two doctrines – theological and biological – were often confused in the early Christian world and the types of conception of both Anne to Mary and Mary to her son Jesus melded into one. Here God's implantation in Mary's womb is germane. Despite posing problems for early churchmen, the incarnation of Christ – Mary's virgin birth – was definitively established in 1483 by Pope Sextus IV and soon after sanctioned by the Council of Trent.[25] A rival alchemical tradition also arose, discussed by Paracelsus and Jacob Boehme, treating the virgin birth in very different terms, which Hill tapped into because he cites it in "Johnson's" 1750 riposte to "Roe" (Sbiroli 1989, 77, 91). *Lucina* did not develop these diverse, incarnate strands, except parenthetically, but few well-read readers in the eighteenth century can have overlooked them. The significance for his panspermist joke is not specifically the theological confusion about Lucina's virgin birth but the biological context, i.e., how it could be that reproduction occurred without the commerce of a man. So many tales about fantastical conception had arisen during Hill's formative years – not just peasant girls giving birth to rabbits, freaks, and other monsters, but the miraculous possibilities and exotic circumstances of each case – that it is unsurprising Hill chose this specific target. In the confused milieu about generation of the 1750s anything seemed possible, even miraculous births (Huet 1993; Wilson 1993; Daston and Park 1998).[26]

French cultural historian Pierre Darmon has demonstrated how the impotent were persecuted in eighteenth-century France – he called them "the damned innocent" – and elsewhere how they were scorned and marginalized (Darmon 1985; Darmon 1986). These practices revealed Darmon's "myths of procreation": perceptions of fertility inherited by the ancien regime yet alien to our ears in an era of over population. Not yet Malthusians, nations suspected what untapped riches they had in their populations as workforces. Recently historian Lisa Cody has demonstrated that human conception was closely allied to the "birthing of nations,"

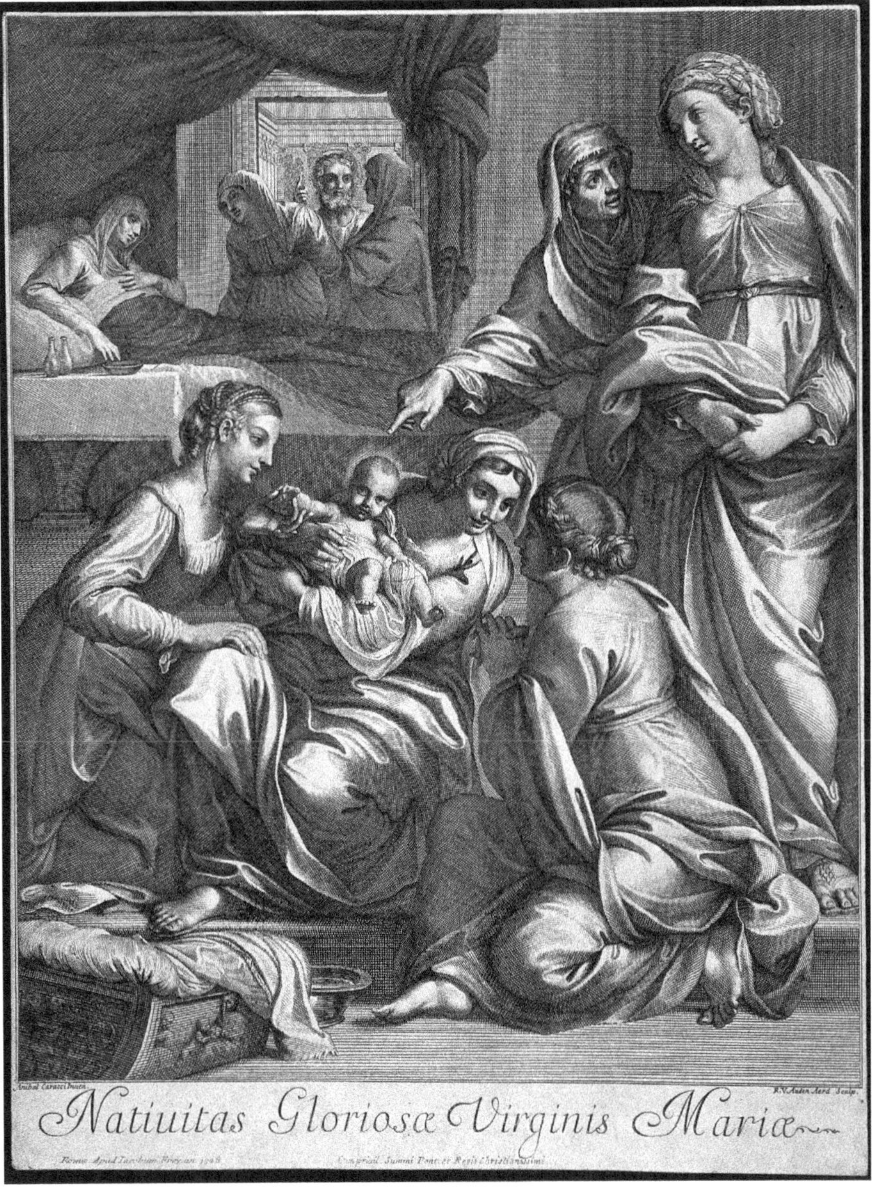

Figure 22.5 Birth of the Virgin Mary, Line engraving by Robert van Audenard after Annibale Carracci, 1728. Courtesy of Wellcome Library, London.

her work following on from Darmon's earlier studies (Cody 2005). Myths about biological conception and reproduction were deeply tied to both views – Darmon's and Cody's – but not their (the views') mythic inversion: passing off biological virgin birth as if it too would assist the nation.

Hill's panspermist message to the world's women insinuated the brashest sequences: seek the wind, suck in the floating embryos from my new technology, forgo heterosexual intercourse as if you are a new, self-sufficient Sapphic race, desist from sexual pleasure, yet become pregnant, conceive, thrive, enlarge the nation.[27] The turn of the screw is that the sequence pretended to act as Christian charity – especially the sacrifice of sexual pleasure. It was a sleight of hand: the dexterity of a deft satirical pen exploiting slippage in jokes.

Lucina on the Continent

Lucina's afterlife was icy, but if frost alone dictated it the post-1750 story would end here. The immediate response in England was predictable. Hill in the guise of "Richard Roe" had published *Lucina*, followed by a swift attack on his own work by one "Abraham Johnson" (Lemay and Rousseau 1978; Rousseau 2012, 68–70). Roe and Johnson, Hill's hack puppets, are natural adversaries. This double-ghosting was a further facet of the panspermist joke: two authors, both sufficiently heated about the biological debates raging over generation, lash out and then tenaciously hold their ground. The fracas was so charged the antagonists could have fought a duel.

The biological future prognosticated something different. Panspermism in both preformation and epigenesis swelled as major topics in Britain and France after mid-century, partly owing to Hill's satiric tract. Put otherwise, the town knew little until its interest was reawakened by an opportunist-chancer-prankster named Hill. Even if it suspected "Roe" to be Hill, it could not have imagined "Johnson" was also Hill. Furthermore, "Johnson" attacked *Lucina* in the bravado of a single rhetorical display of chiasmus: not *Lucina Sine Concubitus* but *Concubitus Sine Lucina* – "conception without fertility" – which Johnson subtitled "pleasure without pain," emphasizing the idea that human life without the joy of sex was incomprehensible (McLaren 1985, 323–41).

Concubitus Sine Lucina appeared within weeks of "Roe's" original work appearing to be a fresh reply, even composed in a different prose style. "Johnson's" substantive arguments were technological – the view that this machine could not capture the embryos in the way "Roe" claimed; besides, even if capable, conception would not follow. Johnson concurred, sounding an alarm about plagiarism, the theft of Réaumur's breeding chickens. What we then have is an author (Hill as Johnson) accusing himself (Hill as Roe) of plagiarism; specifically the notion that he lifted the original design, which he had not. Hence an author accusing himself of plagiarism with impunity because he knows he has not. Chronologically set the dials to mid-1750 and antagonists "Roe and Johnson" are hot properties: read and discussed, their antagonistic positions debated and contested.

To aggravate the debate Hill brought out another edition of "Roe" in 1752, again printed by Mary Cooper, but soon after turned to other projects. Here ended his part in the joke, and he could not have known what *Lucina's* fate would be in Europe apart from possibly having rigged the first French translation in 1750 (Sbiroli 1989: 157).[28] When Hill himself became better known in the 1750s and 1760s, other publishers (Robert Dodsley et al.) continued to reissue "Roe's" work, often followed by "Johnson's" reply.[29] Hill played no known role in the first German translation (1751), as he was not corresponding with Germans.[30] Most French translators probably acted on their own volition, buoyed by the intensity of debates about generation across the Channel in Britain.

Lucina's subsequent life would have astonished even the ingenious chancer-puffer Hill. The crucial phase began a year after his death in 1775; it was one thing for the French translation of 1751 to follow so swiftly on the heels of the English versions, especially if the jester-cum-prankster Hill rigged its appearance, and another for a new translation to appear in 1776, long after the original rumpus fizzled and when Hill himself was dead. Controversy about generation had not, of course, diminished in that quarter century (1750–75), nor did Hill's death play a part in spurring European translations: he may have been a household name in London by 1775 but was not abroad except among the Linnaean naturalists. The reasons for renewed interest now (following 1776) were owing to the topic: conception and fertility, topics increasingly alluring as the century wore on and swiftly gathering political significance. Furthermore, *Lucina* had a different resonance in Catholic countries like France and Italy, where translations also followed. In ancien regime France potency and fertility were slowly becoming politically charged, as Pierre Darmon has shown, not merely his "damning of the innocent" as contributing nothing to the nation –"unproductive" in the word's then double entendre – but now also feeding into the myth about procreation in the political sphere.

This further transformation of a panspermist hoax is the facet Hill could not have predicted. While France remained in the clutches of the ancien regime, fascination for *Lucina* was more or less limited to realms biological.

Once the seeds of revolution – so different from "seeds" blown about by Hill's zephyrs – took hold, *Lucina* assumed new significance as an allegory of the "new birthing" that would catapult into France and eventually Europe.

Revolutionary and Post-Revolutionary *Lucina*

The French translation of 1776 claimed the original *Lucina* contained political content, and the Italian translation of 1781 that, however much the original *Lucina* may have been "una mera burla, un semplice scherzo" – a mere jest – it was ultimately "un scherzo morale" (Sbiroli 1989: 148), an allegory prognosticating Europe's future. Most translators after 1776 combined the procreative and revolutionary tendencies, while others restricted their interpretations to the generative domain. Jean-François Sacombe (1750–1822), a Montpellier-trained French obstetrician who exploited the popular French reading taste for underbelly erotica disguised as reproductive biology, was one. His writings elevated the reproduction debates of the 1790s into something more than biological fact. Sacombe exploited polemics and poetic form in various "luciniades" to explode the nonsense that all species cross over and mix; as commentator Hugues Marchal recently notes, "deriding an [unnamed] British surgeon's theory that every species crosses and mixes ... a rooster can fertilize a female carp, the sole can inseminate a frog, and the oyster a fly" (Carlino and Wenger 76). But most extracted their ideology from the biological sphere, buttressing Thomas Laqueur's view that the new model of female reproductive biology "solved ideological problems inherent in ... social and political practices" (Laqueur 1987, viii).

A favourite tack was nostalgic allusion to the tumultuous events of 1637 in the Dauphine, which lent these translations a venerable antiquity connecting them to a lost France. Even obstetrician Sacombe, who made a name for himself in France attacking abuses in Caesarian births when the whole class of midwives was being challenged, alluded to that key year (Sacombe 1792; Sacombe 1799; Sacombe 1803). He noted how Louis XIII's "Parliament" augured future political catastrophes within Grenoble's courts of justice a century and a half before they occurred. *Lucina's* first French translator (1751) had included a "postscript" imitative of "Roe's" original and citing lists of the court's prognostications; after 1776 translators continued to include these "verdicts," exploiting their relevance to a France being torn asunder by political difference; and by 1791 *Lucina* was said to have allegorically prognosticated the Revolution itself (Sbiroli 1989, 125–58), historically a ridiculous assertion.

Sacombe called his version of 1793 "Lusiniades," which he continued to reprint for a decade (1793–1803); he turned one version into poetry (Sacombe 1792; Sacombe 1799; Sacombe 1803). But now, after a half century, *Lucina's* plot was recast as a metaphor for history's strangest *recent* "birthing": the political Terror with its monstrous queen and her unnatural conceptions (Hunt 1984; Hunt 1993).[31]

The Terror eventually revolutionized the Western world and, as the 1790s rolled on, editors of *Lucina* continued to assert, rather than derive, its political significance – truthfully or not documenting which prior edition they had consulted in which library. Some claimed to have stumbled upon it "accidentally" in the catalogue of a "private library," so intrigued they petitioned to read it.[32] Others went further: the translator of a much-cited 1786 French edition detected veiled allusions to Armand-Thomas Miromésnil (1723–96), Louis XVI's minister for whom a famous boulevard in Paris is named. This translator's apparatus – preface to postscripts – speculates on the reproductive practices of the rich and famous: Madame Pompadour, Madame Nacard (Sbiroli 1989, 136–9), and several others.

Another Italian translation, declared to be based on the 1786 French version, begins contending that the "discoveries" in the original *Lucina* were as important as those of "Martin Bebaimb, Christopher Columbus, and Americo Vespucci" (Sbiroli 1989, 153).[33] These European "luciniades" of the 1790s commingled Eros and Reproduction – Venus and Juno – with the more awesome political "birthing" occurring as heads swung in the Bastille and guillotines massacred innocents. Two generations later, another French version of *Lucina* published in 1865 claimed to be based on a translation of the 1790s edited by a certain "St. Colombe" (not to be confused with the French composer and player of viols who lived in the second half of the seventeenth century). Its editor explained that St Colombe was a late eighteenth-century author of garden books, known to Buffon, who had become preoccupied with Hill-the-botanist (Sbiroli 1989, 149) but no reason exists to believe this fabrication.

Something universal in *Lucina*'s original germ sporadically haunted the Western imagination that could not be reduced to reproductive seed. Some substratum of the deceit, some deep-seated desire to believe such procreation possible, as Freud may have proposed if he could have read Hill's bagatelle, electrified readers' unconsciouses. Hill's original idea had never been an aesthetics of intrigue: "mistakes of the night," mistakes caused by dress, or the risible "errors" of masquerade.[34] Hill's notion of wind-breeding seeds enabled confusion but depended, more fundamentally, on primitive belief, faith in miracle, and transformations between an old biological generation and newer politically charged procreation. One can imagine what eighteenth-century readers of *Lucina* and its translations would have thought if they could have read about the Russian woman, alive in the 1780s, alleged to have given birth to sixty-nine children (Levesque 2004, 6).

These responses fuelled *Lucina*'s periodical returns. Another French edition appeared in 1914 just before the events in Sarajevo plunged Europe into its first "Great War." As dark clouds gathered one wonders whether these wartime readers construed the humble eighteenth-century maid's birthing as a metaphor prognosticating the blitzing to come. Or was the raison-d'etre of this edition fuelled by the nineteenth-century's demonstrations that technology enabled men to dominate medical control of women's bodies?

After 1914 *Lucina* took a few steps to return to its first biological principles, but these were small paces.[35] Its sweep over several centuries was driven by the aim to integrate religion, reproduction, and sexual intercourse – or their lack of integration. Flashing forward closer to our own time, one can imagine Hill's suggestive reproductive technology extending to our frozen embryos and the ethical challenges they pose, even if he neither envisioned the financial benefits to technology of such asexual reproduction nor the huge advantage it would bestow on mothers wishing to conceive at much older ages. Howard W. Jones Jr, an American physician who performed the first successful in vitro fertilization procedure during the 1960s, has offered some of the reasons in *Personhood Revisited: Reproductive Technology, Bioethics, Religion and the Law*. These touch on similar categories to those we have been discussing, especially the way theories of procreation naturally lead to models of identity and personhood. Perhaps *Lucina* may yet be reinvented again.

NOTES

1 This chapter is an expanded version of an essay that appeared in Carole Reeves (ed.), *A Cultural History of the Human Body in the Enlightenment*, vol. 4 (Oxford: Berg, 2010), 53–72. It was enhanced by the late Lynn Salkin Sbiroli's study of the translations of *Lucina* (Sbiroli 1989). My practice refers

readers to the relevant place in her book rather than citing each edition and translation. Her book is not widely available and has never been translated into English. *Lucina* was a much discussed satire in the early 1750s, as the weeklies and monthlies make plain: if not a best-selling work, nevertheless one so often mentioned in extant accounts of London print life during the 1750s that for a while it became canonical; more accurately, inversely canonical as the product of its notorious author then widely flayed and lampooned. *Lucina* was one of three fierce lampoons of the Royal Society (the other two being *A Dissertation on Royal Societies: In Three Letters from a Nobleman on his Travels to a Person of Distinction in Sclavonia* and *A Review of the Works of the Royal Society of London*) Hill published within a few months that prompted this premier national organization dedicated to scientific research to take stock of its practices and reform its procedures later in the decade. These matters are more fully treated in my biography of Hill (Rousseau 2012).

2 For jokes in their eighteenth-century contexts, see Findlen 1990; Critchley 2002; Dickie 2003.

3 This argument has been developed by Judith Halberstam.

4 Halberstam states as much; this passage in my argument is indebted to her.

5 Laqueur also suggested that "the reinterpretation of women's reproductive biology solved ideological problems inherent in eighteenth- and nineteenth-century social and political practices" (Laqueur 1987, viii). Citing Lacan (1988), Laqueur claimed what "devastating attack ... [the] linking of female orgasm to conception had come under" (1987, 2) in the late eighteenth century. Had he known about Hill's *Lucina Sine Concubitu* Laqueur might have used it as further evidence for his model about the newly diminished female orgasm.

6 These views would have surprised Nathaniel Highmore (Highmore 1651), whose view of generation followed the old two-sexes model. For competing theories of reproduction, see Needham 1959.

7 One wonders whether *Lucina* had indeed been informed by the new view of the male sodomitical body described in *Satan's Harvest Home: Reasons for the Growth of Sodomy* (1749), which had been published just as Hill was imagining his joke.

8 Sibly printed the book privately and paid for the print run himself.

9 Sibly had not read Everard Home's publications, especially those appearing in the *Philosophical Transactions* in the 1790s.

10 Every biographer of Hunter has recounted the story of Home's plagiarism from, and subsequent destruction of, Hunter's vast manuscripts over three decades after his death in 1793; a parliamentary committee was formed to investigate it.

11 Home was also interested in human reproductive abnormality (1790).

12 One reconstruction of the historical events is found in Poynter 1968, 97–113.
13 For the different resonance of organs of generation versus the technology of reproduction, see Roger 1997.
14 Printed in December 1749. The *Gentleman's Magazine* and *Monthly Review* reviewed it in their January issues (*GM*, 20 Jan. 1750, 48; *MR*, 2 Jan. 1750, 255–6). The anonymous reviewer in *MR* lists it as "said to be Dr Hill."
15 For his cross-gendered authorial phase and its role in shaping his public profile, see Rousseau 2006, 213–49. They are also discussed in my biography (Rousseau 2012) together with the other frauds described in this paragraph. Combined, they suggest that Hill had gone mad or that the print culture of his day had. How else explain deceit upon deceit, to such a degree that nothing printed or professed could be considered true. This is one of the riddles of metropolitan culture in the 1750s that scholars have yet to take on board. It is well and good to document the facts of print culture then (printers, publishers, the statistics of print runs, print technology, costs, etc.) and quite another to account for its content.
16 Virgil, *Georgics*, III, which Hill read in Dryden's translation and which he made his epigraph in "Roe," together with passages cited below from Ovid and Milton.
17 From early days Hill gravitated to the microscope and was prominent in its eighteenth-century histories (Hill 1752). He subtitled his philosophical ruminations, "Discoveries by the assistance of Microscopes."
18 For jokes about Réaumur's chicken-breeding machines, see Roger 1997, 483. Gena Corea has studied the technologies of female birthing without the assistance of male sperm (Corea 1985; Corea 1987).
19 For Parsons's career in the Royal Society, see Rousseau 2012, 40–50, 76–80. Parsons assisted Hill with his translation of *Theophrastus* (1747), as did da Costa.
20 For a mini-epitome of the history of semen, see Sibly 1796, 20–6.
21 Laqueur's model change is often overlooked when interpreted in light of Roger's panoptic view.
22 Hill was influenced by Needham's treatise in imagining the plot of *Lucina*.
23 It is puzzling why Poynter (1968) omitted any reference to *Lucina*.
24 Perhaps no one more assiduously than chemist-playwright Carl Djerassi in his play about the ethical dilemmas immaculate conception poses (Djerassi 2000).
25 The matter was so sensitive that Pope Pius IX pronounced it infallible only in 1854.
26 Fantastic births were widely discussed in Georgian England partly under the sway of recent translations of *Aristotle's master-piece: or, The secrets of generation displayed* (1694).

27 The work of Angus McLaren (1984) enriches these areas; without including Hill, he has also explored the Freudian implications (1979).
28 A copy is found in the Wellcome Library, London; Hill himself may have been the translator.
29 Printer Robert Dodsley reissued Roe and Johnson bound together at his own expense in 1761, 1762, 1765, and 1771, all during Hill's lifetime.
30 Nothing is known about the German translations and no translator's name appears on the title page. I have been told there were also Dutch and Danish translations.
31 In Lynn Hunt (1993) the suggestion is made that *Lucina* can figure into the traditions of eighteenth-century pornography.
32 For example, see the preface to the 1795 translation (Hill 1795).
33 Bebaimb was a seventeenth-century anatomist and colleague of Malpighi. This translation is titled *Lucine Sine Concubitu: Lettere Diretta alla Società Reale di Londra …* (Venice: Graziosi, 1786). Sbiroli lists the French and Italian translations on pp. 157–8.
34 Several eighteenth-century titles begin with the phrase *Mistakes of …* as in Oliver Goldsmith, *She Stoops to Conquer: Or, the Mistakes of a Night: A Comedy* (London, 1773), then a common trope.
35 Only modern editions have restored *Lucina* to its earlier authenticity, removing layers of allegorical and political significance. For example, the reader of the 1930 "limited edition" (Golden Cockerel Press, Berkshire) never suspected that Hill's revenge-hoax had any political afterlife.

REFERENCES

Badmington, N. 2000. *Posthumanism*. Basingstoke: Palgrave.
Baker, R. 1996. *Sperm Wars: The Science of Sex*. New York: Basic Books.
Bynum, W.F., and R. Porter, eds. 1985. *William Hunter and the Eighteenth-Century Medical World*. Cambridge and New York: Cambridge University Press.
Carlino, A., and A. Wenger, eds. 2007. *Littérature et medicine: Approches et perspectives (XVI–XIX siècle)*. Geneva: Droz.
Cody, L.F. 2005. *Birthing the Nation: Sex, Science, and the Conception of Eighteenth-Century Britons*. Oxford: Oxford University Press.
Corea, G. 1985. *Man-Made Women: How New Reproductive Technologies Affect Women*. London: Hutchinson.
Corea, G. 1987. *The Mother Machine: Reproductive Technologies from Artificial Insemination to Artificial Wombs*. London: Women's Press.

Critchley, S. 2002. *On Humour: Thinking in Action*. London: Routledge.

Darmon, P. 1985. *Trial by Impotence: Virility and Marriage in Pre-Revolutionary France*. London: Chatto & Windus.

Darmon, P. 1986. *Damning the Innocent: A History of the Persecution of the Impotent in Pre-Revolutionary France*. New York: Viking.

Daston, L., and K. Park. 1998. *Wonders and the Order of Nature, 1150–1750*. New York: Zone Books.

Dickie, S. 2003. "Hilarity and Pitilessness in the Mid-Eighteenth Century: English Jestbook Humor." *Eighteenth-Century Studies* 37 (1): 1–22. http://dx.doi.org/10.1353/ecs.2003.0060.

Djerassi, C. 2000. *An Immaculate Misconception: Sex in an Age of Mechanical Reproduction*. London: Imperial College Press. http://dx.doi.org/10.1142/p213.

Dobson, J. 1969. *John Hunter*. Edinburgh: E. & S. Livingstone.

Findlen, P. 1990. "Jokes of Nature and Jokes of Knowledge: The Playfulness of Scientific Discourse in Early Modern Europe." *Renaissance Quarterly* 43 (2): 292–329. http://dx.doi.org/10.2307/2862366.

Finucci, V., and K. Brownlee, eds. 2001. *Generation and Degeneration: Tropes of Reproduction in Literature and History from Antiquity through Early Modern Europe*. Durham, NC: Duke University Press. https://www.dukeupress.edu/Generation-and-Degeneration/.

Foot, J. 1794. *The Life of John Hunter*. London: T. Becket.

Freud, S. 1960. *Jokes and Their Relation to the Unconscious*. London: Routledge & Kegan Paul.

Gallagher, C., and T. Laqueur. 1987. *The Making of the Modern Body: Sexuality and Society in the Nineteenth Century*. Berkeley: University of California Press.

Halberstam, J., and I. Livingston, eds. 1995. *Posthuman Bodies, Unnatural Acts*. Bloomington: Indiana University Press.

Highmore, N. 1651. *The History of Generation*. London: printed by R.N. for J. Martin.

Hill, J. 1750. *Lucina Sine Concubitu. A Letter Humbly Address'd to the Royal Society*. London: M. Cooper.

Hill, J. 1752. *Essays in Natural History and Philosophy: Containing a Series of Discoveries, by the Assistance of Microscopes*. London: J Whiston et al.

Hill, J. 1795. *Lucine affranchie des loix du concours et le plaisir sans peine, ouvrage singulier, dans lequel il est pleinement démontré … nouvelle édition aug. [sic] de plusieurs morceaux qui n'ont pas encore été imprimés*. Paris: Favre.

Hill, J., and G.S. Rousseau. 1982. *The Letters and Papers of Sir John Hill, 1714–1775*. New York: AMS Press.

Home, E. 1786. "An Account of Mr Hunter's Method of Artificial Insemination." *Philosophical Transactions* ns 14:119–27.
Home, E. 1790. "An Account of a Child with a Double Head." *Philosophical Transactions* 80:296–305.
Home, E. 1795. "Observations on the Mode of Generation of the Kangaroo." *Philosophical Transactions* 85:221–38.
Home, E. 1799. "Account of the Dissection of an Hermaphrodite Dog." *Philosophical Transactions* ns 18:157–78.
Huet, M. 1993. *Monstrous Imagination*. Cambridge, MA, and London: Harvard University Press.
Hunt, L. 1984. *Politics, Culture, and Class in the French Revolution*. Berkeley: University of California Press.
Hunt, L. 1993. *The Invention of Pornography: Obscenity and the Origins of Modernity, 1500–1800*. New York: Zone.
Hunter, J., and E. Home, eds. 1835. *The Works of John Hunter. With Notes*. London: Longman.
Hurley, K. 1995. "Postmodern Bodies: Reading Like an Alien." In *Posthuman Bodies, Unnatural Acts*, edited by J. Halberstam and I. Livingstone, 211–29. Bloomington: Indiana University Press.
Jones, H.W. 2012. *Personhood Revisited: Reproductive Technology, Bioethics, Religion and the Law*. Minneapolis, MN: Langton Street Press.
Kerby-Miller, C.K., ed. 1950. *Memoirs of the Extraordinary Life, Works, and Discoveries of Martinus Scriblerus*. New Haven, CT: Yale University Press.
Lacan, J. 1988. *The Seminar of Jacques Lacan*. Edited by J.A. Miller. Cambridge: Cambridge University Press.
Laqueur, T. 1987. "Orgasm, Generation, and the Politics of Reproductive Biology." In *The Making of the Modern Body: Sexuality and Society in the Nineteenth Century*, edited by C. Gallagher and T. Laqueur, 1–42. Berkeley: University of California Press.
Laqueur, T. 1990. *Making Sex: Body and Gender from the Greeks to Freud*. Cambridge, MA, and London: Harvard University Press.
Lemay, J.A.L., and G.S. Rousseau. 1978. *The Renaissance Man in the Eighteenth Century*. William Andrews Clark Memorial Library Seminar Papers. Los Angeles: University of California Press.
Levesque, C. 2004. "Assisted Reproductive Technologies." *BioTeach Journal* 2:6–12.
McLaren, A. 1979. "Contraception and Its Discontents: Sigmund Freud and Birth Control." *Journal of Social History* 12 (4): 513–29. http://dx.doi.org/10.1353/jsh/12.4.513.
McLaren, A. 1984. *Reproductive Rituals: The Perception of Fertility in England from the 16th to the 19th Century*. London and New York: Methuen.

McLaren, A. 1985. "The Pleasures of Procreation: Traditional and Biomedical Theories of Conception." In *William Hunter and the Eighteenth-Century Medical World*, edited by W.F. Bynum and R. Porter, 323–41. Cambridge and New York: Cambridge University Press.

Needham, J.T. 1749. *Observations Upon the Generation, Composition, and Decomposition of Animal and Vegetable Substances*. London.

Needham, J. 1959. *A History of Embryology*. 2nd ed. Cambridge: Cambridge University Press.

Parsons, J. 1741. *A Mechanical and Critical Enquiry into the Nature of Hermaphrodites*. London: J. Walthoe.

Parsons, J. 1745. *The Microscopical Theatre of Seeds: Being a Short View of the Particular Marks, Characters, Contents, and Natural Dimensions of All the Seeds*. London: M. Cooper.

Parsons, J. 1753. "A Letter to the President Concerning the Hermaphrodite Shewn in London." *Philosophical Transactions* 47:1751–2.

Poynter, F.N.L. 1968. "Hunter, Spallanzani, and the History of Artificial Insemination." In *Medicine, Science, and Culture: Historical Essays in Honor of Owsei Tempkin*, edited by Lloyd G. Stevenson and Robert P. Multhauf, 97–113. Baltimore: Johns Hopkins University Press.

Réaumur, A. 1750a. *The Art of Hatching and Bringing up Domestick Fowl of All Kinds, at Any Time of the Year, Either by Means of the Heat of Hot-Beds, or That of Common Fire*. London: C. Davis, A. Millar, and J. Nourse.

Réaumur, A. 1750b. *The Art of Hatching and Bringing up Domestic Fowls, by Means of Artificial Heat*. Translated by A. Trembley. London: printed for C. Davis.

Reaumur, A. 1751. *Pratique de l'art de faire éclorre et d'élever en toute Saison des Oiseaux Domestiques*. Paris.

Roger, J. 1997. *The Life Sciences in Eighteenth-Century French Thought*. Edited by K.R. Benson and translated by R. Ellrich. Stanford: Stanford University Press.

Rousseau, G.S. 1968. "The London Earthquakes of 1750." *Cahiers d'Histoire Mondiale* 11 (3): 436–54.

Rousseau, G.S. 2006. "Curiosity and the *Lusus Naturae*: Proteus Hill." In *Curiosity and Wonder from the Renaissance to the Enlightenment*, edited by R.J.W. Evans and A. Marr, 213–54. Aldershot: Ashgate.

Rousseau, G.S. 2012. *The Notorious Sir John Hill: The Man Destroyed by Ambition in the Era of Celebrity*. Lehigh, PA: Lehigh University Press.

Rousseau, G.S., and D. Haycock. 1999. "'Voices Calling for Reform': The Royal Society in the Mid-Eighteenth Century – Martin Folkes, John Hill, and William Stukeley." *History of Science* 37:377–406.

Rousseau, G.S., and D. Haycock. 2000. "The Jew of Crane Court: Emanuel Mendes Da Costa (1717–1791), Natural History and Natural Excess." *History of Science* 38:127–70.

Sacombe, J.F. (1792) 1793. 2nd ed. *La Luciniade: Ou, l'art Des Accouchemens, Poème Didactique*. Paris: Garnéry.

Sacombe, J.F. 1799. *La Luciniade, Poème en Dix Chants, Sur l'art Des Accouchemens*. Paris: Courcier.

Sacombe, J.F. 1803. *Lucine Francéaise, ou Recueil d'observations Médicales, Chirurgicales, Pharmaceutiques, Historiques, Critiques et Littéraires, Relatives é La Science Des Accouchemens*. Paris: Bidault.

Sbiroli, L.S. 1989. *Libertine O Madre Illibate*. Venice: Marcilio.

Schurig, M. 1780. *Spermatologia Historico-Medica*. Frankfurt.

Shorter, E. 1985. "The Management of Normal Deliveries and the Generation of William Hunter." In *William Hunter and the Eighteenth-Century Medical World*, edited by W.F. Bynum and R. Porter, 371–84. Cambridge and New York: Cambridge University Press.

Sibly, E. 1796. *The Medical Mirror. Or Treatise on the Impregnation of the Human Female: Shewing the Origin of Diseases, and the Principles of Life and Death*. London: printed for the author and sold by Champante and Whitrow.

Sterne, L. 1950. *The Life and Opinions of Tristram Shandy, Gentleman., 1759–1767*. New York: Odyssey.

Terrall, M. 1996. "Salon, Academy, and Boudoir: Generation and Desire in Maupertuis' Science of Life." *Isis* 87 (2): 217–29. http://dx.doi.org/10.1086/357481.

Terrall, M. 2011. "Frogs on the Mantlepiece: The Practice of Observation in Daily Life." In *Histories of Scientific Observation*, edited by Lorraine Daston and Elizabeth Lunbeck, 185–205. Chicago: University of Chicago Press.

Weinstone, A. 2004. *Avatar Bodies*. Minneapolis: University of Minnesota Press.

Wilson, D.B. 1993. *Signs and Portents: Monstrous Births from the Middle Ages to the Enlightenment*. London: Routledge.

Wollaston, W. 1726. *The Religion of Nature Delineated*. Dublin: George Grierson. http://dx.doi.org/10.1037/11734-000.

Zirkle, C. 1936. "Animals Impregnated by the Wind." *Isis* 25 (1): 95–130. http://dx.doi.org/10.1086/347065.

Contributors

Sonja Boon, Department of Gender Studies, Memorial University
Peter J. Bowler, School of History and Anthropology, Queen's University, Belfast
Ivano Dal Prete, History of Science and Medicine Program, Yale University
Sally Frampton, Faculty of English, University of Oxford
Jennifer Golightly, Arts & Culture Program, University of Denver
Christine Lehleiter, German Department, University of Toronto
Susanne Lettow, Institut für Philosophie, Freie Universität Berlin
Pam Lieske, Department of English, Kent State University at Trumbull
Corrinne Harol, Department of English and Film Studies, University of Alberta
Jessica MacQueen, Department of English and Film Studies, University of Alberta
Lianne McTavish, Department of Art and Design, University of Alberta
Heather Meek, Department of Literatures and Languages of the World, Université de Montréal
Staffan Müller-Wille, Department of Sociology, Philosophy and Anthropology, University of Exeter
Donald W. Nichol, Department of English, Memorial University
Marcia D. Nichols, Center for Learning Innovation, University of Minnesota Rochester
Julie Peakman, Department of History, Classics, and Archaeology, Birkbeck, University of London
Sebastian Pranghofer, Department of Humanities and Social Sciences, Helmut Schmidt University, University of the Federal Armed Forces Hamburg

George Rousseau, Faculty of Modern History, University of Oxford
Raymond Stephanson, Department of English, University of Saskatchewan
Sarah Toulalan, Centre for Medical History, University of Exeter
David M. Turner, Department of History and Classics, Swansea University
Corinna Wagner, Department of English/Department of Art History and Visual Culture, University of Exeter
Darren N. Wagner, Department of History and Classical Studies/ Department of Social Studies of Medicine, McGill University
John C. Waller, Department of History, Michigan State University
Sarah Watkins, Department of History, Classics, and Archaeology, Birkbeck, University of London

Index

www.ingramcontent.com/pod-product-compliance
Lightning Source LLC
LaVergne TN
LVHW010354080826
844660LV00015B/965/J

* 9 7 8 1 4 4 2 6 4 6 9 6 4 *